CHEST RADIOLOGY
The Essentials

CHEST RADIOLOGY
The Essentials
SECOND EDITION

Edited By

Jannette Collins, MD, MEd, FCCP

Professor of Radiology and Medicine
Department of Radiology
University of Wisconsin School of Medicine and Public Health
Madison, Wisconsin

Eric J. Stern, MD

Professor of Radiology
Adjunct Professor of Medicine
Adjunct Professor of Medical Education and Bioinformatics
Vice-Chairman for Academic Affairs
Director of Thoracic Imaging, Harborview Medical Center
University of Washington
Seattle, Washington

Wolters Kluwer | Lippincott Williams & Wilkins
Health

Philadelphia · Baltimore · New York · London
Buenos Aires · Hong Kong · Sydney · Tokyo

Acquisitions Editor: Lisa McAllister
Managing Editor: Kerry Barrett
Marketing Manager: Angela Panetta
Project Manager: Fran Gunning
Manufacturing Manager: Ben Rivera
Art Director: Risa Clow
Production Services: Aptara, Inc.

Library of Congress Cataloging-in-Publication Data

Collins, Jannette.
    Chest radiology: the essentials/Jannette Collins, Eric J. Stern.—2nd ed.
        p. ; cm.
    Includes bibliographical references and index.
    ISBN-13: 978-0-7817-6314-1
    1. Chest—Radiography. 2. Chest—Diseases—Diagnosis. I. Stern, Eric J. II. Title.
    [DNLM: 1. Radiography, Thoracic—methods. 2. Lung Diseases—radiography.
    3. Thoracic Diseases—radiography. WF 975 C712c 2007]
    RC941.c68 2007
    617.5′407572—dc22

                                                                              2007018681

Care has been taken to confirm the accuracy of the information presented and to describe generally accepted practices. However, the authors, editors, and publisher are not responsible for errors or omissions or for any consequences from application of the information in this book and make no warranty, expressed or implied, with respect to the currency, completeness, or accuracy of the contents of the publication. Application of this information in a particular situation remains the professional responsibility of the practitioner.

The author, editors, and publisher have exerted every effort to ensure that drug selection and dosage set forth in this text are in accordance with current recommendations and practice at the time of publication. However, in view of ongoing research, changes in government regulations, and the constant flow of information relating to drug therapy and drug reactions, the reader is urged to check the package insert for each drug for any change in indications and dosage and for added warnings and precautions. This is particularly important when the recommended agent is a new or infrequently employed drug.

Some drugs and medical devices presented in this publication have Food and Drug Administration (FDA) clearance for limited use in restricted research settings. It is the responsibility of the health care provider to ascertain the FDA status of each drug or device planned for use in their clinical practice.

To purchase additional copies of this book, call our customer service department at (800) 638-3030 or fax orders to (301) 824-7390. International customers should call (301) 223-2300.

Visit Lippincott Williams & Wilkins on the Internet: http://www.LWW.com. Lippincott Williams & Wilkins customer service representatives are available from 8:30 am to 6:00 pm, EST.

10 9 8 7 6 5 4 3 2 1

To Mom and Dad (my first teachers),
sister Becki (my first playmate),
and husband Ken (my loving partner in
life with whom I would cycle to
the ends of the earth).
—JC

I dedicate this book to my amazing
children, Ethan, Kyra, and Sophie, who keep
my life in perspective.
—EJS

As a teacher of chest imaging I was delighted to see the second edition of *Chest Radiology: The Essentials.* As in its first edition, the book is concise enough to read cover to cover in a short period of time yet comprehensive enough to include the essential aspects of thoracic imaging. The second edition includes needed updates and a large number of new images. It is an improved version of an excellent book.

The book is easy to read and provides the reader with the basic knowledge required to interpret the chest radiograph and the essential CT findings. The first two chapters illustrate normal anatomy and signs of disease. The remaining chapters follow the pattern approach, the optimal approach to reach a radiologic differential diagnosis. The book contains descriptions of the essential patterns, relevant illustrations, and the most important differential diagnostic considerations.

Each chapter starts by delineating the learning objectives. Chapters contain schematic drawings that greatly facilitate the understanding of the various radiologic signs and numerous tables that summarize the most common causes of any given radiographic abnormality. I particularly enjoyed Chapter 20, a self-assessment review that will be particularly helpful to residents and other physicians to evaluate their knowledge of the core aspects of chest imaging.

Both authors have completed the AJR Figley Fellowship in Radiology Journalism and have considerable teaching and publishing experience. In addition, Dr. Collins has a master's degree in education. The authors' backgrounds and talents as writers are reflected in the clear outline of the book's contents and the concise manner in which it provides a comprehensive review of the basics of chest radiology.

Nestor L. Müller, MD, PhD, FRCPC
Professor and Chairman
Department of Radiology
University of British Columbia
Vancouver, British Columbia, Canada

Give me facts but above all give me understanding.
—*Solomon*

The objective of this book is to provide a practical tool for those wanting to quickly acquire a broad base of knowledge in thoracic imaging. The content is limited to the essentials of chest radiology so as not to overwhelm the novice, yet provides enough detail that it can serve as a quick review for residents or practicing radiologists, a guide for those who teach thoracic imaging, and a reference for internists, pulmonologists, thoracic surgeons, critical care physicians, family practitioners, and other health care professionals whose patients undergo thoracic imaging procedures. What sets this book apart from other similar texts are (a) it is compact and of practical size for a resident to read during an initial 4-week chest radiology experience, (b) it closely follows an established cardiothoracic radiology curriculum, and (c) it provides an exercise for self-assessment.

This second edition carries over the pattern approach, use of mnemonics, and emphasis on chest radiograph/CT correlation. However, several changes were made to the first edition to reflect current technology (in particular, the introduction of fast multidetector CT scanning) and updated curricular guidelines. The specific behaviorally based learning objectives at the beginning of each chapter follow the 2005 revised curriculum on cardiothoracic radiology for diagnostic radiology residency developed by the Education Committee of the Society of Thoracic Radiology (1). A new chapter devoted to cardiac imaging reflects the increased cardiac content in the revised curriculum.

Nearly 800 new images were added to the second edition, many replacing those from the first edition that reflected older technology. All of the new figures were acquired and transferred to the publisher in digital format.

The content of the second edition was expanded to include the new classification of the idiopathic interstitial pneumonias, current techniques used to evaluate solitary pulmonary nodules, guidelines for management of small incidental nodules detected on chest CT, new World Health Organization classification of lung tumors, and numerous new imaging cases for self-assessment.

Many comments from readers of the first edition, particularly residents, were considered in preparing the second edition. Those parts of the first edition that were positively regarded, such as the self-assessment chapter, were expanded. A new section was added on "Patterns of Lung Disease" to provide a one-stop guide to the recognition and understanding of the findings of honeycomb lung, cystic lung disease, interstitial nodules, mosaic lung attenuation, ground-glass opacification, and "tree-in-bud" opacities on thin-section chest CT.

To address the inherent limitations in a book of "essentials," selected scientific literature and larger comprehensive textbooks are referenced at the end of each chapter for readers who want to broaden their foundation of knowledge. The interpretation of chest radiographs and CT scans does not always lend itself to a "cookbook" approach, but as much as possible, this book attempts to provide a logical approach to learning that will not only prepare readers for but also stimulate them to pursue lifelong learning in chest radiology.

Reference

1. Collins J, Abbott GF, Holbert JM, et al. Revised curriculum on cardiothoracic radiology for diagnostic radiology residency with goals and objectives related to general competencies. *Acad Radiol.* 2005;12:210–223.

Jannette Collins, MD, MEd, FCCP
Eric J. Stern, MD

CONTENTS

CHAPTER 1

NORMAL ANATOMY OF THE CHEST

LEARNING OBJECTIVES

1. Name and define the three zones of the airways.
2. Define a secondary pulmonary lobule and its appearance on high-resolution computed tomography (CT).
3. List the lobar and segmental bronchi of both lungs.
4. Identify the following structures on the posteroanterior chest radiograph:

   Lungs—right and left; right upper, middle, and lower lobes; left upper (including lingula) and lower lobes
   Pulmonary arteries—main, right, left, right interlobar, left lower lobe
   Airway—trachea, carina, main bronchi
   Fissures—minor, superior accessory, inferior accessory, azygos
   Aorta—ascending, arch ("knob"), descending
   Veins—superior vena cava, azygos, left superior intercostal ("aortic nipple")
   Aortopulmonary window
   Right paratracheal stripe
   Junction lines—anterior, posterior
   Azygoesophageal recess
   Paraspinal lines
   Left subclavian artery
   Heart—right atrium, left atrial appendage, left ventricle, locations of the four cardiac valves
   Bones—spine, ribs, clavicles, scapulae, humeri

5. Identify the following structures on the lateral chest radiograph:

   Lungs—right and left; right upper, middle, and lower lobes; left upper (including lingula) and lower lobes
   Fissures—major, minor, superior accessory
   Aorta—ascending, arch, descending
   Retrosternal clear space
   Veins—inferior and superior vena cavae, left brachiocephalic (innominate), pulmonary vein confluence
   Brachiocephalic (innominate) artery
   Airway—trachea, upper lobe bronchi, posterior wall of bronchus intermedius
   Heart—right ventricle, right ventricular outflow tract, left atrium, left ventricle, locations of the four cardiac valves

   Pulmonary arteries—right, left
   Posterior tracheal stripe
   Hemidiaphragms—right, left
   Bones—spine, ribs, scapulae, humeri, sternum

6. Identify the following structures on chest CT:

   Lungs—right and left; right upper, middle, and lower lobes; left upper and lower lobes
   Fissures—major, minor, accessory (azygos, superior, and inferior)
   Pleura and extrapleural fat
   Airway—trachea, main bronchi, carina, lobar and segmental bronchi
   Heart—left ventricle, right ventricle, left atrium, right atrium, mitral valve, aortic valve, tricuspid valve, pulmonary valve, coronary arteries (left main, left anterior descending, left circumflex, right, posterior descending), coronary sinus
   Pericardium, including pericardial recesses
   Pulmonary arteries—main, right, left, right interlobar, segmental
   Aorta—ascending, arch, descending
   Arteries—brachiocephalic (innominate), common carotid, subclavian, axillary, vertebral, internal mammary, intercostal
   Veins—superior and inferior pulmonary, superior and inferior vena cavae, brachiocephalic, subclavian, axillary, internal jugular, external jugular, azygos, hemiazygos, left superior intercostal, internal mammary
   Bones—ribs, costochondral cartilages, clavicles, scapulae, sternum, spine
   Esophagus
   Thymus
   Thyroid gland
   Muscles—sternocleidomastoid, anterior and middle scalene, infrahyoid, pectoralis major and minor, deltoid, trapezius, infraspinatus, supraspinatus, subscapularis, latissimus dorsi, serratus anterior
   Aortopulmonary window
   Azygoesophageal recess
   Diaphragm

Anatomy is to physiology as geography is to history: it describes the theatre of events.

Jean Ferne (1497–1558), *On the Natural Part of Medicine*

You've heard it before—what's important in real estate holds true for understanding diseases of the chest: "location, location, location." A good radiologist knows the anatomy, so don't skip this chapter! This chapter is an abbreviated review of thoracic anatomy as seen on chest radiographs and computed tomography (CT) of the chest. As a result of differences in patient age, body habitus, positioning, inspiratory effort, exam technique, and many other factors, normal anatomic structures will vary in appearance on chest radiographs from exam to exam, patient to patient, and even breath to breath. Some structures are not seen consistently (posterior junction line), whereas others are seen on most exams (left upper lobe bronchus on lateral view). Showing the myriad different appearances of normal anatomic structures is beyond the scope of this chapter; they are learned by paying close attention to and identifying normal structures on thousands of chest radiographs.

A frequent question of medical students and residents on their first rotation on a chest radiology service is: "How do you look at a chest radiograph?" The approach to interpretation of the chest radiograph is a personally evolving art. A person's approach changes over time after seeing many chest radiographs. That answer doesn't help the beginner, so a few general "chest radiograph rules" are offered in Table 1-1, and reference standards are presented in Table 1-2. Normal anatomic structures are labeled on posteroanterior (PA) and lateral chest radiographs (Figs. 1-1 and 1-2) and axial CT images (Figs. 1-3 and 1-4). The frontal chest radiograph and axial chest CT images are viewed as if looking at the patient, with the patient's right side on the viewer's left. Lateral radiographs are, by convention, viewed with the patient facing to the viewer's left (patient's left side closest to the imaging plate).

ZONES OF THE AIRWAYS

The airways are composed of three zones. The *conductive zone* includes the trachea, bronchi, and nonalveolated bronchioles (air cannot diffuse through the well-developed wall). The *transitory zone* has both conductive and respiratory functions and consists of respiratory bronchioles, alveolar ducts, and alveolar sacs. The *respiratory zone* consists of alveoli. The primary function of this zone is the exchange of gases between air and blood.

LUNG ARCHITECTURE

The *primary pulmonary lobule* consists of all alveolar ducts, alveolar sacs, and alveoli, together with their accompanying blood vessels, nerves, and connective tissues distal to the last respiratory bronchiole. This unit is too small to be seen radiologically. *The secondary pulmonary lobule* is the smallest discrete portion of the lung that is surrounded by connective tissue septae, and it is composed of three to five terminal bronchioles with their accompanying transitory airways and parenchyma (Fig. 1-5). A secondary pulmonary lobule contains 30 to 50 primary lobules, is polyhedral in shape and 1.0 to 2.5 cm in diameter, and can be appreciated on thin-section (1- to 2-mm) images of the lung. A *pulmonary acinus* is also an anatomic unit, defined as that portion of lung distal to the terminal bronchiole, comprising the respiratory bronchioles, alveolar ducts, alveolar sacs, and alveoli. Typically, six to 12 acini are grouped together in a secondary pulmonary lobule (1).

(Text continues on page 7)

TABLE 1-1

INTERPRETATION OF THE CHEST RADIOGRAPH: "RULES" TO FOLLOW

1. When you have them, always look at both views (PA and lateral). To confirm that pathology is within the chest, it must usually be seen in the chest on both views.
2. The right heart border is formed by the right atrium, and it is obscured by medial segment right middle lobe processes (disease limited to the lateral segment will not obscure the right heart border).
3. The left heart border is formed mainly by the left ventricle and is obscured by lingular processes.
4. The right diaphragm is usually 1.5 to 2.0 cm higher than the left.
5. The diaphragm is obscured by lower lobe processes (unless only the superior segment of the lower lobe is involved).
6. Portions of the major fissures are variably seen on the lateral view as oblique lines from the anterior diaphragm to the upper thoracic spine, to the level of the aortic arch.
7. The minor fissure is on the right, separating the right upper lobe from the right middle lobe. It courses from the right hilum to the right lateral anterior chest wall and is variably seen on PA and lateral chest radiographs.
8. Normal hilar opacities are predominantly caused by the pulmonary arteries and should be symmetric in size and density.
9. The aortic arch, or "knob," is above the left hilum. (Watch out for the right aortic arch variant!)
10. The trachea is midline but may be deviated to the right or forward from a tortuous aorta.
11. The costophrenic angles should be sharp on both views (sharp enough to pick your teeth with), except in patients with severe pulmonary emphysema, resulting in flattening of the hemidiaphragms.
12. With good inspiratory effort, the size of the heart on the PA radiograph is normally less than or equal to 50% of the widest diameter of the thoracic cage.
13. Right middle lobe and lingular processes are projected over the heart on the lateral view.
14. A young healthy person can take a breath deep enough to inflate the lungs to the level of the 10th rib posteriorly (or the sixth rib anteriorly).
15. Opacity of the lungs should be symmetric unless the patient is rotated.
16. The stomach bubble is under the left hemidiaphragm. (Watch out for situs inversus.)
17. Don't forget to look at the bones and soft tissues.

TABLE 1-2

SIZE AND DENSITY RATIOS ON THE PA CHEST RADIOGRAPH

Size

Cardiothoracic The heart diameter should be half or less than half of the chest diameter. An easy way to eyeball this—assuming the spine is straight and in the middle of the chest—is to see if the heart to the right of the midline fits between the left heart border and the left ribs.

Aortopulmonary The left pulmonary artery, as it passes over the left main bronchus, should be less than the width of the aortic knob. The aortic arch is approximately 3 cm above the carina in adults until the aorta begins to get tortuous. The left pulmonary artery is approximately 3 cm down the left main bronchus then ascends up and out at approximately 45 degrees.

Azygotracheal The azygos vein, if visualized (at the right tracheobronchial angle), should be no wider than approximately one half the width of the trachea, and its height should be no greater than the width of the trachea.

Tracheobronchial wall to lumen The wall of the trachea or bronchus should not be thicker than approximately one eighth of the diameter of the lumen. The tracheal diameter should be equal on the PA and lateral views and should be less than the width of a vertebral body.

Right lower lobe artery to trachea The right lower lobe pulmonary artery should not be wider than the width of the tracheal lumen.

Hilar height The left hilus should be approximately 2 cm higher than the right, because the left pulmonary artery has to go over the left main bronchus.

Arteriobronchial An artery and its accompanying bronchus should be the same size (seen best "end-on").

Density

Cardiohepatic The heart should be about half as dense as the middle of the liver (it's about half as thick). This reference requires good exposure. Beware the "ivory heart" of left lower lobe collapse.

Intracardiac The heart should be the same density on each side of the spine.

Intrahepatic The top of the liver should be about half as dense as the middle, because it's about half as thick, provided the diaphragm domes normally.

Right paratracheal–aortic The density to the right of the trachea at the level of the aortic arch should never be as great or greater than the density of the aortic knob.

Hilar The hila should be the same density (they are composed of the same vascularity).

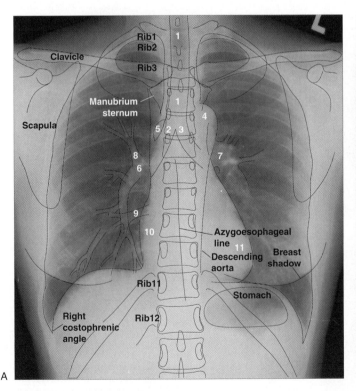
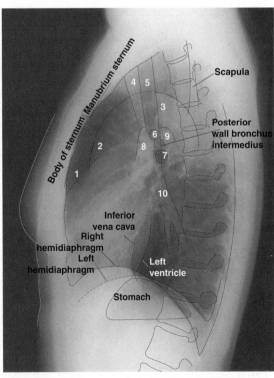

FIGURE 1-1. Normal anatomic structures on posteroanterior (PA) and lateral chest radiographs. A: PA view showing trachea (*1*), right mainstem bronchus (*2*), left mainstem bronchus (*3*), aortic "knob" or arch (*4*), azygos vein emptying into superior vena cava (*5*), right interlobar pulmonary artery (*6*), left pulmonary artery (*7*), right upper lobe pulmonary artery (truncus anterior) (*8*), right inferior pulmonary vein (*9*), right atrium (*10*), left ventricle (*11*), and other structures as labeled. **B:** Lateral view showing pulmonary outflow tract (*1*), ascending aorta (*2*), aortic arch (*3*), brachiocephalic vessels (*4*), trachea (*5*), right upper lobe bronchus (*6*), left upper lobe bronchus (*7*), right pulmonary artery (*8*), left pulmonary artery (*9*), confluence of pulmonary veins (*10*), and other structures as labeled.

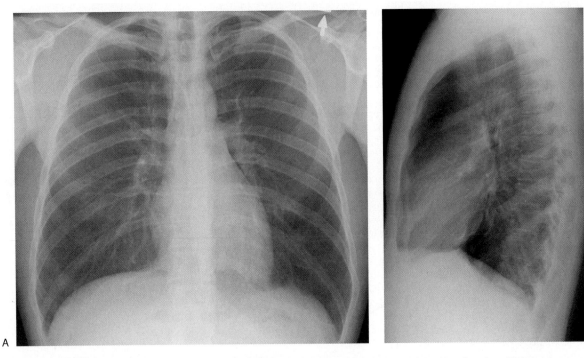

FIGURE 1-2. Normal PA (A) and lateral (B) chest radiographs, showing the structures numbered and labeled in Figure 1-1.

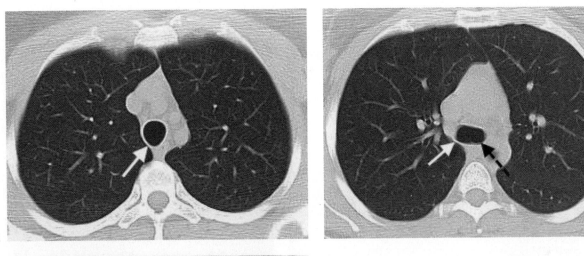

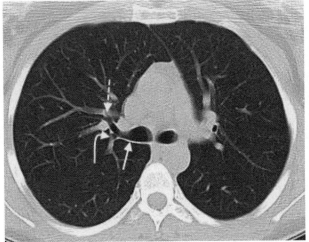

FIGURE 1-3. Axial CT images (1.25-mm reconstructions) of the normal lungs and airways. For all images, the window widths and levels are 1,700 and 500, respectively. **A:** The intrathoracic trachea has a flat or rounded contour posteriorly on inspiration (*arrow*). Pulmonary arteries branch and taper from the central portion of the lungs to the periphery. **B:** Just below the level of the carina, the right (*white arrow*) and left (*black dashed arrow*) mainstem bronchi are visualized. **C:** Image inferior to (**B**) shows right upper lobe bronchus (*arrow*) branching into anterior (*dashed arrow*) and posterior (*curved arrow*) segmental bronchi. (*Continued*)

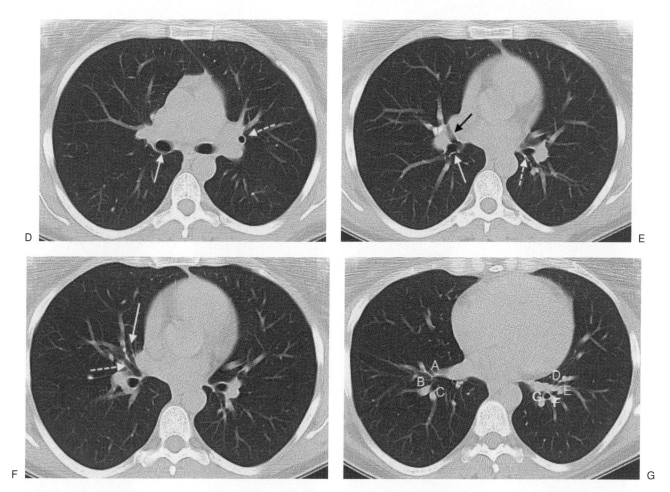

FIGURE 1-3. *(Continued)* **D:** Image inferior to (**C**) shows thin posterior wall of bronchus intermedius (*arrow*) and left upper lobe bronchus (*dashed arrow*). **E:** Image inferior to (**D**) shows right middle lobe bronchus (*black arrow*) and right (*white solid arrow*) and left (*dashed arrow*) lower lobe bronchial trunks. **F:** Image inferior to (**D**) shows right middle lobe medial (*white solid arrow*) and lateral (*white dashed arrow*) segmental bronchi. **G:** Image inferior to (**F**) shows individual lower lobe basilar segmental bronchi: right medial (*A*), anterior (*B*), posterolateral (*C*), and left medial (*D*), anterior (*E*), lateral (*F*), and posterior (*G*). Note that individual left anterior and medial basilar segmental bronchi are seen, which arise from a common anteromedial basilar trunk. Separate right posterior and lateral basilar segmental bronchi are not seen on this image.

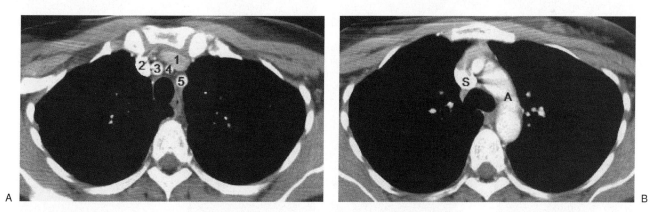

FIGURE 1-4. Axial CT images (5-mm collimation) of the normal mediastinum with intravenous contrast enhancement. For all images, the window widths and levels are 350 and 35, respectively. **A:** The intravenous contrast was injected from a right antecubital vein. Every axial CT scan of the chest (10-mm collimation or less) in patients with standard anatomy will have at least one "five-vessel image" like this, showing the left brachiocephalic vein (*1*), right brachiocephalic vein (*2*), innominate (brachiocephalic) artery (*3*), left common carotid artery (*4*), and left subclavian artery (*5*). **B:** Image inferior to (**A**) shows the aortic arch (*A*) and superior vena cava (*S*) densely enhancing with contrast. *(Continued)*

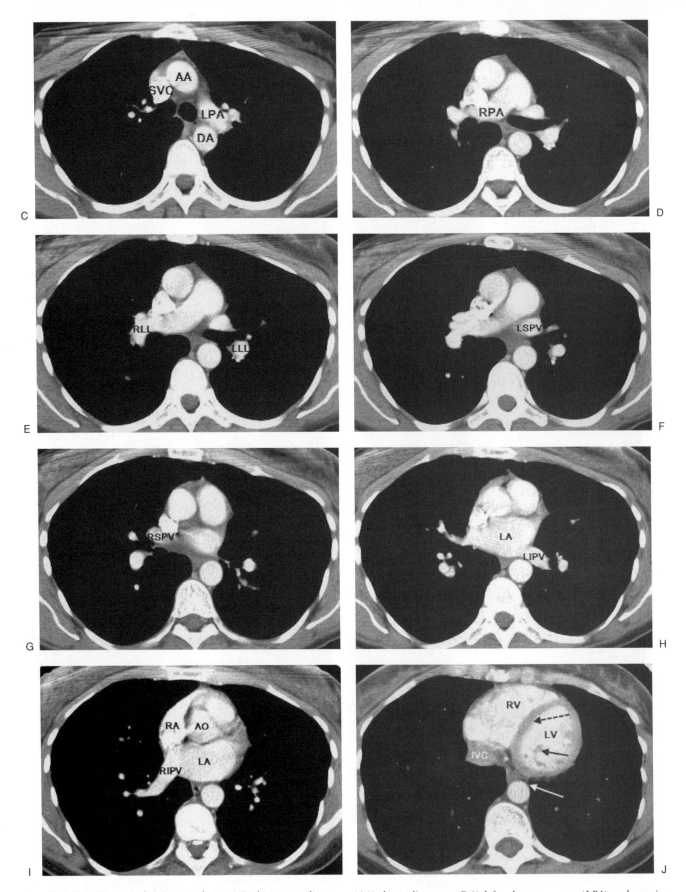

FIGURE 1-4. *(Continued)* **C:** Image inferior to (**B**) shows ascending aorta (*AA*), descending aorta (*DA*), left pulmonary artery (*LPA*), and superior vena cava (*SVC*). **D:** Image inferior to (**C**) shows the right pulmonary artery (*RPA*). **E:** Image inferior to (**D**) shows the right (*RLL*) and left (*LLL*) pulmonary arteries. **F:** Image inferior to (**E**) shows the left superior pulmonary vein (*LSPV*). **G:** Image inferior to (**F**) shows the right superior pulmonary vein (*RSPV*). **H:** Image inferior to (**G**) shows the left atrium (*LA*) and left inferior pulmonary vein (*LIPV*). **I:** Image inferior to (**H**) shows the right atrium (*RA*), aortic outflow (*AO*), left atrium (*LA*), and right inferior pulmonary vein (*RIPV*). **J:** Image inferior to (**I**) shows the right ventricle (*RV*), left ventricle (*LV*), interventricular septum (*dashed black arrow*), papillary muscles (*solid black arrow*), esophagus (*white arrow*), and inferior vena cava (*IVC*).

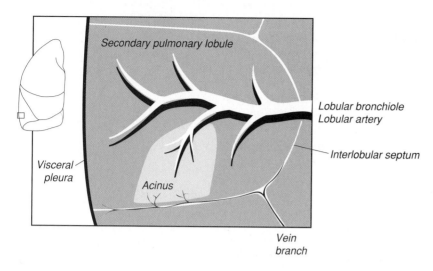

FIGURE 1-5. Secondary pulmonary lobule. Normal visceral pleural thickness is 0.1 mm. Lobular artery and bronchiole diameters are 1.0 mm. The secondary pulmonary lobule has a polyhedral shape and is the smallest discrete portion of lung that is surrounded by connective tissue septae (interlobular septae). Pulmonary veins and lymphatics are within the interlobular septae. A pulmonary acinus is defined as that portion of lung distal to the terminal bronchiole, and up to 12 acini can make up one secondary pulmonary lobule.

TRACHEOBRONCHIAL ANATOMY

The *intrathoracic trachea* is 6 to 9 cm in length (2) and enters the thorax 1 to 3 cm above the level of the suprasternal notch. The upper limits of normal for coronal and sagittal tracheal diameters in adults on chest radiography are 21 and 23 mm, respectively, for women, and 25 and 27 mm for men (3). The trachea has 15 to 20 C-shaped rings of hyaline cartilage (absent in the posterior membranous trachea), which provide the rigidity that prevents the trachea from collapsing (4). The trachea divides into *right* and *left mainstem bronchi* at the carina. The right main bronchus, about 2.5 cm in length, is shorter, wider, and more nearly vertical than the left. Because it is almost in a direct line with the trachea, foreign objects passing through the trachea usually enter the right main bronchus.

The lobar and segmental branching patterns of the mainstem bronchi and pulmonary lobes and segments are shown in Figures 1-6 to 1-8. There are ten *segmental bronchi* on the right. On the left, apicoposterior and anteromedial combinations result in eight left segmental bronchi, although some anatomists refer to ten segments on the left. Segmental bronchi divide, and after six to 20 divisions they no longer contain cartilage in their walls and are referred to as *bronchioles*. The bronchioles divide, and the last of the purely conducting airways is referred to as the *terminal bronchiole*. Beyond the terminal bronchioles lie the acini, the gas exchange units of the lung. Subsegmental bronchi can routinely be identified with thin-section CT.

PULMONARY HILA

On chest radiography, normal hilar opacities are composed of both major bronchi and blood vessels, but most of what you see are pulmonary arteries. The left hilus is higher than the right, as seen on the PA chest radiograph, because the left pulmonary artery is higher than the right. The right upper lobe bronchus is higher than the left upper lobe bronchus, as seen on the lateral chest radiograph, because the right upper lobe bronchus is *eparterial* (above the artery); the left lower lobe bronchus is *hyparterial* (below the artery). The transverse diameter of the lower lobe arteries should normally be 9 to 16 mm (1). Bronchi and pulmonary arteries branch out from the hilum together, whereas pulmonary veins drain to the heart, separate from the bronchi and arteries. In the outer two thirds of the lungs, arteries cannot be distinguished from veins on chest ra-

diography. More centrally, the orientations of the arteries and veins differ. The inferior pulmonary veins draining the lower lobes run more horizontally and are directed toward the left atrium, whereas the lower lobe arteries are oriented more vertically. In the upper lobes, the arteries and veins show a similar gently curving vertical orientation; the upper lobe veins lie lateral to the arteries and can sometimes be traced to the superior pulmonary vein. There are right and left superior and inferior pulmonary veins, which drain into the left atrium. Lymph flows to the hilum via lymphatic channels that are found in a subpleural location and within the interlobular septae.

FISSURES

The major (oblique) fissures run obliquely forward and downward from approximately the level of the fifth thoracic vertebral body to the diaphragm and divide the lungs into upper and lower lobes (Fig. 1-9). The *right major fissure* is more oblique, ends further forward inferiorly (more anterior on the lateral chest radiograph), merges with the right hemidiaphragm, and joins the minor fissure. The *minor (horizontal) fissure* separates the right middle from the right upper lobe and fans out forward and laterally from the right hilus (Fig. 1-10). It is unusual to be able to trace both fissures in their entirety on chest radiographs. Fissures are often "incomplete" and only partially separate lobes.

On CT scans, the region of the major fissures can usually be seen as a band of avascularity. The fissure itself may be invisible, or it may be seen as a poorly defined or well-defined band of density, depending upon slice thickness. The position of the minor fissure can be inferred on CT scans from the large oval deficiency of vessels on one or more sections at the level of the bronchus intermedius.

Numerous *accessory fissures* may be identified as normal variants. Approximately 1% of the population will have an *accessory azygos fissure*, creating an accessory azygos lobe in the right superomedial lung (Fig. 1-11). The azygos fissure contains the azygos vein (which, in the case of an azygos fissure, is always located higher than its usual location in the tracheobronchial angle) within its lower margin, and it is easily seen on chest radiography because it contains four pleural layers (two visceral and two parietal). The *left minor fissure* separates the lingula from the other left upper lobe segments. The *superior accessory fissure* separates the superior segment from the basal segments in either lower lobe, is horizontally oriented, and is seen below the level of the minor fissure on the right. The *inferior accessory fissure* separates the medial basal segment from

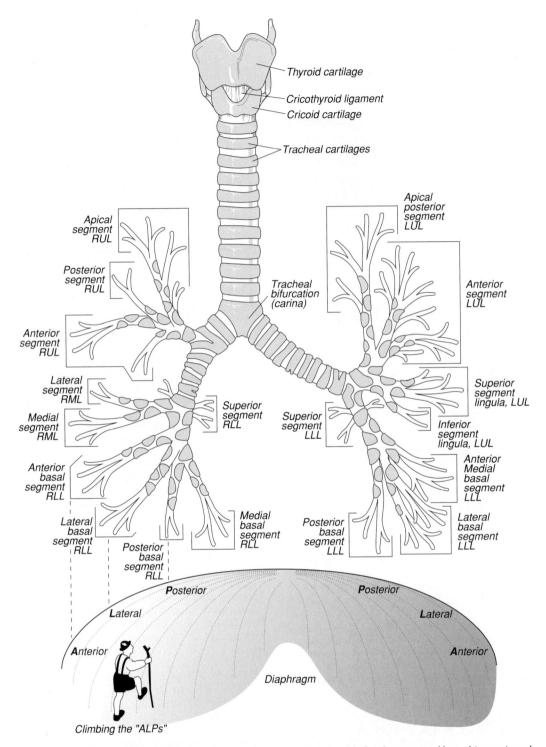

Thyroid cartilage

Cricothyroid ligament
Cricoid cartilage

Tracheal cartilages

Apical
segment
RUL

Apical
posterior
segment
LUL

Posterior
segment
RUL

Tracheal
bifurcation
(carina)

Anterior
segment
LUL

Anterior
segment
RUL

Lateral
segment
RML

Superior
segment
RLL

Superior
segment
lingula, LUL

Medial
segment
RML

Superior
segment
LLL

Inferior
segment
lingula, LUL

Anterior
basal
segment
RLL

Anterior
Medial
basal
segment
LLL

Lateral
basal
segment
RLL

Posterior
basal
segment
RLL

Medial
basal
segment
RLL

Posterior
basal
segment
LLL

Lateral
basal
segment
LLL

Posterior   Posterior

Lateral   Lateral

Anterior   Anterior

Diaphragm

Climbing the "ALPs"

FIGURE 1-6. Diagram of normal airway anatomy, frontal view. Note how the basilar segmental bronchi are oriented from lateral to medial. The anterior basilar segmental bronchus is most lateral (pneumonia confined to the lateral segment of the right lower lobe extends to the periphery of the lung), and the posterior basilar segmental bronchus is medial, just lateral to the right medial basilar segmental bronchus. Climbing the diaphragm from lateral to medial can be thought of as climbing the *ALP*s (*A*nterior, *L*ateral, and *P*osterior basilar segmental bronchi), as a way to remember this orientation. RUL, right upper lobe; RML, right medial lobe; RLL, right lower lobe; LUL, left upper lobe, LLL, left lower lobe.

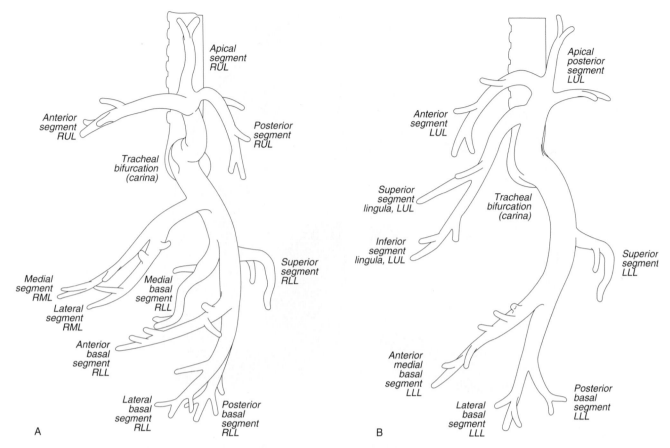

FIGURE 1-7. **Diagrams of normal airway anatomy, lateral views. A:** Right bronchial tree. Note that the middle lobe bronchi are relatively anterior (right middle lobe pneumonia is projected anteriorly over the heart on a lateral chest radiograph). RLL, right lower lobe; RML, right middle lobe; RUL, right upper lobe. **B:** Left bronchial tree. Note that the lingular bronchi are relatively anterior (analogous to the right middle lobe bronchi). LLL, left lower lobe; LUL, left upper lobe.

other basal segments in either lower lobe, and it runs obliquely upward and medially toward the hilus from the diaphragm (Fig. 1-12).

MEDIASTINAL BLOOD VESSELS

The *thoracic aorta* has ascending, transverse (arch), and descending portions. The ascending portion becomes more prominent as a patient ages. On a frontal chest radiograph, the arch is seen to the left of midline as a smooth "knob." The descending portion gradually moves from a position to the left of the vertebral bodies to an almost midline position before exiting the chest through the aortic hiatus in the diaphragm. The three major aortic branches, lying anterior to and to the left of the trachea, are (in order from the patient's right to left) the *brachiocephalic (innominate) artery*, the *left common carotid artery*, and the *left subclavian artery.*

The *superior vena cava* (SVC) is seen in the right paratracheal area, typically representing the right superior mediastinal contour. In 0.3% to 0.5% of people without congenital heart disease, a *left superior vena cava* is present (5). A left SVC arises from the junction of the left jugular and subclavian veins and travels vertically through the left mediastinum, usually emptying into the coronary sinus, which drains into the right atrium.

Patients with a left SVC may also have a right SVC, which is typically smaller than usual.

The *azygos vein* courses anterior to the spine, either behind or to the right of the esophagus, until it arches anteriorly to join the posterior wall of the SVC. The azygos vein usually remains within the mediastinum and occupies the right tracheobronchial angle (in the case of an azygos lobe, the azygos vein traverses the lung before entering the SVC). The *hemiazygos* and *accessory hemiazygos* veins lie against the vertebral bodies, posterior to the azygos vein. The accessory hemiazygos vein drains into the left *superior intercostal vein*, which arches around the aorta at the junction of the arch and the descending portion, and joins the left brachiocephalic vein (this contact with the aorta forms the so-called "aortic nipple" occasionally seen on the PA chest radiograph). Venous anatomy is illustrated in Figure 1-13. In patients with absence of the inferior vena cava (IVC), the azygos vein forms the venous conduit draining the "IVC blood" back to the heart (hepatic veins then drain into the right atrium, not into the IVC). In such cases, the azygos vein will be very large, as seen on the PA chest radiograph in the tracheobronchial angle, and can resemble adenopathy.

The *main pulmonary artery* is anterior and to the left of the ascending aorta. The left pulmonary artery arches higher than the right and passes over the left main bronchus.

(Text continues on page 12)

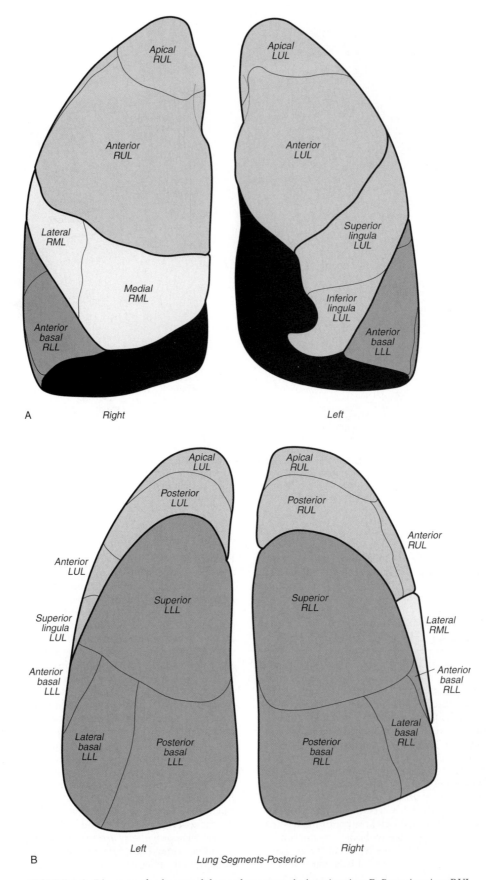

FIGURE 1-8. Diagrams of pulmonary lobes and segments. A: Anterior view. B: Posterior view. RUL, right upper lobe; RML, right middle lobe; RLL, right lower lobe; LUL, left upper lobe, LLL, left lower lobe.

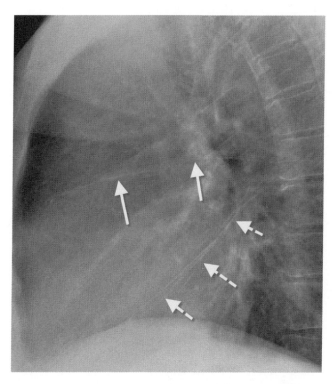

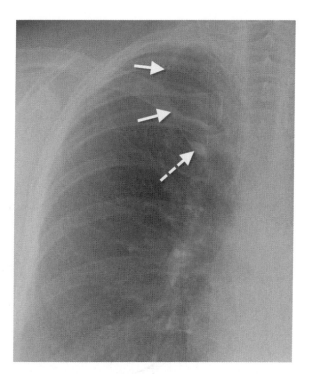

FIGURE 1-11. Accessory azygos fissure. The accessory azygos fissure (*solid arrows*) creates an accessory azygos lobe. The fissure contains the azygos vein (*dashed arrow*), which is higher than its usual location in the tracheobronchial angle.

FIGURE 1-9. Major and minor fissures on lateral chest radiograph. The inferior portions of the major fissures (*dashed white arrows*) and the right minor fissure (*solid white arrows*) are shown. They outline the location of the right middle lobe. The superior portions of the major fissures are not well seen. It is not uncommon that portions of the fissures are not visualized on normal chest radiographs.

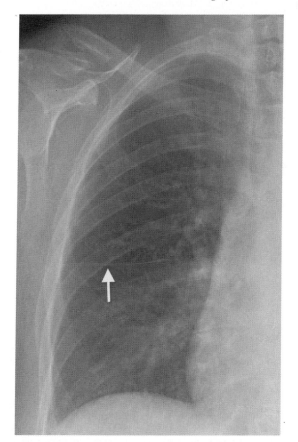

FIGURE 1-10. Minor fissure on PA chest radiograph. The minor fissure has a horizontal course from the right hilum to the periphery of the right lung (*arrow*).

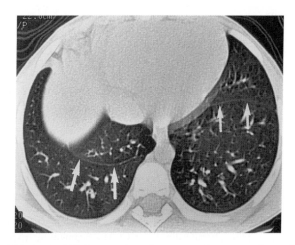

FIGURE 1-12. Inferior accessory fissure. Axial CT scan shows the right inferior accessory fissure (*larger arrows*), which separates the medial from the other basilar segments of the right lower lobe, and the left major fissure (*smaller arrows*).

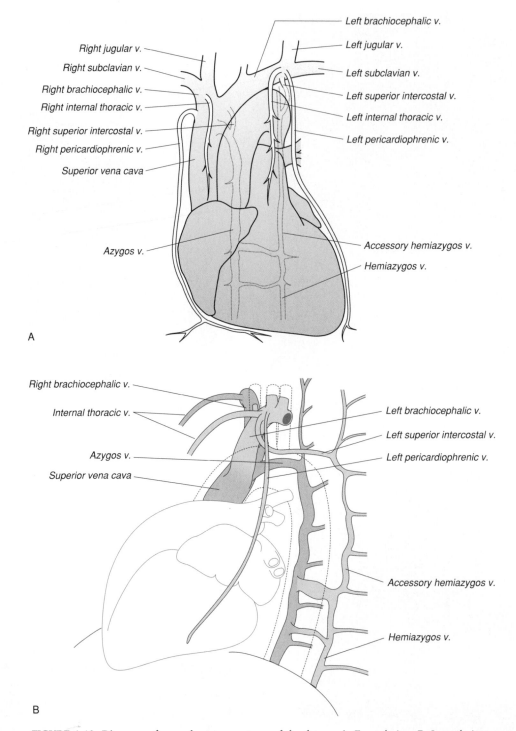

FIGURE 1-13. Diagrams of normal venous anatomy of the thorax. A: Frontal view. B: Lateral view. v, vein.

MEDIASTINAL SPACES, LINES, STRIPES, AND BORDERS

The *aortopulmonary window* is the space under the aortic arch and above the left pulmonary artery. The ligamentum arteriosum (remnant of the ductus arteriosus) and recurrent laryngeal nerve traverse this space (a mass in the aortopulmonary window can involve the recurrent laryngeal nerve and result

in hoarseness). The *subcarinal space* is inferior to the carina, bounded by the main bronchi, and is a site where adenopathy occurs. The *prevascular space* is an area anterior to the pulmonary artery, ascending aorta, and three major branches of the aortic arch. This space lies between the two lungs and is bounded anteriorly by the chest wall. Where the lungs approximate, there is no prevascular space but rather an anterior junction line. Within the prevascular space is the left brachiocephalic vein, internal mammary arteries, lymph nodes,

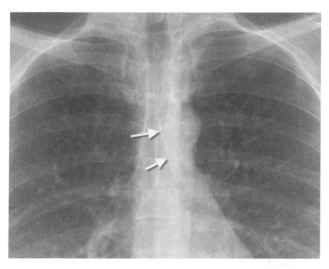

FIGURE 1-14. Anterior junction line on PA chest radiograph (*arrows*). Note that the line does not extend above the level of the clavicles.

thymus, and phrenic nerve. The *retrocrural space* (aortic hiatus) is the space bounded by the diaphragmatic crura and the spine. Structures that pass through this area can be thought of as the "birds of the mediastinum": azygos vein ("azygoose"), hemiazygos vein ("hemiazygoose"), and thoracic duct ("thoracic duck"). The esophagus ("esophagoose") is another of the birds of the mediastinum; however, it passes through the esophageal hiatus.

The *right* and *posterior tracheal stripes* are formed where the lung contacts the trachea to the right and posteriorly, and they are normally 3 mm wide or less. The *anterior junction line* is where the right and left lungs approximate above the level of the heart and below the manubrium (Fig. 1-14). It is composed of four layers of pleura (both the parietal and visceral layers from each hemithorax), may reach the level of the clavicles superiorly, and is not always evident on chest radiography because of intervening fat and/or thymus. Deviation of the anterior junction line suggests a mass or shift of the mediastinum. The *posterior junction line* is where the two lungs meet behind the trachea and heart. Unlike the anterior junction line, it extends to the lung apices, projecting above the clavicles (Fig. 1-15). It is also composed of four pleural layers,

and bulging of the border is normal only in the area of the azygos vein or aortic arch. The *azygoesophageal line*, seen on the frontal chest radiograph below the aortic arch, is where the right lower lobe makes contact with the right wall of the esophagus and the azygos vein as it ascends next to the esophagus. This portion of lung is known as the *azygoesophageal recess* and the interface is known as the azygoesophageal line. The upper few centimeters of the azygoesophageal line are always straight or concave toward the lung in adults; a convex shape indicates a subcarinal mass. *Paraspinal lines* are stripes of soft tissue density, parallel to the left and right margins of the spine, formed by the approximation of the lung with the spine. They are usually less than 1 cm in width. Aortic tortuosity will contribute to the thickness of the left paraspinal line.

Above the aortic arch, the *left paratracheal shadow* is caused by the left carotid and subclavian arteries and the left jugular vein. The outer margin of the left tracheal wall is almost never outlined because the trachea is not contiguous with the lung (it is separated by the aorta and great vessels). Below the arch, the *left mediastinal border* is formed by the aortic pulmonary pleural stripe, the main pulmonary artery, and the heart. The right mediastinal border is formed by the right brachiocephalic vein, SVC, and right atrium. A right paratracheal stripe is seen in approximately two thirds of normal subjects through the right brachiocephalic vein and SVC.

DIAPHRAGM

The diaphragm can normally have a smooth or a scalloped contour. The right hemidiaphragm is higher than the left in approximately 88% of people by 1.5 to 2.0 cm. The left is higher than the right in approximately 3% of people but by less than 1 cm. The hemidiaphragms are at the same level in approximately 9% of people (6). *Eventration* (incomplete muscularization of the diaphragm) refers to a thin membranous sheet replacing what should be muscle, causing a smooth hump on the contour of the diaphragm (frequently the anteromedial right diaphragm). Total eventration, more common on the left than on the right, results in elevation of the whole hemidiaphragm.

LATERAL CHEST RADIOGRAPH

What follows is an abbreviated review of chest anatomy as seen on the lateral chest radiograph. A complete review of the left lateral chest radiograph was published in 1979 by Proto and Speckman (7).

The brachiocephalic (innominate) artery arises anterior to the tracheal air column. Its posterior wall can be seen as a gentle S-shaped interface crossing the tracheal air column. The left brachiocephalic vein often forms an extrapleural bulge behind the manubrium. The posterior border of the right brachiocephalic vein and the SVC can occasionally be identified curving downward in much the same position and direction as the brachiocephalic artery, but they are sometimes traceable below the upper margin of the aortic arch. The convex margin of the innominate artery–right subclavian artery complex projects through the tracheal air column and merges with the posterior aspect of the right brachiocephalic vein–SVC to form a sigmoid-shaped interface.

The course of the trachea is straight or bowed forward in patients with aortic tortuosity. The carina is not visible on the lateral chest radiograph. The anterior wall of the trachea is visible in only a minority of people. The posterior wall of the trachea is usually visible, because lung often passes behind the trachea, forming the posterior tracheal stripe (seen in 50% to 90% of adults). This stripe is normally narrower than 3 to 4 mm. If there is little or no air in the esophagus, this stripe

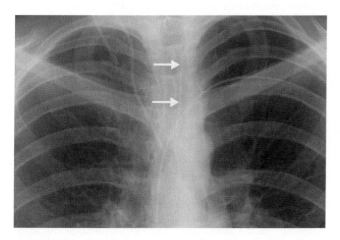

FIGURE 1-15. Posterior junction line on PA chest radiograph (*arrows*). Note that the line extends above the level of the clavicles.

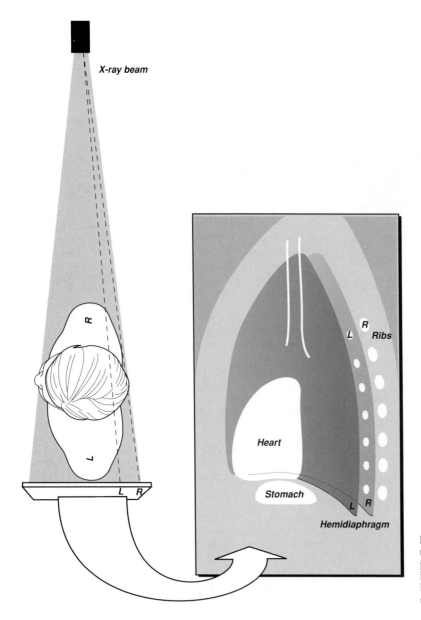

X-ray beam

R

Ribs

Heart

Stomach

Hemidiaphragm

FIGURE 1-16. Diagram illustrating how magnification results in the right (*R*) ribs being larger and projected behind the left (*L*) ribs on a properly positioned left lateral chest radiograph. Note that the stomach bubble is under the left hemidiaphragm. The heart obscures the anterior portion of the left hemidiaphragm.

is formed by the full width of a collapsed esophagus (leading to a band of density 1 cm or wider) and is then called the tracheoesophageal stripe.

The retrosternal line is a bandlike opacity along the lower half or third of the anterior chest wall. Because the left lung does not contact the anterior portion of the left thoracic cavity at this level, the heart with its epicardial fat occupies this space.

The posterior wall of the IVC is visible just before it enters the right atrium. The ascending aorta projects slightly superior and posterior to the right ventricular outflow tract. These structures are distinguished as discrete bulges on approximately 10% of lateral chest radiographs. The right pulmonary artery is seen on end as a round or oval structure anterior to the bronchus intermedius. The left pulmonary artery has an arcuate contour and courses superior and then posterior to the orifice of the left upper lobe bronchus (it can be likened to a miniaturized version of the transverse aortic arch).

At the hilum, the right upper lobe bronchus is superior to the left upper lobe bronchus, and the posterior wall of the

bronchus intermedius is seen as a thin opaque stripe between the two and intersecting the left upper lobe bronchus. Often, only the left upper lobe bronchus (and not the right upper lobe bronchus) is seen on the lateral view. The posterior wall of the bronchus intermedius should be no thicker than 3 mm. The most common causes of thickening are pulmonary edema and variation in patient positioning, but malignancy can also result in thickening.

Several methods can be used to localize the right and left hemidiaphragms on the lateral chest radiograph (Fig. 1-16). On the standard left lateral chest radiograph, the right ribs are projected behind the left and appear larger because of magnification (unless the patient is not in a true left lateral position). Occasionally, the diaphragm can be followed out to its respective ribs. The stomach bubble is under the left hemidiaphragm (unless the patient has situs inversus). Pathologic processes obscuring only one hemidiaphragm on the PA view will confirm which diaphragm is being obscured by the same pathology on the lateral view. The right diaphragm will often be seen extending more anteriorly than the left hemidiaphragm, because the left hemidiaphragm will be partially obscured by the heart anteriorly. In some cases, however, none of these methods work, and which hemidiaphragm is which cannot be determined.

CHEST RADIOLOGY CONCEPTS

The chest radiograph is really more of a "lung radiograph." It is not optimized for examination of the mediastinum or osseous structures. Nonetheless, how do you tell if the chest radiograph is adequately exposed? Ideally, there is a balance between overexposure (good for seeing the mediastinum) and underexposure (good for seeing the lungs). This balance is generally reached when the vertebral disc spaces are just barely visible. On hard-copy film, overexposure is better than underexposure, because you can see the darker areas under a bright light (copy films cannot be bright-lighted, as information has been lost in copying). With underexposure, information is irretrievably lost. With digital radiography systems, this is less of a problem.

Was the film exposed during optimal inspiration? The degree of inspiration is limited in obese patients, or in patients with intra-abdominal mass effect, such as ascites, especially when imaged in the supine position. In general, expiratory films demonstrate more "doming" of the diaphragm, causing the apex of the heart to project below the left lung–diaphragm interface. The lungs are more dense and the blood vessels more crowded together. If you judge that the inspiration is poor or limited, be cautious and do not overinterpret; this is particularly true for patients with suspected mild pneumonia or congestive heart failure.

Extrapericardial fat pads vary in size from patient to patient and may result in relatively radiolucent opacities in the cardiophrenic angles that can obscure the lower inch or so of the heart border(s). When present, they can be visible on either frontal or lateral views or on both views, and they can be very large.

Reference standards are used in making judgments of abnormality either clinically or radiologically. External reference standards are equivalent to experience. If you see enough examples, you will eventually get good at it. This is not much help to the novice. Four types of internal reference standards can be used by the novice: time (interval change, which allows instant judgment as to activity or chronicity); symmetry (paired structures, such as ribs, should look alike); continuum disturbance (similar structures, such as ribs or vertebral bodies, should show a progressive change); and ratios (density and

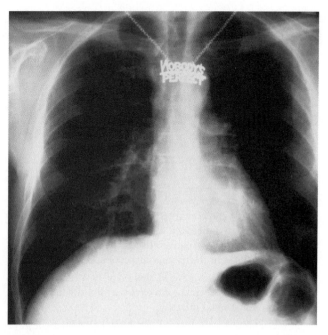

FIGURE 1-17. "Nobody's perfect" (courtesy of June Unger, MD, Scottsdale, AZ).

size—density ratios require a well-exposed film, size ratios do not). Size and density ratios are outlined in Table 1-2. These ratios are for everyday use and will quickly become instinctive. When all else fails, remember that "nobody's perfect" (Fig. 1-17), neither you nor the patient!

References

1. Armstrong P. Normal chest. In: Armstrong P, Wilson AG, Dee P, Hansell DM, eds. *Imaging Diseases of the Chest*. 2nd ed. St. Louis, MO: Mosby; 1995:21.
2. Gamsu G, Webb WR. Computed tomography of the trachea and main bronchi. *Semin Roentgenol.* 1983;18:51–60.
3. Breatnach E, Abbott GC, Fraser RE. Dimensions of the normal human trachea. *Am J Roentgenol.* 1984;142:903–906.
4. O'Rahilly R. The esophagus, trachea, and main bronchi. In: O'Rahilly R. *Gardner–Gray–O'Rahilly Anatomy. A Regional Study of Human Structure.* Philadelphia: WB Saunders; 1986:283.
5. Cha EM, Khoury GH. Persistent left superior vena cava: radiologic and clinical significance. *Radiology.* 1972; 103:375–381.
6. Felson B. *Chest Roentgenology.* Philadelphia: WB Saunders; 1973.
7. Proto AV, Speckman JM. The left lateral radiograph of the chest. Part 1. *Med Radiogr Photogr.* 1979;55:29–74.

CHAPTER 2

SIGNS AND PATTERNS OF LUNG DISEASE

LEARNING OBJECTIVES

1. Recognize the *air bronchogram sign* on a chest radiograph and computed tomographic (CT) scan and that the sign indicates a lung parenchymal process, including nonobstructive atelectasis, as distinguished from pleural or mediastinal processes.

2. Recognize the *air crescent sign* on a chest radiograph and CT scan as a sign of a cavity within the lung, often caused by fungal infection.

3. Recognize the *continuous diaphragm sign* on a chest radiograph and that the sign represents pneumomediastinum.

4. Recognize the *CT angiogram sign* on a CT scan and state the mechanism of how the sign is produced (e.g., enhancing pulmonary vessels against a background of low-attenuation material in the lung).

5. Recognize the *deep sulcus sign* on a supine chest radiograph and that the sign represents pneumothorax.

6. Recognize the *fallen lung sign* on a chest radiograph and CT scan and that the sign represents a fractured bronchus.

7. Recognize the *flat waist sign* on a chest radiograph and that the sign represents lower lobe collapse.

8. Recognize the *finger-in-glove sign* on a chest radiograph and CT scan and that the sign represents bronchial impaction, which is seen in allergic bronchopulmonary aspergillosis.

9. Recognize the *S sign of Golden* on a chest radiograph and that the sign represents lobar collapse, potentially caused by an obstructing endobronchial carcinoma in an adult.

10. Recognize the *halo sign* on a CT scan and that the sign suggests the diagnosis of invasive pulmonary aspergillosis in a leukemic patient.

11. Recognize the *Hampton hump sign* on a chest radiograph and CT scan and that the sign represents hemorrhagic edema or pulmonary infarction as a result of pulmonary embolism.

12. Recognize the *luftsichel sign* on a chest radiograph and that the sign is associated with upper lobe collapse, potentially caused by an obstructing endobronchial carcinoma in an adult.

13. Recognize air around the pulmonary artery on frontal and lateral chest radiographs and CT scan as the *ring around the artery sign* and that the sign represents pneumomediastinum.

14. Recognize loss of the contour of the heart or diaphragm as the *silhouette sign*, and localize a lung parenchymal process by knowing that a process involving the medial segment of the right middle lobe obscures the right heart border, lingular processes obscure the left heart border, and basilar segmental lower lobe processes obscure the diaphragm.

15. Recognize the *split pleura sign* on a CT scan as a sign of empyema or other exudative pleural effusion.

16. Recognize the *Westermark sign* on a chest radiograph and CT scan as a sign of focal oligemia that is potentially caused by pulmonary embolism.

17. Recognize the *honeycomb pattern* on a chest radiograph and CT scan as a sign of pulmonary fibrosis.

18. Recognize the *pattern of septal thickening* on a chest radiograph and CT scan as representing thickening of the interlobular septae (Kerley lines) and suggesting the diagnosis of pulmonary edema with smooth septal thickening and lymphangitic carcinomatosis with beaded septal thickening.

19. Recognize a *cystic pattern* on a chest radiograph and CT scan as suggesting the diagnosis of lymphangioleiomyomatosis in a female patient and Langerhan cell histiocytosis when nodules and an upper lung distribution are seen in a cigarette smoker.

20. Recognize a *nodular pattern* on a CT scan; classify the nodules as perilymphatic, random, centrilobular, or bronchovascular in distribution; and list an appropriate differential diagnosis for each.

21. Recognize a *mosaic pattern of lung attenuation* on a CT scan, which suggests an infiltrative process, small airway disease, or pulmonary vascular disease, depending on the caliber of pulmonary vessels, presence of air trapping on expiration, other associated CT findings, and clinical history.

22. Recognize the *tree-in-bud pattern* on a CT scan and list an appropriate differential diagnosis, indicating infection and aspiration as the most common causes.

A *sign* in chest radiology refers to a radiographic and/or computed tomographic (CT) scan finding that implies a specific pathologic process. Understanding the meaning of a sign indicates comprehension of an important concept related to the radiologic findings. Knowing the name of the sign is not as important as recognizing and understanding the meaning of the radiologic findings, but it will help in communicating with clinicians and radiologists who use the "sign" terminology. A CT "pattern" refers to a nonspecific radiologic finding or collection of findings suggesting one or more specific disease processes. The material that follows is not an all-inclusive list but represents a collection of the more common and useful signs and patterns of focal and diffuse lung disease.

AIR BRONCHOGRAM SIGN

This sign refers to a branching, linear, tubular lucency representing a bronchus or bronchiole passing through airless lung parenchyma (Fig. 2-1). This sign does not differentiate nonobstructive atelectasis from other abnormal parenchymal opacities such as pneumonia. An air bronchogram indicates that the underlying opacity must be parenchymal rather than pleural or mediastinal in location. Although cancers tend to be solid masses, air bronchograms are a characteristic feature of lymphoma and bronchoalveolar cell carcinoma.

AIR CRESCENT SIGN

A mass growing within a pre-existing cavity, or an area of pneumonia that undergoes necrosis and cavitates, may form a peripheral crescent of air between the intracavitary mass and the cavity wall, resulting in the air crescent sign (Fig. 2-2). Intracavitary masses are most often caused by mycetomas. In immunocompromised patients with invasive aspergillosis, the appearance of the air crescent sign, representing necrosis and cavitation, indicates recovery of the immune system and white blood cell response to the infection.

BULGING FISSURE SIGN

Historically, the bulging fissure sign was seen as a result of pneumonia caused by *Klebsiella pneumoniae* involving the right upper lobe (Fig. 2-3). Also called Friedländer pneumonia, the disease is often confined to one lobe, with consolidation spreading rapidly, causing lobar expansion and bulging of the adjacent fissure inferiorly (1). Because of timely antibiotic treatment, pneumonia rarely progresses to this state.

CONTINUOUS DIAPHRAGM SIGN

This sign is seen as a continuous lucency outlining the base of the heart, representing pneumomediastinum (Fig. 2-4). Air in the mediastinum tracks extrapleurally, between the heart and diaphragm (2). Pneumopericardium can have a similar appearance but will show air circumferentially outlining the heart.

CT ANGIOGRAM SIGN

This sign refers to the identification of vessels within an airless portion of lung on contrast-enhanced CT (Fig. 2-5). The vessels are prominently seen against a background of low-attenuation material (3,4). This sign has been associated with bronchoalveolar cell carcinoma and lymphoma, but it can also be seen with other processes, including many infectious pneumonias.

DEEP SULCUS SIGN

This sign refers to a deep, sometimes fingerlike collection of intrapleural air (pneumothorax) in the costophrenic sulcus as seen on the supine chest radiograph (5). In the supine patient, air rises to the nondependent anteromedial basilar pleural space and may not cause displacement of the visceral pleural line laterally or at the apex, as seen on upright chest radiographs (Figs. 2-6 and 2-7). When present, this sign may represent a pneumothorax that is much larger than initially expected.

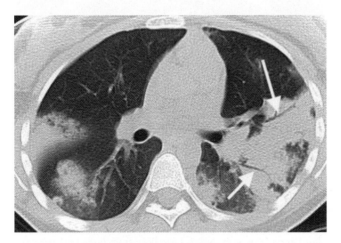

FIGURE 2-1. Air bronchogram sign. CT of the chest shows bilateral subpleural areas of airspace opacity with air bronchograms (*arrows*) resulting from acute eosinophilic pneumonia. Air bronchograms can also be seen with other causes of airspace disease, including infectious pneumonia, hemorrhage, edema, bronchoalveolar cell carcinoma, lymphoma, lipoid pneumonia, "alveolar" sarcoidosis, and alveolar proteinosis and can also be seen in atelectasis not caused by central obstruction. The presence of the sign indicates that the process is parenchymal in location, rather than mediastinal or pleural.

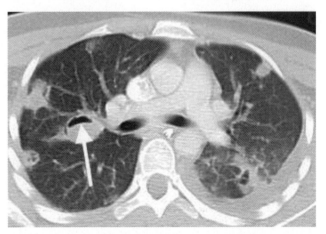

FIGURE 2-2. Air crescent sign. CT of the chest shows bilateral pulmonary nodules in a predominantly subpleural distribution resulting from septic emboli. Some of the nodules are cavitary. A resulting crescent of air (*arrows*) is contained within and outlined by the thin cavity wall.

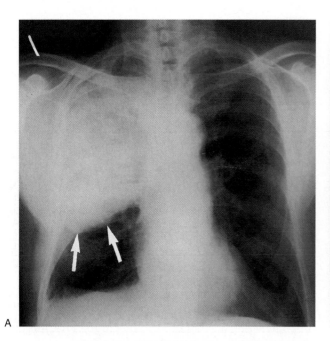

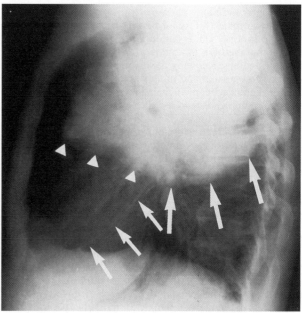

FIGURE 2-3. Bulging fissure sign. A: Posteroanterior (PA) chest radiograph shows dense opacification of the right upper lobe resulting from *Klebsiella* pneumonia. The inflammatory process is extensive and results in expansion of the lobe and bulging of the fissure inferiorly (*arrows*). **B:** Lateral view shows bulging of the superior portion of the major fissure inferiorly (*larger arrows*). The right upper lobe is outlined by the superior portion of the major fissure and the minor fissure (*arrowheads*). The middle lobe is outlined by the inferior portion of the major fissure (*smaller arrows*) and the minor fissure. The right lower lobe is outlined by the major fissure, which is divided into superior and inferior portions by the minor fissure.

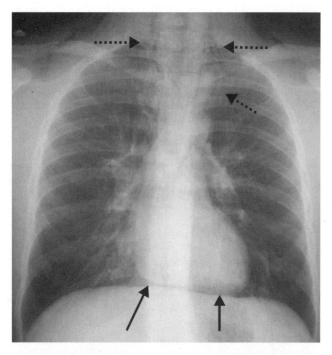

FIGURE 2-4. Continuous diaphragm sign. In this patient with pneumomediastinum, a continuous lucency is seen between the heart and the diaphragm (*solid arrows*). Air in the mediastinum is also seen tracking into the neck bilaterally (*dashed arrows*).

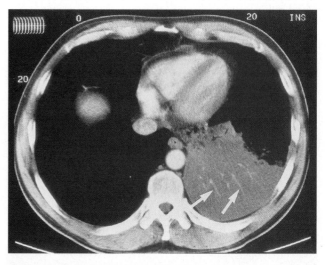

FIGURE 2-5. CT angiogram sign. CT with intravenous contrast shows opacification of the left lower lobe from bronchoalveolar cell carcinoma. The pulmonary vessels (*arrows*) are seen prominently against a background of low-attenuation mucus within the tumor. Other processes producing low-attenuation material within the lung can also produce this sign, including lymphoma, lipoid pneumonia, and bacterial pneumonia.

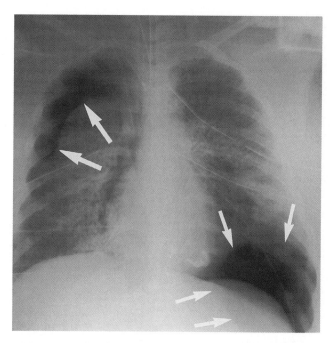

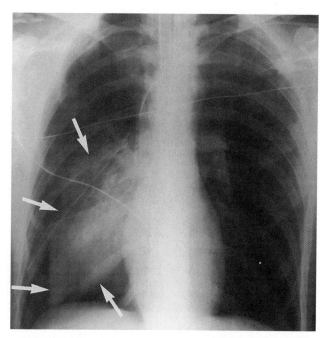

FIGURE 2-6. Deep sulcus sign. Anteroposterior (AP) supine chest radiograph shows bilateral pneumothoraces (intrapleural air) as a result of barotrauma from mechanical ventilation. On the right, the visceral pleura is separated from the parietal pleura by intrapleural air along the apicolateral chest wall (*larger arrows*). On the left, the intrapleural air is collecting at the lung base, expanding the costophrenic sulcus (*smaller arrows*). The stiff lungs do not collapse completely in this patient with acute respiratory distress syndrome.

FIGURE 2-8. Fallen lung sign. AP supine chest radiograph of a man involved in a motor vehicle accident. There is a large pneumothorax on the right, which persists with adequate chest tube placement, as a result of a fractured right mainstem bronchus. The lung has collapsed inferiorly and laterally (*arrows*), instead of toward the hilum, because it is hanging from a fractured pedicle (bronchus).

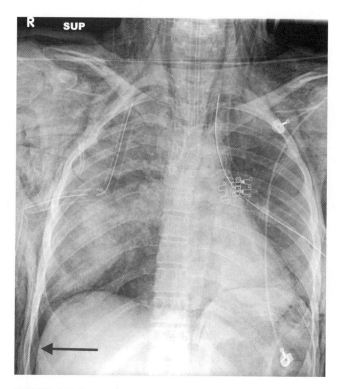

FIGURE 2-7. Deep sulcus sign. AP supine chest radiograph of a patient involved in chest trauma shows a right basilar pneumothorax (*arrow*), which expands the costophrenic sulcus, creating a tonguelike extension of air that continues inferiorly along the right lateral chest wall. Note bilateral lung contusion, pneumomediastinum, and bilateral subcutaneous emphysema.

FALLEN LUNG SIGN

This sign refers to the appearance of the collapsed lung occurring with a fractured bronchus (6). The bronchial fracture results in the lung "falling" away from the hilum, either inferiorly and laterally in an upright patient (Fig. 2-8) or posteriorly, as seen on CT in a supine patient. Normally, a pneumothorax causes a lung to collapse inward toward the hilum.

FLAT WAIST SIGN

This sign refers to flattening of the contours of the aortic knob and adjacent main pulmonary artery (Fig. 2-9). It is seen in severe collapse of the left lower lobe and is caused by leftward displacement and rotation of the heart (7).

FINGER-IN-GLOVE SIGN

In allergic bronchopulmonary aspergillosis, a clinical disorder secondary to *Aspergillus* hypersensitivity, the bronchi become impacted with mucus, cellular debris, eosinophils, and fungal hyphae. The impacted bronchi appear radiographically as opacities with distinctive shapes (Fig. 2-10), variously described as "gloved finger," "Y," "V," "inverted V," "toothpaste," and so forth (8).

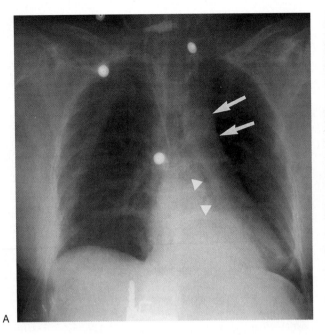
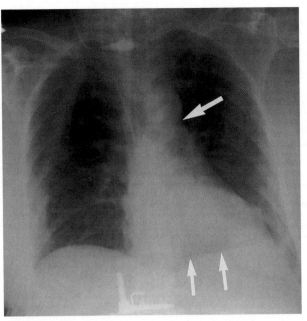

A   B

FIGURE 2-9. **Flat waist sign. A:** Frontal chest radiograph shows left lower lobe opacification from left lower lobe collapse. Note loss of the medial contour of the left hemidiaphragm, which is known as the *silhouette sign.* The left lower lobe bronchus has a more vertical course than normal (*arrowheads*). Leftward displacement and rotation of the heart in left lower lobe collapse results in flattening of the contours of the aortic knob and adjacent main pulmonary artery (*arrows*), termed the *flat waist sign.* **B:** Frontal chest radiograph obtained 1 day later shows partial re-expansion of the left lower lobe. The medial left hemidiaphragm is now visible (*smaller arrows*). There is a notch between the aorta and the pulmonary artery (*larger arrow*) and no flat waist sign.

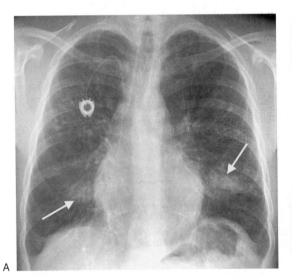
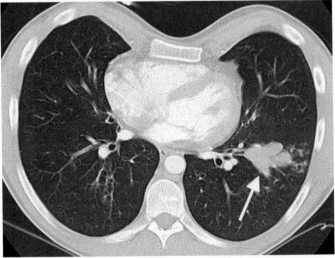

A   B

FIGURE 2-10. **Finger-in-glove sign. A:** PA chest radiograph of a patient with cystic fibrosis and allergic bronchopulmonary aspergillosis. Bronchi impacted and distended with mucus, cellular debris, eosinophils, and fungal hyphae produce tubular or masslike opacities, as seen in both lower lobes (*arrows*). Also shown is diffuse bronchiectasis related to cystic fibrosis. **B:** CT scan of the same patient shows dilated and impacted central bronchi in the left lower lobe (*arrow*).

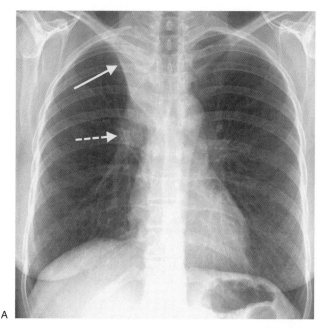

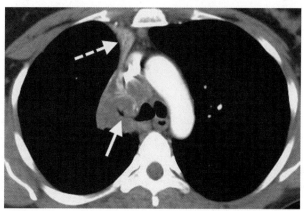

FIGURE 2-11. Golden S sign. A: PA chest radiograph of a man with bronchogenic carcinoma of the right upper lobe. The endobronchial tumor causes collapse of the right upper lobe, and upward displacement of the minor fissure (*solid arrow*). The tumor mass produces a convex margin toward the lung at the right hilum (*dashed arrow*). The contour of the displaced fissure and central mass creates a reverse S shape. Note the elevation of the right hemidiaphragm, another sign of right upper lobe volume loss. B: CT of the chest shows tumor encasing and occluding the right upper lobe bronchus (*solid arrow*) and collapse of the right upper lobe, with superior and medial displacement of the minor fissure (*dashed arrow*).

GOLDEN S SIGN

When a lobe collapses around a large central mass, the peripheral lung collapses and the central portion of lung is prevented from collapsing by the presence of the mass (Fig. 2-11). The relevant fissure is concave toward the lung peripherally but convex centrally, and the shape of the fissure resembles an S or a reverse S (9). This sign is important because it signifies the presence of a central obstructing mass that, in an adult, may represent bronchogenic carcinoma.

HALO SIGN

This sign refers to ground-glass attenuation on CT scanning that surrounds, or forms a halo around, a denser nodule or area of consolidation (Fig. 2-12). Although most hemorrhagic pulmonary nodules produce this sign (10), when seen in patients with acute leukemia, the halo sign suggests early invasive pulmonary aspergillosis (11).

HAMPTON HUMP SIGN

Pulmonary infarction secondary to pulmonary embolism produces an abnormal area of opacification on the chest radiograph, which is always in contact with the pleural surface (Fig. 2-13). The opacification may assume a variety of shapes.

When the central margin is rounded, a "hump" is produced, as described by Hampton and Castleman (12).

JUXTAPHRENIC PEAK SIGN

This sign refers to a small triangular shadow that obscures the dome of the diaphragm (Fig. 2-14), secondary to upper lobe atelectasis (13). The shadow is caused by traction on the lower end of the major fissure, the inferior accessory fissure, or the inferior pulmonary ligament.

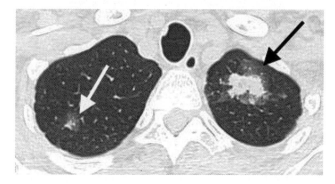

FIGURE 2-12. Halo sign. CT shows nodular consolidation associated with a halo of ground-glass opacity (GGO) in both apices (*arrows*) resulting from invasive pulmonary aspergillosis. This halo represents hemorrhage and, when seen in leukemic patients, is highly suggestive of the diagnosis of invasive pulmonary aspergillosis.

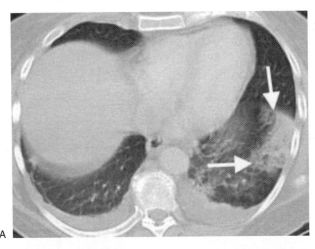
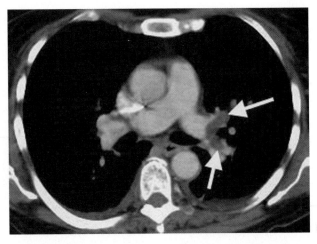

FIGURE 2-13. Hampton hump sign. A: CT with lung windowing shows a focal subpleural area of consolidation in the left lower lobe (*arrows*). This hump-shaped area of opacification represents pulmonary infarction secondary to pulmonary embolism. There are also small bilateral pleural effusions, which are commonly seen with acute pulmonary emboli. **B:** CT with mediastinal windowing shows low-attenuation filling defect, which represents a saddle embolus (*arrows*) bridging the lingular and left lower lobe pulmonary arteries.

LUFTSICHEL SIGN

In left upper lobe collapse, the superior segment of the left lower lobe, which is positioned between the aortic arch and the collapsed left upper lobe, is hyperinflated. This aerated segment of left lower lobe is hyperlucent and shaped like a sickle, where it outlines the aortic arch on the frontal chest radiograph (Fig. 2-15). This peri-aortic lucency has been termed the *luftsichel sign,* derived from the German words *luft* (air) and

sichel (sickle) (14). Although this sign can also be seen on the right, it is more common on the left because of the difference in anatomy and the presence of a minor fissure on the right. This sign and associated findings of upper lobe collapse signify the probable diagnosis of bronchogenic carcinoma in an adult.

MELTING ICE CUBE SIGN

This sign refers to the appearance of a resolving pulmonary infarct on a chest radiograph or CT scan, which looks like an ice cube that is melting peripherally to internally (Fig. 2-16). This is distinguished from the pattern of resolving pneumonia, where the opacification disappears in a patchy fashion (15).

RING AROUND THE ARTERY SIGN

This sign refers to a well-defined lucency encircling the right pulmonary artery (Fig. 2-17), as seen on frontal and lateral chest radiographs, representing pneumomediastinum (16).

SILHOUETTE SIGN

Felson and Felson (17) popularized the term *silhouette sign* to indicate an obliteration of the borders of the heart, other mediastinal structures, or diaphragm by an adjacent opacity of similar density. An intrathoracic lesion not anatomically contiguous with a border of one of these structures will not obliterate that border. Parenchymal processes involving the medial segment of the right middle lobe obliterate the right heart border (Fig. 2-18). If the lingula is involved, the left heart border is obliterated (Fig. 2-19). Lower lobe processes involving one or more basilar segments result in obliteration of all or a part of the border of the diaphragm.

FIGURE 2-14. Juxtaphrenic peak sign. PA chest radiograph of a man treated with mediastinal radiation shows paramediastinal radiation fibrosis (*dashed arrows*) and upward retraction of both hila. There is tenting of the left hemidiaphragm (*solid arrow*), indicating a loss of left upper lobe volume, seen as the juxtaphrenic peak sign.

(Text continues on page 25)

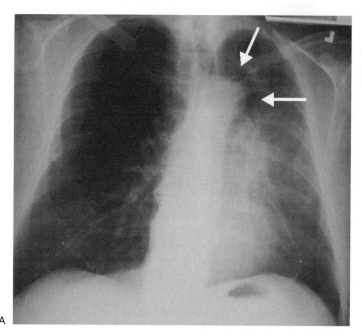
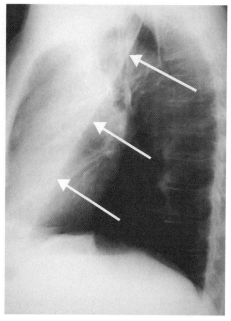

A   B

FIGURE 2-15. Luftsichel sign. A: PA chest radiograph shows a crescentic lucency adjacent to the aortic arch (*arrows*), representing hyperaeration of the superior segment of the left lower lobe, which is positioned between the aortic arch medially and the collapsed left upper lobe laterally. There is hazy opacification of the left lung (sparing the apex and costophrenic angle), elevation of the left hemidiaphragm, and partial obscuration of the left heart border (the silhouette sign), indicating a loss of left upper lobe volume. **B:** Lateral view shows anterior displacement of the major fissure (*arrows*). The superior extent of the displaced fissure indicates extension of the superior segment of the lower lobe to the lung apex. The luftsichel sign is just one sign of upper lobe collapse. The associated signs of volume loss make the diagnosis obvious. In an adult, left upper lobe collapse is highly suggestive of an obstructing bronchogenic carcinoma.

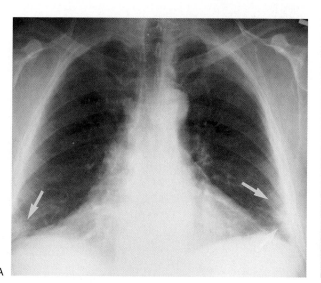
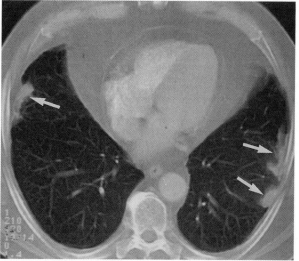

A   B

FIGURE 2-16. Melting ice cube sign. A: PA chest radiograph of a 69-year-old man with a 6-week history of cough, pleuritic chest pain, and hemoptysis shows bilateral, subpleural airspace opacities at the costophrenic angles (*arrows*), representing parenchymal infarcts. **B:** CT scan obtained 2 weeks later shows bilateral peripheral opacities (*arrows*), an appearance typical of resolving pulmonary infarcts. Note that the opacities are not wedge shaped or rounded, as expected with acute infarcts. Infarcts resolve from the periphery inward, like a melting ice cube.

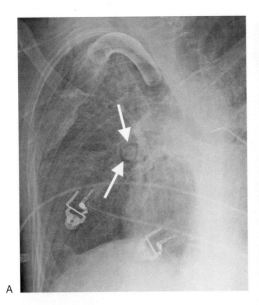
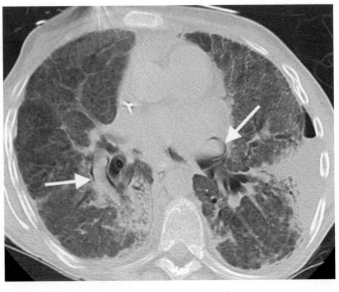

A   B

FIGURE 2-17. **Ring around the artery sign. A:** PA chest radiograph of a patient with acute respiratory distress syndrome shows a ring of lucency around the right pulmonary artery (*arrows*), signifying pneumomediastinum. **B:** CT confirms air surrounding both pulmonary arteries (*arrows*).

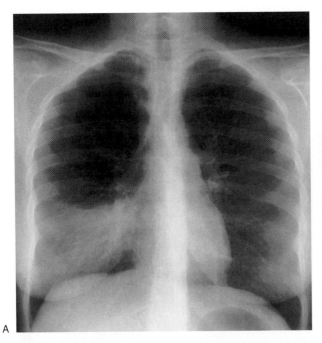
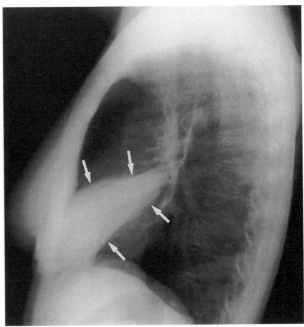

A   B

FIGURE 2-18. **Silhouette sign. A:** PA chest radiograph of a patient with pneumococcal pneumonia shows opacification of the right lower lung, which partially obscures the right heart border (the silhouette sign), indicating a process involving the right middle lobe. **B:** Lateral view shows a triangular opacity over the heart (*arrows*), confirming a right middle lobe process.

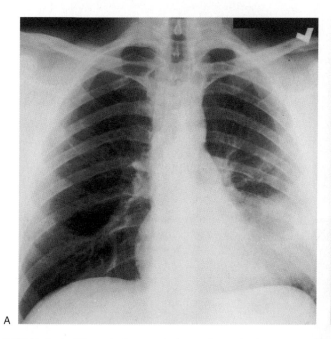
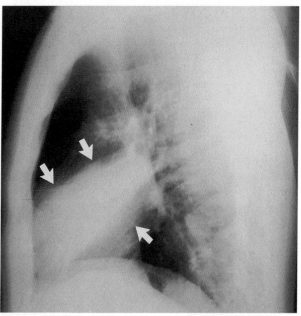

A   B

FIGURE 2-19. Silhouette sign. A: PA chest radiograph of a patient with pneumonia shows opacification of the left lower lung partially obscuring the left heart border (silhouette sign), indicating a lingular process. Note that the left hemidiaphragm is not obscured, as would be seen with a process involving any of the basilar segments of the lower lobe. B: Lateral view shows an opacity over the heart (*arrows*), confirming the lingular location of the pneumonia.

SPLIT PLEURA SIGN

Normally, the thin visceral and parietal pleura cannot be distinguished as two separate structures on CT scanning. With an exudative pleural effusion, such as empyema (Fig. 2-20), the fluid separates or "splits" the thickened and enhancing pleural layers (18).

WESTERMARK SIGN

This sign refers to oligemia of the lung beyond an occluded vessel in a patient with pulmonary embolism (Fig. 2-21) (19).

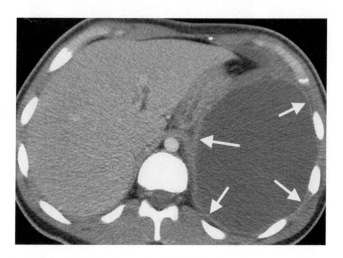

FIGURE 2-20. Split pleura sign. CT with intravenous contrast shows empyema in an intrapleural location with associated thickening, contrast enhancement, and separation of the visceral and parietal pleura (*arrows*).

SPINE SIGN

Lower lobe pneumonia may be poorly visualized on a posteroanterior (PA) chest radiograph. In such cases, the lateral view is often helpful when it shows the spine sign, which is an interruption in the progressive increase in lucency of the vertebral bodies from superior to inferior (Fig. 2-22) (20).

PATTERNS

The following patterns are not always isolated findings on chest radiographs or CT scans. They commonly occur in combination with other patterns and findings and may or may not represent the predominant imaging feature.

Honeycomb Pattern

Honeycombing is characterized by the presence of cystic airspaces with thick, clearly definable fibrous walls lined by bronchiolar epithelium. It results from destruction of alveoli and loss of acinar architecture and is associated with pulmonary fibrosis. The cysts are typically layered along the pleural surface, helping to distinguish them from the nonlayered subpleural lucencies seen with paraseptal emphysema.

Honeycombing produces a characteristic appearance on CT that allows a confident diagnosis of lung fibrosis (Fig. 2-23) (21). On CT, the cystic spaces usually average 1 cm in diameter, although they can range from several millimeters to several centimeters in size. They have clearly definable walls that are 1 to 3 mm thick, they are air-filled, and they appear lucent in comparison to normal lung parenchyma. Honeycombing is usually associated with other findings of lung fibrosis, such as architectural distortion, intralobular interstitial thickening, traction bronchiectasis, and irregular linear opacities. Honeycombing on CT usually represents idiopathic pulmonary fibrosis,

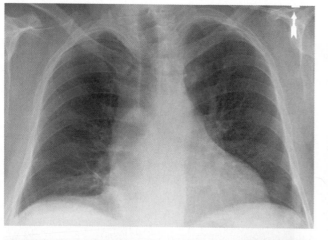

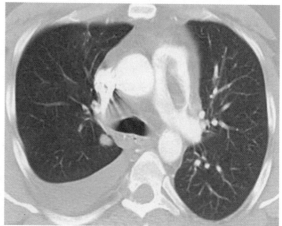

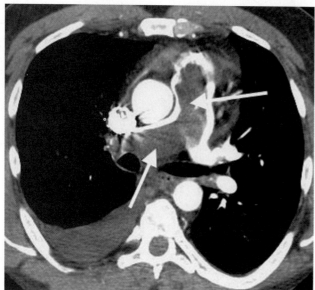

FIGURE 2-21. Westermark sign. A: PA chest radiograph shows oligemia of the right lung, the so-called Westermark sign. Note how the vessels on the right are diminutive compared with those on the left. As a result, the right hemithorax appears hyperlucent. **B:** CT with lung windowing better shows the diminution of vessels on the right compared with the left. There is also a right pleural effusion. **C:** CT with mediastinal windowing shows thrombus expanding and filling the main and right pulmonary arteries (*arrows*).

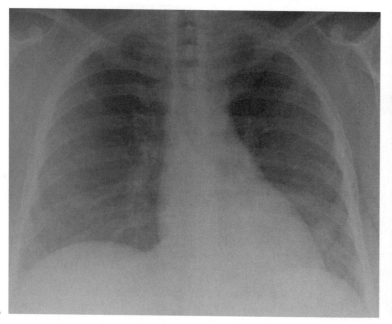

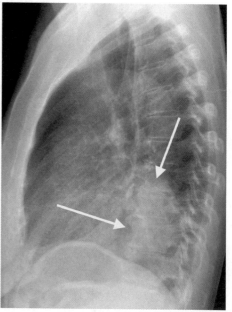

FIGURE 2-22. Spine sign. A: PA chest radiograph of a patient with left lower lobe pneumonia shows abnormal opacity in the left lower lung. **B:** Lateral view shows this opacity projected over the lower spine (*arrows*). Normally, the spine becomes progressively more lucent from the top to the bottom on the lateral view. The presence of increased opacity over the lower spine is an indication of a lower lobe process, typically pneumonia, and is called the spine sign.

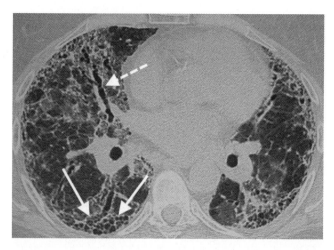

FIGURE 2-23. Honeycomb pattern. CT shows layers of subpleural cysts (*solid arrows*) representing the honeycomb pattern of pulmonary fibrosis. Also shown is traction bronchiectasis (*dashed arrow*), another sign of pulmonary fibrosis.

collagen vascular disease, asbestosis, chronic hypersensitivity pneumonitis, or drug-related fibrosis (Table 2-1).

Septal Thickening

An interlobular septum marginates part of a secondary pulmonary lobule and contains pulmonary veins and lymphatics. These septa measure approximately 0.1 mm in thickness and are occasionally seen on normal thin-section CT scans. Abnormal thickening of interlobular septa is caused by fibrosis, edema, or infiltration by cells or other material. Within the peripheral lung, thickened septa 1 to 2 cm in length may outline part or all of a secondary pulmonary lobule, perpendicular to the pleural surface. They represent the CT counterpart of Kerley B lines seen on chest radiographs.

Interlobular septal thickening can be smooth (Fig. 2-24) or nodular (22) (Table 2-1). Smooth thickening is seen in patients with pulmonary edema or hemorrhage, lymphangitic spread of carcinoma, lymphoma, leukemia, interstitial infiltration associated with amyloidosis, and some pneumonias. Nodular or "beaded" thickening occurs in lymphangitic spread

TABLE 2-1

DIFFERENTIAL DIAGNOSIS OF PATTERNS OF DISEASE ON CT OF THE LUNGS

Honeycomb
Idiopathic pulmonary fibrosis
Collagen vascular diseases
Asbestosis
Chronic hypersensitivity pneumonitis
Drug-related fibrosis

Interlobular septal thickening
<u>Smooth</u>
Pulmonary edema
Pulmonary hemorrhage
Lymphangitic spread of carcinoma
Infectious pneumonia
Lymphoma and leukemia
Amyloidosis

<u>Beaded</u>
Lymphangitic spread of carcinoma
Lymphoma
Sarcoidosis
Silicosis and coal worker's pneumoconiosis
Lymphocytic interstitial pneumonitis
Amyloidosis

Cystic
Langerhan cell histiocytosis
Lymphangioleiomyomatosis
Sarcoidosis
Lymphocytic interstitial pneumonitis
Collagen vascular diseases
Pneumocystis pneumonia
Honeycombing
Centrilobular emphysema

Nodular
<u>Perilymphatic</u>
Sarcoidosis
<u>Random</u>
Silicosis and coal worker's pneumoconiosis

Tuberculosis and fungal infection
Metastases
Langerhan cell histiocytosis
<u>Centrilobular</u>
Subacute hypersensitivity pneumonitis
Respiratory bronchiolitis
<u>Bronchovascular</u>
Lymphoproliferative disorders
Leukemia
Kaposi sarcoma
<u>Cavitating</u>
Metastases
Wegener granulomatosis
Septic emboli
Mycobacterial or fungal infection

Ground-glass opacity
Infectious pneumonia
Pulmonary edema
Pulmonary hemorrhage
Acute or subacute hypersensitivity pneumonitis
Desquamative interstitial pneumonitis
Pulmonary alveolar proteinosis
Inadvertent exhalation

Mosaic lung attenuation
Infiltrative lung processes
Small airway disease
Pulmonary vascular disease

Tree-in-bud
Infection
Aspiration
Allergic bronchopulmonary aspergillosis
Cystic fibrosis
Diffuse panbronchiolitis
Obliterative bronchiolitis
Asthma

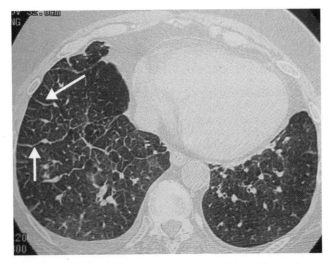

FIGURE 2-24. Smooth septal thickening. CT shows smooth thickening of the interlobular septae (*arrows*) in this patient with pulmonary edema. There are also small pleural effusions and scattered areas of GGO, which support the diagnosis.

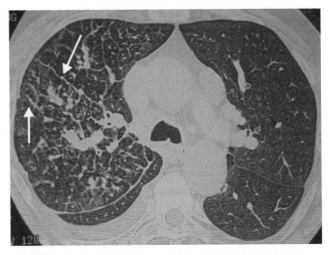

FIGURE 2-25. Nodular septal thickening. CT shows nodular thickening of the septae (*arrows*), other scattered small nodules, and areas of GGO, involving only the right lung. These findings are highly suggestive of this patient's diagnosis: lymphangitic carcinomatosis associated with primary bronchogenic carcinoma involving the right lung. Lymphangitic carcinomatosis from an extrathoracic malignancy usually involves both lungs.

of carcinoma (Fig. 2-25) or lymphoma, sarcoidosis, silicosis or coal worker's pneumoconiosis, lymphocytic interstitial pneumonia, and amyloidosis.

Cystic Pattern

The term "cyst" is nonspecific and refers to a thin-walled (usually less than 3 mm thick), well-defined, well-circumscribed, air- or fluid-containing lesion, 1 cm or more in diameter, that has an epithelial or fibrous wall. A cystic pattern results from a heterogeneous group of diseases that have in common the presence of focal, multifocal, or diffuse parenchymal lucencies and lung destruction (Table 2-1). Pulmonary Langerhan cell histiocytosis, lymphangioleiomyomatosis, sarcoidosis, lymphocytic interstitial pneumonitis, collagen vascular diseases, *Pneumocystis* pneumonia, and honeycombing can manifest a cystic pattern on CT. Although they do not represent true cystic disease, centrilobular emphysema and cystic bronchiectasis mimic cystic disease on chest CT scans.

In cases of Langerhan cell histiocytosis, the cysts are often confluent, usually thin-walled, and often associated with

pulmonary nodules 1 to 5 mm in diameter that may or may not be cavitary (Fig. 2-26). The intervening lung parenchyma is typically normal, without evidence of fibrosis or septal thickening. The distribution of findings is usually upper lungs, with sparing of the costophrenic sulci. The cysts are distributed diffusely throughout the lungs in lymphangioleiomyomatosis (Fig. 2-27), and nodules are not a common feature. The "cystic" spaces seen with centrilobular emphysema often contain a small nodular opacity representing the centrilobular artery (Fig. 2-28). This finding is helpful in distinguishing emphysema from lymphangioleiomyomatosis and Langerhan cell histiocytosis.

Nodular Pattern

A *nodular pattern* refers to multiple round opacities, generally ranging in diameter from 1 mm to 1 cm, that may be very difficult to separate from one another as individual nodules on a

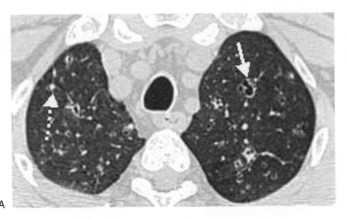
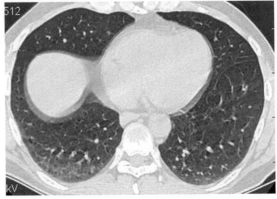

FIGURE 2-26. Cystic pattern. A: CT of this patient with Langerhan cell histiocytosis shows irregular, variably sized cysts with definable walls (*solid arrow*) and scattered small nodules (*dashed arrow*) involving both upper lungs. **B:** CT at a level inferior to A shows normal lower lungs. The sparing of the lower lungs and the combination of cysts and nodules is highly suggestive of Langerhan cell histiocytosis.

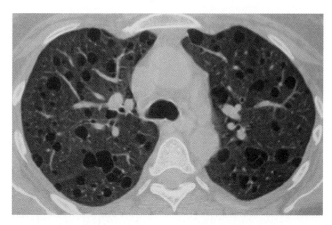

FIGURE 2-27. Cystic pattern. CT scan of a woman with lymphangioleiomyomatosis shows fairly homogeneous thin-walled cysts with normal intervening lung parenchyma. The cysts involve the upper and lower lungs equally (not shown).

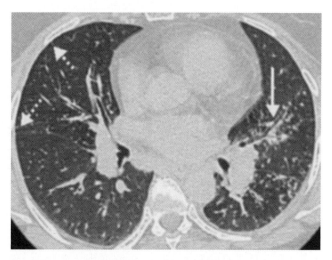

FIGURE 2-29. Perilymphatic nodular pattern. CT scan of a young man with sarcoidosis shows numerous small nodules distributed along the bronchovascular bundles (*solid arrow*) and subpleural lung (*dashed arrows*). This is a perilymphatic distribution, which is typical of sarcoidosis.

chest radiograph because of superimposition but which are accurately diagnosed on CT. Nodular opacities may be described as miliary (1 to 2 mm, the size of millet seeds), small, medium, or large as the diameter of the opacity increases. Nodules can be further characterized according to their margins (e.g., smooth or irregular), presence or absence of cavitation, attenuation characteristics (such as ground-glass opacity [GGO] or calcification), and distribution (e.g., centrilobular, perilymphatic, or random) (23) (Table 2-1).

Multiple small smooth or irregularly margined nodules in a perilymphatic distribution are characteristic of sarcoidosis (Fig. 2-29). The nodules represent the coalescence of microscopic noncaseating granulomas distributed along the bronchoarterial bundles, interlobular septa, and subpleural regions. A similar appearance can be seen with silicosis or coal worker's pneumoconiosis, although with the latter, the distribution of nodules is random, with predominant upper lung zone involvement. Within affected areas, the nodules of silicosis can show a predominantly posterior distribution. As disease progresses, coalescence of the silicotic nodules leads to progressive massive fibrosis. Numerous small nodules of GGO in a cen-

trilobular distribution are characteristic of the acute or subacute stage of extrinsic allergic alveolitis (Fig. 2-30) or respiratory bronchiolitis. The nodules are poorly defined and usually measure less than 3 mm in diameter. A random distribution of miliary nodules can be seen with hematogenous spread of tuberculosis (Fig. 2-31), fungal infection, or metastases from a variety of primary sources. When associated with irregularly shaped, thin-walled cysts, randomly distributed nodules suggest Langerhan cell histiocytosis. Multiple cavitary nodules can be seen with metastases (usually of squamous cell histology), Wegener granulomatosis, rheumatoid lung disease, septic emboli, and multifocal infection (typically of fungal or mycobacterial etiology). Multiple irregular nodules in a bronchovascular distribution are characteristic of benign

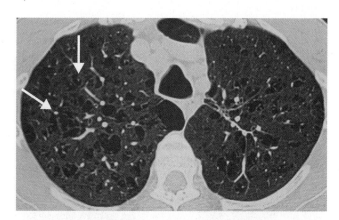

FIGURE 2-28. Cystic pattern look-alike. CT scan shows lucent areas throughout both lungs, which can occasionally be confused with true lung cysts. However, the lucent areas do not have circumferential walls and in some areas, the centrilobular artery is visible within the area of lucency (*arrows*). These findings, along with a distribution that is predominantly in the upper lungs, are typical of centrilobular emphysema.

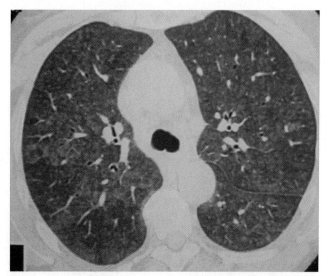

FIGURE 2-30. Centrilobular nodular pattern. CT scan of a man with acute hypersensitivity pneumonitis (also called extrinsic allergic alveolitis) shows numerous ill-defined ground-glass nodules in a centrilobular distribution. This appearance is highly suggestive of the diagnosis but can also be seen in respiratory bronchiolitis. A history of exposure and the presence or absence of cigarette smoking help to make the correct diagnosis.

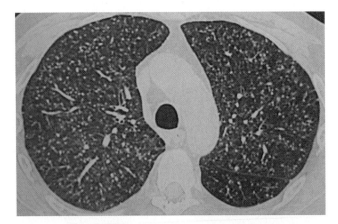

FIGURE 2-31. Random nodular pattern. CT scan of a patient with miliary tuberculosis shows a pattern of diffuse, randomly distributed, well-defined small pulmonary nodules. Some of the nodules appear centrilobular and some are subpleural in location. The same pattern can be seen with fungal infection or pulmonary metastases.

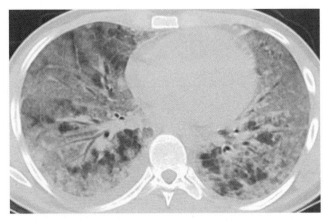

FIGURE 2-33. Ground-glass pattern. CT scan of a patient with diffuse pneumonia shows extensive bilateral GGO. Note that the pulmonary vessels and bronchi are still visible. This is a nonspecific pattern that is also commonly seen with pulmonary hemorrhage and pulmonary edema.

lymphoproliferative disorders (Fig. 2-32), lymphoma, leukemia, and Kaposi sarcoma.

Ground-Glass Pattern

GGO is defined as "hazy increased attenuation of lung, with preservation of bronchial and vascular margins; caused by partial filling of airspaces, interstitial thickening, partial collapse of alveoli, normal expiration, or increased capillary blood volume; not to be confused with consolidation, in which bronchovascular margins are obscured; may be associated with an air bronchogram" (24). GGO is a common but nonspecific finding on CT that reflects the presence of abnormalities below the limit of CT resolution (Table 2-1). In one investigation of patients with chronic infiltrative lung disease in whom lung biopsy was performed in areas of GGO, the pattern was shown to be caused by predominantly interstitial diseases in 54% of cases, equal involvement of the interstitium and airspaces in 32%, and predominantly airspace disease in 14% (25). GGO is an important finding. In certain clinical circumstances, it can suggest a specific diagnosis, indicate a potentially treatable disease, and guide a bronchoscopist or surgeon to an appropriate area for biopsy (26).

Acute lung diseases characteristically associated with diffuse GGO include pneumonia (Fig. 2-33), pulmonary hemorrhage, and pulmonary edema. In patients with acquired immunodeficiency syndrome, the presence of focal or diffuse GGO on CT is highly suggestive of *Pneumocystis* pneumonia. In patients with lung transplants, GGO is very suggestive of Cytomegalovirus pneumonia or acute rejection. When diffuse GGO is seen in the first month after bone marrow transplantation, both infection and diffuse alveolar hemorrhage should be considered.

Diffuse or patchy GGO is frequently the main abnormality seen in the acute or subacute phase of extrinsic allergic alveolitis. It is also the predominant finding in patients with desquamative interstitial pneumonia, in which it reflects the presence of mild interstitial thickening and filling of the airspaces with macrophages. In pulmonary alveolar proteinosis, the areas of GGO usually have a patchy or geographic distribution. Although the abnormality consists mainly of filling of airspaces with proteinaceous material, interlobular septal thickening is frequently identified on CT in the areas of GGO, creating a "crazy paving" pattern (Fig. 2-34). Solitary small areas of GGO can signify early stage bronchioloalveolar carcinoma or atypical adenomatous hyperplasia (AAH).

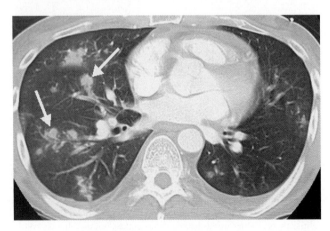

FIGURE 2-32. Bronchovascular nodular pattern. CT scan of a patient with benign posttransplant lymphoproliferative disorder shows multiple ill-defined nodules distributed along the bronchovascular bundles (*arrows*). This appearance can also be seen with malignant lymphoma, leukemia, and Kaposi sarcoma.

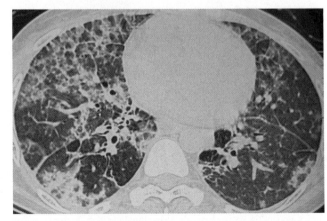

FIGURE 2-34. "Crazy paving" pattern. CT scan of a patient with pulmonary alveolar proteinosis shows patchy areas of GGO associated with septal thickening, so-called "crazy paving." This is a characteristic but not pathognomonic finding of pulmonary alveolar proteinosis.

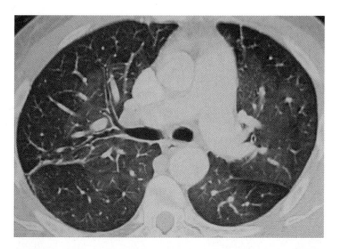

FIGURE 2-35. Mosaic perfusion pattern. CT scan of a patient with sickle cell disease shows a mosaic pattern of lung attenuation. The abnormal lucent areas represent decreased perfusion secondary to microvascular occlusion.

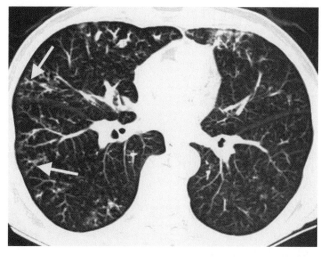

FIGURE 2-37. Tree-in-bud pattern. Maximum-intensity projection axial CT image of a patient with bacterial bronchiolitis shows a pattern of small nodular and linear branching opacities, predominantly in the periphery of the lung (arrows). This is a bronchiolar distribution. The most common etiologies for this pattern are infection and aspiration.

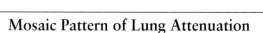

Mosaic Pattern of Lung Attenuation

Lung attenuation normally increases during exhalation. In the presence of airway obstruction and air trapping, lung remains lucent on exhalation and shows little change in cross-sectional area; this is best appreciated when patchy and compared to normal lung. Areas of air trapping are seen as relatively low in attenuation on expiratory CT scans. Areas of air trapping can be patchy and nonanatomic; can correspond to individual secondary pulmonary lobules, segments, and lobes; or may involve an entire lung. Air trapping in a lobe or lung is usually associated with large airway or generalized small airway abnormalities, whereas lobular or segmental air trapping is associated with diseases that affect small airways. Bronchiolectasis is a common associated finding. Pulmonary vessels within the low-attenuation areas of air trapping often appear small relative to vessels in the more opaque normal lung regions (27). This finding is also seen with vascular disease, such as chronic thromboembolic disease, as a result of decreased perfusion to affected areas of lung.

The presence of heterogeneous lung attenuation on inspiratory scans—the so-called mosaic pattern of lung attenuation—can result from infiltrative processes, airway obstruction and

reflex vasoconstriction, mosaic perfusion resulting from vascular obstruction (e.g., chronic thromboembolic disease; Fig. 2-35), or a combination of these (Table 2-1). In patients with GGO from infiltrative processes, expiratory CT shows a proportional increase in attenuation in areas of both increased and decreased opacity. In patients with mosaic attenuation resulting from airway disease, such as obliterative bronchiolitis or asthma, attenuation differences are accentuated or seen only on expiration (Fig. 2-36). In patients with mosaic perfusion caused by vascular disease, air trapping can be seen but is not a dominant feature on expiratory CT.

Tree-in-Bud Pattern

The CT pattern of centrilobular nodular and branching linear opacities has been likened to the appearance of a budding tree. Many disorders can result in this pattern, the most common being infectious processes with endobronchial spread of disease (Fig. 2-37) (28,29) (Table 2-1). The common CT features of all processes producing the tree-in-bud pattern are (a) bronchiolar

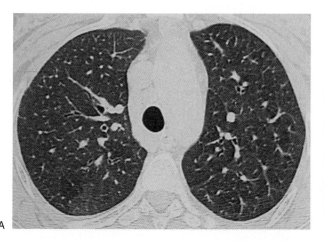

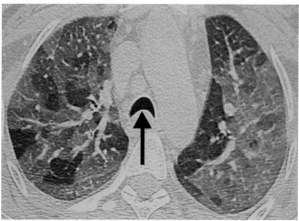

FIGURE 2-36. Mosaic attenuation pattern. A: Inspiratory CT scan of a patient with asthma shows a homogeneous pattern of lung attenuation. B: Expiratory CT scan shows a mosaic pattern of lung attenuation. The abnormal lucent areas represent air trapping related to the patient's asthma. Note the anterior bowing of the posterior membranous trachea (arrow), indicating expiration.

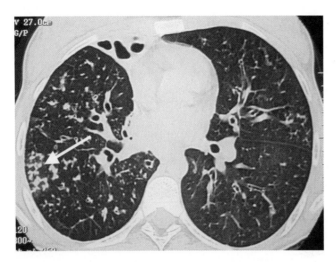

FIGURE 2-38. Tree-in-bud pattern. CT scan of a patient with cystic fibrosis shows bilateral bronchiectasis and bronchiolectasis, along with "tree-in-bud" opacities in the periphery of the right lung (*arrow*). The opacities represent mucoid impaction of the bronchioles.

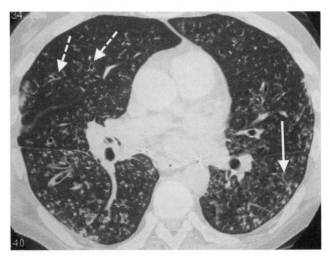

FIGURE 2-40. Tree-in-bud pattern. CT scan of a patient with diffuse panbronchiolitis shows tree-in-bud pattern (*solid arrow*) and dilated, nonimpacted bronchioles (*dashed arrows*).

dilatation and (b) impaction of bronchioles with mucus, pus, or other material. The CT findings are nonspecific, but a specific diagnosis can occasionally be suggested when the findings are correlated with patient history, clinical information, associated CT scan findings, and chronicity of disease.

The term *tree-in-bud* dates back to the bronchogram descriptions of normal respiratory bronchioles by Twining and Kerley (30) but has been more recently popularized by Im et al (31) to describe the CT appearance of the endobronchial spread of *Mycobacterium* tuberculosis.

Numerous noninfectious disorders are associated with the tree-in-bud pattern. In allergic bronchopulmonary aspergillosis, immunologic responses to the endobronchial growth of *Aspergillus* sp result in damage to the bronchial wall, central bronchiectasis, and the formation of mucous plugs that contain fungus and inflammatory cells. The tree-in-bud pattern is seen when the process extends to the bronchioles. In cystic fibrosis, an abnormally low water content of airway mucus is at least partially responsible for decreased mucous clearance, mucous plugging of small and large airways, and an increased incidence of bacterial airway infection. Bronchial wall inflammation pro-

gresses to bronchiectasis, and bronchiolar secretions result in a tree-in-bud pattern (Fig. 2-38). The tree-in-bud pattern can also be seen with aspiration of infected oral secretions or other irritant material (Fig. 2-39), diffuse panbronchiolitis (Fig. 2-40), obliterative bronchiolitis, and asthma.

References

1. Felson LB, Rosenberg LS, Hamburger M. Roentgen findings in acute Friedlander's pneumonia. *Radiology.* 1949; 53:559–565.
2. Levin B. The continuous diaphragm sign: a newly recognized sign of pneumomediastinum. *Clin Radiol.* 1973;24:337–338.
3. Im JG, Han MC, Yu EJ. Lobar bronchioloalveolar carcinoma: "angiogram sign" on CT scans. *Radiology.* 1990;176:749–753.
4. Vincent JM, Ng YY, Norton AJ, et al. CT "angiogram sign" in primary pulmonary lymphoma. *J Comput Assist Tomogr.* 1992;16:829–831.
5. Gordon R. The deep sulcus sign. *Radiology.* 1980;136:25–27.
6. Oh KS, Fleischner FG, Wyman SM. Characteristic pulmonary finding in traumatic complete transection of a main stem bronchus. *Radiology.* 1969;92:371–372.
7. Armstrong P. Basic patterns in lung disease. In: Armstrong P, Wilson AG, Dee P, Hansell DM, eds. *Imaging of Diseases of the Chest.* 2nd ed. St. Louis, MO: Mosby; 1995:89.
8. Gefter WB. The spectrum of pulmonary aspergillosis. *J Thorac Imaging.* 1992;7:56–74.
9. Golden R. The effect of bronchostenosis upon the roentgen-ray shadows in carcinoma of the bronchus. *Am J Roentgenol.* 1925;13:21–30.
10. Primack SL, Hartman TE, Lee KS, Müller NL. Pulmonary nodules and the CT halo sign. *Radiology.* 1994;190:513–515.
11. Kuhlman JE, Fishman EK, Siegelman SS. Invasive pulmonary aspergillosis in acute leukemia: characteristic findings on CT, the CT halo sign, and the role of CT in early diagnosis. *Radiology.* 1985;157:611–614.
12. Hampton AO, Castleman B. Correlations of post mortem chest teleroentgenograms with autopsy findings with special reference to pulmonary embolism and infarction. *Am J Roentgenol.* 1940;43:305–326.
13. Kattan KR, Eyler WR, Felson B. The juxtaphrenic peak in upper lobe collapse. *Semin Roentgenol.* 1980;15:187–193.
14. Burgel E, Oleck HG. Ueber die rechtsseitige paramediastinale Luftsichel bei Oberlappenschrumpfung. *Rofo.* 1960;93:160–163.
15. Woesner ME, Sanders I, White GW. The melting sign in resolving transient pulmonary infarction. *Am J Roentgenol.* 1971;111:782–790.
16. Hammond DI. The "ring around the artery" sign in pneumomediastinum. *J Can Assoc Radiol.* 1984;35:88–89.
17. Felson B, Felson H. Localization of intrathoracic lesions by means of the postero-anterior roentgenogram: the silhouette sign. *Radiology.* 1950;55:363–374.
18. Stark DD, Federle MP, Goodman PC, et al. Differentiating lung abscess and empyema: Radiography and computed tomography. *Am J Roentgenol.* 1983;141:163–167.
19. Westermark N. On the roentgen diagnosis of lung embolism. *Acta Radiol.* 1938;19:357–372.

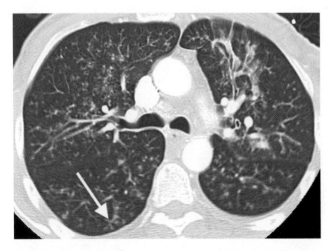

FIGURE 2-39. Tree-in-bud pattern. CT scan of a patient who aspirated shows extensive tree-in-bud pattern (*arrow*) bilaterally.

20. Ely JW, Berbaum KS, Bergus GR, et al. Diagnosing left lower lobe pneumonia: usefulness of the 'spine sign' on lateral chest radiographs. *J Fam Pract*. 1996;43:242–248.

21. Müller NL, Miller RR, Webb WR, et al. Fibrosing alveolitis: CT-pathologic correlation. *Radiology*. 1986;160:585–588.

22. Kang EY, Grenier P, Laurent F, et al. Interlobular septal thickening: patterns at high-resolution computed tomography. *J Thorac Imaging*. 1996;11:260–264.

23. Gruden JF, Webb WR, Naidich DP, et al. Multinodular disease; anatomic localization at thin-section CT: multireader evaluation of a simple algorithm. *Radiology*. 1999;210:711–720.

24. Austin JHM, Müller NL, Friedman PJ, et al. Glossary of terms for CT of the lungs: recommendations of the nomenclature committee of the Fleischner Society. *Radiology*. 1996;200:327–331.

25. Leung AN, Miller RR, Müller NL. Parenchymal opacification in chronic infiltrative lung diseases: CT-pathologic correlation. *Radiology*. 1993;188:209–214.

26. Collins J, Stern EJ. Ground-glass opacity at CT: the ABCs. *Am J Roentgenol*. 1997;169:355–367.

27. Stern EJ, Webb WR. Dynamic imaging of lung morphology with ultrafast high-resolution computed tomography. *J Thorac Imag*. 1993;8:273–282.

28. Collins J, Blankenbaker D, Stern EJ. CT patterns of bronchiolar disease: what is "tree-in-bud"? *Am J Roentgenol*. 1998;171:365–370.

29. Aquino SL, Gamsu G, Webb WR, Kee ST. Tree-in-bud pattern: frequency and significance on thin section CT. *J Comput Assist Tomogr*. 1996;20:594–599.

30. Twining E, Kerley P. *Textbook of X-Ray Diagnosis*. 2nd ed. London: Lewis; 1951:208.

31. Im JG, Itoh H, Shim YS, et al. Pulmonary tuberculosis: CT findings—early active disease and sequential change with antituberculous therapy. *Radiology*. 1993;186:653–660.

CHAPTER 3

INTERSTITIAL LUNG DISEASE

LEARNING OBJECTIVES

1. List and identify on a chest radiograph and computed tomographic (CT) scan the four patterns of interstitial lung disease (ILD): linear, reticular, reticulonodular, and nodular.

2. Make a specific diagnosis of ILD when supportive findings are present in the history or on radiologic imaging (e.g., dilated esophagus and ILD in scleroderma; enlarged heart, pacemaker or defibrillator, prior sternotomy, and ILD in a patient with amiodarone drug toxicity).

3. Identify Kerley A and B lines on a chest radiograph and CT scan and explain their etiology and significance.

4. Recognize the changes of congestive heart failure on a chest radiograph (enlarged cardiac silhouette, pleural effusions, vascular redistribution, interstitial or alveolar edema, Kerley lines, enlarged azygos vein, increased ratio of artery to bronchus diameter).

5. Define "asbestos-related pleural disease" and "asbestosis"; identify each on a chest radiograph and CT scan.

6. Describe what a "B reader" is, as related to the evaluation of pneumoconioses.

7. Identify honeycombing on a chest radiograph and CT scan, state the significance of this finding (end-stage lung disease), and list the common causes of honeycomb lung.

8. Recognize progressive massive fibrosis/conglomerate masses secondary to silicosis or coal worker's pneumoconiosis on a chest radiograph and CT scan.

9. Recognize the typical appearance and upper lobe–predominant distribution of irregular lung cysts or nodules on chest CT of a patient with Langerhan cell histiocytosis.

10. List four causes of unilateral ILD (aspiration, radiation, lymphangitic carcinomatosis secondary to bronchogenic carcinoma, asymmetric edema).

11. List the common causes of lower lobe–predominant ILD (idiopathic pulmonary fibrosis, asbestosis, chronic aspiration, collagen vascular disease).

12. List two causes of upper lobe–predominant ILD (chronic hypersensitivity pneumonitis, sarcoidosis).

13. Recognize the findings of lymphangioleiomyomatosis on a chest radiograph and CT scan.

This chapter on interstitial lung disease (ILD) is followed by a chapter on alveolar lung disease (ALD). When the chest radiograph shows a clear pattern of ILD or ALD, one can render a differential diagnosis based on the pattern of parenchymal disease (Table 3-1). A conundrum arises when widespread small opacities are difficult to categorize into one group or the other on chest radiography, or when ILD and ALD are both present. In these cases, coming up with a differential diagnosis is not as straightforward. One must decide what the *predominant* pattern is, take into consideration the clinical history and any associated radiographic findings, or further define the pattern(s) and distribution of disease with a CT scan of the lungs.

PATTERNS OF INTERSTITIAL LUNG DISEASE

The interstitium of the lung is not normally visible radiographically; it becomes visible only when disease (e.g., edema, fibrosis, tumor) increases its volume and attenuation. The interstitial space is defined as "a continuum of loose connective tissue throughout the lung composed of three subdivisions: (i) the bronchovascular (axial), surrounding the bronchi, arteries, and veins from the lung root to the level of the respiratory bronchiole; (ii) the parenchymal (acinar), situated between the alveolar and capillary basement membranes; and (iii) the subpleural, situated beneath the pleura, as well as in the interlobular septa" (1). Any or all of these three interstitial compartments can be abnormal at any one time.

Interstitial lung disease may result in four patterns of abnormal opacity on chest radiographs and CT scans: linear, reticular, nodular, and reticulonodular (Fig. 3-1). These patterns are more accurately and specifically defined on CT. A *linear* pattern is seen when there is thickening of the interlobular septa, producing Kerley lines. These septal lines were first described by Kerley in patients with pulmonary edema (2). Kerley B lines are short, straight lines (1 to 2 cm) perpendicular to and abutting the lower lateral pleural edge. Kerley A lines are generally longer (2 to 6 cm), they radiate out from the hilum toward the pleura but are not contiguous with the pleura, and they are most obvious in the upper and middle lungs. The interlobular septa contain pulmonary veins and lymphatics. The most common cause of interlobular septal thickening, producing Kerley A and B lines, is pulmonary edema, as a result of pulmonary venous hypertension and distension of the lymphatics (Fig. 3-2). Other causes of Kerley lines are listed in Table 3-2. Anything that causes thickening of the interlobular septa can produce Kerley lines, including edema, inflammation, tumor, or fibrosis. Septal thickening without architectural distortion is more likely to represent pulmonary edema.

TABLE 3-1

DIFFERENTIAL DIAGNOSIS OF INTERSTITIAL LUNG DISEASE

"BADLASH"
Bronchiectasis (ILD "look-alike")
Bugs (especially fungi, mycoplasma, and viruses)
Aspiration, chronic
Amyloidosis
Drug toxicity
Lymphangioleiomyomatosis
Lymphangitic carcinomatosis
Lymphoma
Lymphocytic interstitial pneumonia and other idiopathic interstitial pneumonias
Asbestosis
Sarcoidosis
Scleroderma and other collagen vascular diseases
Silicosis
Hypersensitivity pneumonitis
Heart failure
Histiocytosis (Langerhan cell histiocytosis)

ILD, interstitial lung disease

TABLE 3-2

DIFFERENTIAL DIAGNOSIS OF KERLEY LINES

Pulmonary edema—the most common cause
Mitral stenosis
Lymphangitic carcinomatosis
Malignant lymphoma
Congenital lymphangiectasia
Viral and mycoplasma pneumonias
Idiopathic pulmonary fibrosis
Pneumoconiosis
Sarcoidosis
Late-stage hemosiderosis

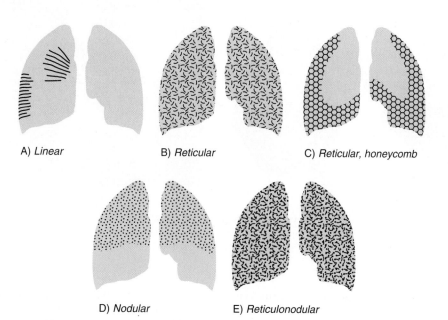

A) *Linear*   B) *Reticular*   C) *Reticular, honeycomb*

D) *Nodular*   E) *Reticulonodular*

FIGURE 3-1. Diagrams illustrating the four types of ILD. A: Linear ILD is seen as Kerley lines. Kerley A lines radiate out from the hila to the periphery of the lung. Kerley B lines are shorter lines that contact and are perpendicular to the lateral pleural edge, predominantly in the lower lungs. Both A and B lines are seen as a result of interlobular septal thickening, most commonly from pulmonary edema. **B:** Reticular ILD is seen as a network of curvilinear opacities. When seen as a result of a reversible process, such as viral pneumonia, sarcoidosis, or hypersensitivity pneumonitis, the distribution can be patchy or diffuse. **C:** When reticular ILD is seen as a result of chronic, irreversible lung disease, such as usual interstitial pneumonia, honeycombing is seen. The curvilinear opacities form small cystic spaces (forming the honeycomb) in a characteristic bibasilar and subpleural distribution. **D:** Nodular ILD will often, but not always, have an upper and middle lung–predominant distribution. This is often the case with sarcoidosis, Langerhan cell histiocytosis, silicosis, and coal worker's lung. The nodules generally range from 1 to 10 mm in size. **E:** Reticulonodular ILD results from a combination of reticular and nodular opacities, or it can be caused by reticular opacities seen end-on. This pattern is often difficult to distinguish from a pure nodular or reticular pattern on chest radiography. The list of diagnostic possibilities to consider when this pattern is seen can be shortened by taking into account the acuity of the disease, the distribution of disease, and associated radiographic abnormalities.

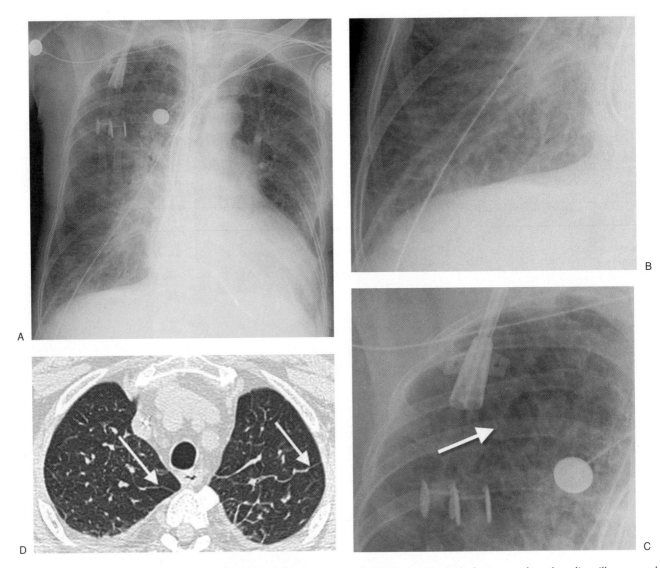

FIGURE 3-2. Kerley lines. This patient presented with cardiogenic edema. **A:** PA chest radiograph shows an enlarged cardiac silhouette and bilateral reticular and linear ILD. **B:** Close-up view of (**A**), lower right lung, shows short linear opacities perpendicular to the lateral pleural edge, representing Kerley B lines. **C:** Close-up of (**A**), right upper lung, shows linear opacities (*arrow*) radiating outward from the hila, representing Kerley A lines. **D:** CT shows interlobular septal thickening (*arrows*), representing Kerley lines.

A *reticular* pattern results from the summation or superimposition of irregular linear opacities. The term *reticular* is defined as meshed, or in the form of a network. Reticular opacities can be described as fine, medium, or coarse, as the width of the opacities increases. A classic reticular pattern is seen with pulmonary fibrosis, in which multiple curvilinear opacities form small cystic spaces along the pleural margins and lung bases (honeycomb lung) (Fig. 3-3).

A *nodular* pattern consists of multiple round opacities, generally ranging in diameter from 1 mm to 1 cm, which may be difficult to distinguish from one another as individual nodules on a chest radiograph. Nodular opacities may be described as miliary (1 to 2 mm, the size of millet seeds), small, medium, or large, as the diameter of the opacities increases (Figs. 3-4 and 3-5). A nodular pattern, especially with an upper lung–predominant distribution, suggests a specific differential diagnosis (Table 3-3).

A *reticulonodular* pattern results from a combination of reticular and nodular opacities, or it can appear when reticular opacities are seen end-on. This pattern is often difficult to distinguish from a purely reticular or nodular pattern, and in such

a case a differential diagnosis should be developed based on the *predominant* pattern. If there is no predominant pattern, causes of both nodular and reticular patterns should be considered. An acute appearance suggests pulmonary edema or pneumonia (Fig. 3-6). A lower lung–predominant distribution with decreased lung volumes suggests idiopathic pulmonary fibrosis, asbestosis, collagen vascular disease, or chronic aspiration. A reticulonodular pattern and larger-than-normal lung volumes can be seen with lymphangioleiomyomatosis and Langerhan cell histiocytosis (LCH). A middle or upper lung–predominant distribution suggests mycobacterial or fungal disease, silicosis, sarcoidosis, LCH, extrinsic allergic alveolitis (hypersensitivity pneumonitis), or, very rarely, ankylosing spondylitis. Kerley lines help limit the differential diagnosis (see Table 3-2). Associated lymphadenopathy suggests sarcoidosis; neoplasm (lymphangitic carcinomatosis, lymphoma, metastases); infection (viral, mycobacterial, or fungal); and silicosis. Associated pleural thickening and/or calcification suggest asbestosis. Associated pleural effusion suggests pulmonary edema, lymphangitic carcinomatosis, lymphoma, collagen vascular disease, or lymphangioleiomyomatosis (especially if the effusion is

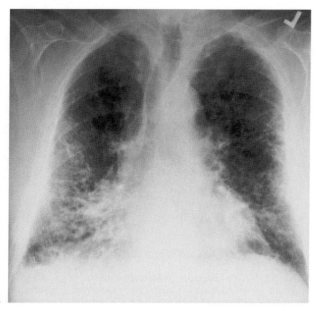
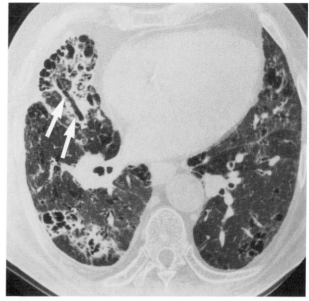

FIGURE 3-3. Farmer's lung and pulmonary fibrosis. This 50-year-old man presented with end-stage lung fibrosis from chronic exposure to inhaled antigens on his farm. **A:** PA chest radiograph shows medium to coarse reticular ILD with a predominant bibasilar and subpleural distribution. **B:** CT scan shows multiple small cysts (honeycombing) involving predominantly the subpleural peripheral regions of lung. Traction bronchiectasis, another sign of end-stage lung fibrosis, is seen in the right middle lobe (*arrows*).

chylous). Associated pneumothorax suggests lymphangioleiomyomatosis or LCH.

PULMONARY EDEMA

Hydrostatic pulmonary edema is defined as abnormal water in the lungs secondary to elevated pulmonary venous pressure from a failing left ventricle, mitral stenosis, increased circulating blood volume (as with anemias), renal failure (causing fluid retention), or overhydration. Interstitial edema is seen on chest radiographs and CT scans as blurring of the margins of the blood vessels and bronchial walls (peribronchial cuffing),

thickening of the fissures (subpleural edema), and thickening of the interlobular septae (Kerley lines) (Fig. 3-7). As capillary pressure rises and interstitial pressure increases, water is forced into the alveolar spaces through the alveolar–capillary membrane; therefore edema is often seen as a combination of both interstitial and alveolar opacities on the chest radiograph. The chest radiograph may also show associated findings of cardiomegaly, pleural effusions, widening of the vascular pedicle, enlargement of the azygos vein, and vascular redistribution (Fig. 3-8). Pulmonary edema is so common, relative to other causes of ILD, that it should often be considered the most likely diagnosis in the differential diagnosis of ILD. An uncommon pattern of edema is more common than an uncommon cause

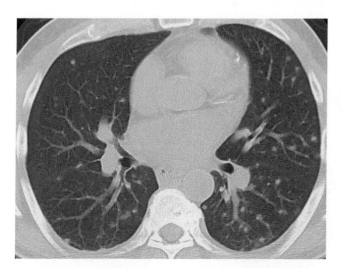

FIGURE 3-4. Disseminated histoplasmosis and nodular ILD. This previously healthy man living in the upper midwestern part of the United States presented with mild symptoms of shortness of breath and cough. CT scan shows multiple bilateral round circumscribed pulmonary nodules.

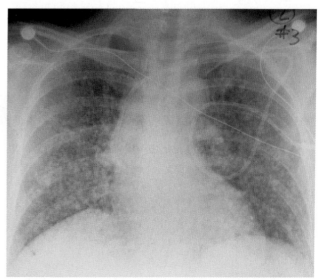

FIGURE 3-5. Hematogenous metastases and nodular ILD. This 45-year-old woman presented with metastatic gastric carcinoma. The PA chest radiograph shows a diffuse pattern of nodules, 6 to 10 mm in diameter.

TABLE 3-3

DIFFERENTIAL DIAGNOSIS OF A NODULAR PATTERN OF INTERSTITIAL LUNG DISEASE

"SHRIMP"
Sarcoidosis
Histiocytosis (Langerhan cell histiocytosis)
Hypersensitivity pneumonitis
Rheumatoid nodules
Infection (mycobacterial, fungal, viral)
Metastases
Microlithiasis, alveolar
Pneumoconioses (silicosis, coal worker's, berylliosis)

This list excludes the relatively uncommon diagnosis of amyloidosis.

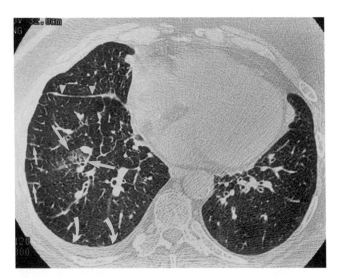

FIGURE 3-7. Cardiogenic pulmonary edema. This 69-year-old woman presented with left ventricular failure and a predominantly interstitial pattern of pulmonary edema. CT scan shows numerous Kerley B lines (*short arrows*), thickening of the right major fissure from subpleural edema (*arrowheads*), patchy areas of ground-glass opacification (*long arrows*), and a right pleural effusion (*curved arrows*).

of ILD. Uncommon patterns of pulmonary edema can result from patient positioning or underlying perfusion abnormalities in the nonedematous lung (e.g., secondary to pulmonary embolism or asymmetric emphysema). Pulmonary edema can be caused by a number of processes other than chronic heart failure, and it may present with a normal-sized heart (Table 3-4).

IDIOPATHIC INTERSTITIAL PNEUMONIAS

The idiopathic interstitial pneumonias (IIPs) are a heterogeneous group of diffuse parenchymal lung diseases that have no well-defined cause (3). The classification is based on histologic criteria, although the diagnosis of IIP is made by correlating the clinical, imaging, and pathologic features. Each IIP "pattern" seen at histologic or CT examination is linked to a specific clinical syndrome. Clinical evaluation must prove that an interstitial pneumonia is idiopathic and exclude a recognizable cause (e.g., collagen vascular disease). Usual interstitial pneumonia (UIP) is the most common of the IIPs. Nonspecific interstitial pneumonia (NSIP) is next most frequent. Cryptogenic organizing pneumonia (COP), desquamative interstitial pneumonia (DIP), respiratory bronchiolitis–associated interstitial lung disease (RB-ILD) and acute interstitial pneumonia (AIP) are less common, and lymphoid interstitial pneumonia (LIP) is rare. Typical CT features of each IIP are distinct, but there is over-

lap (Table 3-5). CT features of UIP and organizing pneumonia may be diagnostic in the correct clinical context, but those of NSIP, DIP, RB-ILD, AIP, and LIP are less specific.

UIP is characterized histologically by a patchy heterogeneous pattern with foci of normal lung, interstitial inflammation, fibroblastic proliferation, interstitial fibrosis, and honeycombing. Temporal heterogeneity is an important histologic feature and helps to distinguish UIP from DIP. Although the terms UIP and idiopathic pulmonary fibrosis (IPF) are often used interchangeably, the term IPF should only be applied to the clinical syndrome associated with the morphologic pattern of UIP. The typical CT features of UIP are a predominantly basal and subpleural reticular interstitial pattern with honeycombing and traction bronchiectasis (Fig. 3-9). Ground-glass opacity and consolidation can be seen but are not dominant features. Architectural distortion, reflecting lung fibrosis, is often prominent. In the correct clinical context, the CT features of UIP are often diagnostic. The presence of honeycombing as a predominant imaging finding is highly specific for UIP and can be used to differentiate it from NSIP, particularly when

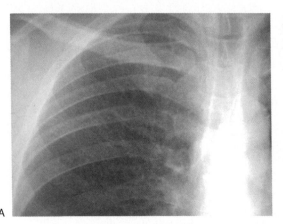
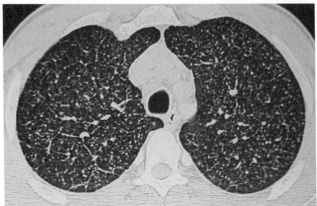

FIGURE 3-6. Disseminated histoplasmosis and reticulonodular ILD. A: PA chest radiograph, close-up of right upper lung, shows reticulonodular ILD. **B:** CT scan shows multiple circumscribed round pulmonary nodules, 2 to 3 mm in diameter.

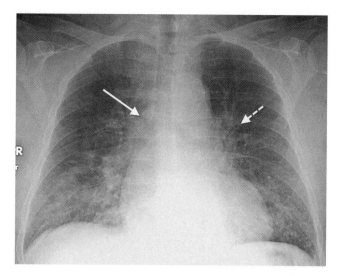

FIGURE 3-8. Cardiogenic pulmonary edema. PA chest radiograph shows enlargement of the cardiac silhouette, bilateral ILD, enlargement of the azygos vein (*solid arrow*), and peribronchial cuffing (*dashed arrow*).

TABLE 3-4

PULMONARY EDEMA WITH A NORMAL-SIZED HEART

"CHIHUAHUAH"
Central nervous system disorders
High-altitude pulmonary edema
Inhalation (e.g., carbon monoxide)
Heroin-induced
Uremia
Acute myocardial infarction
Hypersensitivity reaction
Underwater, near drowning
Aspiration (gastric secretions)
Hemorrhage

the distribution is patchy and subpleural predominant (4). The presence of predominant ground-glass and reticular opacities is highly characteristic of NSIP, but there is a subset of patients with UIP who have this pattern and may require biopsy for differentiation from NSIP. Distinction of UIP from other IIPs is important, because UIP is associated with a poorer prognosis than the other entities.

NSIP is characterized histologically by spatially homogeneous alveolar wall thickening caused by inflammation, fibrosis, or both. The spatial and temporal homogeneity of this pattern is important in distinguishing NSIP from UIP. The prognosis of NSIP is substantially better than that of UIP. Patients with NSIP are more commonly female and generally have a younger mean age than patients with UIP. The typical CT feature of NSIP is predominantly basilar ground-glass and reticular opacities (Fig. 3-10). Consolidation is uncommon and honeycombing is rare. The parenchymal abnormalities of NSIP may be reversible on follow-up CT scanning. Because the CT features of NSIP may overlap with those of organizing pneumonia, DIP, and UIP, a surgical lung biopsy should be considered when the CT pattern suggests NSIP.

DIP is characterized histologically by spatially homogeneous thickening of alveolar septa, which is associated with intra-alveolar accumulation of macrophages. The term *desquamative* refers to an initially incorrect belief that the intra-alveolar macrophages represented desquamated alveolar cells. The majority of patients are cigarette smokers in their fourth

TABLE 3-5

IMAGING FEATURES OF IDIOPATHIC INTERSTITIAL PNEUMONIAS

Morphologic pattern	Imaging features
UIP (clinical diagnosis of IPF)	Basal and subpleural predominant distribution, reticular opacities (often with honeycombing), traction bronchiectasis, and architectural distortion
NSIP (clinical diagnosis of NSIP)	Basal predominant distribution, ground-glass and reticular opacities
DIP (clinical diagnosis of DIP)	Basal predominant distribution, ground-glass opacities, sometimes with cysts
Respiratory bronchiolitis (clinical diagnosis of RB-ILD)	Centrilobular distribution, ground-glass opacity, typically nodular
Organizing pneumonia (clinical diagnosis of COP)	Basal and subpleural predominant distribution, ground-glass opacity and consolidation; bronchovascular distribution is also common
Diffuse alveolar damage (clinical diagnosis of AIP)	Diffuse ground-glass opacity and consolidation
LIP (clinical diagnosis of LIP)	Bronchovascular distribution common, ground-glass and reticular opacities and perivascular cysts

UIP, usual interstitial pneumonia; IPF, idiopathic pulmonary fibrosis; NSIP, nonspecific interstitial pneumonia; DIP, desquamative interstitial pneumonia; RB-ILD, respiratory bronchiolitis–associated interstitial lung disease; COP, cryptogenic organizing pneumonia; AIP, acute interstitial pneumonia; LIP, lymphoid interstitial pneumonia.

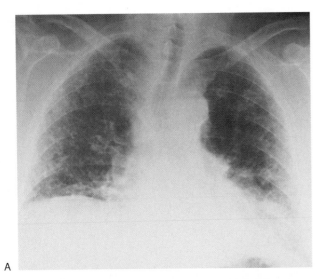

A

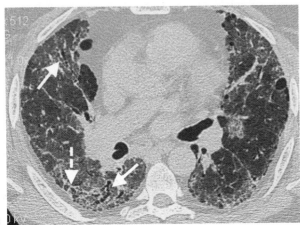

B

FIGURE 3-9. Usual interstitial pneumonia (UIP). A: PA chest radiograph shows medium to coarse reticular ILD with honeycombing, in a predominantly bibasilar and subpleural distribution. Lung volumes are decreased. **B:** CT scan shows bilateral subpleural honeycombing (*dashed arrow*), traction bronchiectasis (*solid arrows*), and a background of ground-glass opacity.

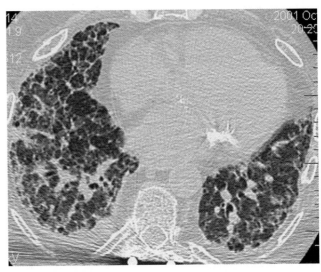

FIGURE 3-10. Nonspecific interstitial pneumonia (NSIP). CT scan shows bibasilar reticular and ground-glass opacities.

glass opacity (Fig. 3-12). In RB-ILD the findings are more extensive (Fig. 3-13) but are at least partially reversible in patients who stop smoking. The imaging features of RB-ILD may be similar to those of hypersensitivity pneumonitis and NSIP. Patients with hypersensitivity pneumonitis often have a history of exposure to an inciting agent and are usually nonsmokers.

Although COP is primarily an intra-alveolar process, it is included in the classification of the IIPs because of its idiopathic nature and because its appearance may overlap with that of the other IIPs. The term *organizing pneumonia* refers to the morphologic imaging or histologic pattern (associated with a wide variety of diseases), whereas COP indicates the associated idiopathic clinical syndrome. Histologically, organizing pneumonia is distinguished by patchy areas of consolidation characterized by polypoid plugs of loose organizing connective tissue with or without endobronchiolar intraluminal polyps. The architecture of the lung is preserved. Patients with COP typically present with cough and dyspnea of relatively short duration. Consolidation is present on CT images in 90% of

or fifth decades of life (5). DIP is more common in men than in women. Most patients improve with cessation of smoking and oral corticosteroids. The histologic features of DIP are similar to those of RB-ILD (a condition seen exclusively in smokers), although the distribution of DIP is diffuse and RB-ILD has a predominantly bronchiolocentric distribution. The typical CT feature of DIP is ground-glass opacity in a predominantly lower lung distribution (Fig. 3-11). Reticulation is frequently seen but is typically limited to the lung bases. Well-defined cysts can occur within the areas of ground-glass opacity.

Respiratory bronchiolitis is a histopathologic lesion found in cigarette smokers and is characterized by the presence of pigmented intraluminal macrophages within respiratory bronchioles (3). It is usually asymptomatic. In rare cases, patients who are heavy smokers may develop RB-ILD, a condition characterized by pulmonary symptoms, abnormal pulmonary function, and imaging abnormalities, with respiratory bronchiolitis being the only histologic lesion identified on lung biopsy. Respiratory bronchiolitis, RB-ILD, and DIP are regarded as a continuum of smoking-related lung injuries. The CT features of patients with asymptomatic respiratory bronchiolitis show ground-glass centrilobular nodules and patchy areas of ground-

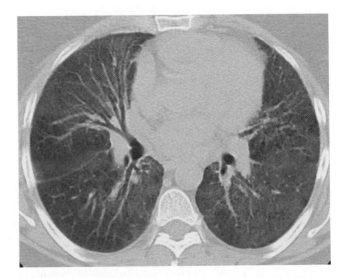

FIGURE 3-11. Desquamative interstitial pneumonia (DIP). CT scan shows bilateral ground-glass opacity in a predominantly lower lung distribution.

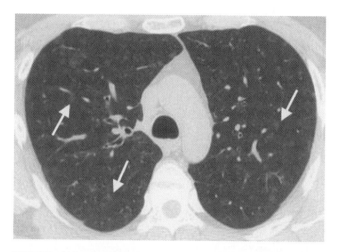

FIGURE 3-12. **Respiratory bronchiolitis.** This patient had a long history of cigarette smoking and no respiratory symptoms. CT scan shows numerous ground-glass nodules in a centrilobular distribution (*arrows*).

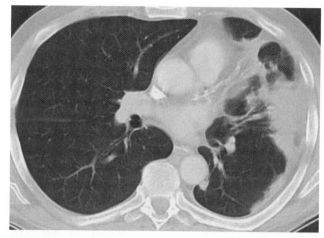

FIGURE 3-14. **Organizing pneumonia.** This patient had a history of rheumatoid arthritis and presented with acute shortness of breath and nonproductive cough. CT scan shows subpleural dense airspace opacity in the left lung.

patients with COP, with a subpleural or peribronchial distribution in up to 50% of cases (3) (Fig. 3-14). Air bronchograms, with mild cylindric bronchial dilatation, are common. Ground-glass opacities are present in about 60% of cases. The lower lungs are more frequently involved. Findings usually improve with steroid treatment. The differential diagnosis of COP includes bronchioloalveolar cell carcinoma, lymphoma, vasculitis, sarcoidosis, chronic eosinophilic pneumonia, and infectious pneumonia.

AIP is a rapidly progressive form of interstitial pneumonia characterized histologically by hyaline membranes within the alveoli and diffuse, active interstitial fibrosis indistinguishable from the histologic pattern found in acute respiratory distress syndrome caused by sepsis and shock. The term *AIP* is reserved for diffuse alveolar damage of unknown origin. Patients with AIP present with respiratory failure developing over days or weeks. Mechanical ventilation is usually required. No etiologic agent is identified. Typical CT features of early stage AIP are ground-glass opacity, bronchiolar dilatation, and dense airspace opacity. Late-stage features are honeycombing, architectural distortion, and traction bronchiectasis.

In adults, LIP is commonly associated with connective tissue disorders (particularly Sjögren syndrome), immunodeficiency syndromes, and Castleman syndrome. Idiopathic LIP is rare. The histologic feature of LIP is alveolar septal interstitial infiltration by lymphocytes and plasma cells. The typical CT findings are ground-glass and reticular opacities, sometimes associated with perivascular cysts (Fig. 3-15). Other findings may include lung nodules, dense airspace opacity, thickening of the bronchovascular bundles, and interlobular septal thickening.

INFECTIOUS INTERSTITIAL PNEUMONIA

Infectious pneumonia resulting in a diffuse interstitial pattern is unusual; however, viral, fungal, mycobacterial, and

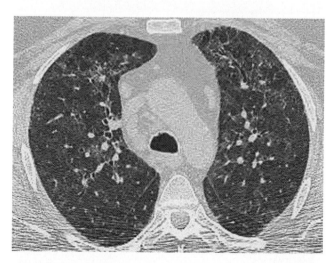

FIGURE 3-13. **Respiratory bronchiolitis-associated interstitial lung disease (RB-ILD).** This patient had a long history of cigarette smoking, chronic cough, and shortness of breath. CT scan shows bilateral reticular and ground-glass opacities in a predominantly upper lung distribution.

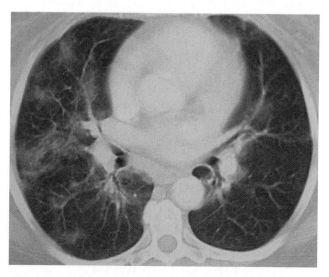

FIGURE 3-15. **Lymphocytic interstitial pneumonia (LIP).** This patient had Sjögren syndrome and new respiratory symptoms. CT scan shows bilateral patchy ground-glass opacities in a peribronchovascular distribution.

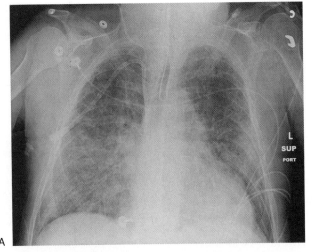

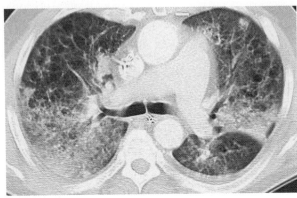

FIGURE 3-16. Influenza pneumonia. This patient had a history of emphysema and acute respiratory symptoms. A: Supine chest radiograph shows bilateral reticular ILD. B: CT scan shows bilateral reticular and ground-glass opacities and areas of consolidation. "Cystic" areas represent pulmonary emphysema.

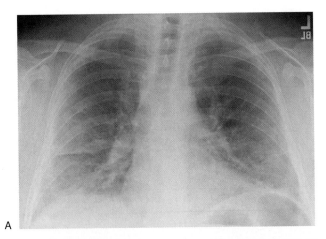

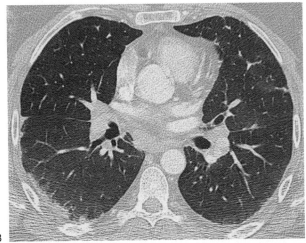

FIGURE 3-17. Methotrexate lung toxicity. A: PA chest radiograph shows bilateral ILD, predominantly in the lower lungs. B: CT scan shows subtle bilateral ground-glass opacity and subpleural reticular and dense airspace opacities.

Mycoplasma pneumonias may be predominantly interstitial or interstitial appearing. Fungal disease is discussed in Chapter 7. *Pneumocystis* pneumonia also produces a fine interstitial pattern on chest radiography and is discussed in Chapter 16.

Mycoplasma pneumoniae usually affects previously healthy individuals between the ages of 5 and 40 years (6). Chest radiographs may show widespread bilateral nodular or reticular opacities, and they may take several weeks to return to normal. Alternatively, dense airspace opacity may be seen involving one or several lobes.

Viruses are the major cause of respiratory tract infection in the community, especially in children. The most common viral pneumonias in infants and young children are caused by respiratory syncytial virus, parainfluenza virus, adenovirus, and influenza; in adults, influenza and adenovirus are most common. Viruses that cause pneumonia in immunocompromised patients include Cytomegalovirus, varicella-zoster, and herpesvirus. The radiographic appearance of viral pneumonias is typically a diffuse interstitial pattern with a diffuse, patchy, often nodular appearance (Fig. 3-16).

DRUG TOXICITY

Numerous drugs can result in transient or permanent lung injury of varying types and severities (Fig. 3-17), some of which are listed in Table 3-6. A more complete list can be found in

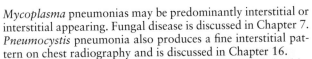

TABLE 3-6

COMMONLY USED DRUGS THAT CAN CAUSE LUNG TOXICITY

Nitrofurantoin
Sulfonamides
Penicillin
Bleomycin
Methotrexate
Azathioprine
Busulfan
Chlorambucil
Cyclophosphamide
Amiodarone
Methysergide
Acetylsalicylic acid
Codeine
Amitriptyline
Interleukin-2
Ornithine-ketoacid transaminase orthoclone
Heroin
Thiazides
Procainamide

the medical literature. The adverse effects of some of the drugs that can cause ILD are discussed below.

Bleomycin is a cytotoxic drug used in the treatment of squamous cell carcinoma, lymphoma, and testicular neoplasms. Toxicity is related to the cumulative dose, and the incidence of pulmonary toxic side effects is between 4% and 15% (7,8). The initial radiographic changes are predominantly basilar reticulonodular interstitial opacities. Progression of disease may result in dense airspace opacity.

Nitrofurantoin is an antibacterial agent used in the treatment of urinary tract infections. An acute reaction produces basilar interstitial or mixed interstitial/alveolar opacities. A chronic reaction develops after months or years of therapy, resulting in pulmonary fibrosis, with a bibasilar and subpleural distribution of reticular ILD and a gradual reduction in lung volume.

Salicylates can alter the capillary permeability of the lung, leading to noncardiogenic pulmonary edema. The radiographic features are indistinguishable from those of cardiogenic edema.

Ornithine-ketoacid transaminase orthoclone (OKT3) is a monoclonal antibody used to treat acute rejection of transplant allografts. OKT3 toxicity manifests as acute pulmonary edema, usually within hours of starting therapy. It is important to ensure that the patient does not have excess pulmonary fluid prior to starting therapy, and pretherapy chest radiographs are commonly ordered for this purpose.

Amiodarone is used to treat refractory cardiac rhythm disturbances. Because of the drug's relatively high incidence of pulmonary toxicity (5%) (9), its potential life-saving benefit must be weighed against the risks of potentially fatal pulmonary toxicity. Amiodarone is concentrated in the lung and has a long tissue half-life, which accounts for the slow appearance of toxic effects and slow clearing following cessation of therapy (months for both). The most common radiographic appearance of amiodarone toxicity is multiple peripheral areas of dense airspace opacity. Another radiographic manifestation is diffuse interstitial opacification leading to pulmonary fibrosis. Amiodarone contains 37% iodine by weight, which can result in high-attenuation pleuroparenchymal, liver, or spleen lesions that are distinctive for amiodarone toxicity on CT scans.

LYMPHANGIOLEIOMYOMATOSIS

Lymphangioleiomyomatosis (LAM) is a disorder characterized by perilymphatic smooth muscle proliferation that later spreads to involve airways, airspaces, arterioles, and venules and that can affect pulmonary, mediastinal, and retroperitoneal lymph nodes. The histologic and radiographic findings of LAM (Table 3-7) are similar to those of tuberous sclerosis, and the two diagnoses are considered to be part of a spectrum of the same disease process. Patients with LAM are female, usually of childbearing age. Spontaneous pneumothorax is the presenting event in more than half of patients and is often recurrent (10) (Fig. 3-18). Other defining events include (a) chylous pleural effusion or ascites and (b) hemoptysis. The earliest radiographic signs of lung disease consist of subtle, diffuse, fine nodular, reticular, or reticulonodular opacities that result from the superimposition of cyst walls. The reticular pattern becomes more coarse and irregular, and cysts, bullae, and honeycombing can develop. During the end-stage of this disease, lung volumes are usually increased. The characteristic findings on CT include multiple thin-walled cysts distributed in a uniform fashion in otherwise essentially normal lung. The cysts are generally rounded and uniform in shape, although when large they can assume polygonal or bizarre shapes.

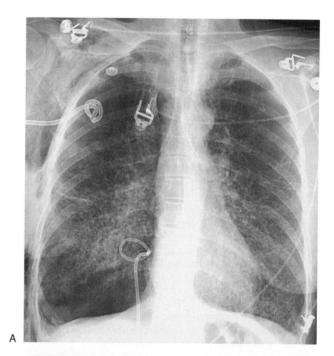

A

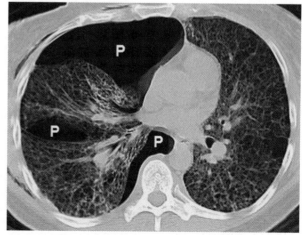

B

FIGURE 3-18. Lymphangioleiomyomatosis (LAM). This 42-year-old woman presented with right chest pain. **A:** PA chest radiograph shows a right basilar pneumothorax and two right pleural drainage catheters. The lung volumes are increased, which is characteristic of LAM, and there is diffuse reticular ILD. **B:** CT scan shows bilateral thin-walled cysts and a loculated right pneumothorax (*P*).

TABLE 3-7
CHEST RADIOGRAPHIC FEATURES OF LYMPHANGIOLEIOMYOMATOSIS

"HER"
Hyperinflation
Effusion (chylous)
Reticulonodular interstitial pattern

"HER" emphasizes that this is a disorder affecting women. The addition of a *P* on the end ("HERP") emphasizes the frequent occurrence of pneumothorax with this disorder.

TUMOR ORIGINS MOST COMMONLY RESULTING IN LYMPHANGITIC CARCINOMATOSIS

"Certain Cancers Spread by Plugging the Lymphatics"
Cervix
Colon
Stomach
Breast
Pancreas
Thyroid
Lung
Larynx

Modified with permission from Dähnert W. *Radiology Review Manual*. Baltimore: Williams & Wilkins; 1991:237.

LYMPHANGITIC CARCINOMATOSIS

Lymphangitic carcinomatosis refers to infiltration of pulmonary lymphatics by neoplastic cells. The most common tumors resulting in lymphangitic carcinomatosis are listed in Table 3-8. Mechanisms of tumor dissemination include (a) blood-borne emboli that lodge in smaller pulmonary arteries, infiltrate the vessel walls, and then spread out into the lymphatic vessels; (b) expansion by way of lymph vessels to hilar nodes and then retrograde into the pulmonary lymphatics; and (c) direct invasion of the pulmonary lymphatics from primary lung neoplasms. Chest radiographs and CT scans show fine reticulonodular opacities and thickened septal lines (Kerley A and B lines). CT scans show interlobular septal thickening and irregular thickening of the bronchovascular bundles (Fig. 3-19). The appearance, especially on chest radiography, may be difficult to distinguish from pulmonary edema. A unilateral distribution suggests primary bronchogenic carcinoma as the underlying tumor; most other tumors result in bilateral lung involvement (Fig. 3-20). Central lymphatic obstruction, with distended lymphatics but no actual carcinomatosis, can have a similar appearance. The septa are usually more irregular and beaded with true carcinomatosis.

PNEUMOCONIOSES

The term *pneumoconiosis* means "dusty lungs" and is used to describe the reactions of the lungs to inhaled dust particles. The notable inorganic dusts involved include coal, silica, and asbestos. Coal worker's pneumoconiosis and silicosis result in similar chest radiographic abnormalities and should not be confused with the findings seen with asbestosis. The reaction of lung tissue to these dusts depends on the sizes of the particles inhaled, the fibrogenicity of the dust, the amount of dust retained in the lungs, the duration of exposure, and the individual immunologic response to the dust.

The International Labour Office (ILO) classification of the radiographic appearances of the pneumoconioses is a standardized, internationally accepted system that is used to codify the roentgenographic changes of the pneumoconioses in a reproducible manner (11). The classification includes a description of small rounded opacities (nodules), irregular linear and reticular opacities, and pleural thickening (diffuse or circumscribed, such as with a plaque). After passing an examination given by the National Institute for Occupational Safety and Health, an individual becomes a "B reader," certified officially to interpret chest radiographs according to the ILO standards.

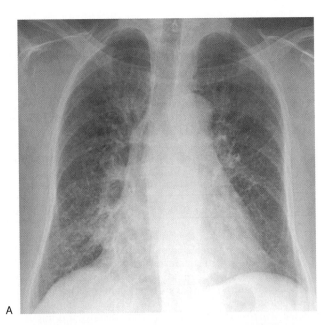

A

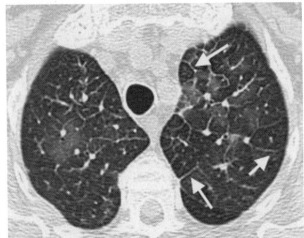

B

FIGURE 3-19. Lymphangitic carcinomatosis. This 68-year-old man had adenocarcinoma of the lung. He developed shortness of breath, which was initially attributed to congestive heart failure. **A:** PA chest radiograph shows bilateral ILD. The cardiac silhouette is chronically enlarged, but there is no pleural effusion or increase in the width of the vascular pedicle. **B:** CT scan shows bilateral patchy ground-glass opacities and thickening of the interlobular septae (*arrows*). The diagnosis of lymphangitic carcinomatosis was confirmed with lung biopsy.

Free silica is present in many rocks in the earth's crust. *Silicosis* refers to lung disease caused primarily by free silica, and it occurs predominantly in individuals who work in quarries, who drill or tunnel in quartz-containing rocks, who cut or polish masonry, who clean boilers or castings in iron and steel foundries, or who are exposed to sandblasting. The chronic form of the disease requires 20 or more years of exposure to high dust concentrations before radiographic changes are visible.

Silica dust particles are ingested by pulmonary macrophages. The macrophages die and release their enzymatic contents, resulting in lung fibrosis. The cycle continues even without ongoing exposure to silica from the environment, as the silica released from the death of macrophages is free to be taken up by other macrophages. Early in the course of silicosis, 1- to 3-mm nodules are seen with an upper

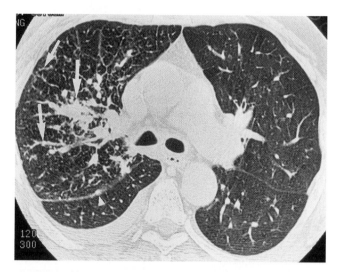

FIGURE 3-20. Lymphangitic carcinomatosis. This 53-year-old man presented with chronic obstructive pulmonary disease, recurrent pneumonia, chronic cough, wheezing, and large-cell bronchogenic carcinoma of the right lung. CT scan shows unilateral nodular thickening of the central and peripheral interstitial compartments (*arrows*) and a malignant right pleural effusion. Note nodular involvement of the subpleural lymphatics adjacent to the right major fissure (*arrowhead*).

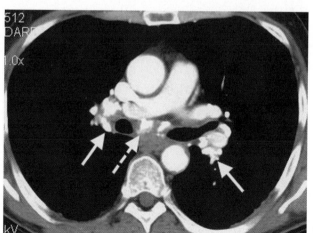

FIGURE 3-21. Complicated silicosis. PA chest radiograph of a male foundry worker shows multiple nodules involving the upper and middle lungs, with coalescence of nodules in the left upper lobe resulting in early "progressive massive fibrosis" (*arrows*).

lung–predominant distribution (12) (Figs. 3-21 and 3-22). As the process advances, the nodules increase in size and number and can calcify. The nodules may coalesce, resulting in larger nodules (greater than 1 cm in diameter), creating masslike opacities referred to as *progressive massive fibrosis*, a stage of "complicated" silicosis (Fig. 3-23). Cavitation of the masses may occur, leading to superinfection with tuberculosis. Contraction of the upper lobes occurs, and cicatricial emphysema and bullae form around the areas of conglomerate masses. The conglomerate masses begin in the periphery of the lungs and slowly migrate toward the hila. Hilar and mediastinal lymph node enlargement is not uncommon, and calcification, sometimes in an "eggshell" pattern, may be seen in the nodes (13). The radiographic signs of coal worker's pneumoconiosis are similar to, and often indistinguishable from, those described for silicosis.

Acute silicosis is a rare condition related to heavy exposure to free silica in enclosed spaces with minimal or no pro-

tection. The disease is rapidly progressive. Chest radiographs show diffuse airspace or ground-glass opacification with a perihilar distribution and air bronchograms (14). A number of connective tissue diseases have been reported to occur with increased prevalence in patients with silicosis. For example, Caplan syndrome consists of the presence of large necrobiotic nodules (rheumatoid nodules) superimposed on a background of simple silicosis. The nodules measure from 0.5 to 5.0 cm, may cavitate and calcify, and may precede the onset of arthritis by months or years.

Asbestos is composed of a group of fibers that can be divided into two principal subgroups based on the physical properties of the fibers: the serpentines and the amphiboles. Serpentine asbestos has long, curly, flexible fibers and accounts for 90% of the asbestos used in the United States. The only serpentine asbestos used commercially is chrysotile. The amphiboles (including crocidolite) have straight, needlelike fibers, which have

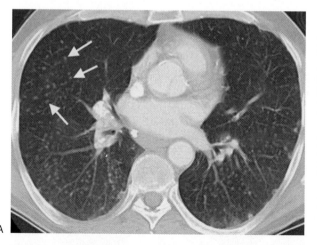

FIGURE 3-22. Simple silicosis. A: CT scan with lung windowing shows numerous circumscribed pulmonary nodules, 2 to 3 mm in diameter (*arrows*). B: CT scan with mediastinal windowing shows densely calcified hilar (*solid arrows*) and subcarinal (*dashed arrow*) nodes.

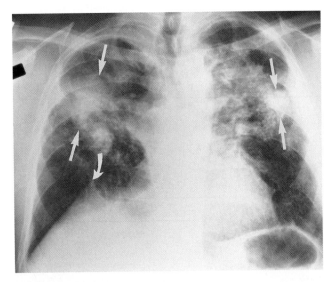

FIGURE 3-23. Complicated silicosis. This 61-year-old man had a 30-year exposure to silica from sandblasting. PA chest radiograph shows conglomerate upper lung masses, referred to as progressive massive fibrosis (*straight arrows*). The masses have a tendency to migrate from the periphery to the hila. There is tenting of the right hemidiaphragm as a result of severe contraction of the right upper lobe (*curved arrow*).

a much greater fibrogenic and carcinogenic potential than the serpentine-form chrysotile. *Benign asbestos-related pleural disease* refers to any or all of the following pleural abnormalities: benign, sometimes recurrent pleural effusions; diffuse pleural thickening; and pleural plaques (with or without calcification) (15). Benign pleural effusion is the most common abnormality seen within 10 years of the onset of asbestos exposure. The amount of fluid is usually small; effusions larger than 500 mL are uncommon. Pleural plaques are usually first identified more than 20 or 30 years after the initial asbestos exposure; they occur on the parietal pleura, in typical locations over the diaphragm and along the posteromedial and anterolateral chest walls. The more benign form of asbestos fiber, chrysotile, is noted for transpleural migration, whereas the more fibrogenic and carcinogenic amphiboles, crocidolite and amosite, tend to get held up in the lung parenchyma. This difference in fiber migration accounts for the finding of asbestos-related pleural disease that can be unassociated with parenchymal fibrosis or intrathoracic malignancy. On chest radiographs, pleural plaques are irregular, smooth elevations of the pleura identified in profile along the margins of the lungs or over the diaphragm. When seen en face, the plaques are flat relative to their width, and the density of the shadow projected over the lungs is less than would be expected for a parenchymal lesion of equivalent size (Fig. 3-24). Plaques are usually multiple and fairly symmetric from side to side.

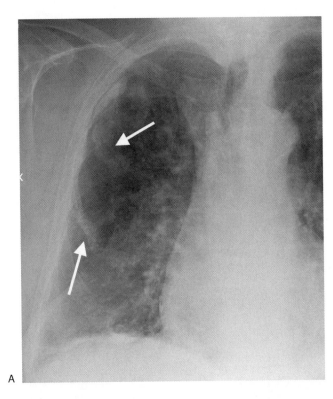

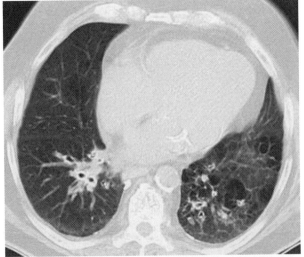

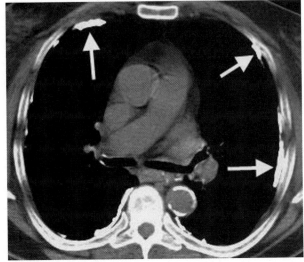

FIGURE 3-24. Asbestos-related pleural disease and asbestosis. A: PA chest radiograph, coned to the right lung, shows curvilinear calcified pleural plaques en face (*arrows*). **B:** CT scan with lung windowing shows bilateral lower lung ground-glass and reticular opacities. The diagnosis of asbestosis was confirmed with lung biopsy. **C:** CT scan with mediastinal windowing shows bilateral calcified pleural plaques (*arrows*). This appearance is virtually diagnostic of previous asbestos exposure.

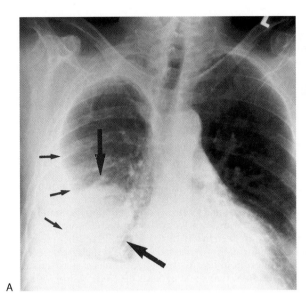

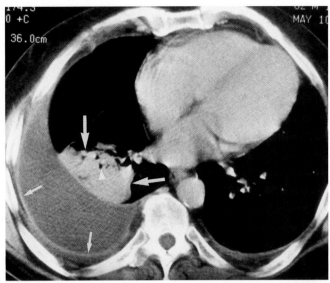

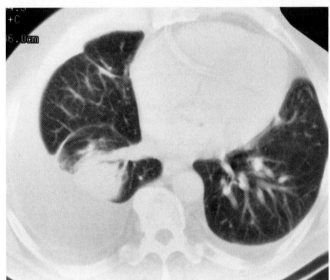

FIGURE 3-25. Asbestos-related pleural disease and rounded atelectasis. This 62-year-old man had a 20-year history of asbestos exposure. A: PA chest radiograph shows a large right lobulated pleural fluid collection (*small arrows*) and a right lower lobe "mass" (*large arrows*). B: CT scan with intravenous contrast enhancement shows thickening and enhancement of the parietal pleura (*small arrows*), indicating a chronic pleural effusion. The parenchymal "mass" (*large arrows*), in contact with the visceral pleural surface, represents collapsed lung. The atelectatic lung has a rounded shape caused by fibrous adhesions and infolding of the visceral pleura. Air bronchograms are seen within the collapsed lung (*arrowhead*). C: CT scan with lung windowing shows the "vacuum cleaner effect" or "comet-tail sign," both descriptions of how the vessels leading toward the atelectatic lung diverge and arc around the undersurface of the atelectatic lung before merging with it.

Calcification in plaques is linear when seen in profile, and when seen en face it may have an irregular, unevenly dense appearance, referred to as a "holly leaf" pattern of calcification. There is no evidence that pleural plaques degenerate into malignant mesothelioma, but there is evidence to support a small but statistically significant increased incidence of mesothelioma in individuals with occupational exposure and radiographically detectable pleural plaques (16). In addition, it was found in one study that occupationally exposed individuals with plaques (but not parenchymal disease) had increased mortality from bronchogenic carcinoma (17).

Rounded atelectasis is a form of juxtapleural lung collapse that can be confused with a neoplasm or pneumonia. Always associated with chronic pleural disease (and therefore commonly associated with asbestos exposure), rounded atelectasis represents an infolding of the visceral pleura as an isolated area of atelectasis. A proposed mechanism of rounded atelectasis is collapsed lung floating on pleural effusion and development of fibrous adhesions suspending the rounded atelectatic area in an elevated and tilted position. The pleural effusion may resolve, but the sequestered atelectatic lung may not re-expand. Rounded atelectasis forms a round or oval mass, usually 2.5 to 5.0 cm in diameter, in contact with the pleural surface. The

vessels leading toward the mass are crowded, and as they reach the mass they tend to diverge and arc around the undersurface of the mass before merging with it. This appearance has been called the *vacuum cleaner effect* and the *comet tail sign* (18) (Fig. 3-25). Rounded atelectasis may slowly resolve or remain unchanged on serial chest radiographs or chest CT scans. To confidently suggest the diagnosis of rounded atelectasis, three criteria must be met: (i) contiguity with chronic pleural effusion/thickening, (ii) typical appearance of crowded vessels and bronchi sweeping into and around the base of the atelectatic lung, and (iii) volume loss in the affected lobe.

The term *asbestosis* refers to asbestos-induced pulmonary fibrosis and is distinguished from asbestos-related pleural disease without pulmonary fibrosis. Time from exposure to evidence of development of asbestosis is generally 20 to 30 years. The chest radiograph shows reticular interstitial disease, often with evidence of honeycombing, in a subpleural and basilar distribution, identical to the UIP pattern. Pleural changes related to asbestos exposure may provide a clue to the underlying diagnosis, but they are not present in all cases. In early or mild stages, chest CT scans can show interlobular septal thickening; subpleural lines (curvilinear opacities paralleling the chest wall in a subpleural location); parenchymal bands (linear structures up to 5 cm in length coursing into the lung from the pleural surface); ground-glass opacities (diffuse, mild alveolar wall fibrosis and edema that cannot be resolved by CT); and centrilobular nodular opacities (peribronchiolar fibrosis). Honeycombing is an end-stage finding. In some cases, when the parenchymal findings are limited to the dependent lung, CT done with prone positioning is helpful to differentiate the findings resulting from asbestosis from the obscuring and confounding effects of gravity-related dependent atelectasis.

Exposure to asbestos increases the incidence of bronchogenic carcinoma, and this risk is multiplied in cigarette smokers. Asbestos exposure also increases an individual's risk of developing malignant mesothelioma, an uncommon and fatal neoplasm of the serosal lining of the pleural cavity, peritoneum, or both. There is usually a latency period of approximately 20 to 40 years between exposure and detection of mesothelioma. This neoplasm is further discussed in Chapter 9.

SARCOIDOSIS

Sarcoidosis is a systemic disease of unknown etiology characterized histologically by noncaseating granulomas. The disease occurs in people of all ages and both sexes but characteristically affects African American women between the ages of 20 and 40. Chest radiographs can be normal or show parenchymal opacities, adenopathy, or both. The most frequent chest radiographic pulmonary abnormality is small rounded or irregular opacities (reticulonodular opacities), with most nodules measuring 2 to 4 mm (19). These opacities are usually bilateral and symmetric, often with a predominant middle or upper and middle lung distribution. Sarcoid granulomas may resolve completely, or they may heal by fibrosis. Chest radiographic findings of sarcoid fibrosis include permanent coarse linear opacities radiating laterally from the hilum into the adjacent upper and middle lungs. The hila are pulled upward and outward, and vessels and fissures are distorted. The fibrosis can be quite extensive, occasionally resembling the progressive massive fibrosis seen with complicated silicosis. Ring opacities can be seen as a result of bronchiectasis or bullae. CT scans of sarcoidosis typically show 1- to 5-mm nodules with irregular margins in a perilymphatic distribution along bronchovascular margins, interlobular septa, and subpleural areas and in the centers of lobules (Fig. 3-26). This distribution of nodules can be identical to the pattern seen with lymphangitic carcinomatosis. Further description of the features of sarcoidosis is provided in Chapter 10.

COLLAGEN VASCULAR DISEASES

Rheumatoid arthritis (RA) is an inflammatory polyarthropathy of unknown cause. The arthritic changes occur more commonly in women, but pulmonary manifestations occur with greater frequency in men. Pleural involvement, typically pleural effusions or pleural thickening, is the most common thoracic manifestation of RA. Pleural effusions are usually unilateral and small to moderate in size but can occasionally be large or bilateral. Pulmonary fibrosis occurs in approximately 10% to 20% of patients with RA, producing radiographic changes similar to those seen in UIP (20) (Fig. 3-27). Another pleuropulmonary abnormality associated with RA is the rare necrobiotic nodule. These nodules are pathologically identical to the subcutaneous nodules that these patients develop. Necrobiotic nodules, which usually occur in patients with established disease, are usually radiologically discrete, rounded or lobulated, and subpleural. They may be single or multiple, and they have a middle and upper lung–predominant distribution. They range in size from a few millimeters to 7 cm, and occasionally a miliary pattern is seen. The nodules cavitate in approximately 50% of cases (21). The nodules may increase in size and number, resolve completely, or remain stable for many years; they may wax and wane with the activity of subcutaneous nodules and arthritis. Systemic vasculitis occurs in patients with RA and can affect the lung in rare cases, resulting in pulmonary arterial hypertension. Other intrathoracic associations with RA include obliterative bronchiolitis, organizing pneumonia, and pericarditis.

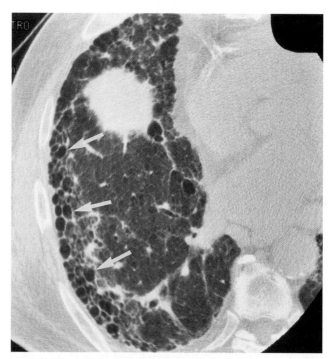

FIGURE 3-27. **Pulmonary fibrosis and rheumatoid arthritis.** CT scan of the right lung shows layers of small cysts in a subpleural location (*arrows*). This pattern of honeycombing is diagnostic of pulmonary fibrosis. The "mass" in the anterior right lung is the liver.

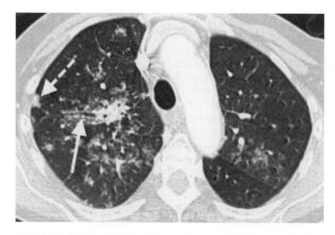

FIGURE 3-26. **Sarcoidosis.** CT scan shows nodular thickening of the bronchovascular bundles (*solid arrow*) and subpleural nodules (*dashed arrow*), illustrating the typical perilymphatic distribution of sarcoidosis.

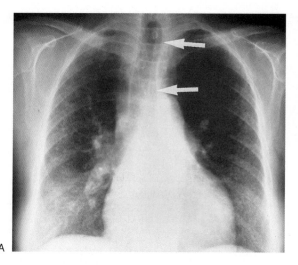
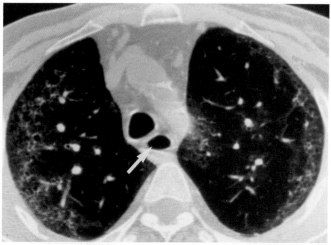

FIGURE 3-28. Systemic sclerosis. This 63-year-old man presented with increasing shortness of breath. **A:** PA chest radiograph shows a bibasilar and subpleural distribution of fine reticular ILD. The presence of a dilated esophagus (*arrows*) provides a clue to the correct diagnosis. **B:** CT scan shows peripheral ILD and a dilated esophagus (*arrow*).

Systemic lupus erythematosus (SLE) is a multisystem collagen vascular disease characterized by widespread inflammatory changes, particularly in the vessels, serosa, and skin. The disease is 10 times more common in women than in men (22), with an increased prevalence among African American women of childbearing age. Pleuritis is found in 40% to 60% of patients with SLE (23). The pleuritis is dry 50% of the time; at other times it is accompanied by a pleural effusion and/or pericardial effusion. The pleural effusion is usually small or moderate in size but may be large, and unilateral and bilateral effusions occur with equal frequency.

Acute lupus pneumonitis is an unusual life-threatening condition resembling infectious pneumonia, pulmonary infarction, and pulmonary hemorrhage, all of which are associated with SLE. The chest radiographic findings in lupus pneumonitis consist of areas of dense airspace opacity, usually bilateral and basal, that represent diffuse alveolar damage mediated by immune complex deposition. Pulmonary hemorrhage is common in patients with SLE, and it is usually manifested radiographically as bilateral and diffuse airspace opacification, similar to the pattern seen with Goodpasture syndrome, another pulmonary–renal syndrome. Pulmonary fibrosis occurs in approximately 3% of patients (24), with a pattern that is radiographically and pathologically identical to that seen in other collagen vascular diseases. Bilateral diaphragm elevation is commonly seen in patients with SLE, and in some reports this has been shown to be the most common radiologic pleuropulmonary abnormality in SLE. As the diaphragm rises, lung volumes decrease, referred to as the "shrinking lungs" sign (25). Pulmonary hypertension and vasculitis, pulmonary embolism (caused by circulating lupus anticoagulant), lymphocytic interstitial pneumonia, obliterative bronchiolitis, and organizing pneumonia are also seen in patients with SLE. Secondary thoracic manifestations of SLE include atelectasis, infectious pneumonia (simple or opportunistic owing to steroid treatment), cardiac failure, pericarditis, and drug-induced changes.

Systemic sclerosis (SS) is a generalized connective tissue disorder characterized by tightening, induration, and thickening of the skin (*scleroderma*); Raynaud phenomenon; musculoskeletal manifestations; and visceral involvement, especially of the gastrointestinal tract, lungs, heart, and kidneys. The pathogenesis is not completely understood. SS occurs more commonly in women in the third to fifth decades of life. The most common radiologic abnormality is pulmonary fibrosis, which causes a symmetric, diffuse, basally predominant reticulonodular pattern with associated loss of lung volume (26) (Fig. 3-28). The CT findings are similar to those of other diseases with a UIP histologic pattern. Pneumonia can occur, particularly after aspiration as a result of esophageal involvement. Esophageal dilatation seen on a chest radiograph or CT scan can provide a clue to the diagnosis of SS.

Sjögren syndrome (sicca syndrome) is an autoimmune disorder characterized by dry eyes (keratoconjunctivitis sicca) and dry mouth (xerostomia). A disease of middle-aged women, it can result in many of the pleural, parenchymal, and diaphragmatic complications associated with other collagen vascular diseases, including pulmonary fibrosis.

LANGERHAN CELL HISTIOCYTOSIS

Also known as *histiocytosis X* and *eosinophilic granuloma of lung*, LCH is a granulomatous disorder of unknown cause characterized by the presence within the granulomas of a histiocyte, the Langerhan cell. LCH represents a spectrum of diseases, with lung involvement seen either in infancy as part of a serious multisystem disorder (Letterer-Siwe disease), in older children as part of a more indolent disorder involving one organ system or a few organs (Hand-Schüller-Christian disease), or as a primary lung disease in adults. LCH is equally prevalent in both sexes, and 95% of adult patients have a history of cigarette smoking (27). Pneumothorax is a classic initial or presenting manifestation of LCH, as it is in LAM. Pneumothoraces occur in 6% to 25% of patients with LCH and are commonly bilateral and recurrent. The characteristic radiographic appearance of LCH is a diffuse, symmetric, reticulonodular pattern or, less commonly, a solely nodular pattern, with a middle and upper lung–predominant distribution (Fig. 3-29). The nodules are usually ill defined, varying in size from 1 to 15 mm, and are usually innumerable. Progression to cystic lung disease results in increased lung volume. The radiographic findings clear in one third of patients, remain stable in one third, and show

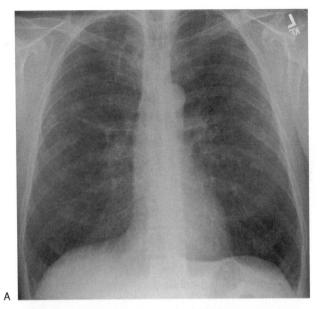

A

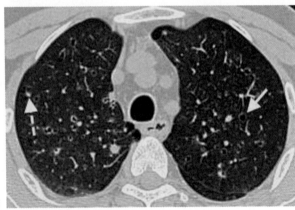

B

FIGURE 3-29. Langerhan cell histiocytosis. This 50-year-old man had a 30 pack-year history of cigarette smoking. **A:** PA chest radiograph shows hyperinflation of the lungs and fine bilateral reticular ILD. **B:** CT scan shows multiple cysts (*solid arrow*) and nodules (*dashed arrow*).

deterioration in one third (28). CT scan findings consist of cysts and nodules, often in combination. When only cysts are seen, the appearance can resemble that of LAM or emphysema. The cysts range in diameter from 1 to 30 mm. Nodule margins tend to be indistinct, and some cavitate. Serial CT scans show progression from nodules, to cavitary nodules, to cysts, to an end stage of destruction resembling generalized emphysema.

UNILATERAL INTERSTITIAL LUNG DISEASE

Most disorders discussed in this chapter result in bilateral chest radiograph changes. The four processes that can characteristically result in unilateral ILD are listed in Table 3-9. Recognizing a unilateral distribution can help narrow the differential diagnosis.

TABLE 3-9

UNILATERAL INTERSTITIAL LUNG DISEASE

"LAX"
Lymphangitic carcinomatosis (primary bronchogenic carcinoma)
Atypical edema (large contralateral pulmonary embolism)
Aspiration pneumonia
X-ray therapy changes

References

1. Tuddenham WJ. Glossary of terms for thoracic radiology: recommendations of the nomenclature committee of the Fleischner society. *Am J Roentgenol.* 1984;143:509–517.
2. Kerley P. Radiology in heart disease. *Br Med J.* 1933;2:594–597.
3. Lynch DA, Travis WD, Müller NL, et al. Idiopathic interstitial pneumonias: CT features. *Radiology.* 2005;236:10–21.
4. Elliot TL, Lynch DA, Newell JD, et al. High-resolution computed tomography features of nonspecific interstitial pneumonia and usual interstitial pneumonia. *J Comput Assist Tomogr.* 2005;29:339–345.
5. Ryu JH, Colby TV, Hartman TE, Vassallo R. Smoking-related interstitial lung diseases: a concise review. *Eur Respir J.* 2001;17:122–132.
6. Mansel JK, Rosenow EC, Martin JW. *Mycoplasma pneumoniae* pneumonia. *Chest.* 1989;95:639–646.
7. White DA, Stover DE. Severe bleomycin-induced pneumonitis: clinical features and response to corticosteroids. *Chest.* 1984;86:723–728.
8. Wolkowicz J, Sturgeon J, Rawji M, et al. Bleomycin-induced pulmonary function abnormalities. *Chest.* 1992;101:97–101.
9. Wood DL, Osborn MJ, Rooke J, et al. Amiodarone pulmonary toxicity: report of two cases associated with rapidly progressive fatal adult respiratory distress syndrome after pulmonary angiography. *Mayo Clin Proc.* 1985;60:601–603.
10. Taylor JR, Ryu J, Colby TV, et al. Lymphangioleiomyomatosis: clinical course in 32 patients. *N Engl J Med.* 1990;323:1254–1260.
11. International Labour Office. *Guidelines for the Use of ILO International Classification of Radiographs of Pneumoconioses.* Geneva: International Labour Office; 1980.
12. Bergin CJ, Müller NL, Vedal S, et al. CT in silicosis: correlation with plain films and pulmonary function tests. *Am J Roentgenol.* 1986;146:477–483.
13. Jacobson GJ, Felson B, Pendergrass EP, et al. Eggshell calcifications in coal and metal miners. *Semin Roentgenol.* 1967;2:276–282.
14. Dee P, Suratt P, Winn W. The radiographic findings in acute silicosis. *Radiology.* 1978;126:359–363.
15. Epler GR, McLoud TC, Gaensler EA. Prevalence and incidence of benign asbestos pleural effusion in a working population. *JAMA.* 1982;247:617–622.
16. Edge JR. Incidence of bronchial carcinoma in shipyard workers with pleural plaques. *Ann N Y Acad Sci.* 1979;330:289–294.
17. Fletcher DE. A mortality study of shipyard workers with pleural plaques. *Br J Ind Med.* 1972;29:142–145.
18. Schneider HJ, Felson B, Gonzalez LL. Rounded atelectasis. *Am J Roentgenol.* 1980;134:225–232.
19. Ellis K, Renthal G. Pulmonary sarcoidosis: roentgenographic observations on course of disease. *Am J Roentgenol.* 1962;88:1070–1083.
20. Doctor L, Snider GL. Diffuse interstitial pulmonary fibrosis associated with arthritis. *Am Rev Respir Dis.* 1962;85:413–422.
21. Martel W, Abell MR, Mikkelsen WM, et al. Pulmonary and pleural lesions in rheumatoid disease. *Radiology.* 1968;90:641–653.
22. Masi AT, Kaslow RA. Sex effects in systemic lupus erythematosus. *Arthritis Rheum.* 1978;21:480–484.
23. Harvey AM, Shulman LE, Tumulty PA, et al. Systemic lupus erythematosus: review of the literature and clinical analysis of 138 cases. *Medicine.* 1954;33:291–437.
24. Eisenberg H, Dubois EL, Sherwin RP, et al. Diffuse interstitial lung disease in systemic lupus erythematosus. *Ann Intern Med.* 1973;79:37–45.
25. Hoffbrand BI, Beck ER. Unexplained dyspnoea and shrinking lungs in systemic lupus erythematosus. *Br Med J.* 1965;1:1273–1277.
26. Gondos B. Roentgen manifestations in progressive systemic sclerosis (diffuse scleroderma). *Am J Roentgenol.* 1960;84:235–247.
27. Marcy TW, Reynolds HY. Pulmonary histiocytosis X. *Lung.* 1985;163:129–150.
28. Lacronique J, Roth C, Battesti J-P, et al. Chest radiological features of pulmonary histiocytosis X: a report based on 50 adult cases. *Thorax.* 1982;37:104–109.

ALVEOLAR LUNG DISEASE

Alveolar lung disease (ALD) refers to filling of the airspaces with fluid or other material (water, pus, blood, cells, or protein). The airspace filling can be partial, with some alveolar aeration remaining, or complete, producing densely opacified, non-aerated lung that obscures underlying bronchial and vascular markings. ALD producing dense airspace opacity is more easily distinguished from interstitial lung disease (ILD) than lesser degrees of alveolar filling. Abnormal "hazy" lung opacification that does not obscure underlying bronchovascular markings is referred to as ground-glass opacification and can represent ILD, ALD, or both. Compared with ILD, ALD tends to produce a homogeneous appearance of parenchymal opacification, with abnormal opacities appearing more confluent. ILD produces linear, reticular, nodular, or reticulonodular opacities. There can be, and often is, overlap in the radiographic appearances of ILD and ALD.

Different causes of ALD often cannot be distinguished based on the radiographic distribution alone, but the clinical history, associated radiographic findings, and chronicity of the process can help to narrow the differential diagnosis. The processes to consider when an ALD pattern is seen are divided into those that are acute and those that are chronic. Recurrence of an acute process can mimic a chronic process (as with recurrent pulmonary hemorrhage in pulmonary–renal syndromes). In these cases, serial chest radiographs can help to show that the process is not caused by bronchoalveolar cell carcinoma, lipoid pneumonia, or lymphoma, for example, because these processes do not typically clear completely and then recur. All causes of acute ALD can resolve completely and subsequently recur, and therefore they should also be considered in the differential diagnosis of chronic ALD when serial chest radiographs or patient history suggests a chronic process with exacerbations and remissions. Although organizing pneumonia and eosinophilic pneumonia often present as ALD, they are discussed in Chapter 12 with other causes of peripheral lung disease.

ACUTE ALVEOLAR LUNG DISEASE

Pulmonary Edema

The four most common processes causing acute ALD are listed in Table 4-1. Pulmonary edema is the most common cause

of ALD on chest radiographs. As mentioned in the previous chapter, on ILD, edema can be (a) hydrostatic (from cardiac failure, renal failure, or overhydration); (b) nonhydrostatic, owing to increased capillary permeability (in acute respiratory distress syndrome [ARDS] and fat embolization syndrome); or (c) inflammatory in etiology (as from chemical pneumonitis or eosinophilic pneumonitis). *Fat embolization syndrome* occurs most commonly after traumatic fracture of long bones, which results in liberated marrow fat entering the pulmonary arterial circulation. Hydrolysis of fat, forming free fatty acids, leads to endothelial damage and increased capillary permeability 12 to 48 hours after trauma. This entity is further discussed in Chapter 8.

The radiographic distinction of pulmonary edema as cardiogenic or noncardiogenic in etiology is not always clear cut (1). Radiographic signs of cardiogenic pulmonary edema include enlargement of the cardiac silhouette (which may be assumed as secondary to cardiomegaly in many cases but is not always distinguishable from pericardial effusion), pleural effusions, pulmonary vascular congestion and redistribution, and interstitial and alveolar opacities. Edema fluid spills into the interstitial spaces and progresses to filling of the airspaces. Often, the chest radiograph shows evidence of interstitial and airspace filling, although occasionally a predominantly interstitial pattern may be seen. Interstitial edema can result in blurring of the margins of blood vessels and hazy thickening of bronchial walls (peribronchial cuffing), thickening of fissures (subpleural edema), and edematous thickening of the interlobular septa (Kerley A and B lines). Subpleural pulmonary edema refers to fluid that accumulates in the loose connective tissue beneath the visceral pleura and is seen radiographically as a thickened fissure; this is sometimes difficult to distinguish from pleural effusion. Chest radiographs are highly sensitive for the diagnosis of pulmonary edema and can show edema in patients who have not yet developed symptoms; conversely, pulmonary edema may be visible radiographically for hours or even days after the hemodynamic factors have returned to normal (2).

The distribution of airspace opacities in alveolar edema is usually patchy, bilateral, and widespread, and the opacities tend to coalesce. Air bronchograms may be evident, particularly when the edema is confluent. Often, alveolar accumulation of fluid in pulmonary edema is most pronounced centrally near the hila, resulting in a "bat's wing" or "butterfly" configuration. A clue to the diagnosis of pulmonary edema, instead

TABLE 4-1

ACUTE ALVEOLAR LUNG DISEASE

"HEAP"
Hemorrhage
Edema
Alveolar proteinosis/Aspiration
Pneumonia (includes infectious, organizing, and eosinophilic pneumonias)

TABLE 4-2

STAGES OF ACUTE RESPIRATORY DISTRESS SYNDROME

Stage 1 (first 24 hours): Capillary congestion and extensive microatelectasis with minimal fluid leakage. The chest radiograph may be normal, or it may show minimal interstitial edema or decreased lung volume.

Stage 2 (1 to 5 days): Fluid leakage and fibrin deposition and hyaline membranes develop. Alveolar consolidation by hemorrhagic fluid becomes extensive. The chest radiograph shows lung opacity (usually bilateral and symmetric), similar in appearance to cardiogenic pulmonary edema or pneumonia, which may start out patchy but rapidly coalesces.

Stage 3 (after 5 days): Alveolar cell proliferation, collagen deposition, and microvascular destruction. The chest radiograph shows a developing interstitial pattern that may result in honeycomb lung.

Reproduced with permission from Greene R. Adult respiratory distress syndrome: acute alveolar damage. *Radiology.* 1987;163:57–66.

of pneumonia, for example, is rapid change on radiographs taken over short time intervals (several hours); rapid clearing is particularly suggestive of the diagnosis. Edema fluid can also change distribution or shift from one lung to the other as a result of the effect of gravity, as when a patient has been lying on one side.

ARDS is the result of increased pulmonary vascular permeability and develops in response to lung injury. The more common of the many lung insults leading to ARDS include sepsis, pneumonia, aspiration of gastric contents, circulatory shock, trauma, burns, and drug overdose. Often there are multiple overlapping inciting events. The clinical syndrome of ARDS is characterized by acute, severe, progressive respiratory distress, usually requiring mechanical ventilation; widespread pulmonary opacity on chest radiographs; hypoxia despite high inspired oxygen concentration; and decreased compliance of the lungs ("stiff lungs"). Damage to the alveolar capillary membrane leads to increased capillary permeability and leakage of proteinaceous fluid into the alveoli. Eventually, alveolar disruption and hemorrhage occur, surfactant is reduced, and the alveoli tend to collapse. The stages of ARDS are outlined in Table 4-2. The radiographic features may be delayed by up to 12 hours or more following the onset of clinical symptoms—an important difference from cardiogenic pulmonary edema, in which the chest radiograph is frequently abnormal before or coincident with the onset of symptoms. Findings on chest radiography include bilateral, widespread, patchy, ill-defined opacities resembling cardiogenic pulmonary edema, but without cardiomegaly, vascular redistribution, or pleural effusion (Fig. 4-1). Although the lungs appear diffusely involved on chest radiographs, computed tomographic (CT) scanning often shows a more patchy distribution with preservation of normal lung regions (3). If an endotracheal tube is not present on the chest radiograph, the diagnosis of ARDS is unlikely, except in the later stages of healing.

Patients with ARDS typically require mechanical ventilation, sometimes with high positive end expiratory pressure because of stiff, noncompliant lungs. This predisposes to barotrauma, with rupture of alveolar walls and subsequent dissection of air into the perivascular bundle sheaths and interlobular septa, resulting in pulmonary interstitial emphysema. Discrete air-filled cysts, or "pneumatoceles," may form in both central and subpleural locations (Fig. 4-2). These air collections can dissect into the mediastinum, causing pneumomediastinum, and can rupture into the pleural space, causing pneumothorax. The lung may be so stiff that it does not collapse easily, even when a pneumothorax is present. Air may dissect from the mediastinum into the neck and chest wall, retroperitoneum, or

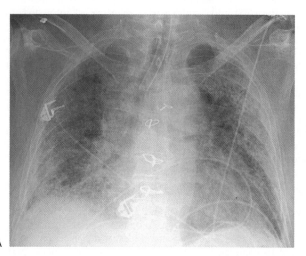 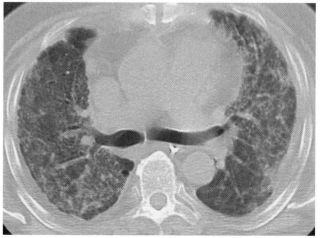

A   B

FIGURE 4-1. Acute respiratory distress syndrome (ARDS). This 69-year-old man had undergone a liver transplant several years earlier and developed ARDS as a result of herpes simplex virus pneumonia. **A:** Anteroposterior (AP) recumbent chest radiograph shows an endotracheal tube and bilateral interstitial and alveolar lung disease. **B:** Computed tomographic (CT) scan shows bilateral diffuse ground-glass and reticular opacities.

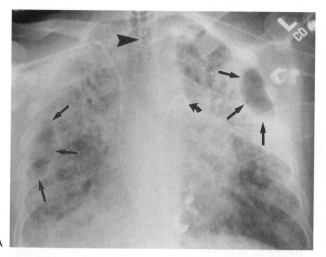

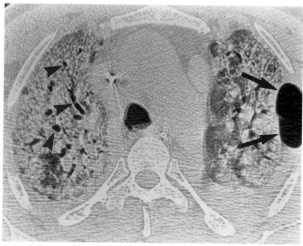

A

B

FIGURE 4-2. **Acute respiratory distress syndrome.** This 38-year-old man with a primary brain neoplasm developed severe respiratory distress requiring mechanical ventilation. **A:** AP recumbent chest radiograph shows bilateral ALD. An endotracheal tube is in place (*arrowhead*). Oval collections of air are present in the periphery of the lungs, representing pneumatoceles from barotrauma (*arrows*). A right subclavian pulmonary artery catheter was placed to measure pulmonary capillary wedge pressure. The pressure was low, consistent with noncardiogenic pulmonary edema of ARDS. The tip of the catheter is projected over the left lower lobe pulmonary artery (*curved arrow*). **B:** CT shows bilateral ALD, multiple abnormal rounded and tubular air collections within the lung representing dilated airways (*arrowheads*), and a peripheral pneumatocele on the left (*arrows*).

peritoneal cavity. The long-term outlook for survivors of ARDS is poorly documented. Mortality is related mainly to multiple organ failure rather than pulmonary dysfunction (4). One study of 109 survivors of ARDS showed that survivors had persistent functional disability 1 year after discharge from intensive care. Most had extrapulmonary conditions, with muscle wasting and weakness being the most prominent (5). Chest radiographs may return to normal or show varying degrees of interstitial lung disease, including pulmonary fibrosis.

Pulmonary Hemorrhage

Bleeding into the lung parenchyma occurs as the result of a variety of disorders (Table 4-3). A triad of features suggesting pulmonary hemorrhage is hemoptysis, anemia, and airspace opacities on chest radiography. Bleeding into the lung, however, does not always lead to hemoptysis (6). When bleeding into the lung is widespread, the pattern is referred to as *diffuse pulmonary hemorrhage* (DPH). The pulmonary features

TABLE 4-3

CAUSES OF PULMONARY HEMORRHAGE

Pulmonary–renal syndromes
Wegener granulomatosis (usually older men)
Systemic lupus erythematosus (younger women)
Goodpasture syndrome (younger men)
Other vasculitides (e.g., polyarteritis nodosa,
  Henoch-Schönlein purpura)
Without renal disease
Anticoagulation
Pulmonary infection or neoplasm
Pulmonary embolism
Idiopathic pulmonary hemosiderosis (childhood disease—rare
  in adult)
Trauma (including iatrogenic, e.g., biopsy)
Bone marrow transplantation (diffuse pulmonary hemorrhage)

of all DPH syndromes are the same, and chest radiographs are generally not helpful in distinguishing among them. Lung opacities range from patchy airspace opacities to widespread confluent opacities with air bronchograms. The lung opacities show a perihilar or middle to lower lung predominance, and they tend to be more pronounced centrally, with sparing of the costophrenic angles and apices. In general, in cases of acute pulmonary hemorrhage (if there are no complicating factors), rapid clearing in 2 to 3 days can be expected. This can aid in narrowing the differential diagnosis when chest radiography shows diffuse ALD (7). When the airspace disease clears, interstitial opacities are often seen on chest radiography, as the result of by-products of blood breakdown being taken up by the septal lymphatics.

Goodpasture syndrome, one of the pulmonary–renal syndromes and the most common cause of DPH, is an anti–basement membrane antibody disease manifesting as DPH and glomerulonephritis. It is a disease of young white men and is only occasionally reported in children (8). The presence of antiglomerular basement membrane antibodies in the serum is a sensitive and specific indicator of the disease. Renal biopsy shows evidence of subacute proliferative glomerulonephritis with linear IgG deposition in the glomeruli. The chest radiograph usually shows bilateral, relatively central, and symmetric ALD, but this is a nonspecific pattern (Fig. 4-3).

Many collagen vascular disorders and systemic vasculitides are associated with DPH, with or without renal disease. The association is most commonly seen with systemic lupus erythematosus (Fig. 4-4) and systemic necrotizing vasculitides of the polyarteritis nodosa type (9).

Wegener granulomatosis (WG) is characterized pathologically by necrotizing granulomatous vasculitis of the upper and lower respiratory tracts, a disseminated small-vessel vasculitis involving both arteries and veins, and a focal, necrotizing glomerulonephritis (10). Mean age at presentation is 50, and there is a slight male predominance. Upper airway involvement with sinusitis, rhinitis, and otitis is the most common clinical presentation. More than 90% of patients with active multiorgan WG have a positive test for cytoplasmic antineutrophil cytoplasmic antibodies (11). There are two characteristic pulmonary radiologic findings: (i) nodules, multiple

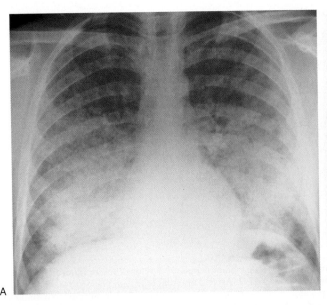
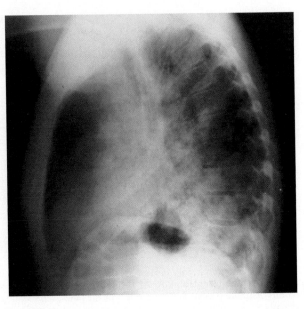

FIGURE 4-3. Goodpasture syndrome. This 21-year-old man presented with recurrent pulmonary hemorrhage. PA (**A**) and lateral (**B**) chest radiographs show bilateral ALD involving predominantly the middle and lower lungs.

or single, ranging from 3 mm to 10 cm in diameter, which may cavitate; and (ii) diffuse areas of lung opacity, representing pulmonary hemorrhage (Fig. 4-5). Occasionally, ill-defined nodular opacities may be present, sometimes appearing as areas of pleural-based, wedge-shaped consolidation, resembling pulmonary infarcts.

DPH can occur as a result of various coagulopathies, including thrombocytopenia (such as in leukemia or after bone marrow transplantation), anticoagulation, coronary thrombolysis, and diffuse intravascular coagulation. Infectious hemorrhagic necrotizing pneumonias or hemorrhagic neoplasms can result in diffuse, focal, or multifocal patchy areas of pulmonary hemorrhage. Pulmonary hemorrhage related to chest trauma is discussed in Chapter 8.

Alveolar Proteinosis

Alveolar proteinosis typically presents in a patient who feels relatively well, in striking contrast to the markedly abnormal radiograph, which shows bilateral diffuse or multifocal patchy opacities. The opacities represent a phospholipoproteinaceous material that fills the alveolar spaces and clears after bronchioalveolar lavage (12). Recurrence of disease can result in a chronic pattern of ALD, with serial chest radiographs showing varying patterns of recurrent ALD with interval clearing (Fig. 4-6). Alveolar proteinosis is associated with an increased incidence of lymphoma and infection with *Nocardia* (13,14).

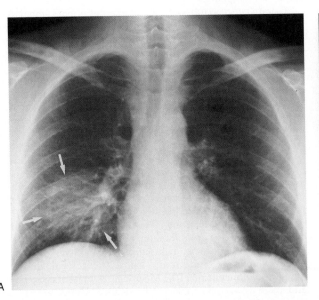
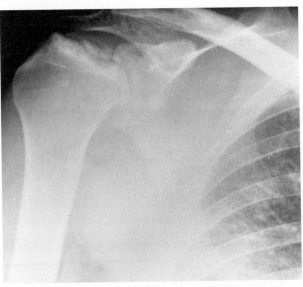

FIGURE 4-4. Systemic lupus erythematosus (SLE) with recurrent pulmonary hemorrhage. This 25-year-old woman presented with hemoptysis. **A:** PA chest radiograph shows focal ALD at the right lung base, with a rounded configuration (*arrows*), suggesting rounded pneumonia. Bronchoalveolar lavage showed evidence of pulmonary hemorrhage and no infectious organisms. The radiographic abnormality cleared in 4 days, consistent with hemorrhage. **B:** Radiograph of the right shoulder, providing a clue to the diagnosis, shows flattening, sclerosis, and collapse of the right humeral head as a result of avascular necrosis, a complication of chronic steroid treatment for SLE.

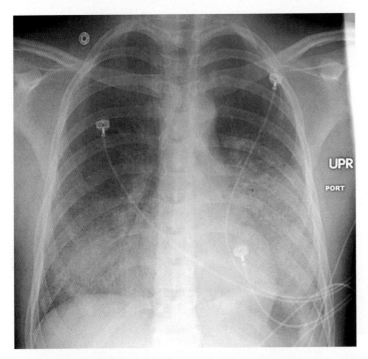

FIGURE 4-5. Wegener granulomatosis. This 19-year-old man, rather young in view of the age group in which this disorder most commonly appears, presented with hemoptysis and shortness of breath. AP chest radiograph shows a nonspecific pattern of bilateral ALD, predominantly involving the middle and lower lungs.

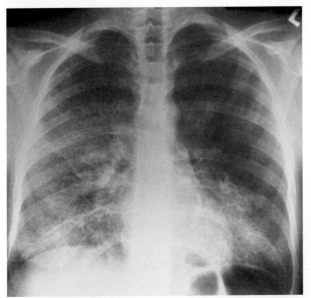

A

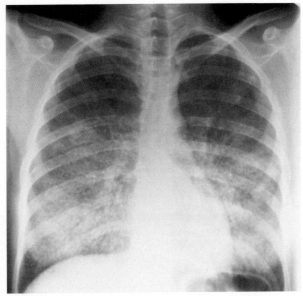

B

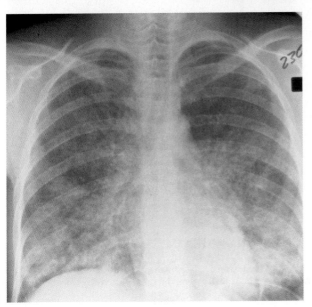

C

FIGURE 4-6. Pulmonary alveolar proteinosis. This 27-year-old man presented with recurrent alveolar proteinosis, which was treated with bronchoalveolar lavage. A: PA chest radiograph shows bilateral mixed interstitial and alveolar opacities involving predominantly the right middle and both lower lungs. Alveolar proteinosis is often associated with a prominent component of interstitial opacities, especially on CT. These opacities cleared after bronchoalveolar lavage. B: PA chest radiograph obtained 1 year later shows recurrent diffuse bilateral ALD, which cleared after treatment with bronchoalveolar lavage. C: PA chest radiograph 1 year after (B) shows recurrent diffuse bilateral ALD, which cleared after treatment with bronchoalveolar lavage. (Continued)

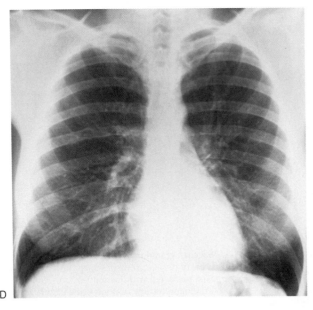

D

FIGURE 4-6. (*Continued*) D: PA chest radiograph obtained 2 years after (C) shows clearing of both lungs.

Infectious Pneumonia Causing Alveolar Lung Disease

Infectious pneumonia is the most common cause of focal ALD, and bacteria are the most common inciting agents. Fungal, mycobacterial, parasitic, and even viral pneumonias can all produce focal or diffuse airspace opacities on chest radiography (Figs. 4-7 to 4-9). Opacity of more than half a lobe with no loss of volume is virtually diagnostic of pneumonia, and common

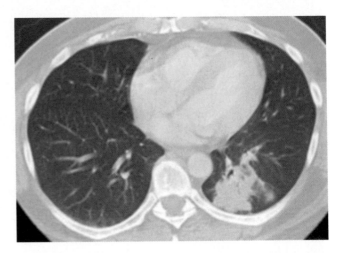

FIGURE 4-8. Pulmonary blastomycosis. This 43-year-old man presented with an infected finger and an abnormal chest radiograph (not shown). CT scan shows focal airspace opacity in the left lower lobe.

causes are *Streptococcus pneumoniae* or *Mycoplasma pneumoniae* (Figs. 4-10 and 4-11). Lobar consolidation with expansion of the lobe, although uncommon, strongly suggests bacterial pneumonia (particularly *S. pneumoniae*, *Klebsiella pneumoniae*, *Pseudomonas aeruginosa*, and *Staphylococcus aureus* pneumonias). A round consolidative process is likely to be caused by pneumonia (Fig. 4-12). Organisms most likely to cause round pneumonia are *S. pneumoniae*, *S. aureus*, *K. pneumoniae*, *P. aeruginosa*, *Legionella pneumophila* or *L. micdadei*, *Mycobacterium tuberculosis*, and several fungi. The development of air–fluid levels within an area of consolidation that is known or presumed to be pneumonia strongly suggests necrotizing pneumonia with abscess formation, and likely pathogens include *S. aureus*, *Klebsiella* sp, *Proteus* sp, and *Pseudomonas*

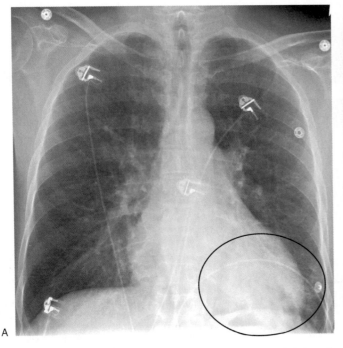

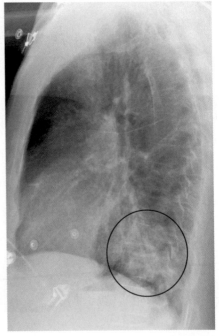

A   B

FIGURE 4-7. Bacterial pneumonia. This 58-year-old man presented with diabetic ketoacidosis, fever, cough, and elevated white blood cell count. A: PA chest radiograph shows ALD in the left lower lobe (*circle*). B: Lateral view shows ALD overlying the spine posteriorly (the so-called "spine sign"; *circle*).

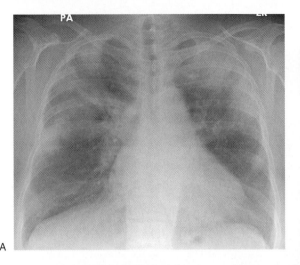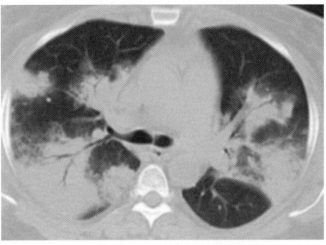

FIGURE 4-9. *Legionella* pneumonia. This 53-year-old woman with rheumatoid arthritis presented with fever, cough, shortness of breath, nausea and vomiting, and an elevated white blood cell count. **A:** PA chest radiograph shows bilateral peripheral ALD in the upper and middle lungs. The appearance was suggestive of organizing pneumonia. **B:** CT scan confirms bilateral subpleural areas of dense airspace opacity with air bronchograms.

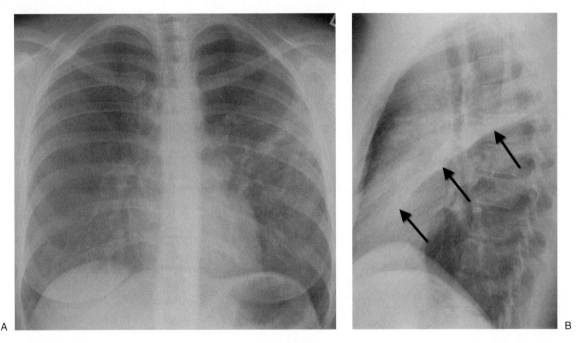

FIGURE 4-10. Pneumococcal pneumonia. This 22-year-old man presented with cough and fever. **A:** PA chest radiograph shows patchy ALD in the left lung, sparing the apex. **B:** Lateral view shows ALD confined to the left upper lobe, outlined posteriorly by the left major fissure (*arrows*).

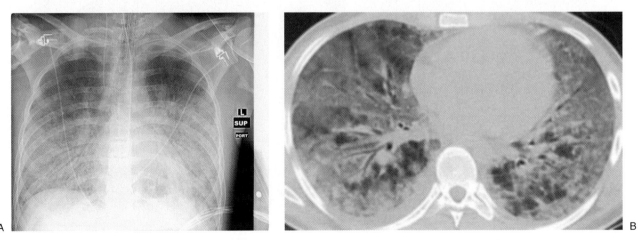

FIGURE 4-11. *Mycoplasma* pneumonia. This 22-year-old man presented with cough, fever, shortness of breath and hypoxemia. **A:** PA chest radiograph shows diffuse, nonspecific bilateral ALD. **B:** CT scan shows diffuse, nonspecific bilateral ground-glass opacity and areas of dense airspace opacity.

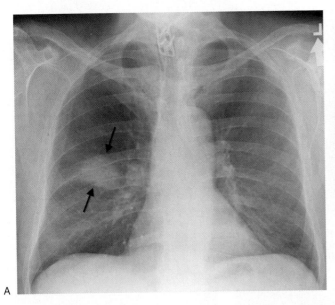
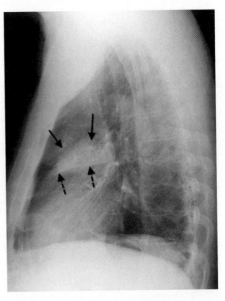

FIGURE 4-12. **Pneumococcal pneumonia. A:** PA chest radiograph shows a rounded area of ALD in the right middle lung (*arrows*). **B:** Lateral view shows that the ALD (*solid arrows*) is confined to the right upper lobe, as outlined by the minor fissure (*dashed arrows*).

sp, as well as mixed infections (Fig. 4-13). Multifocal pneumonia can be caused by numerous organisms, but the "bat's wing pattern" in the immunocompetent patient should suggest aspiration pneumonia, Gram-negative bacterial pneumonia (Fig. 4-14), and nonbacterial pneumonias such as mycoplasma, viral, and rickettsial pneumonia. Pneumonia in the immunocompromised host often results in the bat's wing pattern from opportunistic organisms such as *Pneumocystis jiroveci* and various fungi.

Aspiration

The radiologic manifestation of aspirated material into the lungs is dependent on the type and volume of material aspirated, the immune status of the patient, and the presence or absence of pre-existing lung disease. Aspiration of bland substances such as blood or neutralized gastric contents does not incite an inflammatory process, and associated lung opacities clear rapidly with ventilation therapy or coughing. Aspiration of acidic gastric contents and other irritating substances causes inflammation of the lung. Within several hours of aspirating such substances, chest radiographs usually show progressive airspace opacity in the gravitationally dependent regions of the lungs (Fig. 4-15). Radiologic improvement is generally seen within a few days unless the patient develops superimposed infection or ARDS.

Nasogastric or endotracheal intubation, diminished levels of consciousness, and supine positioning predispose patients to aspirate. Acute aspiration may be accompanied by fever, shortness of breath, and hypoxemia, which can make aspiration difficult to distinguish from bacterial pneumonia.

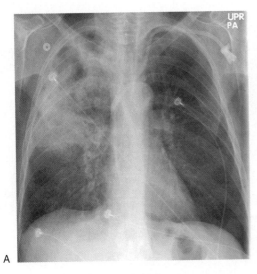
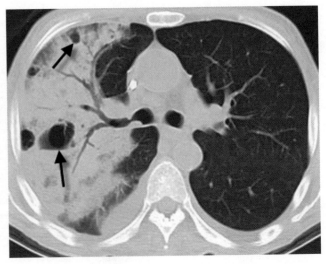

FIGURE 4-13. **Necrotizing *Pseudomonas* pneumonia. A:** PA chest radiograph shows ALD in the right upper and middle lung. **B:** CT shows numerous lucent areas with air–fluid levels (*arrows*) within the densely opacified lung, consistent with lung necrosis. Also shown are prominent air bronchograms.

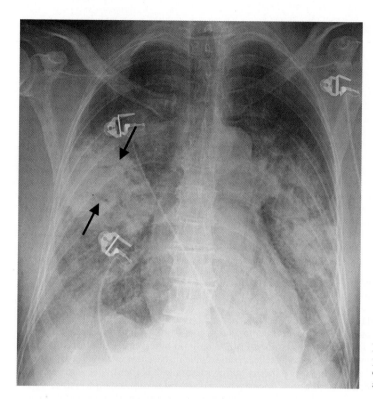

FIGURE 4-14. *Legionella* **pneumonia.** This 57-year-old woman presented with severe shortness of breath and hypoxemia. PA chest radiograph shows bilateral ALD in a "bat's wing" pattern and prominent air bronchograms (*arrows*).

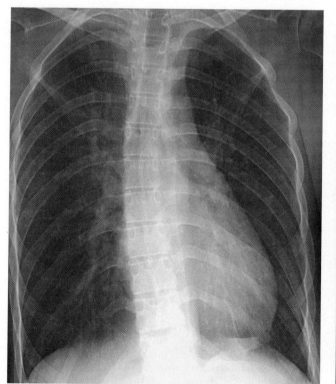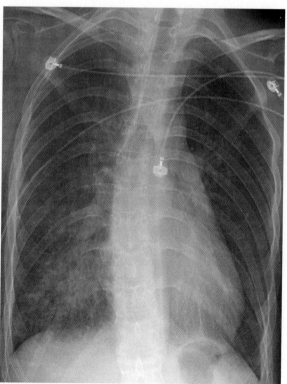

FIGURE 4-15. **Aspiration.** This 21-year-old quadriplegic man had a gastric bleed and aspirated blood. **A:** Baseline PA chest radiograph prior to aspiration shows clear lungs. **B:** PA chest radiograph obtained 1 day later, after aspiration, shows ALD in the right lung base.

TABLE 4-4

CAUSES OF CHRONIC ALVEOLAR LUNG DISEASE

"BALLS"
Bronchoalveolar cell carcinoma
Alveolar proteinosis
Lymphoma
Lipoid pneumonia
Sarcoidosis

CHRONIC ALVEOLAR LUNG DISEASE

Processes that result in a chronic pattern of ALD are listed in Table 4-4. Determining that the process is chronic requires serial chest radiographs showing a static appearance or progression of ALD, typically over several months. Two neoplastic processes should be considered in the differential diagnosis of chronic ALD: *lymphoma* (Figs. 4-16 and 4-17) and *bronchoalveolar cell carcinoma* (a type of primary bronchogenic adenocarcinoma) (Figs. 4-18 and 4-19). These are discussed in Chapters 6 and 15, respectively. *Alveolar proteinosis* has been discussed along with other causes of acute ALD, but it can be recurrent. *Sarcoidosis* can result in myriad chest radiographic patterns, both typical and atypical. Chronic ALD, although not a common pattern of sarcoidosis, should be considered in a young, relatively asymptomatic patient (Fig. 4-20). Although the chest radiographic appearance mimics ALD, sarcoidosis involves only the interstitial compartment of the lung. Areas of airspace opacity, so-called "alveolar sarcoidosis," represent a conglomeration of interstitial granulomas. This disorder is discussed further in Chapter 10.

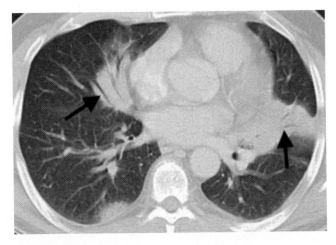

FIGURE 4-16. Pulmonary lymphoma. Chest CT shows bilateral foci of ALD, with prominent air bronchograms (*arrows*).

Lipoid pneumonia results from aspiration of vegetable, animal, or mineral oil, usually in elderly or debilitated patients, patients with neuromuscular disease or swallowing abnormalities, or patients taking mineral oil as therapy for chronic constipation. Most patients are relatively asymptomatic. Chest radiographs show homogeneous segmental areas of lung opacification, or circumscribed masses ("paraffinomas") that remain stable or slowly progress over a period of months and can be similar in appearance to bronchogenic carcinoma. Because of the lipid content, these areas of opacification may be of relatively low attenuation on CT scans of the chest, which may help suggest the correct diagnosis. Dilated colon and chronic stool retention seen on chest or abdominal radiographs may also provide clues to a patient who chronically aspirates mineral oil.

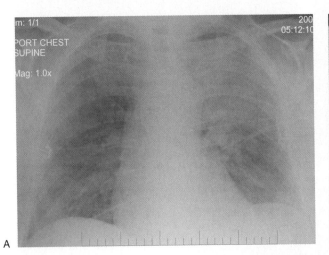

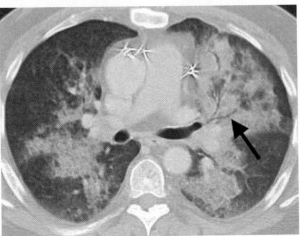

FIGURE 4-17. Burkitt lymphoma. A: PA chest radiograph shows bilateral ALD, most prominent on the left. B: CT scan shows bilateral ALD with prominent air bronchograms (*arrow*).

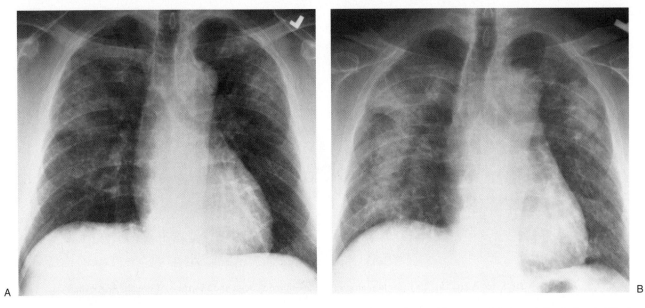

FIGURE 4-18. Bronchoalveolar cell carcinoma. This 56-year-old man presented with chronic ALD on serial chest radiographs. A: PA chest radiograph shows bilateral ALD, which appears "hazy" in some areas and is difficult to discern as interstitial or alveolar. The opacity in the left upper lobe is more confluent. B: PA chest radiograph obtained 16 months later shows progression of ALD.

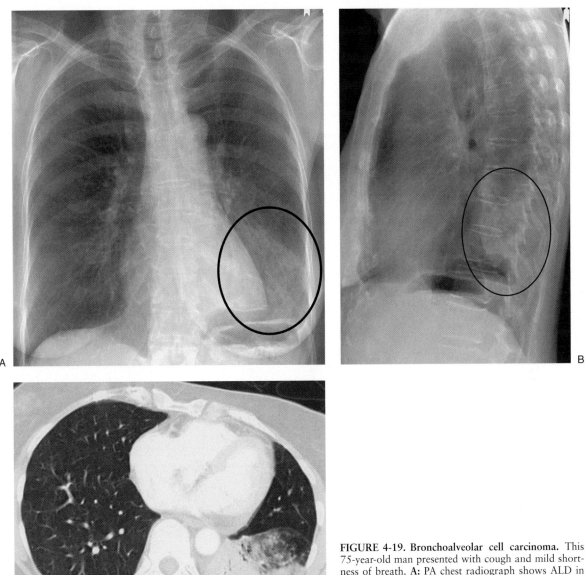

FIGURE 4-19. Bronchoalveolar cell carcinoma. This 75-year-old man presented with cough and mild shortness of breath. A: PA chest radiograph shows ALD in the left lower lobe (circle). B: Lateral view shows that the ALD is posterior, in the left lower lobe (circle). C: CT shows focal ALD in the left lower lobe and prominent air bronchograms.

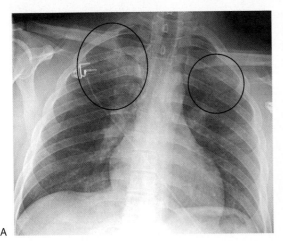
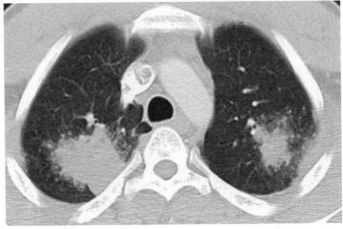

A

B

FIGURE 4-20. **Sarcoidosis.** This 29-year-old man presented with mild cough and shortness of breath. **A:** AP chest radiograph shows patchy ALD in the upper lungs (*circles*). **B:** CT shows bilateral upper lobe ALD. Although the appearance on imaging is that of ALD, sarcoidosis involves only the interstitial space. When the disease is profuse, as in this case, the interstitial granulomas compress and obliterate the adjacent alveolar spaces.

References

1. Sprung CL, Rackow EC, Fein IA, et al. The spectrum of pulmonary edema: differentiation of cardiogenic, intermediate and non-cardiogenic forms of pulmonary edema. *Am Rev Respir Dis.* 1981;124:718–722.
2. Pistolesi M, Miniati M, Milne ENC, et al. The chest roentgenogram in pulmonary edema. *Clin Chest Med.* 1985;6:315–344.
3. Maunder RJ, Shuman WP, McHugh JW, et al. Preservation of normal lung regions in the adult respiratory distress syndrome: analysis by computed tomography. *JAMA.* 1986;255:2463–2465.
4. Montgomery AB, Stager MA, Carrico CJ, Hudson L. Causes of mortality in patients with the adult respiratory distress syndrome. *Am Rev Respir Dis.* 1985;132:485–489.
5. Herridge MS, Cheung AM, Tansey CM. One-year outcomes in survivors of the acute respiratory distress syndrome. *Indian J Crit Care Med.* 2003;7: 53–54.
6. Soergel KH, Sommers SC. Idiopathic pulmonary hemosiderosis and related syndromes. *Am J Med.* 1962;32:499–511.
7. Bowley NB, Steiner RE, Chin WS. The chest x-ray in antiglomerular basement membrane antibody disease (Goodpasture's syndrome). *Clin Radiol.* 1979;30:419–429.
8. Benoit FL, Rulon DB, Theil GB, et al. Goodpasture's syndrome. *Am J Med.* 1964;37:424–444.
9. Bradley JD. The pulmonary hemorrhage syndromes. *Clin Chest Med.* 1982; 3:593–605.
10. Leavitt RY, Fauci AS. Pulmonary vasculitis. *Am Rev Respir Dis.* 1986; 134:149–166.
11. Hoffman GS, Kerr GS, Leavitt RY, et al. Wegener's granulomatosis: an analysis of 158 patients. *Ann Intern Med.* 1992;116:488–498.
12. Prakash UBS, Barham SS, Capenter HA. Pulmonary alveolar phospholipoproteinosis: experience with 34 cases and a review. *Mayo Clin Proc.* 1987;62:499–518.
13. Carnovale R, Zornoza J, Goldman A, Luna M. Pulmonary alveolar proteinosis: its association with hematologic malignancy and lymphoma. *Radiology.* 1977;122:303–306.
14. Palmer DL, Harvey RL, Wheeler JK. Diagnostic and therapeutic considerations in *Nocardia asteroides* infections. *Medicine.* 1974;53:391–401.

CHAPTER 5

MONITORING AND SUPPORT DEVICES—"TUBES AND LINES"

LEARNING OBJECTIVES

1. Describe and identify on chest radiography the normal appearance and complications associated with each of the following:

   - Endotracheal tube
   - Central venous catheter
   - Peripherally inserted central venous catheter
   - Pulmonary artery catheter
   - Enteric drainage and feeding tubes
   - Chest tube
   - Intra-aortic balloon pump
   - Pacemaker generator and leads
   - Automatic implantable cardiac defibrillator

   - Ventricular assist device
   - Intraesophageal manometer, temperature probe, and pH probe

2. Explain how an intra-aortic balloon pump works.

3. Describe how a ventricular assist device works and three indications for placement.

4. Describe the venous anatomy and expected course of veins from the axillary vein to the right atrium relative to anatomic landmarks.

5. Recognize the difference between a skin fold or chest tube track and pneumothorax on a frontal chest radiograph.

One of the most useful and cost-effective functions of chest radiography is the evaluation of complications related to the placement of monitoring and support tubes and lines. This is especially true for chest radiographs of patients in intensive care units, who usually have several support devices in place at one time. The placement of tubes and lines is often the first thing a radiologist interprets on a chest radiograph from the intensive care unit. Because this is such an important, common, and useful function of the chest radiograph, frequently resulting in a change in patient management (thus often requiring a call to the physician who ordered the radiograph), it is important for the interpreting radiologist to understand the function, normal radiographic appearance, and complications of the more commonly placed tubes and lines. The specific appearances of these devices vary by manufacturer and local practice, so it is important to become familiar with the specific characteristics of the devices used in a particular work setting.

CENTRAL VENOUS CATHETERS ("LINES")

Central venous catheters, often referred to as CVP (central venous pressure) lines, are used to monitor CVP and administer fluids intravenously. A centrally placed catheter ensures more consistent venous flow than does a route through the peripheral veins, which may vasoconstrict, particularly during periods of cardiovascular collapse. The internal jugular, subclavian, and femoral veins constitute the three most common access sites for CVP catheter placement.

The origins of the brachiocephalic veins (BCV) are demarcated by the sternoclavicular joint. Catheters within the left BCV show an anterior curve on the lateral chest radiograph because the left BCV crosses anteriorly to join the right BCV (Fig. 5-1). The subclavian veins drain the upper extremities and are a continuation of the axillary veins at a point demarcated by the lateral aspect of the first rib. The internal and external jugular and vertebral veins also contribute to the origin of each BCV. The left superior intercostal vein drains the second through fourth posterior intercostal veins and arches anteriorly to join the left BCV. It courses along the aortic arch, occasionally forming a rounded projection on the frontal chest radiograph referred to as the "aortic nipple."

The preferred position of a CVP line tip is central to the venous valves, at the origin of the superior vena cava (SVC). The SVC is formed by the junction of the right and left BCVs. This junction lies to the right of midline at the level of the first intercostal space. The SVC is the preferred location for measuring CVP and avoiding catheter complications. The SVC is joined by the azygos vein posteriorly, just prior to entering the pericardium. Posterior orientation of the catheter tip suggests that it enters the azygos vein (Fig. 5-2).

Peripherally inserted central catheters (PICCs) are small-caliber tubes that can be left in place for long durations. The preferred position of these catheters is reported to be the SVC (1,2); however, at some institutions, these catheters are placed in the radiology department, under direct fluoroscopic guidance, into the right atrium. There is little or no risk of atrial rupture or dysrhythmia with this placement, and there is a decreased incidence of peritip thrombus, which occurs with SVC placement in up to 90% of patients (3).

A left-sided SVC, a normal anatomic variant, is found in 0.3% of normal individuals (Fig. 5-3). Eighty percent of such patients also have a right-sided SVC and 60% have a left BCV connecting the right and left SVCs (4). When a left SVC is present, both the right SVC and the left BCV are usually diminutive. The left SVC most commonly drains into the right atrium via a dilated coronary sinus.

Many potential complications of CVP catheter placement can be recognized on chest radiography (Table 5-1). As many as one third of CVP catheters are placed incorrectly at the time of initial insertion (5) (Figs. 5-4 and 5-5). The most common

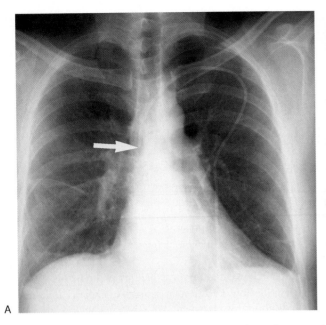
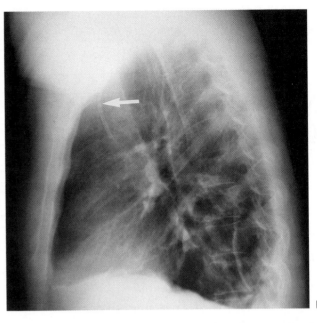

A   B

FIGURE 5-1. Left subclavian vein, central venous catheter placement. A: Posteroanterior (PA) chest radiograph shows the catheter entering the left subclavian vein under the left clavicle, crossing the midline as it courses to the right and descending, with the tip positioned over the expected area of the superior vena cava (SVC) (*arrow*). **B:** Lateral chest radiograph shows the catheter curving anteriorly (*arrow*), where it crosses from the left brachiocephalic vein to join the right brachiocephalic vein. This anterior curve makes it possible to determine on a lateral radiograph that a catheter has been placed from the left side.

aberrant locations include the internal jugular vein, the right atrium or ventricle, the opposite subclavian vein, the corresponding artery, the inferior vena cava, and various extrathoracic locations. Placement within the right atrium can lead to cardiac perforation by the catheter (although this is less of a risk with some of the commonly used, peripherally placed, flexible, small-bore PICC lines) (6). Positioning in the area of the tricuspid valve can cause dysrhythmias. Aberrant positioning will interfere with accurate measurement of central venous pressure and can lead to infusion of potentially toxic substances directly into the liver or heart rather than into the central venous system, where rapid dilution can take place. Catheter tips that are directed against the lateral wall of the SVC can produce excess focal pressure on the venous wall, leading (although rarely) to venous perforation (7).

Pneumothorax occurs with 6% of CVP catheter placements (8). In evaluating for pneumothorax, the entire pleural surface should be evaluated bilaterally, since a failed attempt at placement of a CVP catheter on one side may have gone undetected clinically before successful placement on the opposite side. Every chest radiograph should be evaluated for pneumothorax when a CVP catheter is present. This is because the initial radiograph, especially if supine, may not demonstrate the pneumothorax, and pneumothorax can persist several days after

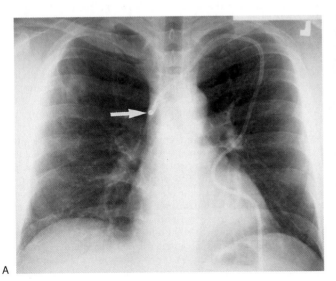
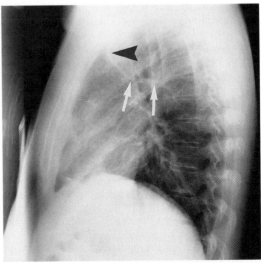

A   B

FIGURE 5-2. Azygos vein placement of central venous catheter. A: PA chest radiograph shows that the catheter tip is positioned over the expected area of the SVC. The tip is seen on end (*arrow*), however, which is a clue to azygos vein placement. The SVC is joined by the azygos vein posteriorly. **B:** Lateral chest radiograph shows the catheter coursing posteriorly, along the expected course of the azygos vein (*arrows*). Note how the more proximal portion of the catheter curves anteriorly (*arrowhead*), confirming placement from the left.

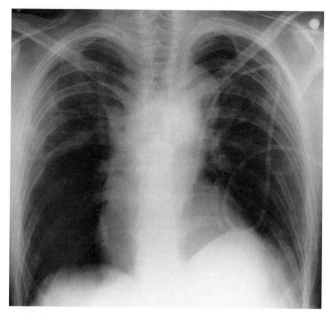

FIGURE 5-3. Left superior vena cava placement of central venous catheter. PA chest radiograph shows that, instead of crossing the midline to enter the SVC on the right, the catheter courses inferiorly to the left of the aortic arch, which is typical of placement within a persistent left SVC. This placement should be confirmed on a lateral chest radiograph to exclude aberrant positioning of the catheter within another venous or arterial structure.

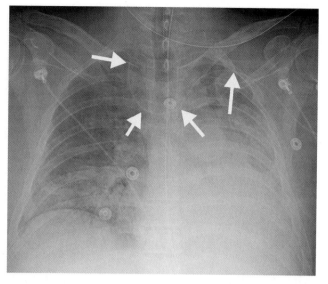

FIGURE 5-4. Malpositioned left peripherally inserted central venous catheter (PICC). AP chest radiograph shows a PICC (arrows) placed from the left side, crossing the midline, with the tip directed cephalad over the expected right jugular vein.

line placement (9). Skin folds, commonly seen on supine chest radiographs, may produce a thin radiopaque line that mimics a pneumothorax. Repeating the exam after repositioning the patient usually solves the dilemma.

Also occurring with CVP catheters placed via the subclavian vein is the complication of ectopic infusion of fluid into the mediastinum or pleural space (10) (Fig. 5-6). The rapid accumulation of fluid opacifying the mediastinum or pleural space after insertion of a subclavian catheter should suggest the diagnosis of ectopic infusion, which can be confirmed by injection of contrast through the catheter or thoracentesis if the fluid is accumulating in the pleural space.

Laceration of the catheter by the insertion needle, catheter fracture at a point of stress, or detachment of the catheter from its hub can result in catheter embolization. The catheter fragment can lodge in the SVC, inferior vena cava, right side of the heart, or pulmonary artery and can cause thrombosis, infection, or perforation (11).

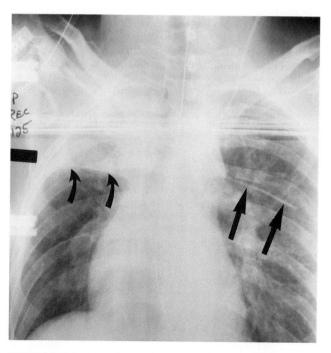

FIGURE 5-5. Intercostal vein placement of central venous catheter. Anteroposterior (AP) recumbent chest radiograph shows the left jugular central venous catheter crossing to the left and coursing horizontally, inferior to the left fifth posterior rib, typical of intercostal vein placement (straight arrows). The intercostal vessels and nerves are inferior to the rib; when performing thoracentesis, the needle should be inserted along the top of the rib to avoid puncturing these vessels. Note collapse of the right upper lobe, with superior displacement of the minor fissure (curved arrows).

TABLE 5-1

COMPLICATIONS RESULTING FROM CENTRAL VENOUS CATHETER PLACEMENT

Malposition
    Opposite subclavian vein
    Internal jugular vein with tip directed cephalad
    Corresponding artery
    Right atrium
    Right ventricle
    Extrathoracic location
Pneumothorax—usually immediate, may be delayed
Ectopic infusion of fluid into mediastinum or pleural space
Catheter breakage and embolization
Inadvertent puncture of subclavian artery
Air embolization
"Pinch-off" syndrome between the clavicle and first rib
Venous perforation
Thrombosis

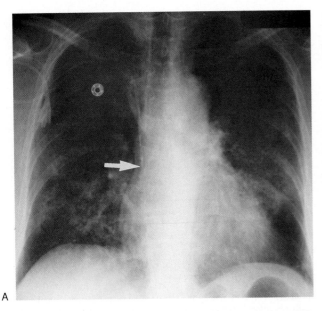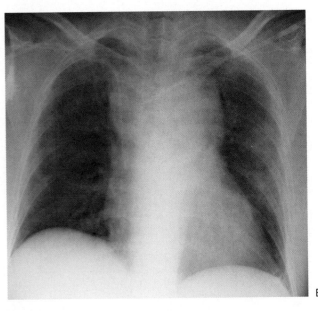

FIGURE 5-6. **Malpositioned catheter resulting in ectopic fluid administration. A:** PA chest radiograph obtained prior to left catheter placement. The right subclavian central venous catheter tip is positioned over the expected junction of the SVC and right atrium (*arrow*). **B:** PA chest radiograph after placement of a new left subclavian central venous catheter shows acute widening of the mediastinum from extravascular placement of the catheter and ectopic infusion of fluid into the mediastinum. The extravascular location of the catheter is not obvious on the radiograph, but the change in mediastinal width should prompt further investigation to confirm catheter position.

Inadvertent puncture of the subclavian artery during subclavian vein CVP catheter placement can result in localized bleeding, which may be self-limiting but is rarely severe enough to require surgical intervention (Figs. 5-7 and 5-8). Air embolization can occur during venipuncture or intravenous contrast injection. When this occurs, air may be visible in the pulmonary artery on a chest radiograph or computed tomographic (CT) scan, signifying this usually asymptomatic but potentially fatal complication. Clot frequently forms around the catheter tip with prolonged catheter placement, resulting in malfunctioning of the catheter. If thrombus progresses, venous occlusion and even pulmonary embolus can result. "Pinch-off" syndrome refers to compression of a CVP catheter between the clavicle and the first rib. This compression can lead to catheter fracture or fragmentation (12).

PULMONARY ARTERY CATHETERS

Pulmonary artery catheters consist of a central channel to monitor left atrial pressure and a second channel connected to

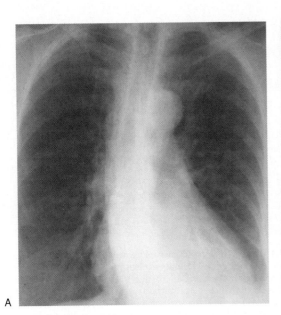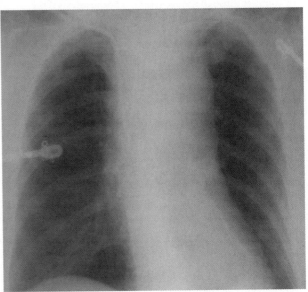

FIGURE 5-7. **Mediastinal hematoma from subclavian artery perforation. A:** PA chest radiograph prior to catheter placement shows a normal upper mediastinal width. **B:** PA chest radiograph after placement of right subclavian central venous catheter shows acute widening of the mediastinum.

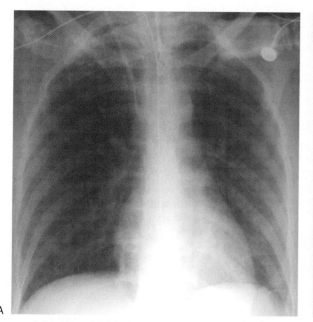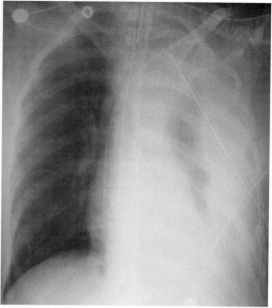

FIGURE 5-8. Hemothorax as a complication of central venous catheter placement. A: PA chest radiograph shows a normally positioned right jugular central venous catheter. B: PA chest radiograph after removal of the right catheter and placement of left subclavian central venous catheter shows a new large left pleural effusion. A chest tube was placed, which drained bright red blood.

an inflatable balloon at the catheter tip (13). A third channel measures CVP and cardiac output. The catheter is usually inserted from a subclavian vein approach, but jugular and femoral vein approaches are also used through a sheath called a *cordis*. The sheath allows easy advancement and withdrawal of the catheter and serves as short-term venous access after the pulmonary artery catheter has been removed. The purpose of the pulmonary artery catheter is to measure pulmonary capillary wedge pressure, which reflects left atrial pressure and left ventricular end-diastolic volume. Measurements of pulmonary capillary wedge pressure help to differentiate cardiogenic from noncardiogenic pulmonary edema. The ideal catheter tip position is within the right or left pulmonary artery or within the proximal interlobar artery. Inflation of the balloon causes the catheter to float into a peripheral pulmonary artery branch, in a wedged position, and deflation of the balloon results in the catheter resuming its more central position.

An important complication associated with the pulmonary artery catheter is pulmonary infarction distal to the catheter tip (14). This occurs when the catheter tip is placed too distally within the pulmonary artery. As the diameter of the catheter approaches the diameter of the pulmonary artery in which the catheter resides, occlusion of the artery by the catheter occurs. Clot can also form around the tip of the catheter and occlude the pulmonary artery, occasionally leading to pulmonary infarction (seen as patchy airspace opacification, often wedge shaped and in a subpleural location).

The pulmonary artery catheter balloon appears radiographically as a 1-cm rounded radiolucency at the tip of the catheter (Fig. 5-9). The balloon should be inflated for only a very short period of time, during measurement of pressure, and it should not be inflated while chest radiography is performed. If the balloon is left inflated, it can obstruct a major pulmonary artery and lead to pulmonary infarction.

Coiling or redundancy of pulmonary artery catheter tubing in the right side of the heart can irritate the myocardial conduction bundle and result in dysrhythmias (Fig. 5-10). Other potential complications of pulmonary artery catheter placement

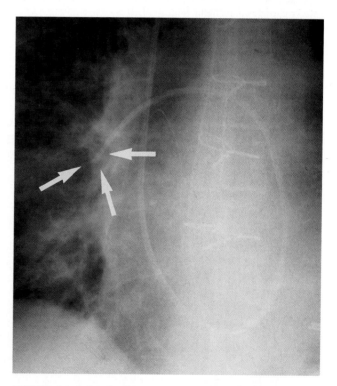

FIGURE 5-9. Inflated pulmonary artery catheter balloon. AP recumbent intraoperative chest radiograph, taken during measurement of pulmonary capillary wedge pressure, shows the inflated radiolucent balloon at the tip of the catheter (*arrows*). Normally, the balloon should not be inflated during the time of radiographic exposure. The balloon should be inflated for only a short period while measurements are obtained and then immediately deflated; when left inflated for longer periods, blood flow distal to the balloon is interrupted, resulting in pulmonary infarction.

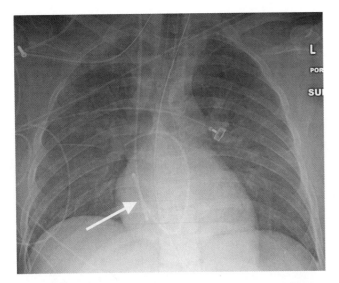

FIGURE 5-10. Looping of pulmonary artery catheter tubing. AP chest radiograph shows looping of the pulmonary artery catheter tubing (*arrow*) over the expected right atrium. This redundancy of catheter tubing can lead to dysrhythmias.

include pulmonary artery rupture (leading to pulmonary hemorrhage), pulmonary artery pseudoaneurysm (Figs. 5-11 and 5-12), fistulae between the pulmonary artery and the bronchial tree, intracardiac knotting of the catheter, and balloon rupture (Table 5-2). Complications that can occur with CVP catheter placement can also occur with pulmonary artery catheter placement (Fig. 5-13).

INTRA-AORTIC BALLOON PUMP

The intra-aortic balloon pump (IABP) (also called an intra-aortic counterpulsation balloon) is used in some centers to improve cardiac function in the setting of cardiogenic shock. The device consists of a long inflatable balloon (26 to 28 cm in length) that surrounds the distal end of a centrally placed catheter. The catheter is placed via a femoral artery retrograde to the thoracic aorta. The balloon is inflated during diastole (increasing diastolic pressure to the coronary arteries and increasing oxygen delivery to the myocardium) and is forcibly deflated during systole (decreasing left ventricular afterload and oxygen requirements). A commonly used IABP is radiolucent, except for a radiopaque marker that defines its tip. The balloon can be seen as a long tubular radiolucency (Fig. 5-14), following the expected course of the descending thoracic aorta to the left of the thoracic spine, if the radiograph is exposed during diastole when the balloon is inflated. The ideal location of the tip is just distal to the left subclavian artery (projecting at the level of the aortic arch on a frontal chest radiograph), allowing maximal augmentation of diastolic pressures in the proximal aorta. Even with appropriate positioning, the mesenteric and renal artery ostia are crossed by the long balloon (15). If the IABP is advanced too far, it may obstruct the left subclavian artery (Fig. 5-15) or cause cerebral embolus. If the IABP is not advanced far enough, less effective counterpulsation can result (Fig. 5-16).

Aortic dissection can occur during IABP insertion, which may result in death (16). Other potential complications include reduction of platelets, red blood cell destruction, peripheral emboli, balloon rupture with gas embolus, renal failure, and vascular insufficiency of the catheterized limb (17) (Table 5-3).

VENTRICULAR ASSIST DEVICE

Ventricular assist devices (VADs) are surgically implanted mechanical devices used in some medical centers to perform the work of the right (RVAD), left (LVAD), or bilateral (BVAD) ventricles in patients with intractable congestive heart failure. VADs can be implanted to support the failing heart and serve as a "bridge to transplant." In some patients with reversible

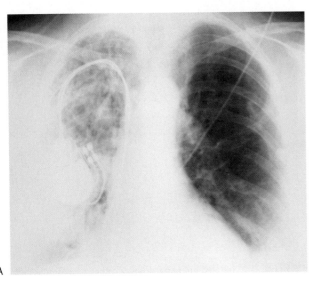

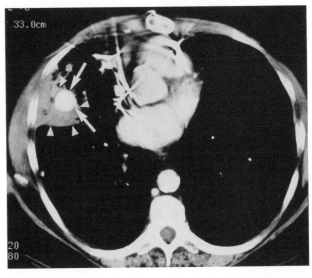

FIGURE 5-11. Pulmonary artery pseudoaneurysm as a complication of pulmonary artery catheter placement. A: AP recumbent chest radiograph in a 66-year-old woman with a history of chronic obstructive pulmonary disease and prior lung volume reduction surgery. The film was taken shortly after right heart catheterization, during which time a pulmonary artery catheter was placed into the right pulmonary artery to measure pulmonary capillary wedge pressure. The radiograph shows diffuse airspace disease in the right lung, consistent with acute pulmonary hemorrhage, which was new compared with a precatheterization radiograph. **B:** CT scan obtained after administration of intravenous contrast material, performed the same day as the chest radiograph in (**A**), shows an enhancing peripheral pulmonary artery pseudoaneurysm (*arrows*), with surrounding pulmonary hemorrhage (*arrowheads*). The pseudoaneurysm was embolized with coils by interventional radiologists, and the bleeding stopped.

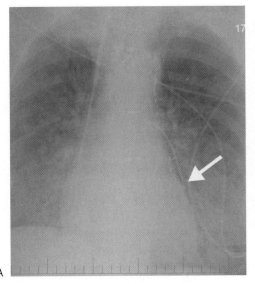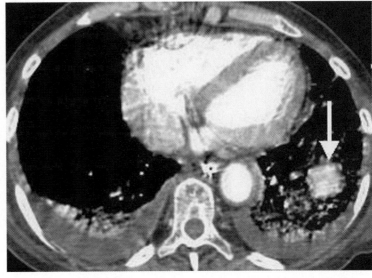

FIGURE 5-12. Pulmonary artery pseudoaneurysm as a complication of pulmonary artery catheter placement. A: AP chest radiograph shows pulmonary edema and the tip of a pulmonary artery catheter projected over an expected left lower lobe segmental pulmonary artery branch (*arrow*). B: The distal placement of the catheter tip resulted in perforation of a subsegmental pulmonary artery and development of a pulmonary artery pseudoaneurysm, shown as an enhancing mass in the left lower lobe on CT (*arrow*).

forms of cardiac failure, a VAD can be implanted with the hope that it will allow the heart to recover; the assist device can be removed later. This indication is known as "bridge to recovery" (18). In selected patients who are not good candidates for cardiac transplantation because of other medical complications, VADs can be implanted as a means of supporting circulation over a period of years. This indication is known as "destination therapy." The new generation of pumps is designed for chronic, out-of-hospital use so that most patients can return home after the VAD is implanted. Reported complications from VAD placement, recognized on chest radiographs and CT scans, include pneumothorax, hemothorax, infection, thromboembolism, bowel obstruction, and mechanical failure (19). On chest radiography, the TCI Heartmate LVAD pump (Thermocardiosystems Inc., Woburn, MA) is identified in the left upper quadrant of the abdomen. The inflow cannula of the pump inserts into the left ventricular apex, directed at the mitral valve, drawing blood from the heart into the pump, and the polymer graft outflow cannula, usually 12 to 15 cm in length, carries blood from the pump to the ascending aorta (Fig. 5-17).

Much of the outflow cannula is radiolucent. The inflow and outflow conduits contain porcine bioprosthetic valves, which are located outside the pump. A drive line, which exits through a fascial tunnel in the left lower quadrant of the abdomen, connects the device to an external portable console, which provides either pneumatic or electric power to the device.

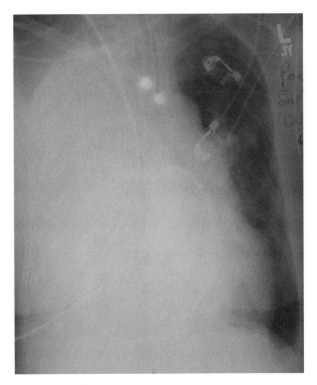

FIGURE 5-13. Hemothorax as a complication of pulmonary artery catheter placement. AP chest radiograph shows appropriate placement of a right jugular pulmonary artery catheter. However, there is complete opacification of the right hemithorax, representing acute and massive hemothorax.

TABLE 5-2

COMPLICATIONS RELATED TO PULMONARY ARTERY CATHETER PLACEMENT

Complications associated with central venous catheter placement (see Table 5-1)
Pulmonary infarction
  Distal placement of catheter tip
  Failure to deflate catheter balloon
Dysrhythmias
  Catheter tip in right atrium or right ventricle
Excessive coiling or redundancy of catheter tubing in right heart
Pulmonary artery pseudoaneurysm
Pulmonary artery rupture and pulmonary hemorrhage
Pulmonary artery to bronchial tree fistula
Intracardiac knotting of catheter
Balloon rupture

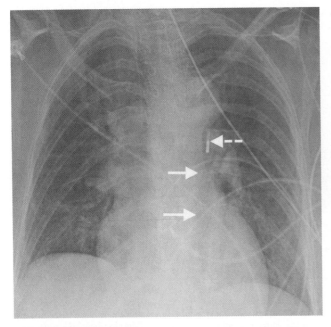

FIGURE 5-14. Inflated balloon of intra-aortic balloon pump. AP chest radiograph shows the radiopaque tip of an intra-aortic balloon pump (*dashed arrow*) and its radiolucent air-filled balloon (*solid arrows*). The balloon is inflated during diastole and deflated during systole. The tip is slightly low, with the desired location at the level of the aortic arch.

TRANSVENOUS PACEMAKERS

Numerous types of single- and dual-lead pacemakers and combination pacer–defibrillators are available. They are used to treat a variety of dysrhythmias. Accurate interpretation of their appearance on chest radiography requires knowledge of the specific type of pacemaker placed. The three major approaches

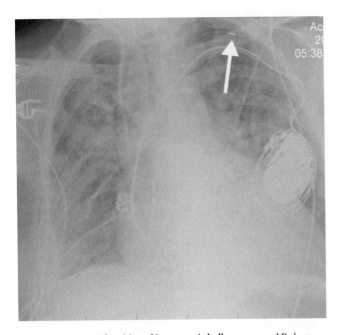

FIGURE 5-15. Malpositioned intra-aortic balloon pump. AP chest radiograph shows the radiopaque tip of an intra-aortic balloon pump projected over the expected left subclavian artery (*arrow*). This positioning can result in cerebral embolism and partial occlusion of blood flow to the left upper extremity.

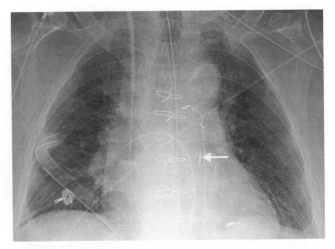

FIGURE 5-16. Malpositioned intra-aortic balloon pump. AP chest radiograph shows that the tip of the intra-aortic balloon pump (*arrow*) is below the desired level of the aortic arch.

to insertion of a pacemaker electrode into the heart include epicardial, subxiphoid, and transvenous implantations; transvenous is the most common. With single-lead pacers, the wire is placed into the right ventricle by way of the cephalic, subclavian, or jugular vein. When the lead is wedged into the myocardial trabeculae near the cardiac apex, the lead will be stable and have maximal contact with the endocardial surface. With dual-lead pacers, one lead is generally placed into the right atrium and the other into the right ventricle. It is important to know where the desired placement of leads is for each patient, because placement within the coronary sinus may be accidental or purposeful. After the electrodes are positioned, the generator is placed in a pouch in the subcutaneous tissues of the chest wall or beneath the pectoralis muscle. Biventricular pacemakers are used to treat congestive heart failure. Leads are placed in the right atrium and right ventricle, and a third lead is placed in the coronary sinus for pacing the left ventricle (Fig. 5-18).

Failure of the pacemaker to elicit a ventricular response may be caused by (a) exit block, (b) lead fracture, (c) electrode dislodgment, (d) electrode malposition, (e) myocardial perforation, (f) thrombosis, (g) infection, or (h) battery failure (20). Of these, malpositioning, fracture, and perforation may be recognized on chest radiographs. The leads can be malpositioned within the coronary sinus, and in this case the catheter often appears to be ideally positioned on the frontal radiograph but

TABLE 5-3
COMPLICATIONS RELATED TO INTRA-AORTIC BALLOON PUMP PLACEMENT

Balloon advanced too far
   Obstruction of the left subclavian artery
   Cerebral embolus
Balloon not advanced far enough
   Inadequate counterpulsation during diastole
Aortic dissection
Reduction of platelets
Red blood cell destruction
Emboli
Balloon rupture with gas embolus
Renal failure (balloon occlusion of renal artery)
Vascular insufficiency of catheterized limb

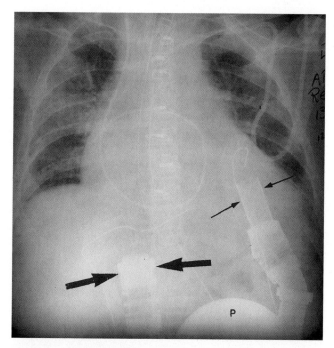

FIGURE 5-17. Left ventricular assist device. AP recumbent chest radiograph shows the inflow cannula (*small arrows*) within the left ventricle and directed toward the mitral valve, the pump (*P*), and the radiopaque portion of the outflow cannula (*large arrows*). The outflow cannula carries blood from the pump to the ascending aorta (the distal portion of the outflow cannula is nonradiopaque). The cardiac silhouette is markedly enlarged in this patient with end-stage heart disease.

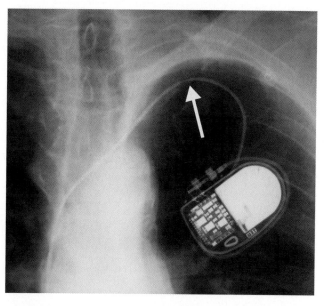

FIGURE 5-19. Fractured insulation covering pacer lead. PA chest radiograph shows a short segment of pacer lead that is less opaque (*arrow*). Note that the lead is not completely fractured. Even so, disruption of the insulation can result in pacer malfunction.

is directed posteriorly rather than anteriorly on the lateral projection. Approximately 2.7% of electrodes will fracture (21), generally near the pulse generator, at sharp bends in the lead wires, at the point of venous entry, or where the lead is embedded in the cardiac muscle (Figs. 5-19 to 5-21). If the insulating sheath holds the ends of a fractured lead in close proximity, the fracture may not be readily visible on a radiograph. Tight an-

choring ligatures at the venous entry site can produce lucency of the lead, giving the false appearance of a fracture.

Electrode dislodgment occurs in 3% to 14% of patients (22), generally during the first weeks following insertion. Late displacement is uncommon because of the fibrin sheath that develops between the electrode and the endocardium. *Twiddler's syndrome* is a rare complication seen in patients with implanted pacemakers or defibrillators; it is a result of the patient either consciously or unconsciously twisting and rotating the implanted device in its pocket, resulting in torsion, dislodgment, and often fracture of the implanted lead (23,24). The diagnosis is confirmed by a chest radiograph, which will reveal a twisted, entangled, and dislodged pacing lead. A small amount of catheter play should be present during systole, but

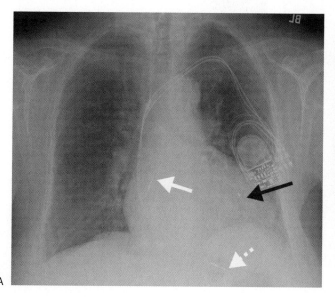

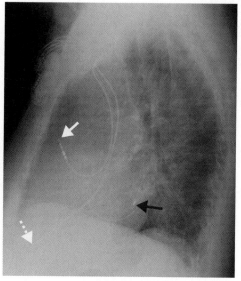

FIGURE 5-18. Biventricular pacer. PA (A) and lateral (B) chest radiographs show normal positioning of lead tips in the right atrium (*solid white arrow*), right ventricle (*dashed white arrow*), and coronary sinus (*solid black arrow*).

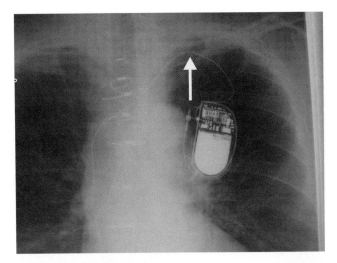

FIGURE 5-20. Fractured pacer lead. PA chest radiograph shows complete separation of lead fragments at the site of pacer lead fracture (*arrow*).

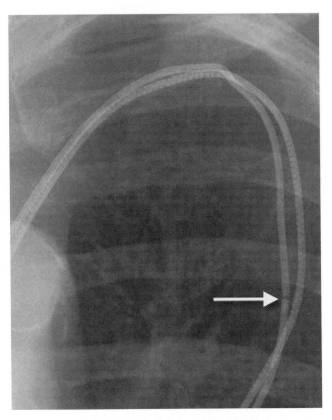

FIGURE 5-21. Fractured pacer lead. PA chest radiograph shows a fractured lead (*arrow*) and minimal distraction of the fracture fragments.

none should be present during diastole. If the catheter is short, dislodgment may occur, and the catheter may enter the right atrium, pulmonary artery, SVC, or coronary sinus. If the lead is too long, a bend in the wire may occur, causing lead fracture (Fig. 5-22). A redundant lead may also perforate the myocardium; this complication generally occurs at the time of or within a few days after insertion. The frontal or lateral radiograph will show the catheter tip outside or within 3 mm of the edge of the cardiac silhouette (Fig. 5-23). Perforation can lead to cardiac tamponade or postcardiotomy syndrome. Inflammation and infection can occur within the vein or the generator pocket; the latter occurs in up to 5% of patients (20). Major vein thrombosis and pulmonary embolism are additional complications of pacemaker insertion.

There are several models of implantable cardioverter-defibrillators, which are used for treatment of life-threatening ventricular tachyarrhythmia, generally using a combination of two transvenously placed electrodes and one subcutaneous electrode. A thoracotomy may or may not be required for placement, although most are now placed transvenously. These devices can be combined with a preexisting pacemaker. It is important that the radiologist be familiar with the normal appearance, variations, and complications of these devices, such

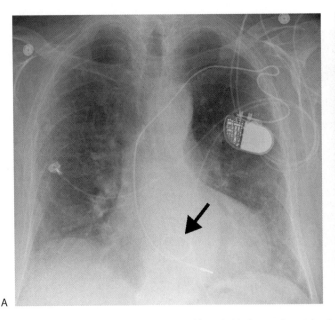

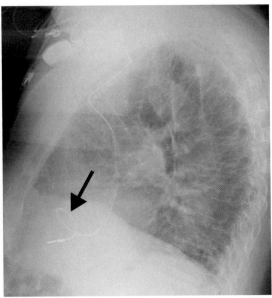

FIGURE 5-22. Looped pacer lead. PA (A) and lateral (B) chest radiographs show looping of the pacer lead over the area of the expected tricuspid valve (*arrow*). This positioning can result in dysrhythmia, lead fracture, or myocardial perforation.

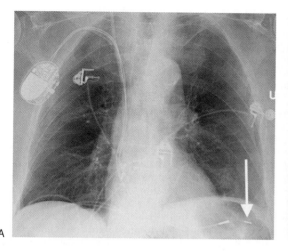
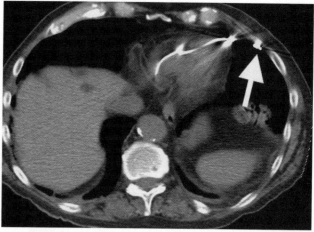

FIGURE 5-23. Displacement of pacer lead. A: PA chest radiograph shows that the tip of the pacer lead (*arrow*) is beyond the expected right ventricular wall. B: CT shows the lead outside of the myocardium (*arrow*). A more inferior image (not shown) showed that the lead tip was within the anterior chest wall.

as deformity of the subcutaneous patch electrode, lead fracture, and electrode malposition and migration (25).

ENDOTRACHEAL AND TRACHEOSTOMY TUBES

Patients require mechanical ventilation for any of three reasons: (i) airway obstruction, (ii) disorders of gas exchange, and (iii) failure of the airway's protective mechanisms. Intubation can be performed with an oral or a nasal endotracheal tube (ETT), cricothyroidotomy, or tracheotomy. Most ETTs are opaque or have an opaque strip demarcating the tip of the tube. When the head and neck of an adult are in the neutral position, the ETT tip should ideally be in the midtrachea, approximately 4 to 7 cm from the carina. On portable radiographs, the carina projects over T5, T6, or T7 in 95% of patients, and therefore if the carina is not visible, it should be assumed to be at the level of the T4-5 interspace (26). Flexion and extension of the neck

can result in 2 cm of descent or ascent of the ETT, respectively. In other words, the "hose goes where the nose goes." When the head and neck are flexed, the ETT should ideally be 2 to 4 cm from the carina; with extension, it should be 7 to 9 cm from the carina. Therefore, it is very important to check or know the position of the head/neck before recommending tube repositioning. The inflated ETT cuff (balloon) should fill but not bulge the lateral tracheal walls (Fig. 5-24).

The most frequent complications of ETT placement include difficulty in sealing the airway, self-extubation, right main bronchus intubation, esophageal intubation, and aspiration of gastric contents (27) (Table 5-4). With right main bronchial intubation, the left lung usually collapses (Figs. 5-25 and 5-26). If the ETT is placed in the pharynx or is dislodged from the trachea, mechanical ventilation is disrupted, the stomach may distend with air, and gastric contents may be aspirated. An ETT tip placed just beyond the vocal cords may cause vocal cord injury when the cuff is inflated. Inadvertent placement of the ETT into the esophagus can be life threatening. When this occurs, the ETT may be visualized lateral to the tracheal air shadow on chest radiography, the lungs appear hypoventilated, and the stomach appears markedly distended with air. A rare complication of ETT placement is tracheal laceration; in this case, the chest radiograph may show pneumothorax, pneumomediastinum, or both. The ETT cuff may appear overdistended, as the cuff herniates through the tracheal tear. Other causes of an overdistended cuff include inadvertent cuff hyperinflation, intraesophageal cuff location, chronic intubation,

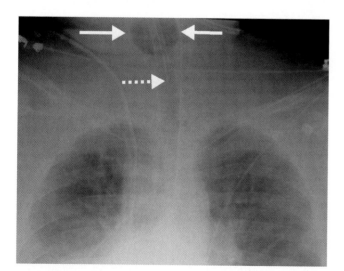

FIGURE 5-24. Overdistended endotracheal tube cuff. AP chest radiograph, coned to the neck and upper chest, shows that the tip of the ETT (*dashed arrow*) is above the thoracic inlet. The ETT balloon is overdistended (*solid arrows*). If left in this position long enough, the cuff could cause permanent damage to the vocal cords.

TABLE 5-4
COMPLICATIONS RELATED TO ENDOTRACHEAL OR TRACHEOSTOMY TUBE PLACEMENT
Malposition
Right mainstem endotracheal tube intubation leading to hypoventilation or collapse of left lung
Dislodgment from trachea
Placement just beyond vocal cords
Placement within esophagus
Tracheal or laryngeal laceration
Tracheostenosis
Tracheomalacia

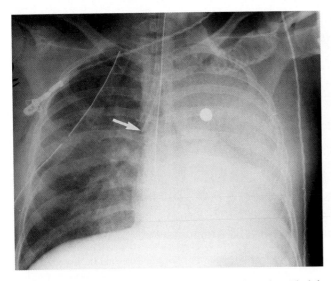

FIGURE 5-25. Endotracheal tube within right main bronchus. The left lung is radiopaque, and there is a shift of the mediastinum to the left because of malpositioning of the ETT within the right main bronchus (*arrow*); atelectasis of the left lung has resulted.

and tracheomegaly. ETT placement increases the incidence of sinusitis owing to mucosal edema and obstruction of sinus drainage.

Tracheostomy is usually performed 1 to 3 weeks after ETT placement in patients who require long-term mechanical ventilation or tracheal suctioning. The tracheostomy tube is inserted through a stoma at the level of the third tracheal cartilage, and it should be positioned with the tip several centimeters above the carina. Unlike the ETT, motion of the head and neck has little influence on the position of the tube in relation to the carina. The cuff should not extend to the tracheal wall. Following tracheostomy, subcutaneous air in the neck and up-

per mediastinum is common and is usually an unimportant consequence of the surgery (28). Massive air collections are caused most often by paratracheal insertion of the tube or perforation of the trachea. Pneumothorax is usually caused by inadvertent entry into the apical pleural space during surgery but may also be the result of tracheal perforation.

The incidence of serious tracheal injuries has decreased since the introduction of high-volume, low-pressure cuffs. Mucosal irritation from the tube and bacterial colonization lead to varying degrees of mucosal injury in every patient. In a small percentage of patients, the injury progresses to ulceration, which may lead to cartilage necrosis. After extubation, mucosal edema, erythema, and superficial ulcerations usually heal spontaneously. Deep ulcerations may result in permanent laryngeal scarring, tracheal stenosis, and tracheomalacia. Symptoms caused by permanent airway compromise usually appear several weeks to many months after extubation. Following extubation, all chest radiographs should be studied for the possibility of laryngeal or tracheal narrowing.

Pulmonary injury and air leak caused by mechanical ventilation occur in 5% to 50% of patients, with a higher incidence seen in patients with acute respiratory distress syndrome (29). Barotrauma develops when the alveoli are hyperdistended and rupture. The air dissects medially along the bronchovascular connective tissue to the mediastinum. Air can decompress cephalad into the visceral compartment of the neck or follow the esophagus caudad into the retroperitoneum. Retroperitoneal gas may continue along the anterior and posterior perirenal space into the properitoneal fat, and it can track along the anterior abdominal wall and chest wall and into the scrotum in men. Air may rupture into the peritoneum. If these routes do not adequately decompress the mediastinum, air ruptures the mediastinal parietal pleura and enters the pleural space.

CHEST TUBES

Pleural drainage tubes are used for evacuation of pleural fluid and air (hydrothorax and pneumothorax, respectively). Several types and sizes of tubes are used, and all should be evaluated by chest radiography for proper placement of the tip and side holes. A side hole is marked by an interruption of the radiopaque identification line; it should be medial to the inner margin of the ribs (Fig. 5-27). Placement of the tube tip in the

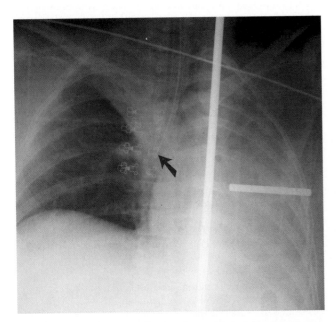

FIGURE 5-26. Endotracheal tube within bronchus intermedius. AP recumbent chest radiograph of a 29-year-old woman after a motor vehicle accident. The patient was intubated emergently outside the hospital. Malpositioning of the ETT within the bronchus intermedius (*arrow*) resulted in aeration of the right middle and lower lobes, with associated collapse of the right upper lobe and the entire left lung.

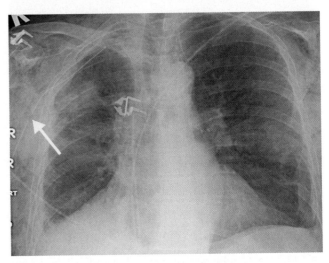

FIGURE 5-27. Malpositioned chest tube. AP chest radiograph shows that the side hole of the right chest tube (*arrow*) is outside of the pleural space. Note bilateral subcutaneous emphysema, seen as mottled lucencies within the soft tissues of the chest wall.

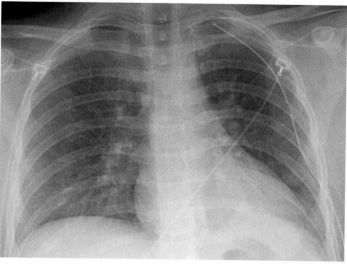

FIGURE 5-28. Chest tube track mimicking pneumothorax. A: PA chest radiograph, coned to the left upper hemithorax, shows a thin curvilinear opacity paralleling the chest wall (*arrows*). B: AP chest radiograph obtained 1 day earlier shows a chest tube following the course of the opacity seen in (A).

subcutaneous tissues, a fissure, or the lung parenchyma can be diagnosed with chest radiography or CT scanning. CT scans can also be used to identify loculated pleural collections and direct the placement of drainage tubes. Location within a fissure can be suspected when the tube reproduces the anatomy of the minor or major fissure, or when the tube takes more of a horizontal rather than a vertical course as seen on a frontal chest radiograph. Tubes within fissures may become occluded by the surrounding lung. Tubes can be inadvertently advanced into the mediastinum or through the lung parenchyma, liver, spleen, or diaphragm, resulting in bronchopleural fistula, hemorrhage, and infection (20,30). After removal of a

thoracostomy tube, a residual pleural or parenchymal line from the tube track is often identified on the chest radiograph (Fig. 5-28); this should not be mistaken for the visceral pleural edge of a pneumothorax. If a large amount of pleural fluid is removed at one time (e.g., >1.5 L), rapid lung re-expansion can, rarely, result in so-called "re-expansion" pulmonary edema.

ESOPHAGEAL/GASTRIC TUBES

Standard nasogastric tubes are used for suctioning gastric contents as well as for tube feeding. These tubes should be placed such that the tip is within the stomach, with the side port beyond the gastroesophageal junction. The most frequent misplacements are (a) incomplete insertion and (b) tube coiling within the esophagus (Figs. 5-29 to 5-31) (31). Small-bore

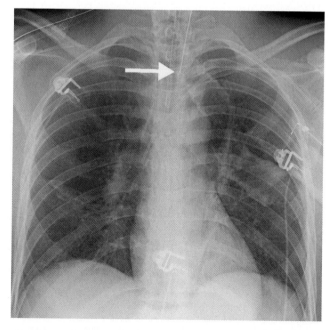

FIGURE 5-29. Malpositioned nasogastric tube. AP chest radiograph shows that the tip of the nasogastric tube (*arrow*) is well above the gastroesophageal junction. Note the distinctive morphology of the tip, which assists in recognizing its placement.

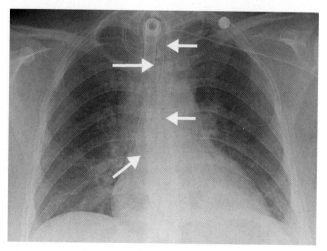

FIGURE 5-30. Looped nasogastric tube. AP chest radiograph shows the nasogastric tube (*arrows*) looped over the expected location of the esophagus.

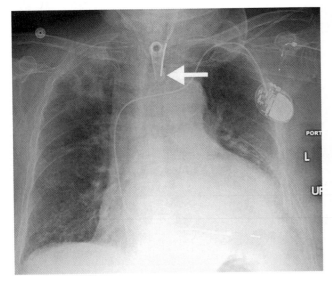

FIGURE 5-31. Malpositioned feeding tube. AP chest radiograph shows that the radiopaque tip of the feeding tube (*arrow*) is well above the gastroesophageal junction. The distinctive morphology of the tip aids in recognizing its placement.

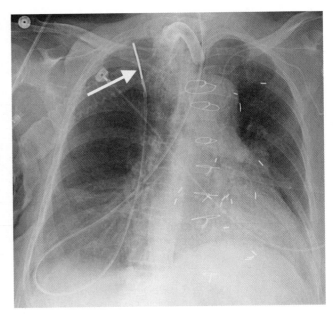

FIGURE 5-33. Malpositioned feeding tube in the lung. AP chest radiograph shows a feeding tube outside the expected course of the esophagus, with the tip projected over the right lung apex (*arrow*).

feeding tubes, ideally placed within the distal stomach or proximal small bowel, may be inadvertently placed into the lungs (Figs. 5-32 to 5-34), into the pleura (Fig. 5-35), or even through the diaphragm. Administration of tube feedings into the tracheobronchial tree may result in fatal pneumonia (32–34). Esophageal perforation can be caused by feeding tube placement. Radiographic findings secondary to the rare event of iatrogenic esophageal perforation include pleural effusion,

pneumomediastinum, extraesophageal location of the tube, mediastinal widening, and mediastinal air–fluid levels.

Several different types of esophageal measurement probes may be placed in the esophagus to measure intrathoracic pressure, temperature, and pH. The tips of pressure and temperature probes are usually placed in the distal esophagus. pH probes are usually positioned with the tip 5 cm above the lower esophageal sphincter (35).

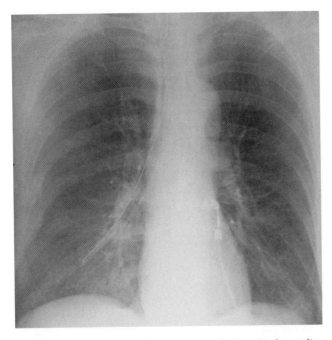

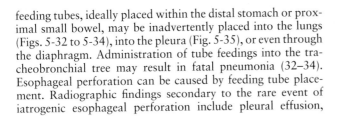

FIGURE 5-32. Nasogastric tube placement in the lung. AP chest radiograph shows the course of the nasogastric tube following the expected course of the right main bronchus and out into the lung.

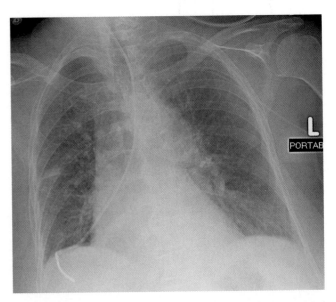

FIGURE 5-34. Malpositioned feeding tube in the lung. AP chest radiograph shows a feeding tube projected over the right lung base. If not recognized before feeding the patient, such a placement can result in chemical pneumonitis.

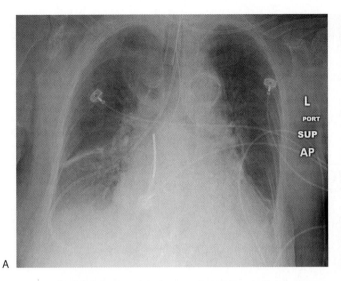
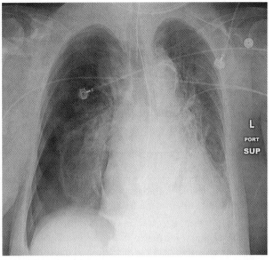

FIGURE 5-35. Malpositioned feeding tube. A: AP chest radiograph shows the feeding tube outside the expected course of the esophagus. **B:** After removal of the tube, the patient developed a large right pneumothorax as a result of the tube having penetrated the pleural space.

References

1. Hadaway LC. An overview of vascular access devices inserted via the antecubital area. *J Intraven Nurs.* 1990;13:297–305.
2. James L, Bledsoe L, Hadaway L. A retrospective look at tip location and complications of peripherally inserted central catheter lines. *J Intraven Nurs.* 1993;16:104–109.
3. Ahmed N, Payne RF. Thrombosis after central venous cannulation. *Med J Aust.* 1976;1:217–220.
4. Cha EM, Khoury GH. Persistent left superior vena cava. *Radiology.* 1972;103:375–381.
5. Langston CS. The aberrant central venous catheter and its complications. *Radiology.* 1971;100:55–59.
6. Huyghens L, Sennesael J, Verbeelen D, et al. Cardiothoracic complications of centrally inserted catheters. *Acute Care.* 1985;11:53–56.
7. Tocino IM, Watanabe A. Impending catheter perforation of superior vena cava: radiographic recognition. *Am J Roentgenol.* 1986;146:487–490.
8. Gibson RN, Hennessy OF, Collier N, et al. Major complications of central venous catheterization: a report of five cases and a brief review of the literature. *Clin Radiol.* 1985;36:205.
9. Sivak SL. Late appearance of pneumothorax after subclavian venipuncture. *Am J Med.* 1986;80:323.
10. Aulenbacher CE. Hydrothorax from subclavian vein catheterization. *JAMA.* 1970;214:372.
11. Blair E, Hunziker R, Flanagan ME. Catheter embolism. *Surgery.* 1970;67:457.
12. Hinke DH, Zandt-Stastny DA, Goodman LR, et al. Pinch-off syndrome: a complication of implantable subclavian venous access devices. *Radiology.* 1990;177:353–356.
13. Swan HJC, Ganz W. Use of a balloon flotation catheter in critically ill patients. *Surg Clin North Am.* 1975;55:501.
14. Sise MJ, Hollinsworth P, Brimm JE, et al. Complications of the flow-directed pulmonary artery catheter: a prospective analysis of 219 patients. *Crit Care Med.* 1981;9:315.
15. Barnett MG, Swartz MT, Peterson GJ, et al. Vascular complications from intraaortic balloons; risk analysis. *J Vasc Surg.* 1994;19:81–87.
16. Pace PD, Tilney NL, Lesch M, et al. Peripheral arterial complications of intra-aortic balloon counterpulsation. *Surgery.* 1977;82:685.
17. Vail CM, Ravin CE. Cardiovascular monitoring devices. In: Goodman LR, Putman CE, eds. *Critical Care Imaging.* 3rd ed. Philadelphia: WB Saunders; 1992:73.
18. Mayo Clinic. Ventricular assist devices. Available at: http://www.mayoclinic.org/heart-transplant/vad.html. Accessed March 7, 2006.
19. Knisely BL, Collins J, Jahania SA, et al. Imaging of ventricular assist devices and their complications. *Am J Roentgenol.* 1997;169:385–391.
20. Wechsler RJ, Steiner RM, Kinori I. Monitoring the monitors: the radiology of thoracic catheters, wires, and tubes. *Semin Roentgenol.* 1988;23:61–84.
21. Ehrlich I. Cardiac pacemakers. In: Teplick G, Haskin ME, eds. *Surgical Radiology.* Philadelphia: WB Saunders; 1981.
22. Steiner RM, Tegtmeyer CJ. The radiology of cardiac pacemakers. In: Morse D, Steiner RM, Parsonnet V, eds. *A Guide to Cardiac Pacemakers.* Philadelphia: Davis; 1983.
23. Bayliss CE, Beanlands DS, Baird RJ. The pacemaker twiddler's syndrome: a new complication of implantable transvenous pacemakers. *Can Med Assoc J.* 1968;99:371–373.
24. de Buitleir M, Canver CC. Twiddler's syndrome complicating a transvenous defibrillator lead system. *Chest.* 1996;109:1391–1394.
25. Takasugi JE, Godwin JD, Bardy GH. The implantable pacemaker-cardioverter-defibrillator: radiographic aspects. *RadioGraphics.* 1994;14:1275–1290.
26. Goodman LR, Conrardy PA, Laing F, et al. Radiographic evaluation of endotracheal tube position. *Am J Roentgenol.* 1976;127:433.
27. Stauffer JL, Olson DE, Petty TL. Complications and consequences of endotracheal intubation and tracheotomy: a prospective study of 150 critically ill adult patients. *Am J Med.* 1981;70:65.
28. Goodman LR. Pulmonary support and monitoring apparatus. In: Goodman LR, Putman CE, eds. *Critical Care Imaging.* 3rd ed. Philadelphia: WB Saunders; 1992:45.
29. Petersen GW, Baier H. Incidence of pulmonary barotrauma in a medical ICU. *Crit Care Med.* 1983;11:67.
30. Tocino I. Chest imaging in the intensive care unit. *Eur J Radiol.* 1996;23:46–57.
31. Fraser RG, Pare JAP. *Diagnosis of Diseases of the Chest.* 2nd ed. Philadelphia: WB Saunders; 1977.
32. Muthuswamy PP, Patel K, Rajendran R. "Isocal pneumonia" with respiratory failure. *Chest.* 1982;81:390.
33. Torrington KG, Bowman MA. Fatal hydrothorax and empyema complicating a malpositioned nasogastric tube. *Chest.* 1981;79:240–242.
34. Vaughan ED. Hazards associated with narrow bore naso-gastric tube feeding. *Br J Oral Surg.* 1981;19:151–154.
35. Richard B, Colletti RB, Christie DL, et al. Indications for pediatric esophageal pH monitoring: a medical position statement of the North American Society for Pediatric Gastroenterology and Nutrition. *J Pediatr Gastroenterol Nutr.* 1995;21:253–262.

MEDIASTINAL MASSES

The mediastinum includes the organs located between the two lungs. Because the mediastinum is invested by the medial parietal pleura, a mass isolated to the mediastinum will generally have a smooth contour (created by the pleural surface). Lung parenchymal masses, on the other hand, are not surrounded by pleura and may therefore have an irregular contour. Mediastinal masses can be recognized on chest radiographs when there is an abnormal contour to the normal mediastinal structures. On the right, these normal structures include, from superior to inferior, the brachiocephalic vessels, superior vena cava, azygos arch, ascending aorta, and right atrium. On the left, the mediastinal contour, from superior to inferior, is made up of the brachiocephalic vessels, aortic arch, main pulmonary artery, and left ventricle. On the lateral chest radiograph, the mediastinum extends from the inner margin of the sternum to the inner margins of the posterior ribs.

The mediastinum can be divided into compartments, and many classification systems have been devised to simplify the differential diagnosis when an abnormality is seen in one or more compartments. A system based on anatomic subdivisions (the superior, anterior, middle, and posterior mediastinal compartments) will be used in this chapter (Fig. 6-1). Approximately 60% of all mediastinal masses arise in the anterior mediastinum, 25% appear in the posterior mediastinum, and 15% occur in the middle mediastinum (1). When an abnormality is not isolated to one mediastinal compartment, as is often the case with large mediastinal masses, the list of diagnostic possibilities can be determined by localizing the abnormality to the mediastinal compartment serving as the "epicenter" of the abnormality or by considering all abnormalities that occur in the compartments involved. Associated radiologic findings can also help to narrow the list of diagnostic possibilities; these include deviation of the trachea (commonly seen with thyroid masses); presence of axillary, abdominal, and retroperitoneal adenopathy (suggesting the diagnosis of lymphoma); or posterior rib erosion or destruction (consistent with a posterior mediastinal mass, such as a neurogenic tumor).

SUPERIOR MEDIASTINUM

The superior mediastinum is bounded above by the thoracic inlet and below by a line from the sternomanubrial joint to the fourth thoracic vertebral body. The other mediastinal compartments lie inferior to this line. Abnormalities in the superior mediastinum include masses that extend down into the upper

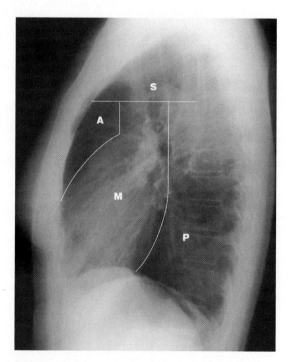

FIGURE 6-1. Mediastinal compartments. Lateral chest radiograph shows the boundaries delineating the superior (*S*), anterior (*A*), middle (*M*), and posterior (*P*) mediastinal compartments.

mediastinum from the neck, such as thyroid goiters or cystic hygromas; mediastinal adenopathy; and vascular abnormalities, such as aneurysms.

ANTERIOR MEDIASTINUM

Also referred to as the *prevascular space*, the anterior mediastinum is bounded above by the superior mediastinum, laterally by pleura, anteriorly by the sternum, and posteriorly by pericardium and great vessels. This compartment contains areolar tissue, lymph nodes, lymphatic vessels, thymus gland, thyroid gland, parathyroid glands, and internal mammary arteries and veins.

Masses occurring in the anterior mediastinum are listed in Table 6-1. In addition to the "4 Ts" (*t*hymoma, *t*hyroid mass, *t*eratoma, and *t*errible lymphoma), which account for the great majority of lesions, there are many other less common causes of an anterior mediastinal mass. These include vascular tortuosity or aneurysm, cardiac tumors or prominent pericardiac fat (Fig. 6-2), cystic hygroma, bronchogenic cyst, pericardial cyst, hemangioma, lymphangioma, parathyroid adenoma (Fig. 6-3), various other mesenchymal tumors (e.g., fibroma or lipoma), sternal tumor, primary lung tumor invading the anterior mediastinum, Morgagni hernia (Fig. 6-4), abscess (Fig. 6-5), and mediastinal lipomatosis (Fig. 6-6).

TABLE 6-1
ANTERIOR MEDIASTINAL MASSES
"4 Ts"
Thymoma (generally over age 40)
Teratoma (and other germ cell tumors, generally under age 40)
Thyroid (goiter or neoplasm, look for tracheal deviation)
Terrible lymphoma

An intrathoracic *thyroid* mass is usually a benign multinodular goiter that originates in the neck and extends downward into the mediastinum through the thoracic inlet. This continuity is an important diagnostic feature on chest radiography. Many thyroid masses displace or narrow the trachea (Fig. 6-7). Another useful sign of a thyroid mass is the relative high attenuation value of the thyroid tissue, at least 20 Hounsfield units above that seen in adjacent muscles on both precontrast and postcontrast computed tomographic (CT) images (2). CT scans can show cystic components. Calcification is common and usually caused by benign disease when it is dense, amorphous, and well defined with a nodular, curvilinear, or circular configuration. Distinguishing between benign and malignant thyroid masses on chest radiography or CT scanning is not possible unless the tumor has clearly spread beyond the

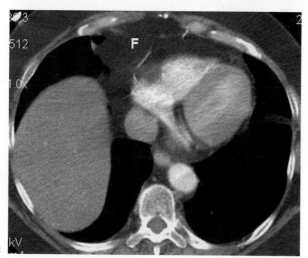

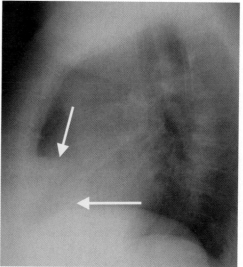

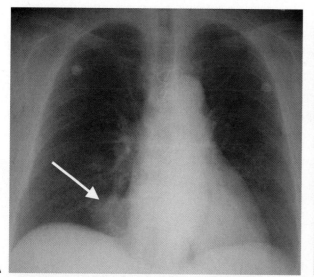

FIGURE 6-2. Prominent pericardial fat. A: Posteroanterior (PA) chest radiograph shows a round mass at the right cardiophrenic angle (*arrow*) that is less opaque than the adjacent heart. **B:** Lateral view shows that the mass is projected over the anterior inferior heart (*arrows*) in the typical location of pericardiac fat. **C:** CT shows this mass to be of fat attenuation (F), similar to that of the subcutaneous fat.

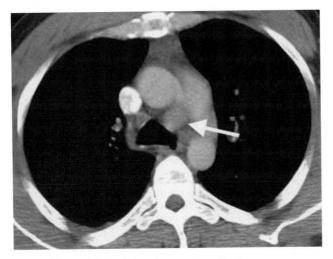

FIGURE 6-3. Parathyroid adenoma. CT shows a nonspecific enhancing mass (*arrow*) in the aortopulmonary window. Although commonly an anterior mediastinal mass, parathyroid adenomas can occur in any mediastinal compartment.

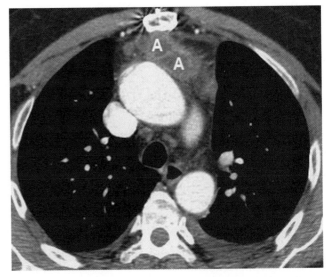

FIGURE 6-5. Anterior mediastinal abscess. CT scan of a 54-year-old man who recently underwent aortic valve replacement shows a loculated fluid collection (*A*) with an enhancing rim anterior to the ascending aorta and posterior to the sternum.

thyroid gland (indicating malignancy). Malignant thyroid masses can also have calcifications, generally with a configuration of fine dots grouped in a cloudlike formation (3–5). However, the patterns of benign and malignant calcifications serve as general guidelines, and malignant medullary thyroid carcinoma can contain well-defined, occasionally ring-shaped, dense calcifications that are similar in appearance to the calcifications seen with benign thyroid goiter. Radionuclide imaging is a very sensitive and specific method of determining the thyroid nature of an intrathoracic mass (Fig. 6-8), but CT provides more information about the mass.

Thymomas are tumors consisting of thymic epithelial cells and reactive lymphocytes, with noninvasive or invasive patterns of growth (6). The presence or absence of tumor spread beyond the capsule (usually determined surgically), rather than the histologic appearance within the thymus, determines whether a tumor is benign or malignant. Thymomas occur at an average age of 50 years and with equal frequency in men and women (6). They are associated with a variety of autoimmune diseases, most notably myasthenia gravis. Approximately 40% of patients with thymoma have myasthenia gravis, and the incidence of thymoma in patients with this disease is approximately 15% (7). Most thymomas arise in the upper anterior mediastinum, anterior to the ascending aorta above

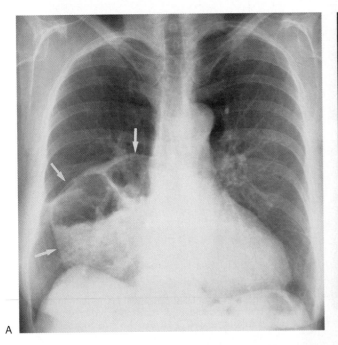

A

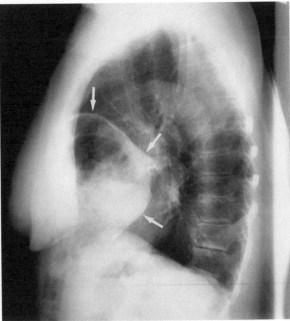

B

FIGURE 6-4. Morgagni hernia. PA (A) and lateral (B) chest radiographs show colon, filled with air and stool (*arrows*), herniating into the anterior mediastinum through a congenital defect in the anteromedial diaphragm.

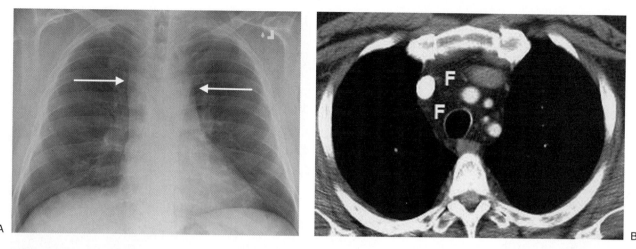

FIGURE 6-6. Mediastinal lipomatosis. A: PA chest radiograph shows an abnormally wide upper mediastinum with straight margins (*arrows*). **B:** CT scan shows abundant mediastinal fat (*F*).

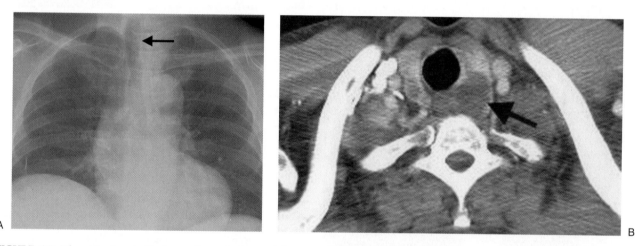

FIGURE 6-7. Thyroid goiter. A: PA chest radiograph shows a left paratracheal mass and deviation of the trachea to the right (*arrow*). **B:** CT scan shows a heterogeneous left thyroid mass with cystic components (*arrow*). There is also a smaller cyst within the right lobe.

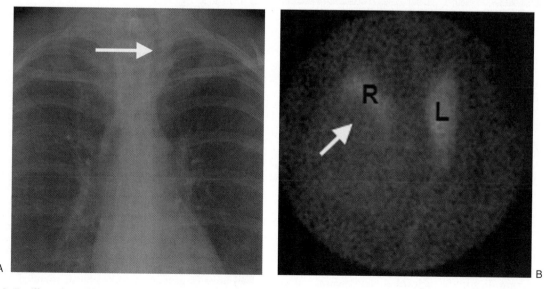

FIGURE 6-8. Papillary thyroid carcinoma. A: PA chest radiograph of a 48-year-old woman shows a right paratracheal mass and deviation of the trachea to the left (*arrow*). **B:** Technetium pertechnetate–enhanced thyroid scan shows a "cold" nodule in the right lobe of the thyroid gland (*arrow*). Nearly all thyroid cancers are nonfunctioning or "cold" nodules on nuclear medicine thyroid scans. R, right lobe of thyroid; L, left lobe of thyroid.

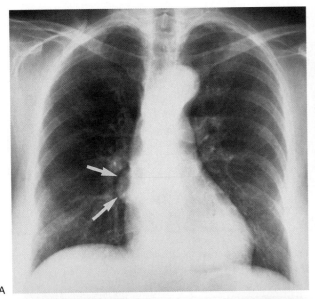

A

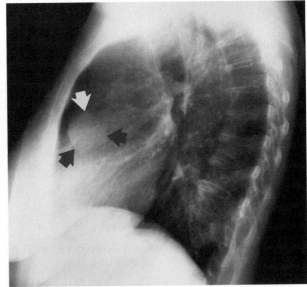

B

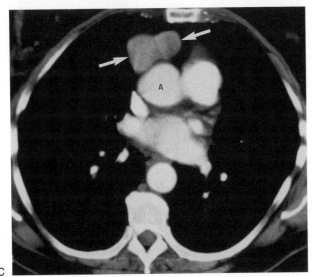

C

FIGURE 6-9. Benign thymoma. A: PA chest radiograph of a 70-year-old woman shows a rounded mass overlying the right heart border. The visualized margins are well circumscribed (*arrows*). **B:** Lateral chest radiograph suggests that the mass is located in the anterior mediastinum (*arrows*). **C:** CT scan shows a peanut-shaped mass of fairly homogeneous attenuation (*arrows*). The mass is located anterior to the ascending aorta (*A*), above the right ventricular outflow tract, a typical location for thymomas.

the right ventricular outflow tract and main pulmonary artery (Fig. 6-9). They can extend into the adjacent middle or posterior mediastinum, and they can occur or extend into the lower third of the mediastinum, as low as the cardiophrenic angles. Punctate, curvilinear, or ringlike calcification is common in both benign and invasive thymomas (8). On a CT scan, thymomas are usually of homogeneous attenuation and show uniform enhancement, but rarely they can appear cystic with discrete nodular components (Figs. 6-10 and 6-11). In patients under age 40, diagnosing a small thymoma can be difficult because the normal gland is variable in size. A normal thymus, in contrast to a thymic mass, conforms to the shape of the adjacent great vessels on CT and magnetic resonance imaging (MRI). A mass gives rise to focal thymic enlargement, usually with its center away from the midline, whereas a normal gland is approximately symmetric and maintains a somewhat triangular shape on axial imaging. Invasive thymomas inhabit the mediastinal fat, spreading to the pericardium and pleura. Unless mediastinal invasion has occurred, distinguishing benign from invasive thymoma is not possible with CT scanning. Transpleural spread may manifest as so-called "drop metastases" at a site distant from the primary lesion (Fig. 6-12), and imaging of the entire pleural space and upper abdomen is therefore im-

portant. Extensive pleural involvement may mimic malignant mesothelioma. Other less common thymic masses include cyst (Fig. 6-13), abscess, thymolipoma, malignant lymphoma (most notably Hodgkin lymphoma), thymic carcinoid, germ cell tumors, and thymic carcinoma (Fig. 6-14).

A *teratoma* is a neoplasm derived from more than one embryonic germ layer. Other germ cell tumors include benign dermoid cyst, malignant seminoma (the most common germ cell tumor), teratocarcinoma, embryonal carcinoma, endodermal sinus tumor (yolk sac tumor), choriocarcinoma, and mixtures of these types. Germ cell tumors in the mediastinum arise from primitive rest cells and generally are not metastatic from gonadal tumors. Some malignant germ cell tumors secrete beta-human chorionic gonadotropin and alpha-fetoprotein, which can be used to diagnose and monitor progression of disease.

Benign teratomas are found in patients of all ages but are most common in adolescents and young adults (Fig. 6-15). They usually produce a well-defined, rounded, or lobulated mass in the anterior mediastinum. They grow slowly, although rapid increase in size may occur as a result of hemorrhage, producing imaging features suggestive of a malignant mass.

(Text continues on page 86)

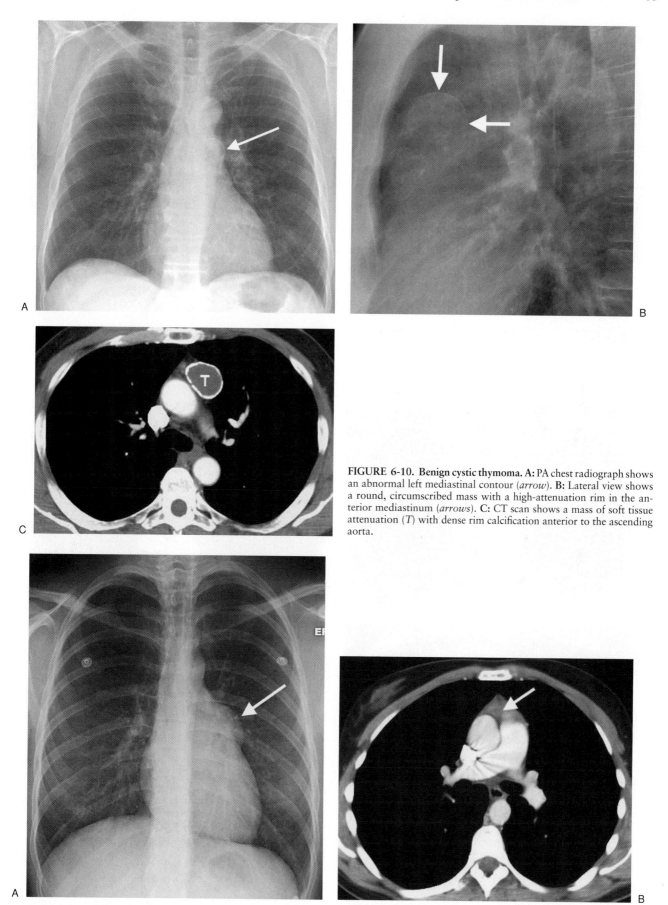

FIGURE 6-10. Benign cystic thymoma. A: PA chest radiograph shows an abnormal left mediastinal contour (*arrow*). **B:** Lateral view shows a round, circumscribed mass with a high-attenuation rim in the anterior mediastinum (*arrows*). **C:** CT scan shows a mass of soft tissue attenuation (*T*) with dense rim calcification anterior to the ascending aorta.

FIGURE 6-11. Benign thymoma. A: PA chest radiograph shows an abnormal left mediastinal contour (*arrow*). **B:** CT scan shows soft tissue anterior to the ascending aorta in the expected location of the thymus gland (*arrow*). (*Continued*)

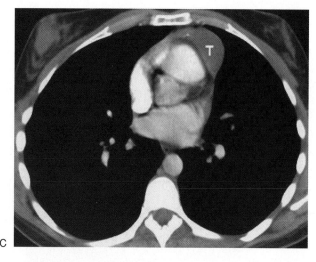

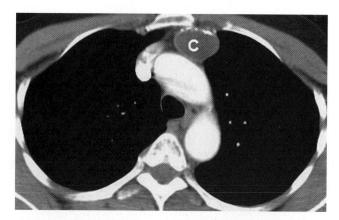

FIGURE 6-13. Thymic cyst. CT scan of a 60-year-old man shows a circumscribed, rim-calcified oval mass of homogeneous fluid attenuation (*C*) in the expected location of the thymus gland.

FIGURE 6-11. (*Continued*) C: CT scan inferior to (**B**) shows that the thymic soft tissue (*T*) is focally enlarged on the left.

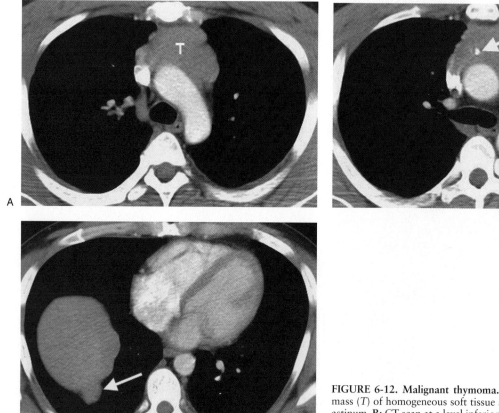

FIGURE 6-12. Malignant thymoma. A: CT scan shows a lobulated mass (*T*) of homogeneous soft tissue attenuation in the anterior mediastinum. B: CT scan at a level inferior to (**A**) shows course calcification (*arrow*) within the mass. C: A "drop" metastasis (*arrow*) is seen along the right hemidiaphragm.

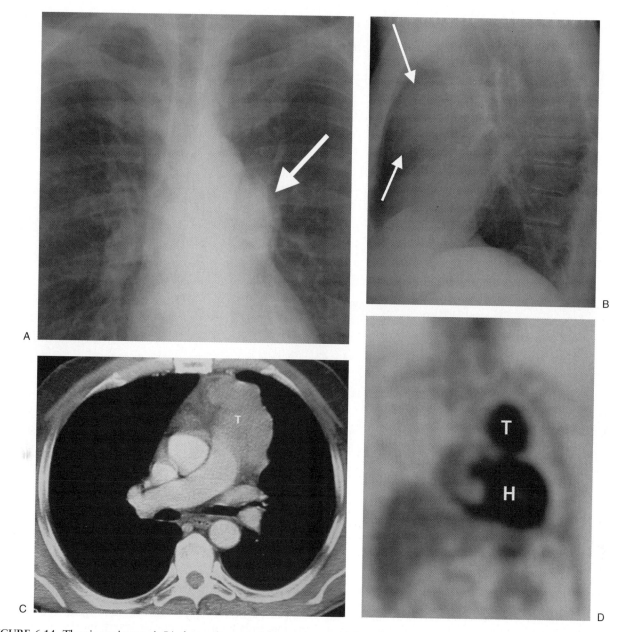

FIGURE 6-14. Thymic carcinoma. A: PA chest radiograph shows an abnormal left mediastinal contour (*arrow*). **B:** Lateral view shows abnormal opacity in the retrosternal area (*arrows*). **C:** CT scan shows a lobulated mass of homogeneous soft tissue attenuation (*T*) in the anterior mediastinum. **D:** Coronal positron emission tomographic scan shows normal activity in the heart (*H*) and abnormal activity in the thymic mass (*T*).

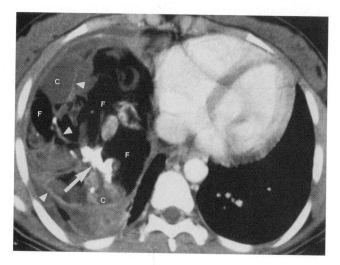

FIGURE 6-15. Benign teratoma. CT scan of a 16-year-old girl shows a large mass containing fat (*F*), cystic areas (*C*), and rudimentary "teeth" (*arrow*). Septations are present within the mass (*arrowheads*). At this windowing, fat appears similar in attenuation to air. Unequivocal fat within the mass confirms the diagnosis of teratoma. Note that large mediastinal masses can appear to fill an entire hemithorax.

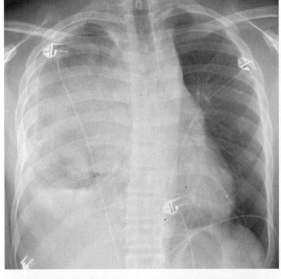

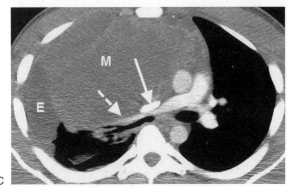

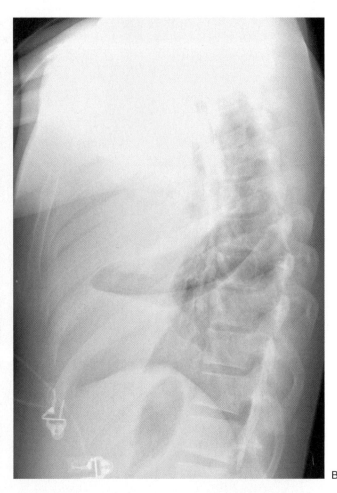

FIGURE 6-16. Benign teratoma. A: PA chest radiograph shows abnormal opacity in the right hemithorax, some of which is caused by pleural effusion, and mediastinal shift to the left. **B:** Lateral view shows abnormal opacity in the retrosternal area. **C:** CT scan shows an anterior mediastinal mass of homogeneous soft tissue attenuation (*M*), compressing a narrowed superior vena cava (*solid arrow*) and right pulmonary artery (*dashed arrow*), and right pleural effusion (*E*).

Calcification, ossification, teeth, or fat may be visible on a chest radiograph and on CT scans. CT scans may show cystic components and/or a fat–fluid level. A cyst wall with curvilinear calcification is often present. Unequivocal fat within the mass confirms the diagnosis of teratoma, but the absence of fat or calcium does not exclude a teratoma (Fig. 6-16).

Imaging features of malignant germ cell tumors are similar to those of benign teratoma except that fat density is not noted and calcification is rare. The malignant tumors grow rapidly, and metastases may be seen in the lungs, bones, or pleura. The adjacent mediastinal fat planes may be obliterated. The tumors may be of homogeneous attenuation or show areas of contrast enhancement interspersed with rounded areas of decreased attenuation from necrosis and hemorrhage. Rarely, coarse tumor calcification may be seen (9).

Lymphoma often extends beyond the anterior mediastinal compartment, involving a variety of lymph node chains, and is discussed along with middle mediastinal masses (see following). When lymphoma is isolated to the anterior mediastinum, the CT appearance can be similar to that of thymoma and germ cell neoplasms.

MIDDLE MEDIASTINAL MASSES

Also referred to as the *vascular space*, the middle mediastinum is bounded in front by the anterior mediastinum and posteri-

orly by the posterior mediastinum. The middle mediastinum contains the heart and pericardium, ascending and transverse aorta, superior vena cava and azygos vein that empties into it, phrenic nerves, upper vagus nerves, trachea and its bifurcation, main bronchi, pulmonary artery and its two branches, pulmonary veins, and adjacent lymph nodes. The esophagus is variably described as a middle or posterior mediastinal structure. The main categories of abnormalities occurring in the middle mediastinum include adenopathy, aneurysm/vascular abnormalities, and abnormalities of development (Table 6-2). Less common middle mediastinal abnormalities include giant lymph node hyperplasia (Castleman disease; Fig. 6-17); neural tumor (involving the vagus or phrenic nerve); abscess; fibrosing mediastinitis; hiatal hernia (Fig. 6-18); primary tumors of the trachea or esophagus (namely, leiomyoma, leiomyosarcoma, or carcinoma; Figs. 6-19 and 6-20); and hematoma.

Adenopathy

There are many causes of mediastinal and hilar lymph node enlargement (adenopathy). Three main categories to consider are neoplasm, infection, and noninfectious granulomatous disease (i.e., sarcoidosis). Neoplastic causes include malignant lymphoma, lymphoproliferative disorders, leukemia, and metastatic carcinoma (most notably from the lung, esophagus, breast, kidney, testis, and head and neck).

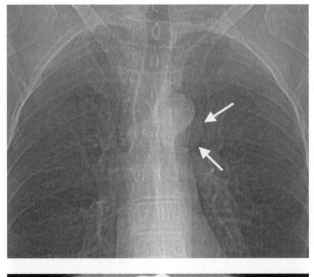

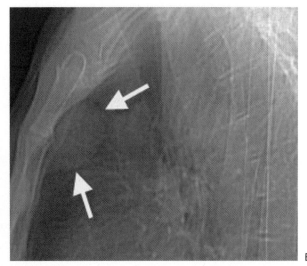

A

B

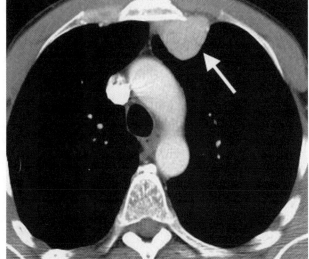

C

FIGURE 6-17. Castleman disease. A: PA chest radiograph of a 48-year-old man shows an abnormal left mediastinal contour (*arrows*). B: Lateral view shows a circumscribed oval retrosternal mass (*arrows*). C: CT scan shows an enhancing retrosternal mass (*arrow*). Pathology confirmed Castleman disease involving the left internal mammary node. Prominent enhancement is a characteristic feature of Castleman disease. Although the example shown is in the anterior mediastinum, Castleman disease most commonly occurs in the middle mediastinum.

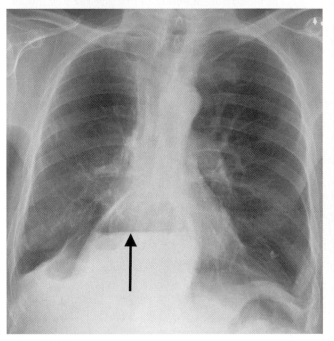

A

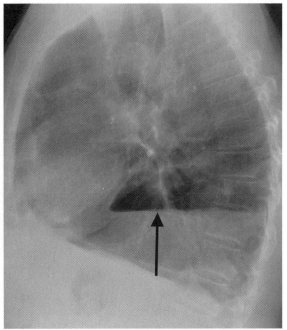

B

FIGURE 6-18. Hiatal hernia. A: PA chest radiograph shows a mediastinal mass containing an air–fluid level (*arrow*). B: Lateral view confirms herniation of stomach through the esophageal hiatus and again shows an air–fluid level (*arrow*).

TABLE 6-2

MIDDLE MEDIASTINAL MASSES

"3 As"

Adenopathy
  Infection (fungal and mycobacterial)
  Neoplasm (bronchogenic carcinoma, metastases,
    lymphoma, leukemia)
  Sarcoidosis

Aneurysm/vascular

Abnormalities of development
  Bronchogenic cyst
  Pericardial cyst
  Esophageal duplication cyst
  (Neurenteric cyst—posterior mediastinum)

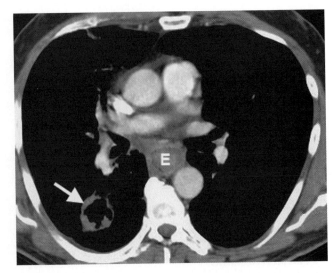

FIGURE 6-20. Esophageal carcinoma. CT scan of a 63-year-old man shows a distal esophageal mass (*E*). The man also had a cavitary squamous cell carcinoma in the right lower lobe (*arrow*).

Lymphoma is classified as either Hodgkin or non-Hodgkin lymphoma (Figs. 6-21 and 6-22). The onset of Hodgkin lymphoma most commonly occurs in the second or third decade, with a secondary peak in the fifth or sixth decades of life. Non-Hodgkin lymphoma occurs in all age groups. The main feature of malignant lymphomas on chest radiography or CT scanning is mediastinal and hilar lymphadenopathy, in some cases with accompanying pulmonary, pleural, or chest wall involvement. The enlarged nodes can calcify, especially after therapy, in irregular, eggshell, or diffuse patterns. The appearances of intrathoracic adenopathy on chest radiographs and CT scans are similar in Hodgkin and non-Hodgkin lymphoma, but the frequencies and distributions of the abnormalities differ. Any intrathoracic nodal group may be enlarged in patients with lymphoma. In general, the anterior mediastinal and paratracheal nodes are the most frequently involved, with tracheobronchial and subcarinal nodes also commonly enlarged. The majority of cases of Hodgkin lymphoma show enlargement of two or more nodal groups, whereas only one nodal group is involved in about half the cases of non-Hodgkin lymphoma. Hilar adenopathy is rare without accompanying mediastinal adenopathy. The enlarged nodes may be discrete or matted together, and the margins can be well defined or ill defined. Low-density areas can be seen, resulting from cystic degeneration. Hodgkin lymphoma can arise primarily in the thymus. Parenchymal involvement of the lung at initial presentation is unusual. Parenchymal involvement in Hodgkin disease is almost always accompanied by intrathoracic adenopathy (except after irradiation), whereas in non-Hodgkin lymphoma, isolated pulmonary involvement occurs more than 50% of the time (10). The most common pattern of parenchymal involvement is one or more discrete nodules, which can cavitate. Another common pattern is round or segmental, focal or patchy areas of dense airspace opacity often with air bronchograms, mimicking pneumonia.

Pleural effusions are seen on CT scans in 50% of patients with lymphoma (11). Most pleural effusions are unilateral exudates, occasionally chylous in nature, and they can be large. Both pleural and pericardial effusions can occur and have nodular solid components. Chest wall invasion and rib destruction are seen on occasion.

The most frequent *infections* that give rise to intrathoracic adenopathy are caused by mycobacterial disease (most notably tuberculosis) and fungal disease (particularly histoplasmosis; Fig. 6-23), each of which can occur without evident pneumonia. Some patients develop a chronic progressive immune

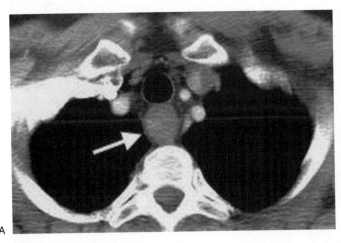

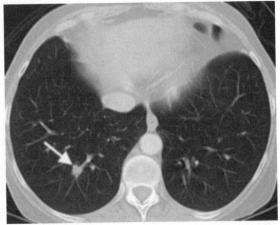

A   B

FIGURE 6-19. Esophageal carcinoma. A: CT scan of a 54-year-old woman with dysphagia shows a circumferential mass involving the upper esophagus (*arrow*). Note the lack of air within the thick-walled esophagus. **B:** CT scan at a level inferior to (**A**), with lung windowing, shows a parenchymal metastasis (*arrow*).

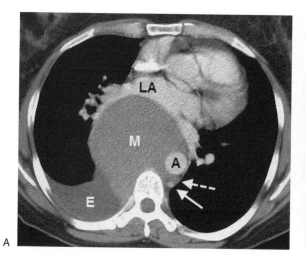

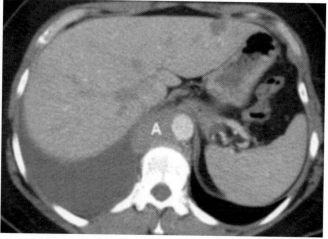

FIGURE 6-21. Hodgkin lymphoma. **A:** CT scan of a 59-year-old man with shortness of breath shows a homogeneous mass of soft tissue attenuation (*M*) compressing the left atrium (*LA*), nearly encasing the aorta (*A*), and abutting the esophagus (*dashed arrow*) and azygous vein (*solid arrow*). There is also a right pleural effusion (*E*). **B:** CT scan at a more inferior level shows retrocrural lymphadenopathy (*A*).

response to dead *Histoplasma* capsular antigens, resulting in a condition known as fibrosing mediastinitis. In this condition, nonmalignant fibrous tissue encases and obliterates vasculature (arteries, veins, lymphatics) and airways in the mediastinum (Fig. 6-24). Subcarinal and right paratracheal nodes are most commonly involved. Calcification of nodes and simultaneous encasement of airways and vasculature are characteristic CT findings of this disease. Intrathoracic nodal enlargement can also be seen in tularemia, whooping cough, anthrax, plague, and mycoplasmal, viral, and other more common bacterial infections.

Sarcoidosis is a frequent cause of intrathoracic adenopathy in young adults. When multiple node groups are involved and adenopathy is symmetrically distributed in the hila and mediastinum in young asymptomatic adults, sarcoidosis is the likely cause. The hilar lymph nodes are frequently potato shaped and clear of the cardiac borders, a feature that is often useful in distinguishing sarcoidosis from lymphoma (Fig. 6-25).

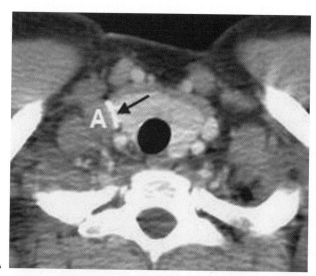

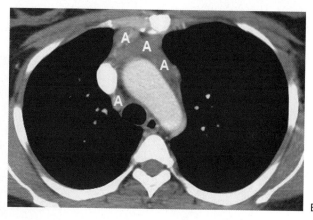

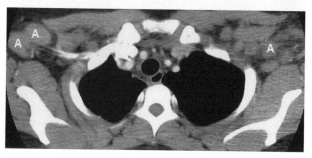

FIGURE 6-22. Hodgkin lymphoma. **A:** CT scan shows right supraclavicular lymphadenopathy (*A*) compressing the right jugular vein (*arrow*). **B:** CT scan at a more inferior level shows confluent anterior mediastinal and right paratracheal lymphadenopathy (*A*). **C:** Another CT scan shows bilateral axillary lymphadenopathy (*A*).

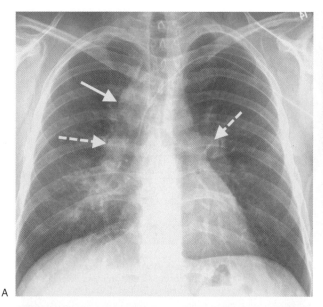

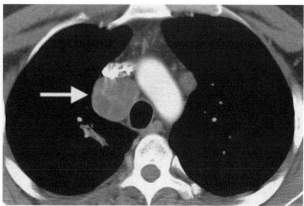

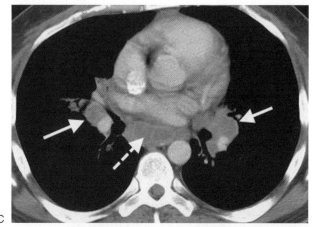

FIGURE 6-23. Pulmonary histoplasmosis. A: PA chest radiograph shows right paratracheal (*solid arrow*) and bilateral hilar (*dashed arrows*) lymphadenopathy. B: CT scan shows bulky right paratracheal lymphadenopathy (*arrow*). C: CT scan at a more inferior level shows bilateral hilar (*solid arrows*) and subcarinal (*dashed arrow*) lymphadenopathy. The appearance is indistinguishable from that of sarcoidosis.

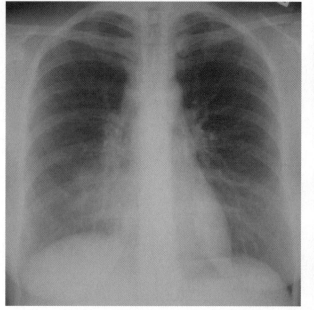

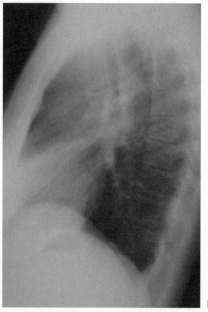

FIGURE 6-24. Fibrosing mediastinitis. A: PA chest radiograph of a 26-year-old woman with dysphagia, dilated chest and neck veins, dyspnea on exertion, and fatigue shows abnormal opacity obliterating the right heart margin (indicating a right middle lobe process) associated with elevation of the right hemidiaphragm and abnormal right paratracheal opacity. B: Lateral view confirms abnormal opacity in the right middle lobe. (*Continued*)

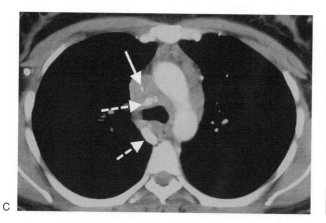
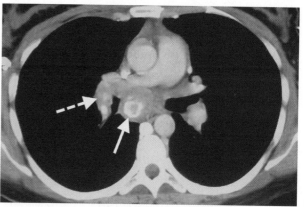

FIGURE 6-24. (*Continued*) **C:** CT scan shows fibrous tissue encasing and almost obliterating the superior vena cava (*solid arrow*) and coarse mediastinal calcifications (*dashed arrows*). **D:** CT scan of a more inferior level shows calcified fibrous tissue (*dashed arrow*) encasing the right lower lobe pulmonary artery, along with densely calcified subcarinal fibrous tissue (*solid arrow*).

Enlargement of paratracheal and bilateral hilar lymph nodes (the Garland triad, or the "1-2-3 sign") is a nonspecific pattern of adenopathy that is common in patients with sarcoidosis (Fig. 6-26).

Adenopathy is more easily identified and quantified via CT scanning than chest radiography. The CT signs of adenopathy are (a) an increase in size of individual nodes, (b) invasion of surrounding mediastinal fat, (c) nodal masses, and (d) diffuse soft tissue density throughout the mediastinum obliterating the mediastinal fat. There are numerous studies regarding normal lymph node size on CT scans (12–14). In general, nodes greater than 10 mm in short-axis diameter are considered abnormal although nonspecific and not necessarily malignant. Likewise, nodes less than 10 mm in short-axis diameter can be pathologic.

Aneurysm/Vascular Abnormalities

As a structure in the middle mediastinum, the aorta can also give rise to abnormalities in this compartment. It is very important to distinguish an aortic aneurysm from other mediastinal masses, particularly if biopsy is being considered. The aorta commonly becomes atherosclerotic and ectatic with advancing

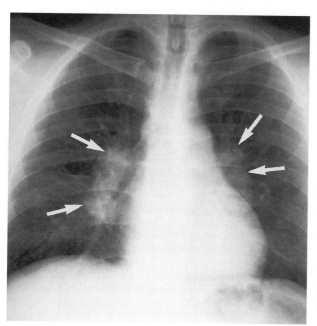
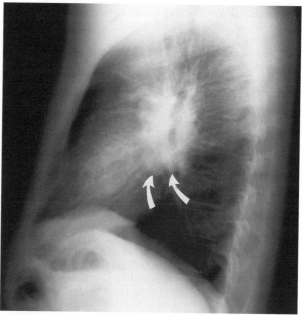

FIGURE 6-25. Sarcoidosis. PA (**A**) and lateral (**B**) chest radiographs of an asymptomatic 25-year-old man show bilateral hilar adenopathy (*straight arrows*). The enlarged nodes are potato shaped and clear of the cardiac borders, a feature that can help distinguish them from lymphomatous enlargement of hilar nodes. On the lateral view, subcarinal adenopathy is also seen (*curved arrows*).

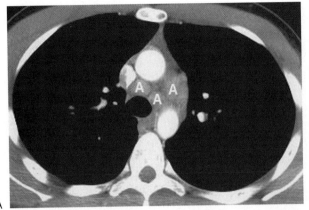

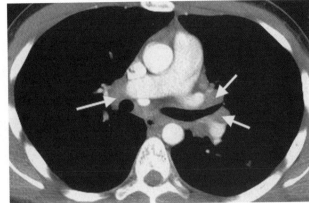

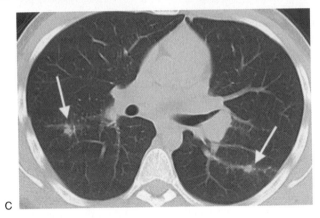

FIGURE 6-26. Sarcoidosis. A: CT scan of a 20-year-old man shows enlarged paratracheal and aortopulmonary lymph nodes (*A*). B: CT scan at a more inferior level shows bilateral hilar (*arrows*) lymphadenopathy. Enlargement of paratracheal and bilateral hilar lymph nodes is commonly seen with sarcoidosis and is referred to as the "1-2-3" sign or Garland triad. C: CT scan with lung windowing shows small, ill-defined nodules in a bronchovascular distribution (*arrows*); this is typical of the parenchymal findings seen with sarcoidosis.

age, and it can become aneurysmal. Rupture is the feared complication of aortic aneurysm (Fig. 6-27). Most atherosclerotic aneurysms are fusiform in shape, although some are saccular. Fusiform aneurysms usually arise in the aortic arch or descending thoracic aorta. Saccular aneurysms usually arise from the descending aorta, or occasionally from the aortic arch, but they are unusual in the ascending aorta. Aortic aneurysms can be distinguished from other mediastinal masses by recognizing their conformity to the aorta and by the presence of curvilinear calcification in the wall of the aneurysm. Traumatic aortic pseudoaneurysm is discussed in Chapter 8. Mycotic aneurysms of the aorta occur in patients with predisposing causes: intravenous drug abusers, patients with valvular disease or congenital disorders of the heart or aorta, patients who have undergone previous cardiac or aortic surgery, patients with adjacent pyogenic infection, and those who are immunocompromised. Mycotic aneurysms are usually saccular in shape, enlarge rapidly, and lack calcification of the wall.

Aortic dissections are collections of blood within the media of the aortic wall that communicate with the true aortic lumen through one or more tears in the intima. Most dissections begin within an intimal tear, and bleeding splits the aortic media. Two classification systems are used to describe aortic dissection. The DeBakey classification divides aortic dissection into three types (15). Type I refers to dissections that start in the ascending aorta and extend into the descending aorta; type II, to dissections confined to the ascending aorta; and type III, to dissections that start just beyond the left subclavian artery and are confined to the descending aorta. The Stanford classification refers to type A (involving the ascending aorta) and type B (confined to the descending aorta) (16). The diagnostic feature of aortic dissection on contrast-enhanced CT scanning is two lumina separated by an intimal flap (Fig. 6-28). The in-

timal flap is seen as a curvilinear low-attenuation area within the opacified aorta. A false lumen usually fills and empties in a delayed fashion compared with a true lumen. The false lumen may be partially or totally filled by thrombus and therefore may not opacify. The true lumen is usually compressed by the false lumen. Displacement of calcified atheromatous plaques by the dissection can be demonstrated on precontrast CT scans when contrast enhancement of the two lumina cannot be achieved (as with a thrombosed false lumen). Aortic dissection is further discussed along with other aortic pathology in Chapter 19.

Abnormalities of Development

Developmental mediastinal cysts include bronchogenic cysts, esophageal duplication cysts, neurenteric cysts, and pericardial cysts. The first three are also referred to as bronchopulmonary foregut malformations, signifying their origin from the embryologic foregut as the result of abnormal ventral budding of the tracheobronchial tree (17). Mediastinal cysts containing cartilage are classified as bronchogenic, and those with gastric epithelium as enteric. Neurenteric and some esophageal duplication cysts arise within the posterior mediastinum, but they will be discussed here with middle mediastinal masses.

Bronchogenic cysts have a fibrous capsule, often contain cartilage, are lined with respiratory epithelium, and contain mucoid material. Most arise in the mediastinum or hilar areas, but they can also arise within the lung parenchyma. These cysts can rapidly increase in size as a result of hemorrhage, infection, or distension with air, indicating communication with the airways. They are seen on chest radiographs as well-defined

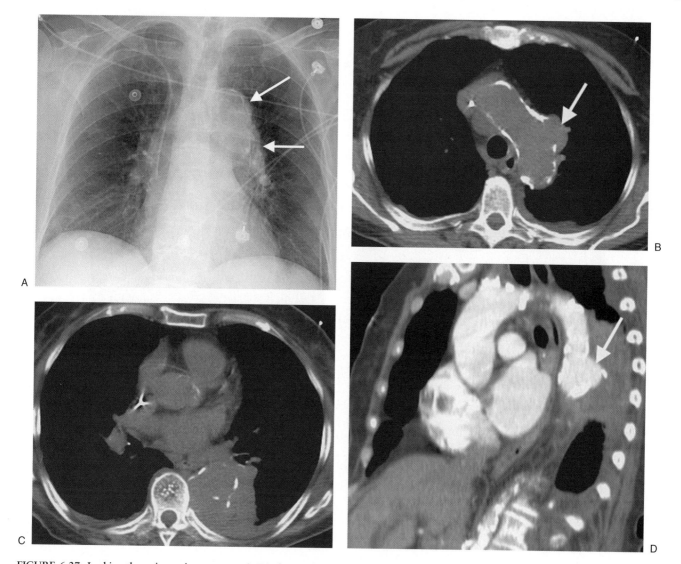

FIGURE 6-27. **Leaking thoracic aortic aneurysm. A:** PA chest radiograph of a 77-year-old man with chest pain shows a widened mediastinum and abnormal left mediastinal contour (*arrows*). **B:** CT scan shows a focal aneurysm of the aortic arch (*arrow*). Note the interruption in dense mural calcification. **C:** CT scan at a more inferior level shows obliteration of the normal aortic contours and adjacent left pleural effusion. **D:** Sagittal reformatted CT scan shows the focal aneurysm (*arrow*) and adjacent fluid collection.

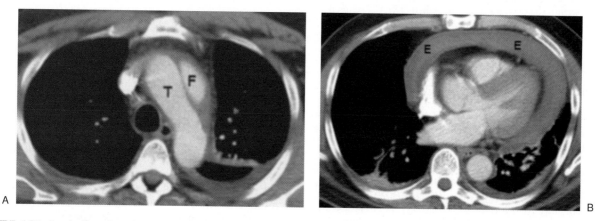

FIGURE 6-28. **Aortic dissection. A:** CT scan shows two aortic lumina—a false lumen (*F*) and a true lumen (*T*)—separated by an intimal flap. **B:** CT scan at a more inferior level shows a pericardial effusion (*E*) that is of high attenuation, indicating hemorrhage.

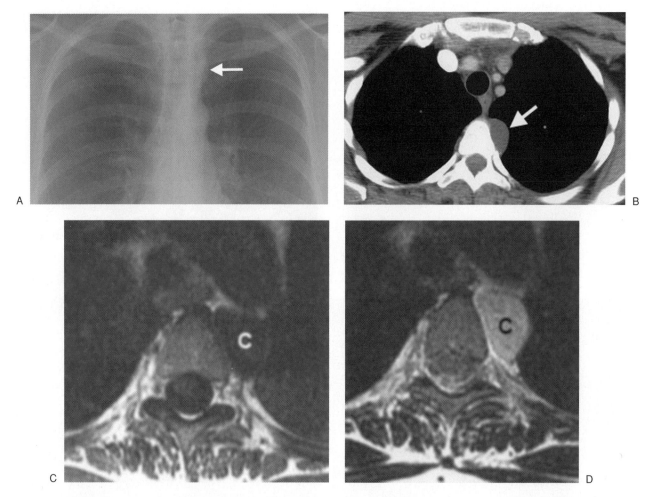

FIGURE 6-29. Bronchogenic cyst. A: PA chest radiograph shows an abnormal left superior mediastinal contour (*arrow*). **B:** CT scan shows a nonenhancing left paraspinal mass of homogeneous fluid attenuation with an imperceptible wall (*arrow*). **C:** T1-weighted MRI shows the mass to have low signal intensity (C). **D:** The mass has high signal intensity on T2-weighted MRI (C), consistent with a cyst.

solitary masses in the mediastinum or hilum (Figs. 6-29 and 6-30) and are usually found in close proximity to the major airways. The single most frequent site is between the carina and the esophagus. Calcification, either rim calcification or milk of calcium within the cyst, has been described (18). CT scans usually show a simple cystic mass with an imperceptible or thin smooth wall. The CT attenuation is generally that of water (−10 to +10 Hounsfield units) but can be higher (as high as 120 Hounsfield units) when filled with milk of calcium or proteinaceous material that accumulates after infection or hemorrhage (Fig. 6-31). The cysts can be unilocular or multilocular. Curvilinear calcification of the wall can be seen.

The imaging features of *esophageal duplication cysts* may be identical to those seen with bronchogenic cysts, except that an esophageal duplication cyst will always have a peri-esophageal location (Fig. 6-32). Neurenteric cysts are posterior mediastinal cystic lesions connected to the meninges through a midline defect in one or more vertebral bodies. Associated vertebral anomalies suggest the diagnosis. *Pericardial cysts* arise most frequently in the right cardiophrenic angle as a result of anomalous outpouching of the parietal pericardium. The cysts typically contact the heart, diaphragm, and anterior chest wall (Fig. 6-33). The majority are sharply marginated, some-

what triangular, and of near-water attenuation on CT scans (Fig. 6-34).

POSTERIOR MEDIASTINAL MASSES

Also referred to as the *postvascular space*, the posterior mediastinum lies behind the heart and pericardium and contains the thoracic descending aorta, esophagus, thoracic duct, azygos and hemiazygos veins, lymph nodes, sympathetic chains, and inferior vagus nerves. Neural tumors are the most common tumors to develop in the posterior mediastinum, but a variety of uncommon abnormalities can occur in this compartment, as listed in Table 6-3 (Figs. 6-35 to 6-38).

Neural tumors can be differentiated into nerve sheath tumors and ganglion cell tumors. Nerve sheath tumors comprise schwannomas, neurofibromas, and their malignant counterparts. The schwannoma is the most common intrathoracic

(Text continues on page 99)

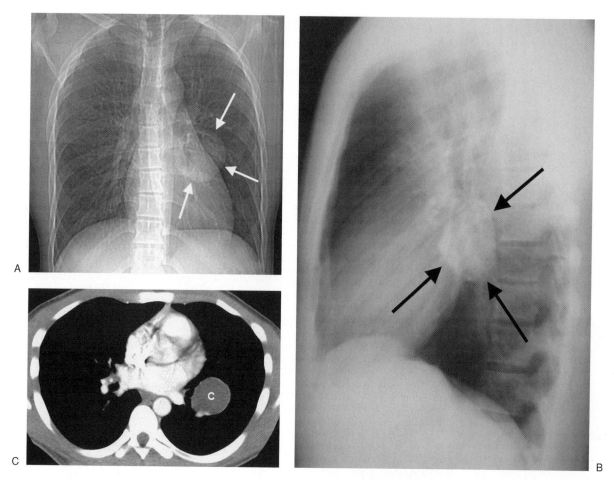

FIGURE 6-30. Bronchogenic cyst. PA (A) and lateral (B) chest radiographs of a 23-year-old man show a round mass in the left medial hemithorax (*arrows*). C: CT scan shows that the nonenhancing left hilar mass is of homogeneous fluid attenuation, consistent with a cyst (C).

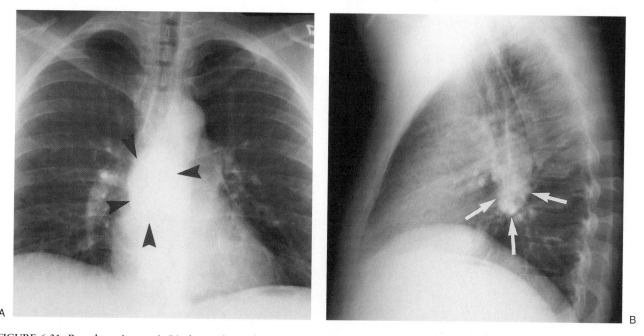

FIGURE 6-31. Bronchogenic cyst. A: PA chest radiograph of a 36-year-old woman shows an ovoid mass in the subcarinal area (*arrowheads*), a typical location for a bronchogenic cyst. B: Lateral view confirms the mass to be in a subcarinal location (*arrows*). (*Continued*)

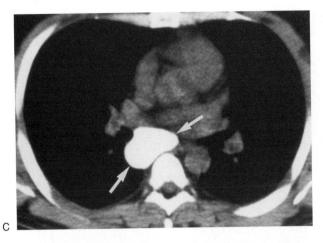

C

FIGURE 6-31. (*Continued*) C: CT scan shows that the mass is extremely dense throughout, consistent with milk of calcium (*arrows*).

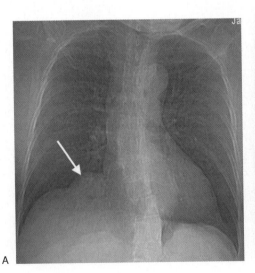

FIGURE 6-32. **Esophageal duplication cyst.** CT scan of a 45-year-old woman shows a subcarinal cystic structure (C) of homogeneous fluid attenuation in contact with the esophagus (*arrow*). The appearance is indistinguishable from that of a bronchogenic cyst.

TABLE 6-3

POSTERIOR MEDIASTINAL MASSES

Common
    Neural tumors
        Neurogenic (neuroblastoma, ganglioneuroma, ganglioneuroblastoma)
        Nerve root tumors (schwannoma, neurofibroma, malignant schwannoma)
Less common
    Paraganglionic cell tumors (chemodectoma, pheochromocytoma)
    Spinal tumor (metastases, primary bone tumor)
    Lymphoma
    Invasive thymoma
    Mesenchymal tumor (fibroma, lipoma, leiomyoma, hemangioma, lymphangioma)
    Abscess
    Pancreatic pseudocyst
    Esophageal varices
    Hematoma
    Traumatic pseudomeningocele
    Bochdalek hernia
    Extramedullary hematopoiesis
    Descending thoracic aortic aneurysm

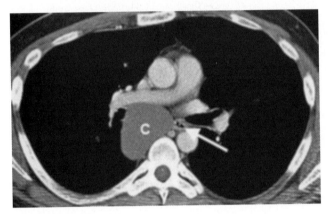

A   B

FIGURE 6-33. **Pericardial cyst.** A: PA chest radiograph shows a round opacity (*arrow*) at the right cardiophrenic angle. B: CT scan shows the mass (*PC*) to be of homogeneous fluid attenuation with rim calcification.

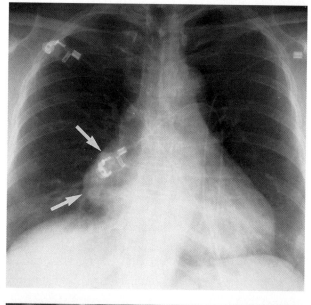

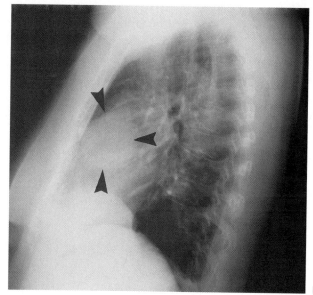

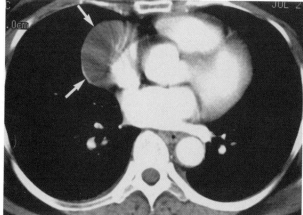

FIGURE 6-34. Pericardial cyst. A: PA chest radiograph shows a smoothly marginated, rounded mass adjacent to the right heart border (*arrows*). B: Lateral chest radiograph shows the mass to be in the anterior or middle mediastinum (*arrowheads*). C: CT scan shows a mass of homogeneous fluid attenuation abutting the right pericardial border, typical of the appearance of a pericardial cyst (*arrows*).

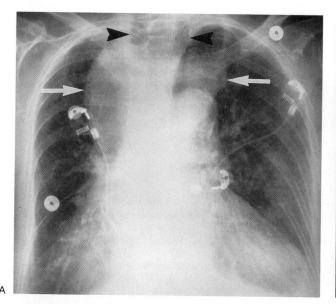

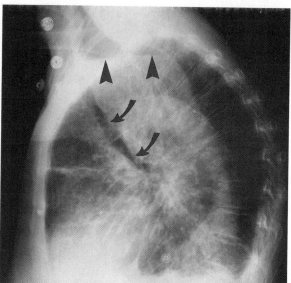

FIGURE 6-35. Achalasia. A: PA chest radiograph of an 86-year-old woman with dysphagia shows a widened contour to the upper mediastinum (*arrows*) and air within the dilated air-filled esophagus (*arrowheads*). B: Lateral chest radiograph shows an air–fluid level within the dilated esophagus (*arrowheads*) and anterior deviation of the trachea (*curved arrows*).

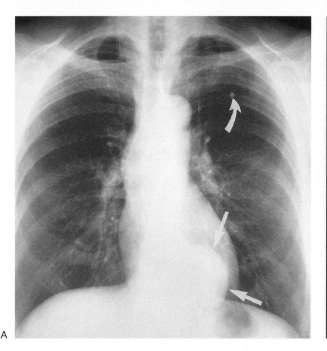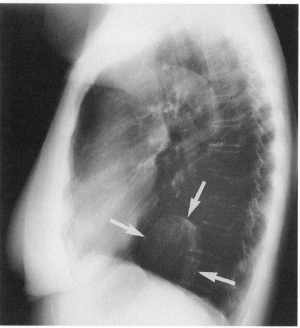

FIGURE 6-36. **Descending thoracic aortic aneurysm. A:** PA chest radiograph of a 69-year-old woman shows a rounded mass in continuity with the descending aorta (*straight arrows*). Incidental note of calcified granuloma in the left upper lobe (*curved arrow*). **B:** Lateral chest radiograph shows curvilinear rim calcification within the wall of the aneurysm (*arrows*).

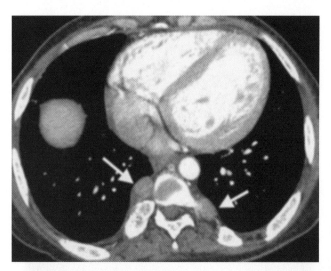

FIGURE 6-37. **Extramedullary hematopoiesis.** CT scan of a 20-year-old woman with thalassemia shows bilateral paraspinal soft tissue masses (*arrows*) and expansion of the adjacent ribs.

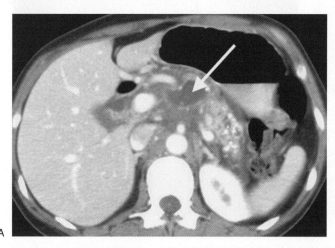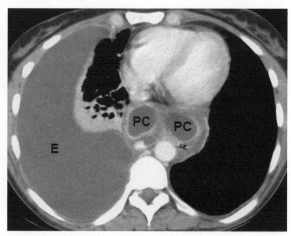

FIGURE 6-38. **Mediastinal pancreatic pseudocysts. A:** CT scan of a 39-year-old man with acute and chronic pancreatitis shows cystic areas within the pancreas (*arrow*) and pancreatic calcifications. **B:** CT scan at a more superior level shows rim-enhancing pancreatic pseudocysts (*PC*) within the posterior mediastinum and a large right pleural effusion (*E*).

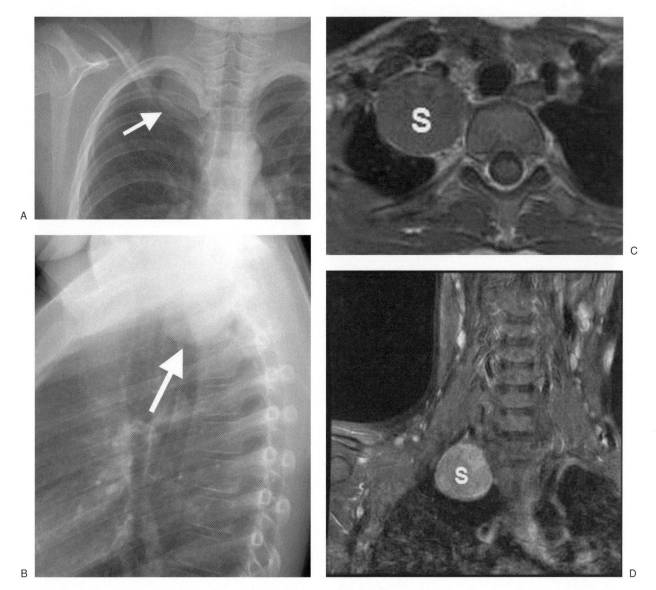

FIGURE 6-39. Benign schwannoma. PA (**A**) and lateral (**B**) chest radiographs of a 9-year-old girl show a circumscribed mass in the right apex (*arrow*). **C:** Axial T1-weighted MRI shows the mass (*S*) is paraspinal in location and has no continuity with the spinal canal. **D:** Coronal MRI, with intravenous contrast, shows that the mass (*M*) has high signal intensity.

nerve sheath tumor (Fig. 6-39). Both schwannomas and neurofibromas are derived from Schwann cells and occur most commonly in patients in their 30s and 40s. Almost all intrathoracic nerve sheath tumors arise from either the intercostal or sympathetic nerves.

The ganglion cell tumors include neuroblastoma (malignant), ganglioneuroma (benign), and ganglioneuroblastoma (intermediate between benign and malignant). The adrenal gland is the most common primary site for these tumors, with the mediastinum being the second most common site. Ganglioneuroma can occur between the ages of 1 and 50, while neuroblastoma and ganglioneuroblastoma occur during childhood, generally under the age of 20 (19).

Nerve sheath and ganglion cell tumors are seen as well-defined masses with a smooth or lobulated outline on imaging studies. Some are very large and can occupy most of a hemithorax. Calcification can be seen in all types. In neuroblastoma, the calcification is usually finely stippled, whereas in ganglioneuroblastoma and ganglioneuroma it is denser and coarser. The bone adjacent to the tumor shows a scalloped

edge, with preservation but thickening of the bony cortex. The ribs can be thinned and splayed apart, and the intervertebral foramina can appear widened. On CT scans, many tumors have mixed attenuation, including low-attenuation regions, that enhance on images taken after administration of intravascular contrast material.

Paragangliomas are tumors of the paraganglionic cells and can be benign or malignant chemodectomas or pheochromocytomas. Mediastinal paragangliomas are rare, comprising only 2% of the large series of neural tumors of the thorax (19). Paragangliomas occur in the area of the aortic arch and are classified as aortic body tumors. They form rounded soft tissue masses that are extremely vascular and enhance brightly on CT scans after administration of intravenous contrast material.

References

1. Rubush JL, Gardner IR, Boyd WC, et al. Mediastinal tumors: review of 186 cases. *J Thorac Cardiovasc Surg.* 1973;65:216–222.

2. Morris UL, Colletti PM, Ralls PW, et al. CT demonstration of intrathoracic thyroid tissue. *J Comput Assist Tomogr.* 1982;6:821–824.

3. Margolin FR, Winfield J, Steinbach HL. Patterns of thyroid calcification: roentgenologic-histologic study of excised specimens. *Invest Radiol.* 1967;2:208–212.

4. Park CH, Rothermel FJ, Judge DM. Unusual calcification in mixed papillary and follicular carcinoma of the thyroid gland. *Radiology.* 1976;119: 554.

5. Wallace S, Hill CS, Paulus DD, et al. The radiologic aspects of medullary (solid) thyroid carcinoma. *Radiol Clin North Am.* 1970;8:463–474.

6. LeGolvan DP, Abell MR. Thymomas. *Cancer.* 1977;39:2142–2157.

7. Lewis JE, Wick MR, Scheithauer BW, et al. Thymoma: a clinicopathological review. *Cancer.* 1987;60:2727–2743.

8. Harper RAK, Guyer PB. The radiological features of thymic tumours: a review of sixty-five cases. *Clin Radiol.* 1965;16:97–100.

9. Levitt RG, Husband JE, Galzer HS. CT of primary germ-cell tumors of the mediastinum. *AJR Am J Roentgenol.* 1984;142:73–78.

10. Jenkins PF, Ward MJ, Davies P, et al. Non-Hodgkin's lymphoma, chronic lymphocytic leukaemia and the lung. *Br J Dis Chest.* 1981;75:22–30.

11. Lewis ER, Caskey CI, Fishman EK. Lymphoma of the lung: CT findings in 31 patients. *AJR Am J Roentgenol.* 1991;156:711–714.

12. Genereux GP, Howie JL. Normal mediastinal lymph node size and number: CT and anatomic study. *AJR Am J Roentgenol.* 1984;142:1095–1100.

13. Glazer BH, Gross BH, Quint LE, et al. Normal mediastinal lymph nodes: Number and size according to American Thoracic Society mapping. *AJR Am J Roentgenol.* 1985;144:261–265.

14. Ingram CE, Belli AM, Lewars MD, et al. Normal lymph node size in the mediastinum: A retrospective study in two patient groups. *Clin Radiol.* 1989;40:35–39.

15. DeBakey ME, Henly WS, Cooley DA, et al. Surgical management of dissecting aneurysms of the aorta. *J Thorac Cardiovasc Surg.* 1965;49:130–149.

16. Appelbaum A, Karp RB, Kirklin JW. Ascending vs descending aortic dissection. *Ann Surg.* 1976;183:296–300.

17. Fitch SJ, Tonkin ILD, Tonkin AK. Imaging of foregut duplication cysts. *RadioGraphics.* 1986;6:189–201.

18. Bergstrom JF, Yost RV, Ford KT, et al. Unusual roentgen manifestations of bronchogenic cysts. *Radiology.* 1973;107:49–54.

19. Reed JC, Haller KK, Feigin DS. Neural tumours of the thorax: subject review from the AFIP. *Radiology.* 1978;126:9–17.

CHAPTER 7

SOLITARY AND MULTIPLE PULMONARY NODULES

LEARNING OBJECTIVES

1. Name the three most common causes of a solitary pulmonary nodule.
2. Name four important considerations in the evaluation of a solitary pulmonary nodule.
3. Define the terms *pulmonary nodule* and *pulmonary mass*.
4. Name six common causes of cavitary nodules.
5. Name four common causes of multiple pulmonary nodules.
6. Describe the indications for percutaneous biopsy of a solitary pulmonary nodule.
7. Describe the most frequent complications related to percutaneous lung biopsy using computed tomographic or fluoroscopic guidance.
8. Describe the role of positron emission tomography in the evaluation of a solitary pulmonary nodule.
9. Describe an appropriate imaging algorithm to evaluate a solitary pulmonary nodule.
10. Describe an appropriate algorithm for management of small incidental pulmonary nodules detected on computed tomography.

A *pulmonary nodule* is defined as "any pulmonary or pleural lesion represented in a radiograph by a sharply defined discrete, nearly circular opacity 2 to 30 mm in diameter" (1). A pulmonary *mass* is distinguished from a nodule based on size and is defined as "any pulmonary or pleural lesion represented in a radiograph by a discrete opacity greater than 30 mm in diameter (without regard to contour, border characteristics, or homogeneity), but explicitly shown or presumed to be extended in all three dimensions" (1). Some authors, however, use the terms *nodule* and *mass* interchangeably (2). A nodule seen on computed tomography (CT) is defined as a "small, approximately spherical, circumscribed focus of abnormal tissue" (3). Definitions are helpful but imprecise; in practice, there is variability in what is termed a pulmonary nodule or mass. The differential diagnoses are different for solitary and multiple pulmonary nodules, and thus each will be discussed separately in this chapter.

SOLITARY PULMONARY NODULES

Solitary pulmonary nodules (SPNs) are very common. A radiologist in an active practice may see one or more per day. Many more are not perceived. At chest radiography, an SPN is seldom evident until it is at least 9 mm in diameter (4), and nearly 90% of newly discovered SPNs on chest radiographs may be visible in retrospect on prior radiographs (5). The importance of an SPN derives from the frequency with which it represents a primary bronchogenic cancer. The causes of an SPN are many (Table 7-1), but more than 95% fall into one of three groups: (i) malignant *neoplasms*, either primary or metastatic; (ii) infectious *granulomas*, either tuberculous or fungal (Fig. 7-1); and (iii) benign tumors, notably *hamartoma* (2). In addition to specific radiologic features, clinical history is important in considering the likely cause of an SPN (Fig. 7-2). Bronchogenic carcinoma is rare in patients under 30 years of age and is more common in cigarette smokers than nonsmokers. History of a

TABLE 7-1

CAUSES OF SOLITARY PULMONARY NODULES

Neoplastic: Malignant
  Bronchogenic carcinoma
  Solitary metastasis
  Lymphoma
  Carcinoid tumor

Neoplastic: Benign
  Hamartoma
  Benign connective tissue and neural tumors (e.g., lipoma, fibroma, neurofibroma)

Inflammatory
  Granuloma
  Lung abscess
  Rheumatoid nodule
  Inflammatory pseudotumor (plasma cell granuloma)

Congenital
  Arteriovenous malformation
  Lung cyst
  Bronchial atresia with mucoid impaction

Miscellaneous
  Pulmonary infarct
  Intrapulmonary lymph node
  Mucoid impaction
  Hematoma
  Amyloidosis
  Normal confluence of pulmonary veins

Mimics of SPN
  Nipple shadow
  Cutaneous lesion (e.g., wart, mole)
  Rib fracture or other bone lesion
  "Vanishing pseudotumor" of congestive heart failure (loculated pleural effusion)

SPN, solitary pulmonary nodule.

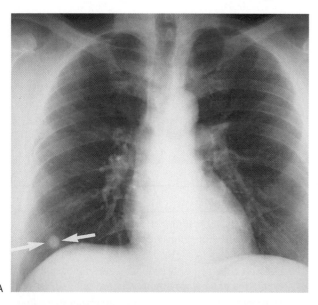
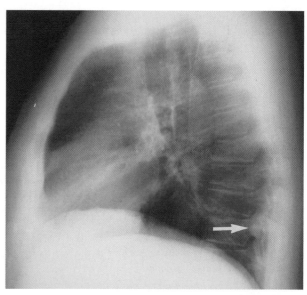

FIGURE 7-1. Granuloma. A: PA chest radiograph shows a small, well-circumscribed, round opacity at the right lung base (*arrows*). B: Lateral view shows that the opacity is within the lung on two views (posterior segment of the right lower lobe) and thus represents a pulmonary nodule (*arrow*). The high density of the nodule relative to its small size indicates that it is densely calcified. The appearance is characteristic of a benign calcified granuloma, and no further evaluation of the nodule is needed (an exception would be in a patient with a known calcium-producing primary tumor, such as osteosarcoma, which can lead to calcified pulmonary metastases; in this case, older radiographs confirmed over 2 years of stability of the granuloma).

known primary tumor makes a metastasis more likely than a new (or second) primary tumor. Certain regions of the country are endemic for fungal disease and therefore have a higher prevalence of benign nodules than other regions.

Management options with an SPN include further imaging workup, declaration of benign etiology and no further evaluation, follow-up (usually with CT), or tissue diagnosis (either with percutaneous or transbronchial biopsy or via surgical resection). Management algorithms should take into account radiologic and clinical factors. Such additional information may obviate further workup (Fig. 7-3).

Two rules must be remembered when evaluating an SPN: first, a "nodule" is not confirmed to be within the lung unless it is seen in the lung on both posteroanterior (PA) and lateral chest radiographs or it is seen in the lung on a chest CT. Second, the current radiograph or CT scan should be compared with prior radiologic studies, when available, to confirm the chronicity of the nodule. Following these two basic rules will, on occasion, prevent unnecessary further workup and concern.

Four important considerations in the evaluation of an SPN are (i) attenuation characteristics, (ii) rate of growth, (iii) shape, and (iv) size. Each of these will be discussed separately; however, it should be noted that no single radiologic feature or combination of features is entirely specific for lung carcinoma or other primary malignant tumors.

The presence or absence of calcium is the most important feature that distinguishes benign from malignant nodules. Unfortunately, 45% of benign nodules are not calcified (6). Benignity can be confirmed confidently if the lesion is smaller than 3 cm in diameter, is smoothly margined, and exhibits one

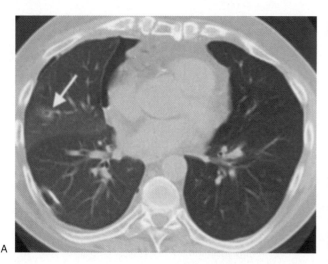
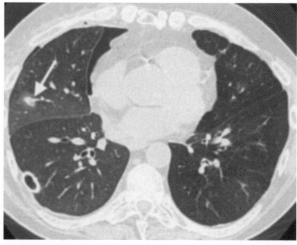

FIGURE 7-2. Postbiopsy hematoma. This 62-year-old man underwent transbronchial biopsy of the right middle lobe 11 days after lung transplantation. The history supports hematoma as the cause of the nodule in the right lung. A: CT scan shows a ground-glass nodule with central cavitation (*arrow*) in the right middle lobe. B: At a more inferior level, the nodule (*arrow*) appears more solid.

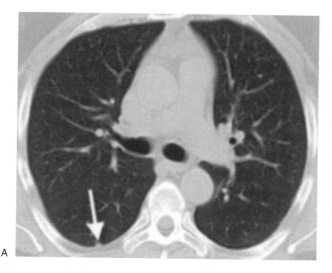
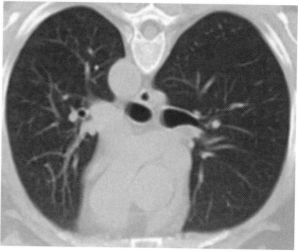

FIGURE 7-3. Dependent atelectasis. A: Supine CT image shows a small rounded opacity (*arrow*) in the dependent right lower lobe. B: The "nodule" disappears on prone imaging, confirming the etiology to be focal atelectasis.

of the following patterns of calcification: large central nidus, laminated, popcorn, or diffuse. All other patterns of calcification are less specific, as further described later. SPNs smaller than 9 mm in diameter are rarely visible on chest radiographs, and a nodule of this size that is clearly seen is likely to be diffusely calcified and benign (Fig. 7-1). Dual-energy subtraction chest radiography can better depict calcification in pulmonary nodules compared with conventional chest radiography (7). So-called popcorn calcifications, which are randomly distributed, often overlapping rings of calcium, are seen when cartilage is present, such as with a hamartoma (Fig. 7-4). Large areas of dystrophic calcium are essentially diagnostic of benign nodules, usually granulomas, and the exceptions are extremely rare. Any calcium in a nodule makes the nodule more likely to be benign. When calcium is detected on thin-section CT (≤3-mm

sections), even when not diffuse and not obviously benign in nature, the likelihood of benignity is high enough to warrant follow-up imaging. This management is recommended, however, only for nodules that are otherwise smoothly marginated, 3 cm or smaller in diameter, and not increasing in size at a rate compatible with bronchogenic carcinoma (Fig. 7-5) (8). The presence of eccentric calcium in a nodule occasionally represents a sign of "scar carcinoma," where the cancer has arisen from a granuloma or engulfed a fibrotic, calcified granuloma. Central calcification in a spiculated SPN should be viewed with suspicion, because most benign SPNs have smooth or minimally lobulated margins. Calcifications in lung cancers may appear amorphous, stippled, or diffuse, and some can have dense foci of calcification or be entirely calcified, with a pattern resembling that of benign disease. These last two patterns

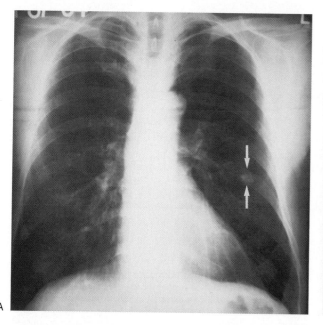
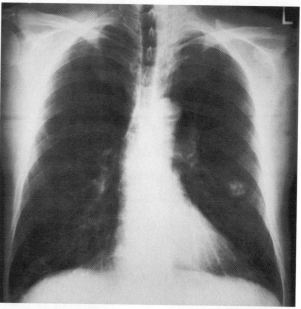

FIGURE 7-4. Hamartoma. A: PA chest radiograph shows a rounded opacity in the left middle lung with calcification (*arrows*). B: PA chest radiograph obtained 5.5 years later shows enlargement of the nodule, which has doubled in volume. The randomly distributed calcifications, arranged in overlapping rings, now have the typical "popcorn" appearance described with hamartomas. It is not unusual for hamartomas to enlarge; unlike malignant nodules, however, the growth rate is slow, with doubling occurring in more than 18 months' time.

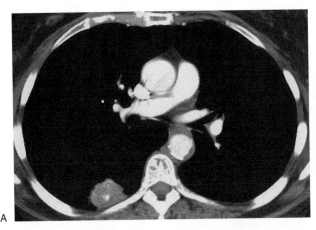

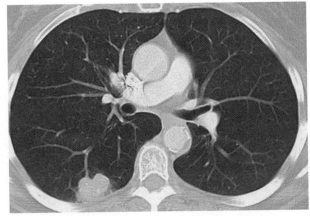

FIGURE 7-5. Small-cell carcinoma. A: CT image shows an irregular, calcified, round nodule in the right lower lobe. The pattern of calcification is not definitely benign and the nodule's irregular margin makes it suspicious for neoplasm. **B:** CT scan with lung windowing shows the nodule to have a lobulated contour.

can be seen in carcinoid tumors, metastatic osteosarcoma, and chondrosarcomas. Stippled calcification can be seen in metastases from mucin-secreting tumors such as colon or ovarian cancers.

If fat is present within a nodule, the most likely diagnosis is hamartoma, and less likely diagnoses are lipoma or myelolipoma. Exceptions include metastatic liposarcoma or re-

nal cell carcinoma, which rarely present as fat-containing nodules on CT. Pulmonary *hamartomas* are benign lesions consisting of an abnormal mixture of the normal constituents of the lung. Most pulmonary hamartomas contain masses of cartilage and may also contain fat or cystic collections of fluid (Figs. 7-6 and 7-7). They grow slowly and are usually solitary (see Fig. 7-4). More than 90% are peripheral in location

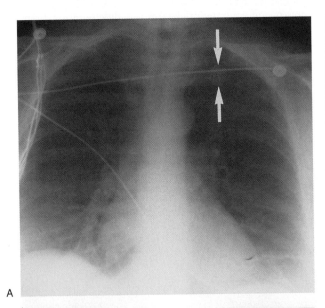

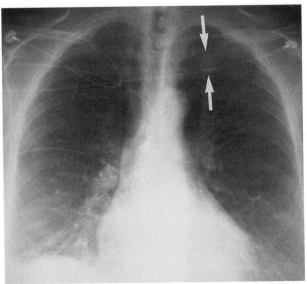

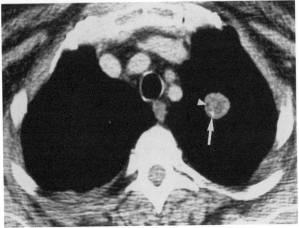

FIGURE 7-6. Hamartoma. A: PA chest radiograph shows an approximately 2-cm round nodule superimposed over the left first rib end that is partially obscured by an external electrocardiogram lead (*arrows*). This nodule was not recognized at the time the radiograph was taken because it was "hiding" among the shadows of overlapping bones in the upper lung. **B:** PA chest radiograph obtained 3 years later shows that the nodule has not changed (*arrows*). This period of stability is consistent with benign etiology. **C:** CT scan shows calcification (*arrow*) and fat (*arrowhead*) within the nodule, characteristic of a benign hamartoma.

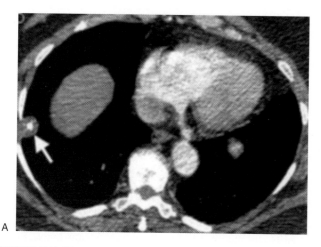

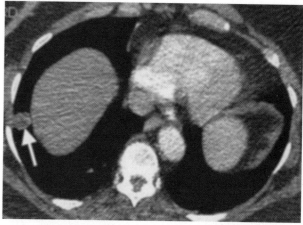

FIGURE 7-7. Hamartoma. A: CT scan shows a round, circumscribed nodule with coarse central calcification in the periphery of the right lower lobe (*arrow*). **B:** CT scan at a more inferior level shows central low attenuation (–40 Hounsfield units) (*arrow*) consistent with fat.

(9). Pulmonary hamartomas can range up to 10 cm in diameter, although most are less than 4 cm, and are usually spherical, lobulated, or notched with a very well-defined edge. In patients without prior malignancy, focal fat attenuation (–40 to –120 Hounsfield units) is a reliable indicator of a hamartoma (10).

On CT, nodules can be described as solid, partly solid, or nonsolid. Aerated lung is visible through a nonsolid (ground-glass) nodule. Whereas most cancerous nodules are solid, partly solid nodules are most likely to be malignant and are often caused by bronchioloalveolar cell carcinoma (Figs. 7-8 to 7-10). Air bronchograms and bronchiolograms are seen more commonly in pulmonary carcinomas than in benign nodules.

An SPN that exhibits no growth for at least 2 years is generally considered benign (11). However, even benign lesions, such as granulomas, can grow slowly. Therefore, growth alone cannot be used to predict malignancy. Bronchogenic carcinomas usually take between 1 and 18 months to double in volume (12). A volume doubling is a change in diameter of about 1.25 times the previous diameter. Doubling times that are faster than 1 month suggest infection, infarction, histiocytic lymphoma, or a fast-growing metastasis from tumors such as germ cell tumor, lymphoma, melanoma, and soft tissue sarcoma (Table 7-2) (13). Doubling times slower than 18 months suggest

granuloma, hamartoma, bronchial carcinoid, salivary gland adenoid cystic carcinoma, thyroid carcinoma metastases, and round atelectasis. However, there are exceptions, and cancerous tumors with doubling times of more than 730 days may appear stable during a 2-year observation period. Growth is more accurately assessed on CT than on chest radiography, and diameters measured with electronic calipers are preferable to diameters measured manually. However, many factors, including size of the nodule and determination of the nodule margin, can limit the accuracy of measurement. It is difficult to reliably show changes in size that are smaller than 2 mm, and even a substantial increase in volume may be missed with small nodules.

Edge characteristics indicative of malignancy include irregularity, spiculation, and lobulation (Fig. 7-11) (14). A *corona radiata*, described as numerous strands radiating from the nodule into the surrounding lung, is very suggestive of bronchogenic carcinoma, although there are exceptions in which a corona radiata is seen in benign lesions such as infectious granulomas and other chronic inflammatory lesions (15). The "tail sign" consists of a linear opacity that extends from a peripheral nodule to the visceral pleura; for some years this sign was regarded as a reliable sign of malignancy. Studies have shown, however,

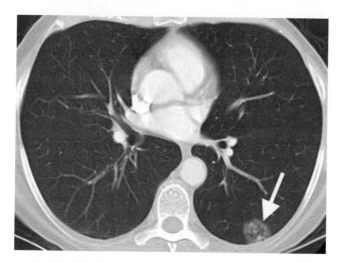

FIGURE 7-8. Bronchioloalveolar cell carcinoma. CT scan shows a mixed solid/ground-glass nodule in the periphery of the left lower lobe (*arrow*). Internal "bubble" lucencies are a characteristic feature of this type of neoplasm.

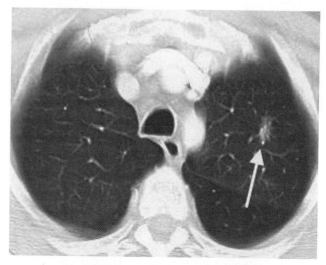

FIGURE 7-9. Bronchioloalveolar cell carcinoma. CT scan shows a mixed solid and ground-glass nodule in the left upper lobe (*arrow*).

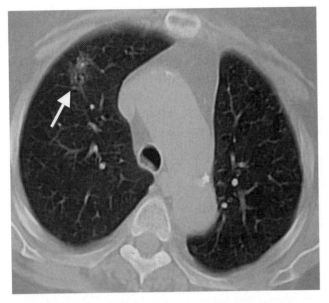

FIGURE 7-10. Bronchioloalveolar cell carcinoma. CT scan shows a poorly defined ground-glass nodule in the right upper lobe (*arrow*).

that up to half of nodules showing the tail sign represent benign granulomas (16), and therefore the tail sign is a nonspecific feature of peripherally located pulmonary lesions that cannot be used to distinguish a benign from a malignant lesion. Lobulation and notching are seen with both benign and malignant nodules and are not very useful discriminating features (Figs. 7-12 and 7-13). A well-defined, smooth, nonlobulated edge is most compatible with hamartoma, granuloma, or metastasis. However, a smooth margin does not indicate benignity, as up to one third of malignant lesions have smooth margins

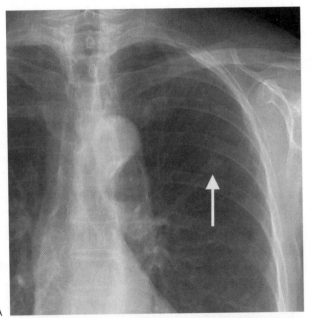

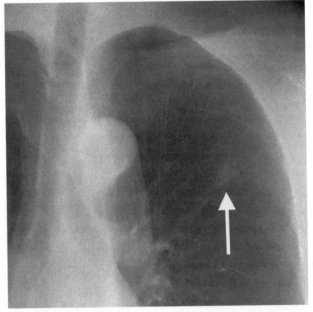

A

B

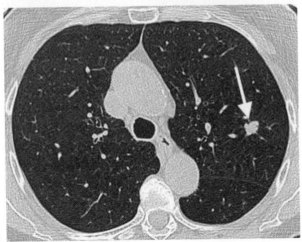

C

FIGURE 7-11. Primary adenocarcinoma. A: Preoperative chest radiograph of an asymptomatic 68-year-old woman with an abdominal aortic aneurysm shows a subtle, small nodule (*arrow*) in the left upper lobe. B: The nodule (*arrow*) is more apparent on dual-energy chest radiography, optimized for lung evaluation. C: CT scan shows that the nodule has irregular margins (*arrow*).

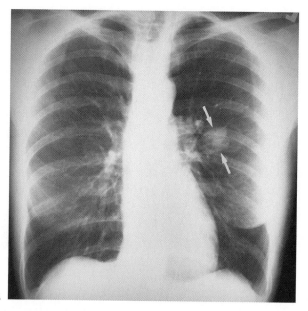

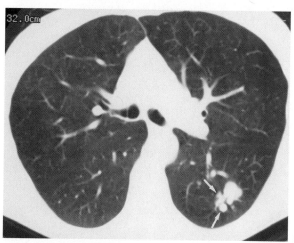

FIGURE 7-12. Coccidioidomycosis. A: PA chest radiograph of a 38-year-old woman living in California with a remote history of pneumonia shows a slightly lobulated, 3-cm nodule in the superior segment of the left lower lobe (*arrows*), which had enlarged compared with chest radiograph from 3 months earlier (not shown). B: CT scan shows a dominant nodule, slightly lobulated and notched, and adjacent smaller satellite nodules (*arrows*). Satellite nodules are more commonly seen with benign entities, but they can be seen with malignant neoplasms and therefore cannot be used to distinguish benign from malignant nodules. Coccidioidomycosis occurs in the southwest United States and was the suspected diagnosis.

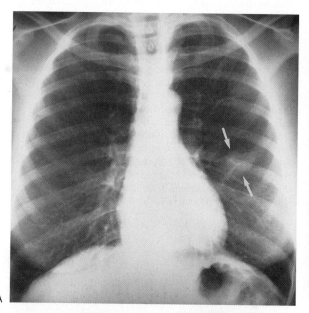

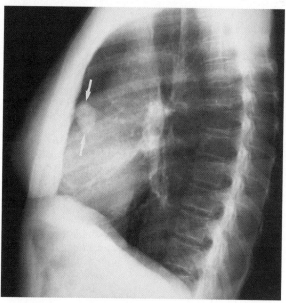

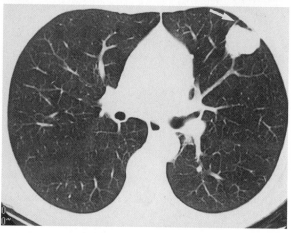

FIGURE 7-13. Large-cell bronchogenic carcinoma. A: PA chest radiograph of a 45-year-old cigarette smoker with a cough for 3 months shows an approximately 3-cm nodule in the left upper lobe (*arrows*), which was new compared to prior chest radiographs. Note the similarity between the appearance of this nodule and the nodule in Figure 7-12. B: Lateral view confirms the location of the nodule in the anterior left upper lobe (*arrows*), with no visible calcification. C: CT scan shows that the nodule is slightly lobulated but fairly well circumscribed. The tail sign is present (*arrow*); this is a nonspecific feature of peripherally located pulmonary lesions that does not distinguish a benign from a malignant lesion.

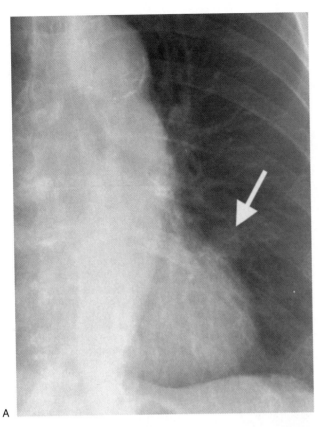

A

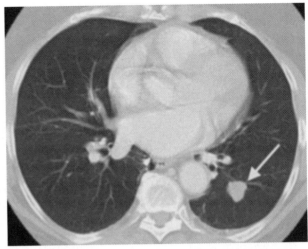

B

FIGURE 7-14. Non–small-cell bronchogenic carcinoma. A: Chest radiograph shows a subtle nodular opacity adjacent to the left heart border (*arrow*). B: CT scan shows a slightly lobulated nodule with smooth margins in the left lower lobe (*arrow*).

(Fig. 7-14) (17). Therefore, the previously mentioned signs are more helpful in their absence. Adjacent tiny nodules, called *satellite nodules*, are strongly associated with benignity (Fig. 7-12) but do not allow a confident diagnosis of benignity, as 10% of dominant nodules with satellite nodules will be malignant (Fig. 7-15) (6).

SPNs with irregular-walled cavities thicker than 16 mm tend to be malignant, whereas benign cavitated lesions usually have thinner, smoother walls. However, because there is considerable overlap, cavity wall characteristics cannot be used to confidently differentiate benign and malignant SPNs (Figs. 7-16 and 7-17) (18).

Sequential thin-section CT (1- to 3-mm section width) performed through an entire nodule with a single breath hold provides information regarding nodule size, attenuation, edge characteristics, and the presence of calcification, cavitation, or fat. In some cases, the findings will provide evidence that the nodule is benign. However, the cause of many SPNs will remain undetermined. If the nodule is at least 10 mm in diameter, a contrast–enhanced CT may be performed. The nodule is examined with 3-mm collimation before and after administration of intravenous contrast material. Contrast-enhanced images are acquired at 1-minute intervals up to 4 minutes after injection of contrast material. Nodule enhancement of less than 15 Hounsfield units after administration of contrast material is strongly indicative of benignity. Although enhancement

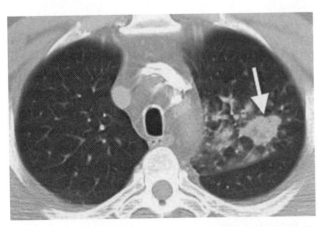

FIGURE 7-15. Primary squamous cell carcinoma. CT scan shows a dominant nodule (*arrow*) with adjacent smaller irregular nodules and ground-glass opacities.

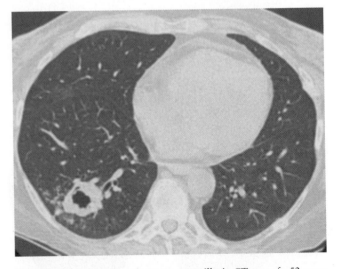

FIGURE 7-16. Invasive pulmonary aspergillosis. CT scan of a 52-year-old woman with a liver transplant shows a thick-walled, irregular, cavitary mass in the right lower lobe.

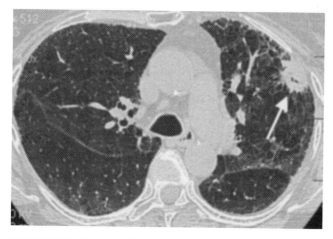

FIGURE 7-17. Primary adenocarcinoma. CT scan of a 66-year-old woman with idiopathic pulmonary fibrosis shows a cavitary spiculated nodule in the left upper lobe (*arrow*).

of more than 15 Hounsfield units is more likely to represent malignancy, the false-positive rate is high and is caused by active inflammatory disease such as granulomas or organizing pneumonias. Therefore, nodule enhancement is a sensitive but nonspecific indicator of malignancy (19).

Positron emission tomography (PET) with fluorine-18-fluorodeoxyglucose of SPNs larger than 1 cm in diameter is

being used with increased frequency to determine whether a lesion is malignant or benign (20). For SPNs 1 to 3 cm in diameter, sensitivity and specificity are approximately 94% and 83%, respectively (21). False-positive PET findings are associated with focal infections, inflammation, and granulomatous diseases such as tuberculosis and sarcoidosis. False-negative PET findings are seen with carcinoid and bronchioloalveolar cell carcinoma, tumors that have a low metabolic rate. Sensitivity and specificity of PET decreases with nodules smaller than 1 cm in diameter.

Radiologists are frequently asked to perform percutaneous fine-needle aspiration biopsy (FNAB) of pulmonary nodules. CT allows for biopsy of many nodules as small as 5 mm in diameter. In patients who are not candidates for surgery, FNAB can be performed to confirm and determine the histologic type of malignancy. In patients who are candidates for surgery, FNAB can confirm benign disease. Contraindications to FNAB include inability of the patient to hold the breath, lie immobile on the CT table for more than 30 minutes, or refrain from coughing. Relative contraindications include bleeding diatheses, previous pneumonectomy, severe emphysema, severe hypoxemia, pulmonary artery hypertension, or nodules in which successful biopsy cannot be performed because of their small size or location. FNAB has a sensitivity of 86% and a specificity of 98.8% in the diagnosis of malignancy (22). Sensitivity decreases for nodules 5 to 7 mm in diameter and in patients with lymphoma. When the FNAB sample is interpreted as malignant or if a specific benign condition is diagnosed (Fig. 7-18), further decisions regarding care are dictated by the

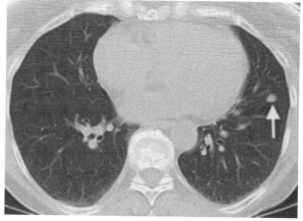

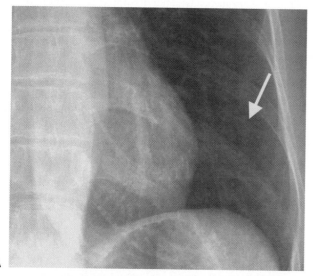

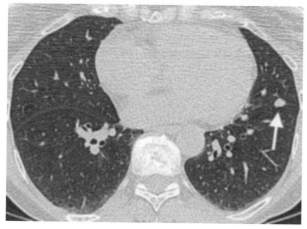

FIGURE 7-18. Benign lymph node. A: Chest radiograph shows a subtle nodule (*arrow*) in the left lower lobe. **B:** CT scan (5-mm slice thickness) shows that the nodule has smooth margins (*arrow*). **C:** Thin-section CT scan (1.25 mm thickness) shows that the nodule (*arrow*) is along the left major fissure, consistent with a benign subpleural lymph node. Although the CT findings were highly suggestive of the diagnosis, fine-needle aspiration biopsy was performed and the diagnosis was confirmed.

TABLE 7-3

SUGGESTED RECOMMENDATIONS FOR FOLLOW-UP AND MANAGEMENT OF
NODULES DETECTED INCIDENTALLY ON CT IN PATIENTS 35 YEARS OF AGE
OR OLDER WITHOUT KNOWN CANCER

Size of nodule	Nonsmoker	Smoker
≤4 mm	No F/U	12/stop
5 to 6 mm	12/stop	12/24/stop
7 to 8 mm	6/12/24/stop	6/12/24/stop
≥9 mm	3/9/24/stop or PET or Bx	3/9/24/stop or PET or Bx

CT, computed tomography; F/U, follow-up, with intervals shown in months; "stop" refers to no
additional F/U in nodules that have shown no change in the interval recommended; Bx, biopsy; PET,
positron emission tomography; mm refers to average of nodule length and width.

diagnosis. When a nonspecific benign condition is diagnosed, such as atypical bronchioloalveolar hyperplasia or inflammation without organisms on a smear or a culture, further evaluation with core-needle biopsy or clinical and radiologic follow-up is required. The most common complications of FNAB are pneumothorax and hemorrhage, with pneumothorax occurring in 25% of patients.

The ability to detect very small nodules improves with each new generation of CT scanner. The majority of cigarette smokers who undergo thin-section CT have been found to have small lung nodules, most of which are smaller than 7 mm in diameter (23). Guidelines for follow-up and management of noncalcified nodules detected on nonscreening CT scans were developed before widespread use of multidetector row CT and still indicate that every indeterminate nodule should be followed with serial CT for a minimum of 2 years. Recently, the Fleischner Society published guidelines for management of SPNs that are detected incidentally on CT scans (24). The Fleischner Society recommendations apply only to adult patients (35 years of age or older) with nodules that are "incidental in the sense that they are unrelated to known underlying disease." In patients under age 35, unless they have a known primary cancer, the guidelines suggest that a single low-dose follow-up CT in 6 to 12 months be considered. Patients with a cancer that may be a cause of lung metastases should be cared for according to the relevant protocol or specific clinical situation. Longer follow-up intervals are recommended for nonsolid (ground-glass) and very small opacities. An abbreviated set of recommendations for nodule follow-up, based on the Fleischner guidelines, is shown in Table 7-3.

MULTIPLE PULMONARY NODULES

The differential diagnosis for multiple pulmonary nodules is different from that for SPNs (Table 7-4), although there is some overlap. In more than 95% of patients with multiple pulmonary nodules, the etiology of the nodules is (a) metastases or (b) tuberculous or fungal granulomas (Fig. 7-19) (2). Determining that the nodules are cavitary is useful in narrowing the list of diagnostic possibilities (Figs. 7-20 to 7-22; Table 7-5) (25). A cavity is defined as a gas-filled space within a zone of pulmonary consolidation or within a mass or nodule that is produced by the expulsion of a necrotic part of the lesion via the bronchial tree; the lucent portion is surrounded by a wall of varied thickness, and there may or may not be an accompanying fluid level (1). Those disorders that can result in cavitary nodules can also result in nodules that are not cavitary or that are not appreciated as cavitary on a chest radiograph; therefore, the mnemonic for cavitary nodules, "CAVITY"

(Table 7-5), can be remembered as a guide for all cases of multiple pulmonary nodules.

The great majority of patients who have multiple noncalcified nodules on chest radiographs have *metastases*. This is even more likely to be the diagnosis when the patient has a known or suspected primary malignancy. The larger and more variable in size that the nodules are, the more likely they are to be neoplastic. Metastases are usually spherical with well-defined margins; as a rule, they vary considerably in size. In autopsy series, the most common sources of metastases from extrathoracic malignancies to the lungs include tumors of the breast, colon (Figs. 7-23 and 7-24), kidney, uterus, prostate, head, and neck (26). Other tumors that have a high incidence of pulmonary metastases, but are not as prevalent in the population and therefore not encountered as frequently, include choriocarcinoma, osteosarcoma, Ewing sarcoma, testicular tumors (Fig. 7-25), melanoma (Fig. 7-26), and thyroid carcinoma. The most common sites of origin of cavitary metastases are the uterine cervix (Fig. 7-27), colon, and head and neck (Fig. 7-28) (27). Squamous cell carcinoma cavitates twice as often as adenocarcinoma (27). Calcification of metastases is seen most commonly with osteosarcoma and chondrosarcoma (Fig. 7-29) or after successful treatment of metastases (28). A miliary nodular pattern of metastases is seen most commonly with thyroid or renal carcinoma, bone sarcoma, trophoblastic disease,

TABLE 7-4

CAUSES OF MULTIPLE PULMONARY NODULES

Neoplastic
  Metastases
  Malignant lymphoma/lymphoproliferative disorders

Inflammatory
  Granulomas
  Fungal and opportunistic infections
  Septic emboli
  Rheumatoid nodules
  Wegener granulomatosis
  Sarcoidosis
  Langerhan cell histiocytosis

Congenital
  Arteriovenous malformations (Osler-Weber-Rendu
    Syndrome)

Miscellaneous
  Hematomas
  Pulmonary infarcts
  Occupational (silicosis)

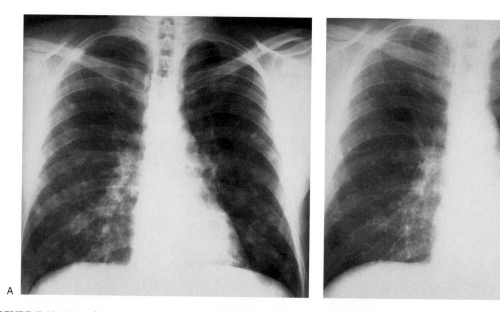

FIGURE 7-19. Acute histoplasmosis. A: PA chest radiograph of a 41-year-old man with cough and fever shows multiple ill-defined nodular opacities bilaterally. **B:** PA chest radiograph obtained 9 years later shows numerous bilateral small calcified granulomas, the residua of prior fungal infection. The nodules are all less than 1 cm in diameter but are seen very well because they are densely calcified.

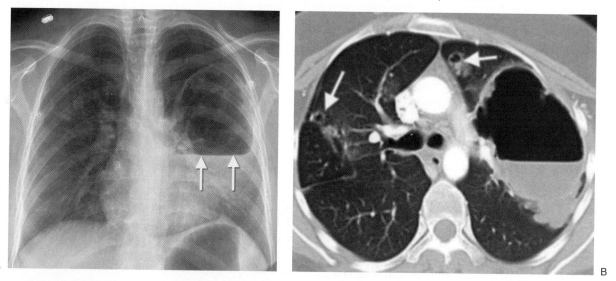

FIGURE 7-20. Wegener granulomatosis. A: PA chest radiograph shows a large cavitary mass in the left lung, demonstrating an air–fluid level (*arrows*). **B:** CT image shows the large left cavitary mass and numerous smaller cavitary nodules (*arrows*).

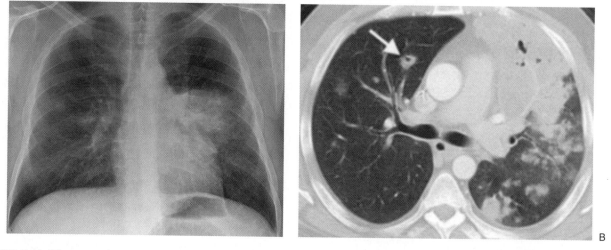

FIGURE 7-21. Blastomycosis. A: PA chest radiograph shows focal airspace opacity in the left lung and a small nodule in the right mid lung. **B:** CT scan shows a cavitary nodule in the right upper lobe (*arrow*), several other irregular nodules, and dense airspace disease in the left upper lobe.

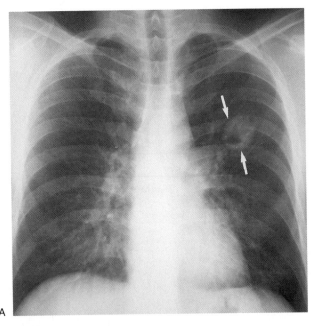

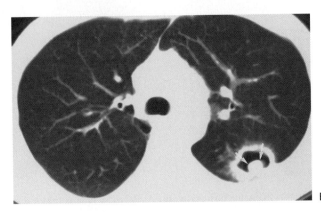

A   B

FIGURE 7-22. Coccidioidomycosis. A: PA chest radiograph of a 40-year-old man with cough and fever shows a 3-cm cavitary nodule in the superior segment of the left lower lobe (*arrows*). **B:** CT image shows a soft tissue mass within the cavity (*arrows*), characteristic of a "fungus ball." On occasion, bronchogenic cancer (especially one of squamous cell histology) can cavitate, and bleeding can result in an intracavitary hematoma, with an appearance similar to that of a fungus ball. A fungus ball will usually roll around inside the cavity with changes in patient positioning.

or melanoma. On occasion, an SPN will be seen in a patient with a known primary tumor. In a patient over age 35 with a squamous cell cancer elsewhere in the body, the solitary lung lesion is usually a separate primary tumor. If the patient has adenocarcinoma elsewhere, there is an equal chance that the solitary nodule is a primary lung cancer or a solitary metastasis. Cancer of the colon is the most common source of a solitary pulmonary metastasis. If there is a soft tissue or skeletal sarcoma or a melanoma elsewhere, the solitary lung lesion is most often a metastasis (29).

The most common sources of *septic emboli* are infected venous catheters (including pacemaker wires) (Fig. 7-30), valvular endocarditis, septic thrombophlebitis, and indwelling prosthetic devices. Septic embolism is a well-known complication of intravenous drug abuse. The diagnosis of septic emboli is usually established by positive blood cultures, although the radiologic findings, especially those on CT of the chest, may be visible before blood cultures become positive (30). The usual radiographic and CT appearance consists of multiple periph-

eral pulmonary opacities that occur in any portion of the lungs but more prevalent in the lower lungs because of the greater pulmonary blood flow to this region. The lesions are usually either round or wedge shaped, as with a pulmonary infarct. Approximately 50% of the lesions cavitate (30). The presence of a distinct vessel leading to the apex of a peripheral area

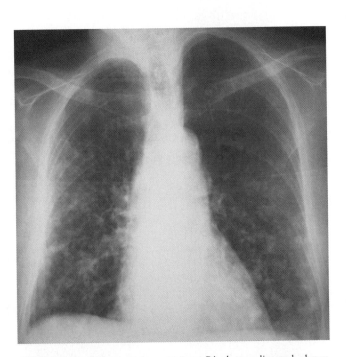

FIGURE 7-23. Colon cancer metastases. PA chest radiograph shows multiple bilateral pulmonary nodules of varying sizes. The nodules do not appear well circumscribed, but their appearance does not exclude the likely diagnosis of metastases in a patient with known colon cancer, a tumor that is a common source of metastases to the lungs.

TABLE 7-5

CAUSES OF CAVITARY PULMONARY NODULES

"CAVITY"
Carcinoma (bronchogenic, metastases—especially squamous cell)
Autoimmune (Wegener granulomatosis, rheumatoid nodules)
Vascular (bland and septic emboli)
Infection (especially mycobacterial and fungal)
Trauma (pneumatocele)
Young—i.e., congenital (sequestration, diaphragmatic hernia, bronchogenic cyst)

Reproduced with permission from Dähnert W. *Radiology Review Manual.* Baltimore: Williams & Wilkins; 1991.

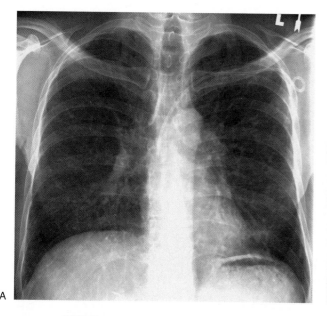

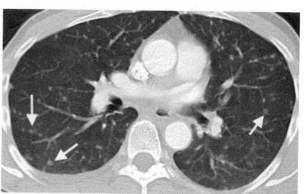

FIGURE 7-24. Colon cancer metastases. A: PA chest radiograph shows small bilateral pulmonary nodules. **B:** CT scan shows numerous small circumscribed pulmonary nodules (*arrows*). The nodule margins are better defined on CT compared with chest radiography.

of consolidation, seen in bland and infected infarcts, has been termed the *feeding vessel sign* (31). This sign is not specific for but is more commonly seen with pulmonary emboli than in other conditions. The combination of multiple peripheral nodules or wedge-shaped consolidations, some of which are cavitated, and a distinct feeding vessel in the appropriate clinical setting is highly suggestive of the diagnosis of septic emboli (Fig. 7-31) (30).

Pulmonary *arteriovenous malformations* (AVMs) are fistulous vascular communications between a pulmonary artery and vein (95%) (Fig. 7-32) or a systemic artery and pulmonary vein (5%) that can be single or multiple. When multiple, nearly 90% of cases are associated with Osler-Weber-Rendu disease (hereditary hemorrhagic telangiectasis), a syndrome of epistaxis, telangiectasia of skin and mucous membranes, and gastrointestinal bleeding. AVMs are usually a congenital defect of

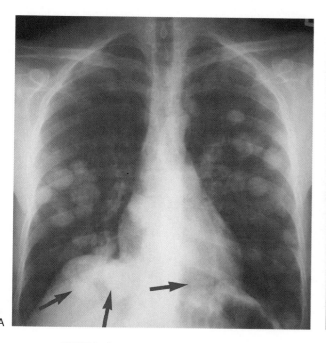

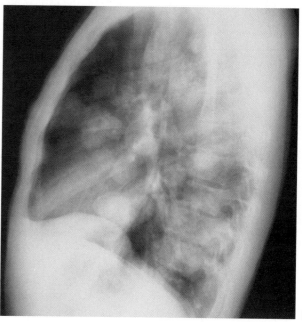

FIGURE 7-25. Metastatic testicular carcinoma. PA (**A**) and lateral (**B**) chest radiographs show numerous bilateral well-circumscribed pulmonary nodules of varying sizes, typical of pulmonary metastases. Testicular carcinoma has a high incidence of pulmonary metastases. Note on the PA view that some of the nodules are "hiding" under the diaphragm (*arrows*) in the posterior lung bases. It is important to always look carefully in this area for nodules, as they are more difficult to see when they are not contrasted with the lucency of the air-filled anterior lung.

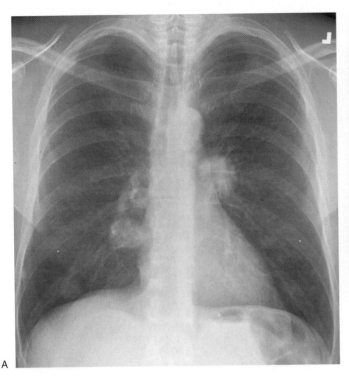
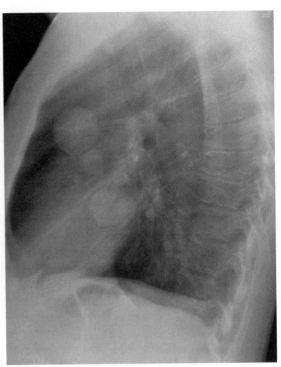

FIGURE 7-26. Metastatic melanoma. A: PA chest radiograph shows multiple bilateral well-circumscribed pulmonary nodules and masses of varying size. The appearance has given rise to the term "cannonball" metastases. **B:** Lateral view confirms the presence of the nodules and masses in the lungs.

capillary structure, but they can be acquired in cirrhosis, cancer, trauma, surgery, or certain infections. The typical radiographic appearance of an AVM is a sharply defined, lobulated oval/round mass, from less than 1 cm to several centimeters in size, associated with an enlarged feeding artery and draining vein. On CT, AVMs will typically demonstrate marked contrast enhancement (Fig. 7-33). Shunting from the fistula can result in hypoxia, systemic abscesses, or infarction, notably of the brain, because the right-to-left shunting of blood bypasses the filtering capacity of the lung (32). Multiple AVMs can be confused with metastases if the enlarged feeding vessels are overlooked.

(Text continues on page 118)

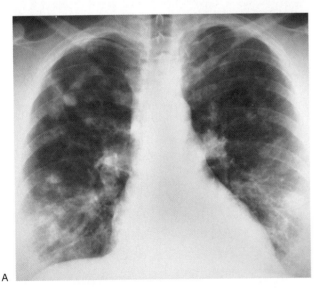
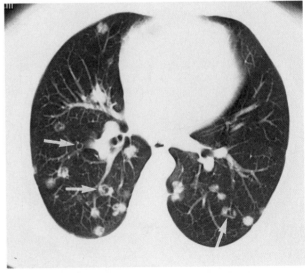

FIGURE 7-27. Cervical carcinoma metastases. A: PA chest radiograph shows multiple bilateral pulmonary nodules, some of which are fairly well circumscribed. The periphery of the lungs "fades out" because of the patient's large body habitus and abundant soft tissues of the chest wall. **B:** CT image shows that many of the nodules are cavitary (*arrows*), and all are well circumscribed. The uterine cervix is one of the most common sites of origin of cavitary pulmonary metastases.

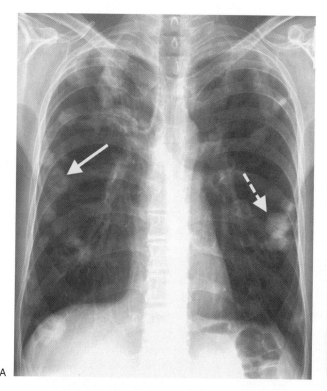

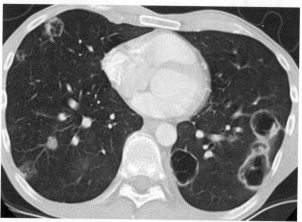

FIGURE 7-28. Tonsillar squamous cell carcinoma metastases. A: PA chest radiograph of a 50-year-old man with a 20–pack-year history of cigarette smoking shows multiple bilateral cavitary (*solid arrow*) and noncavitary (*dashed arrow*) nodules. **B:** CT scan shows that the cavitary nodules have thin walls.

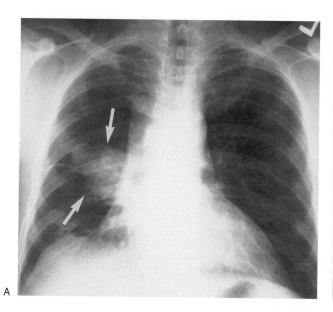

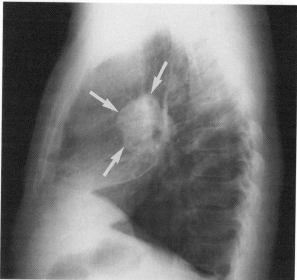

FIGURE 7-29. Metastatic osteosarcoma. A: PA chest radiograph of a 57-year-old man with cough and hemoptysis and a history of mandibular resection for chondroblastic osteosarcoma 7 years prior shows a large lobulated right hilar mass (*arrows*). **B:** Lateral view confirms the hilar location (*arrows*). (*Continued*)

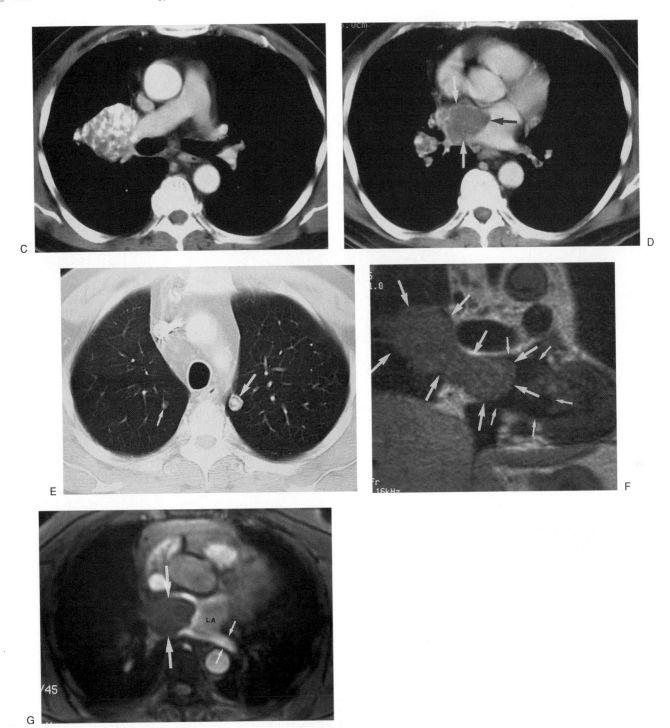

FIGURE 7-29. (*Continued*) **C:** CT scan shows coarse areas of calcification within the mass. **D:** CT at a level inferior to (**C**) shows that the tumor extends into the left atrium (*arrows*). **E:** CT with lung windowing shows a small pulmonary metastasis in the right upper lobe (*small arrow*) and a larger, densely calcified metastasis in the left upper lobe (*large arrow*). **F:** Magnetic resonance (MR) imaging, coronal view, shows that the tumor (*large arrows*) is growing through the right superior pulmonary vein into the left atrium (*small arrows*). **G:** MR axial view, shows low-signal tumor (*large arrows*) invading the normal high-signal-intensity left atrium (*LA*). Note high signal within left inferior pulmonary vein (*small arrows*).

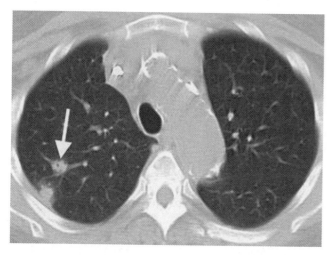

FIGURE 7-30. Septic emboli. CT scan of a 51-year-old woman on hemodialysis for end-stage renal disease and elevated white blood cell count shows nodules, one of which is cavitary (*arrow*), in the right upper lobe. The patient's hemodialysis catheter was the source of the septic emboli.

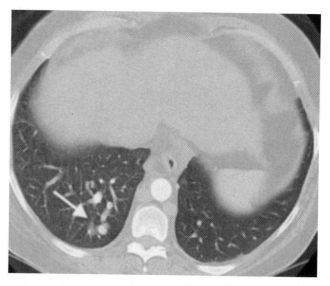

FIGURE 7-32. Arteriovenous malformation. CT scan of a 36-year-old woman with hemoptysis shows a tubular structure in the right lower lobe (*arrow*), representing a large feeding artery and draining vein.

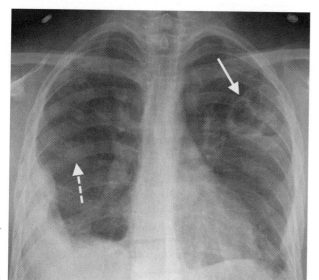

A

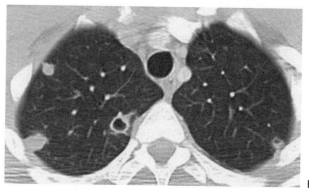

B

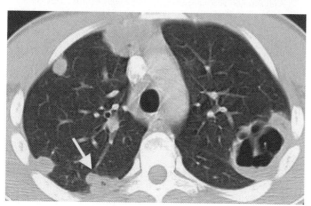

C

FIGURE 7-31. Septic emboli. A: PA chest radiograph shows numerous cavitary (*solid arrow*) and noncavitary (*dashed arrow*) nodules and masses in the lung and bilateral pleural effusions. **B:** CT image shows multiple nodules, some cavitary, in the periphery of the lungs, a common location for septic emboli to appear. **C:** CT at a level inferior to (**B**) shows multiple nodules in the right lung, the feeding vessel sign (*arrow*), and a dominant cavitary mass in the left lung.

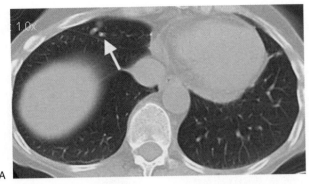
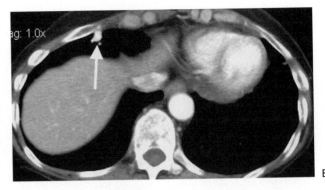

FIGURE 7-33. Arteriovenous malformation. A: CT image of a 62-year-old woman with Osler-Weber-Rendu syndrome shows a tubular structure in the inferior right middle lobe (*arrow*). **B:** CT with soft tissue windowing shows that the structure enhances densely with intravenous contrast (*arrow*).

Pneumatoceles are cystic air collections within the lung that result from infection (most notably *Streptococcus pneumoniae*, *Escherichia coli*, *Klebsiella*, and *Staphylococcus*); blunt or penetrating trauma to the chest; or hydrocarbon inhalation (as from furniture polish or kerosene). In the case of trauma, the pneumatocele represents a laceration that evolves from a lung opacity to a thin-walled cystic structure to a linear scar. Depending on the stage of evolution, a pneumatocele may resemble a cavitary mass, and when multiple they may resemble and be misdiagnosed as metastases or multifocal lung abscesses if the clinical history is not taken into consideration.

Congenital lesions, including sequestration, diaphragmatic hernia, and bronchogenic cyst, can appear as cavitary nodules or masses on chest radiography and are therefore included in the differential diagnosis of cavitary nodules. These entities are discussed further in Chapters 6 and 16.

References

1. Fleischner Society. Glossary of terms for thoracic radiology: recommendation of the nomenclature committee of the Fleischner Society. *AJR Am J Roentgenol.* 1984;143:509–517.
2. Armstrong P. Basic patterns in lung disease. In: Armstrong P, Wilson AG, Dee P, Hansell DM, eds. *Imaging of Diseases of the Chest.* 2nd ed. St. Louis, MO: Mosby-Year Book; 1995:96–107.
3. Austin JH, Müller N, Friedman PJ, et al. Glossary of terms for CT of the lungs: recommendations of the nomenclature committee of the Fleischner Society. *Radiology.* 1996;200:327–331.
4. Kundel HL. Predictive value and threshold detectability of lung tumors. *Radiology.* 1981;139(1):25–29.
5. Muhm JR, Miller WE, Fontana RS, et al. Lung cancer detected during a screening program using 4-month chest radiographs. *Radiology.* 1983;148:609–615.
6. Zerhouni EA, Stitik FP, Siegelmann SS, et al. CT of the pulmonary nodule: a cooperative study. *Radiology.* 1986;160(2):319–327.
7. Kuhlman JE, Collins J, Brooks GN, et al. Dual-energy subtraction chest radiography: what to look for beyond calcified nodules. *RadioGraphics.* 2006;26:79–92.
8. Siegelman SS, Khouri NF, Leo FP, et al. Solitary pulmonary nodules: CT assessment. *Radiology.* 1986;160:307–312.
9. Poirier TJ, Van Ordstrand HS. Pulmonary chondromatous hamartoma: report of seventeen cases and review of the literature. *Chest.* 1971;59:50–55.
10. Siegelman SS, Khouri NF, Scott WW, et al. Pulmonary hamartoma: CT findings. *Radiology.* 1986;160:313–317.
11. Gurney JW, Lyddon DM, McKay JA. Determining the likelihood of malignancy in solitary pulmonary nodules with Bayesian analysis. II. Application. *Radiology.* 1993;186:415–422.
12. Garland LH, Coulson W, Wollin E. The rate of growth and apparent duration of untreated primary bronchial carcinoma. *Cancer.* 1963;16:694–707.
13. Collins VP, Loeffler RK, Tivey H. Observations of growth rates in human tumors. *AJR Am J Roentgenol.* 1956;76:988–1000.
14. Zwirewich CV, Vedal S, Miller RR, et al. Solitary pulmonary nodule: high-resolution CT and radiologic–pathologic correlation. *Radiology.* 1991;179:469–476.
15. Huston J, Muhm JR. Solitary pulmonary opacities on plain tomography. *Radiology.* 1987;163:481–485.
16. Webb WR. The pleural tail sign. *Radiology.* 1978;127:309.
17. Bateson EM. An analysis of 155 solitary lung lesions illustrating the differential diagnosis of mixed tumors of the lung. *Clin Radiol.* 1965;16:51–65.
18. Woodring JH, Fried AM. Significance of wall thickness in solitary cavities of the lung: a follow up study. *AJR Am J Roentgenol.* 1983;140:473–474.
19. Swensen SJ, Viggiano RW, Midthun DE, et al. Lung nodule enhancement at CT: multi-center study. *Radiology.* 2000;214:73–80.
20. Winer-Muram HT. The solitary pulmonary nodule. *Radiology.* 2006;239:34–49.
21. Gould MK, Maclean CC, Kuschner WG, et al. Accuracy of positron emission tomography for diagnosis of pulmonary nodules and mass lesions: a meta-analysis. *JAMA.* 2001;285:914–924.
22. Wallace MJ, Krishnamurthy S, Broemeling LD, et al. CT-guided percutaneous fine-needle aspiration biopsy of small (≤1-cm) pulmonary lesions. *Radiology.* 2002;225:823–828.
23. Swensen SJ, Silverstein MD, Ilstrup DM, et al. The probability of malignancy in solitary pulmonary nodules: application to small radiologically indeterminate nodules. *Arch Intern Med.* 1997;157:849–855.
24. MacMahon H, Austin JH, Gamsu G, et al. Guidelines for management of small pulmonary nodules detected on CT scans: a statement from the Fleischner Society. *Radiology.* 2005;237:395–400.
25. Dähnert W. *Radiology Review Manual.* Baltimore: Williams & Wilkins; 1991:198.
26. Coppage L, Shaw C, Curtis AM. Metastatic disease of the chest in patients with extrathoracic malignancy. *J Thorac Imaging.* 1987;2:24–37.
27. Dodd GD, Boyle JS. Excavating pulmonary metastases. *AJR Am J Roentgenol.* 1961;85:277–293.
28. Maile CW, Rodan BA, Godwin JD, et al. Calcification in pulmonary metastases. *Br J Radiol.* 1982;55:108–113.
29. Cahan WG, Castro EG, Hajdu SI. The significance of a solitary lung shadow in patients with colon carcinoma. *Cancer.* 1974;33:414–421.
30. Kuhlman JE, Fishman EK, Teigen C. Pulmonary septic emboli: diagnosis with CT. *Radiology.* 1990;174:211–213.
31. Huang RM, Nadich DP, Lubat E, et al. Septic pulmonary emboli: CT-radiographic correlation. *AJR Am J Roentgenol.* 1989;153:41–45.
32. Gibbons JR, McIlrath TE, Bailey IC. Pulmonary arteriovenous fistula in association with recurrent cerebral abscess. *Thorac Cardiovasc Surg.* 1985;33:319–321.

CHEST TRAUMA

1. Identify a widened mediastinum on a posttrauma chest radiograph and state the differential diagnosis (including aortic/arterial injury, venous injury, and fracture of sternum or thoracic spine).

2. Identify and describe the indirect and direct signs of aortic injury on contrast-enhanced chest computed tomography (CT).

3. Identify, describe the features of, and state the significance of chronic traumatic pseudoaneurysm of the aorta on a chest radiograph, CT, or magnetic resonance imaging.

4. Identify fractured ribs, clavicle, spine, sternum, and scapula on a chest radiograph or CT.

5. Name five common causes of abnormal lung opacification on a posttrauma chest radiograph or CT.

6. Identify an abnormally positioned diaphragm or loss of definition of a diaphragm on a posttrauma chest radiograph and suggest the diagnosis of ruptured diaphragm.

7. Recognize and describe the signs of diaphragmatic rupture on a chest CT.

8. Identify pneumothorax, pneumopericardium, and pneumomediastinum on a chest radiograph or CT.

9. Identify the fallen lung sign on a chest radiograph or CT and suggest the diagnosis of tracheobronchial tear.

10. Identify a cavitary lesion on a posttrauma chest radiograph or CT and suggest the diagnosis of laceration with pneumatocele formation.

11. Recognize and distinguish between laceration and contusion on a chest radiograph or CT.

Each year in the United States, more than 300,000 patients are hospitalized and 25,000 people die as a direct result of chest trauma (1). Thoracic injury accounts for 25% of all traumatic deaths, and substantial chest trauma is a factor in 50% of fatal traffic accidents (2). Most of the chest trauma seen in civilian populations is blunt chest trauma (90%), usually a result of motor vehicle crashes and falls (3). The incidence of penetrating trauma is stabilizing or decreasing, and many penetrating wounds to the chest can be treated by tube thoracostomy alone (4).

After a patient has been clinically evaluated and stabilized, a chest radiograph is usually obtained. These radiographs are often compromised by limited exposure capability, low lung volumes, poor or absent patient cooperation, obscuration of thoracic anatomy by portions of external monitoring and support devices overlying the patient, suboptimal patient positioning, and magnification and distortion of the mediastinum. In one study, computed tomography (CT) was superior to supine chest radiography in showing findings of chest trauma, and the CT findings influenced patient management in a significant number of patients (5). This chapter reviews the chest radiographic and CT findings of blunt trauma to the chest.

AORTIC AND GREAT VESSEL INJURY

Traumatic rupture of the aorta alone accounts for 16% of fatalities resulting from motor vehicle crashes, and 85% to 90% of patients with traumatic aortic rupture die before reaching a medical facility (6). In clinical series, 90% of aortic ruptures occur at the aortic isthmus, just distal to the origin of the left subclavian artery (7–10) (Fig. 8-1). A few aortic injuries (1% to 3%) involve the descending thoracic aorta, typically at the level of the diaphragm (Fig. 8-2). Chest radiographic signs of

aortic injury lack sensitivity and specificity. The most sensitive (but not specific) radiographic signs are widening of the mediastinum and loss of definition of the aortic arch (Table 8-1) (11). A normal chest radiograph has a high negative predictive value (98%) but a low positive predictive value for aortic injury.

At many institutions, contrast-enhanced, thin-section CT scanning (3 mm collimation or less with overlapping reconstructions) has replaced conventional aortography in evaluating patients for aortic injury. If mediastinal hemorrhage is present, unless it is minimal and not centered around the aorta (Fig. 8-3), without any direct signs of aortic injury, and if no other explanation for the hemorrhage is shown on CT, the patient is generally referred for conventional angiography. If any direct signs of aortic injury are confirmed on CT, including (a) aortic caliber change at the site of injury (pseudoaneurysm or pseudocoarctation), (b) abnormal or irregular aortic wall or contour, (c) intraluminal irregularities or areas of low attenuation (clot, linear intimal flap), (d) intramural hematoma or dissection, and (e) active extravasation of contrast, the patient may or may not proceed to confirmatory conventional angiography at the discretion of the surgeon (Fig. 8-4). Not only is CT useful for detecting direct signs of aortic injury, but CT can also show other causes of a wide mediastinum, including excessive mediastinal fat (Fig. 8-5), paramediastinal atelectasis or pleural effusion, residual thymic tissue, adjacent lung injury (Fig. 8-6), artifact caused by supine positioning, vascular tortuosity, vascular anomalies, lymphadenopathy, and persistent left-sided superior vena cava (12).

Potential pitfalls in CT interpretation include hemomediastinum caused by sternal or vertebral body fracture, left pleural effusion with left lower lobe subsegmental atelectasis "surrounding" the aorta, pulsation artifacts, atherosclerotic plaques, prominent ductus arteriosus, and pseudointimal flaps secondary to volume averaging of the left brachiocephalic vein

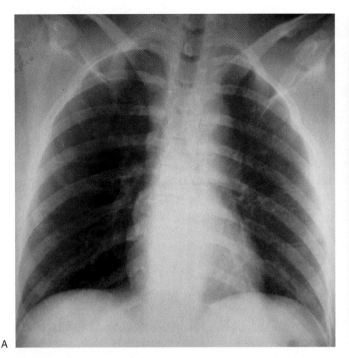

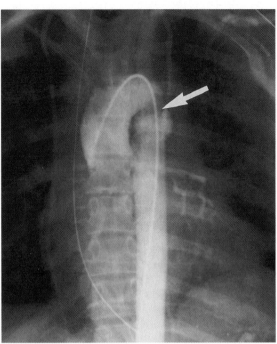

A   B

FIGURE 8-1. Aortic laceration. **A:** Anteroposterior (AP) supine chest radiograph of a young woman after a motor vehicle crash shows nonspecific widening of the mediastinum. **B:** Aortogram shows aortic laceration at the aortic isthmus (*arrow*), the most common site of aortic injury in patients who survive to reach a medical facility. (Reprinted with permission from Collins J. Chest trauma imaging in the intensive care unit. *Respir Care.* 1999;14(9):1044–1063.)

as it crosses in front of the aortic arch. These pitfalls have become less of a problem with the use of multidetector CT and fast scanning techniques.

Occasionally, a chronic pseudoaneurysm can pose diagnostic difficulties. Fewer than 5% of patients will survive long term with an unrepaired pseudoaneurysm (13). Calcification of the wall of the aneurysm and a history of prior thoracic trauma indicate an old aortic injury (Fig. 8-7).

Great vessel injuries (with or without concomitant aortic tear) occur in 1% to 2% of patients with blunt chest trauma (14). A perivascular superior mediastinal or low cervical hematoma, especially in the presence of upper rib fractures or posterior sternoclavicular dislocation, should prompt concern for great vessel injury and injury to other structures in the thoracic inlet (Fig. 8-8).

LUNG PARENCHYMAL INJURY

Abnormal lung parenchymal opacification in trauma patients can result from atelectasis, aspiration, edema, pneumonia, and lung injury (contusion and laceration) and is commonly multifactorial in etiology. Pulmonary contusion ("lung bruise") results in leakage of blood and edema fluid into the interstitial and alveolar spaces. Pulmonary laceration is a more severe injury that causes disruption of the lung architecture.

CT is more sensitive than radiography in demonstrating contusions and lacerations (15–22). On both chest radiography and CT, pulmonary contusions present as areas of airspace opacity, ground-glass opacification, or both, which tend to be peripheral, nonsegmental, and geographic in distribution (Fig. 8-9). Isolated pulmonary contusion in young, healthy patients is not associated with increased mortality (23). Contusions are evident at presentation or within 6 hours after trauma, and they resolve, usually without permanent sequelae, within 5 to 7 days. Pulmonary laceration, on the other hand, may initially be masked by coexistent contusion and other forms of chest

injury on the initial radiograph or CT scan, and it generally takes weeks to months to resolve, sometimes with residual scarring (Fig. 8-10). Lung laceration results in tearing of the lung parenchyma and formation of a cavity filled with blood (hematoma), air (pneumatocele), or both. The radiographic or CT diagnosis of lung laceration is based on the presence of a localized air collection within an area of airspace opacity in the setting of acute chest trauma (20) (Fig. 8-11). Both contusions and lacerations tend to occur adjacent to solid structures, such as the ribs and vertebral bodies (Fig. 8-12).

Fat embolization syndrome is characterized by abnormal diffuse lung opacification on chest radiography, dyspnea, mental status changes, and a petechial rash occurring 12 to 72 hours after trauma. Occurring most commonly after long bone fractures, fat embolization syndrome results when fat droplets

TABLE 8-1
CHEST RADIOGRAPHIC SIGNS OF AORTIC INJURY

Widening of the mediastinum
Obscuration of the aortic arch
Abnormal aortic contour
Hemothorax
Rib fractures
Tracheal shift to the right
Left apical cap
Depression of the left mainstem bronchus below 40 degrees
Nasogastric tube displacement to the right
Pneumothorax
Pulmonary contusion
Widened left paraspinous line

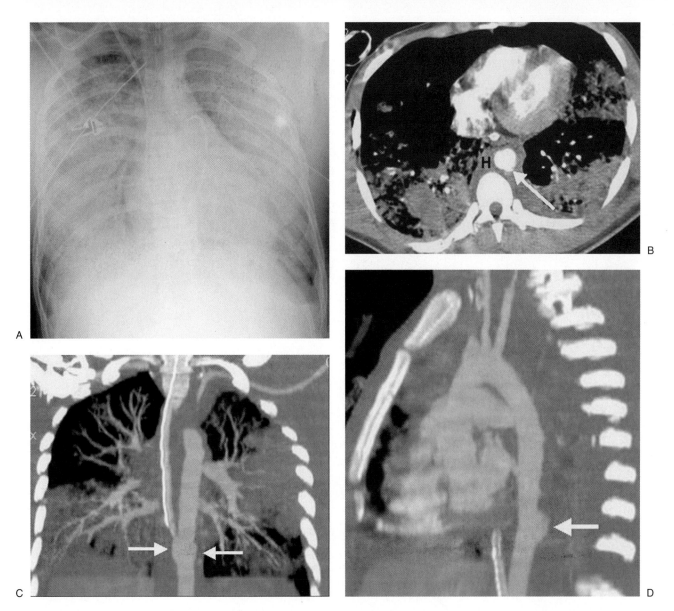

FIGURE 8-2. Descending aortic laceration. A: AP supine chest radiograph shows diffuse opacity of both hemithoraces. B: CT image shows periaortic hematoma (*H*) and irregular contour of the descending aorta (*arrow*). Coronal (C) and sagittal (D) reformatted CT images show a pseudoaneurysm of the descending aorta (*arrows*).

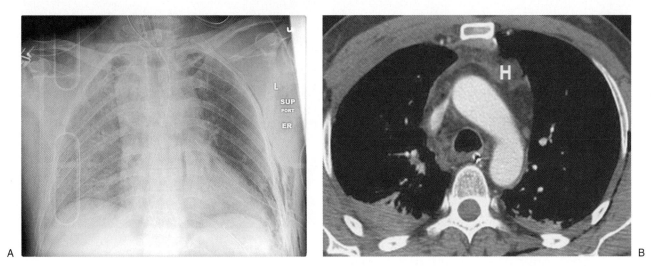

FIGURE 8-3. Mediastinal hematoma. A: AP supine chest radiograph of a patient involved in a motor vehicle crash shows nonspecific widening of the mediastinum. B: CT scan shows blood in the mediastinum (*H*). Note the preservation of a fat plane between the mediastinal blood and the normal aorta, which in the absence of sternal or spine fracture indicates that the bleeding was venous and not arterial.

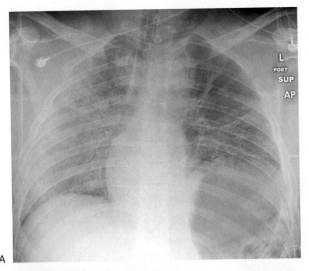

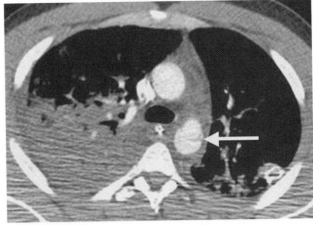

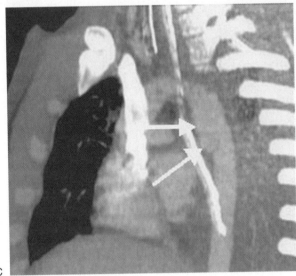

FIGURE 8-4. Aortic laceration. A: AP supine chest radiograph of a patient involved in a motor vehicle crash shows a wide mediastinum and an abnormal aortic contour. The trachea is displaced to the right. B: CT scan shows blood surrounding the aorta, along with disruption of the aorta at the level of the isthmus (*arrow*). C: Sagittal reformatted CT shows an aortic pseudoaneurysm (*arrows*).

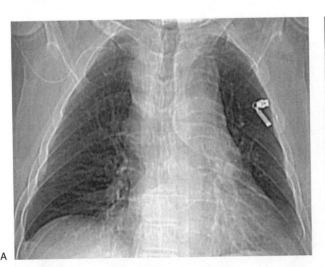

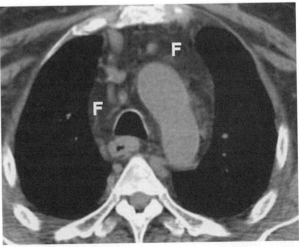

FIGURE 8-5. Mediastinal fat. A: CT chest scout view shows a wide mediastinum. B: Axial CT shows abundant mediastinal fat (*F*), some normal lymph nodes, and no aortic injury or mediastinal mass.

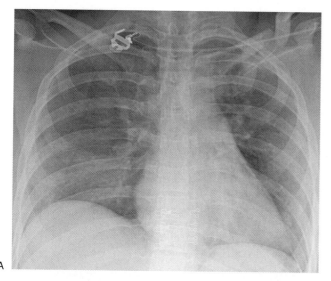

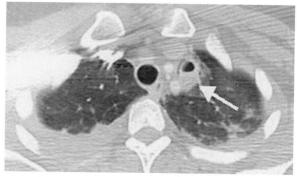

FIGURE 8-6. Lung laceration. A: AP supine chest radiograph of a patient involved in a motor vehicle crash shows a wide upper mediastinum and lack of definition of the aortic arch. **B:** CT shows airspace opacity with central lucency, consistent with laceration and pneumatocele formation, adjacent to the upper mediastinum (*arrow*).

from bone marrow are released into the circulation and occlude capillaries. The patient's symptoms are caused by the decrease in perfusion to various organs from capillary occlusion. In the lungs, chemical pneumonitis ensues as a result of lipolysis and release of free fatty acids, which does not occur immediately after trauma and accounts for the 12- to 72-hour delay in clinical signs and symptoms. The chest radiograph initially appears normal but develops patchy opacities and then widespread diffuse opacity within 72 hours of injury. The pulmonary opacity resembles alveolar pulmonary edema from other causes, with perihilar and basilar predominance and sparing of the lung apices (24) (Fig. 8-13). With fat embolization syndrome, the pulmonary opacity does not clear with diuresis. Contusion is generally seen earlier than fat embolization syndrome on the chest radiograph, and it clears more rapidly (5 to 7 days). Pul-

monary opacity from fat embolization syndrome can take 7 to 10 days to clear.

TRACHEOBRONCHIAL INJURY

The incidence of tracheobronchial injury (TBI) is reported as 0.4% to 1.5% in clinical series of major blunt trauma (25). Blunt trauma must be severe to cause airway rupture, and injury to other structures such as the thoracic cage, lungs, and great vessels is likely. When the intrathoracic trachea or bronchi are injured, the aorta is the most commonly associated injured structure (26). TBI is associated with a 30% overall mortality

(Text continues on page 126)

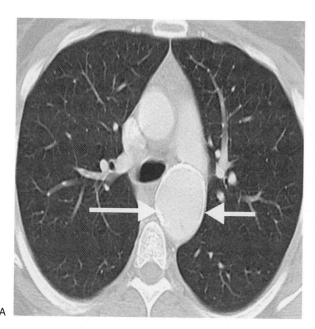

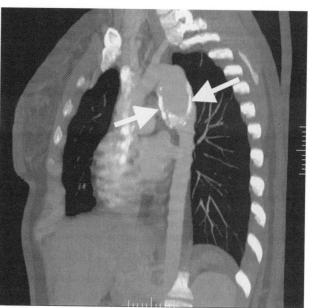

FIGURE 8-7. Chronic pseudoaneurysm. A: CT with lung windowing of a patient with a remote history of chest trauma shows a dilated descending aorta that is densely calcified at the rim (*arrows*). **B:** Sagittal reformatted CT scan shows a densely calcified aortic pseudoaneurysm (*arrows*) at the level of the isthmus.

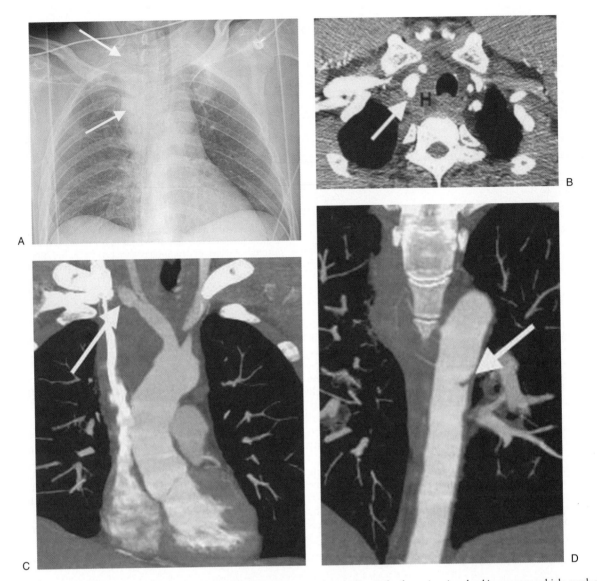

FIGURE 8-8. Concurrent subclavian artery and aortic injuries. A: AP supine chest radiograph of a patient involved in a motor vehicle crash shows a wide upper mediastinum (*arrows*) and leftward shift of the trachea. **B:** CT scan shows mediastinal hematoma (*H*) and pseudoaneurysm of the right subclavian artery (*arrow*). **C:** Coronal reformatted CT scan shows a right subclavian artery pseudoaneurysm (*arrow*) just beyond its origin from the right brachiocephalic artery. **D:** A more posterior coronal reformatted image shows an acute laceration of the aorta (*arrow*).

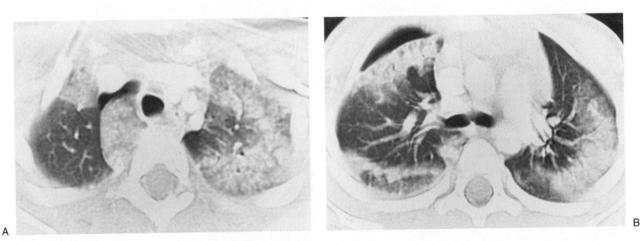

FIGURE 8-9. Pulmonary contusion. A: CT scan of a 4-year-old boy after a motor vehicle crash shows bilateral peripheral areas of airspace opacity, an opacified accessory azygos lobe, and a right pneumothorax. **B:** CT at a level inferior to (**A**) shows bilateral peripheral, nonsegmental areas of airspace opacity typical of pulmonary contusions. (Reprinted with permission from Collins J. Chest trauma imaging in the intensive care unit. *Respir Care.* 1999;14(9):1044–1063.)

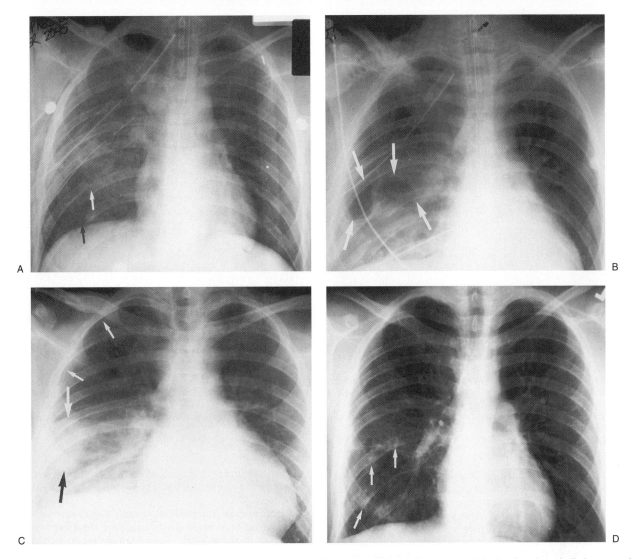

FIGURE 8-10. Pulmonary laceration. A: AP supine chest radiograph of a 16-year-old boy who was struck in the chest by a bull shows patchy opacities in the right lung and several right rib fractures (*arrows*). B: AP supine chest radiograph obtained 4 days later shows numerous rounded lucencies within opacified right lung (*arrows*), consistent with laceration and development of pneumatoceles. C: AP upright chest radiograph 1 week after (B) shows opacification of one of the pneumatoceles (*large arrows*), consistent with hemorrhage and formation of a hematoma. Infection can also result in opacification of a previously air-filled pneumatocele. The patient had no clinical signs or symptoms of infection, and the laceration resolved with minimal residual scarring, without specific treatment. The right chest tubes were removed, and there is a small right pneumothorax (*small arrows*). D: PA upright chest radiograph obtained 2 months after (C) shows small, poorly defined areas of opacification in the right lung (*arrows*), representing residual scarring.

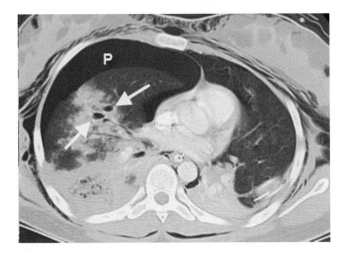

FIGURE 8-11. Pulmonary laceration. CT scan of a patient involved in a motor vehicle crash shows dense opacity in the right lung with central lucencies (*arrows*), consistent with laceration and pneumatocele formation and surrounding hemorrhage. Note a large right pneumothorax (P).

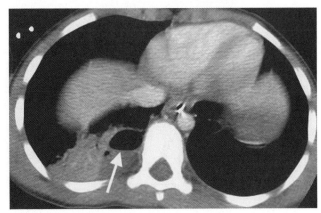

FIGURE 8-12. Pulmonary laceration. CT scan shows a low-density area with an air–fluid level in the right paravertebral area (*arrow*), typical of a shearing type of pulmonary laceration. This should not be confused with a loculated pneumothorax.

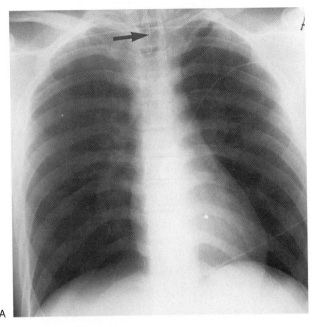

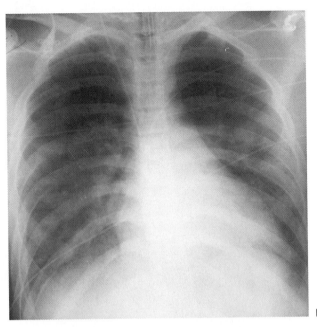

FIGURE 8-13. Fat embolization syndrome. A: AP supine chest radiograph of a young woman shortly after a motor vehicle crash shows clear lungs. The patient sustained multiple long bone fractures that required open reduction and internal fixation. Note the high position of the endotracheal tube (*arrow*). B: AP supine chest radiograph obtained 72 hours later shows bilateral airspace opacities, with a perihilar and basilar predominance, and sparing of the lung apices. (Reprinted with permission from Collins J. Chest trauma imaging in the intensive care unit. *Respir Care.* 1999; 14(9):1044–1063.)

rate, mostly from associated injuries (27). Failure to recognize TBI may result in death or allow cicatrization to occur at the site of injury, with airway obstruction arising days or months after initial injury (Fig. 8-14). More than 80% of TBIs occur within 2.5 cm of the carina (28,29).

Rupture of the cervical trachea may occur as a "clothes-line injury" when the neck is extended on high-speed contact with ropes, wires, or cables by individuals riding many types of recreational vehicles or running. Tracheal laceration may also occur in a motor vehicle crash when the neck of a driver strikes the top of the steering wheel, compressing the airway against the spine.

Pathologically, tracheal injury most commonly presents as a transverse tear between the tracheal rings or a longitudinal tear in the posterior membranous segment. Complete separation of the trachea may occur, but airway continuity can still be maintained by peritracheobronchial tissue. Injury to the mediastinal trachea or major bronchi produces

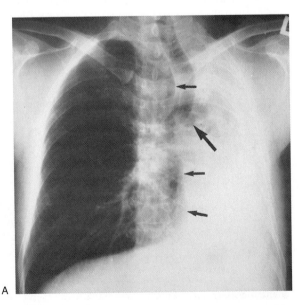

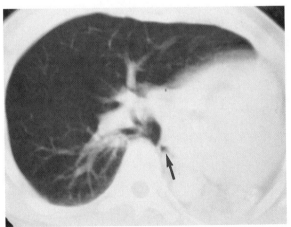

FIGURE 8-14. Remote bronchial fracture. A: PA upright chest radiograph of an asymptomatic man with a remote history of trauma to the chest shows collapse of the left lung, mediastinal shift to the left (note the position of the trachea), and "cut-off" of the left main bronchus (*large arrow*). The right lung is hyperinflated (*small arrows*). B: CT shows collapse of the left lung, cut-off of the left bronchus (*arrow*), and hyperinflation of the right lung. The fractured bronchus was not recognized at the time of injury, and scarring resulted in total occlusion of the bronchus.

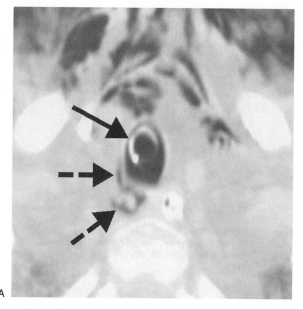

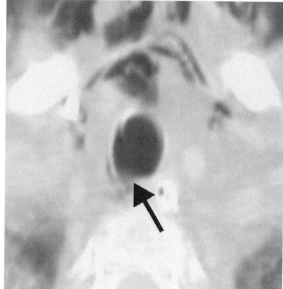

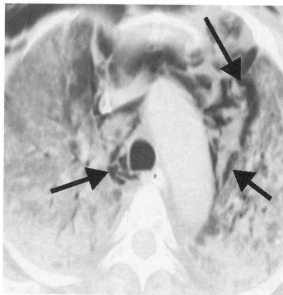

FIGURE 8-15. Acute tracheal injury. A: CT scan of a patient involved in a motor vehicle crash shows an endotracheal tube within the trachea (*solid arrow*) and a curvilinear collection of air posterior to the trachea (*dashed arrows*). B: CT scan at a more inferior level shows the collection of air originating from the posterior trachea (*arrow*) at the site of tracheal tear. C: CT scan at a level inferior to (B) shows air throughout the mediastinum (pneumomediastinum; *arrows*).

pneumomediastinum that rapidly extends into the neck and face, shoulders, and chest wall (Fig. 8-15). Pneumomediastinum is a more specific sign of TBI than is pneumothorax, since pneumothorax is commonly seen with rib fractures. Pneumothorax is seen in 60% to 100% of cases of TBI (30), but it may not be present if the outer adventitial sleeve of the bronchus remains intact and there is no air leak (31). In most cases, pneumothoraces will respond to chest tube placement, so re-expansion of the lung does not exclude tracheobronchial injury. However, a pneumothorax that does not resolve with functioning tube drainage is the sine qua non of mediastinal airway injury (32).

An indication of tracheal tear is elevation of the hyoid bone above the level of C3, as seen on a lateral radiograph of the cervical spine (33). This occurs as a result of injured infrahyoid musculature, causing unopposed elevation of the hyoid bone by suprahyoid musculature. Another sign of tracheal transection is acute overdistension of the endotracheal tube cuff, to the point where it exceeds the normal diameter of the trachea (Fig. 8-16). In tracheal rupture, the balloon may approach the endotracheal tube tip as a result of distal expansion of the balloon in the tear, with partial herniation of the balloon in the tear as the tube moves in the airway or is repositioned (34) (Fig. 8-17).

The "fallen lung sign" (35) is a rarely seen but highly suggestive sign of *bronchial* tear that can be seen on chest radiographs and CT (Figs. 8-18 and 8-19). This sign refers to the lung falling laterally and posteriorly in supine positioning and falling inferiorly away from the hilum in the upright position. Normally with a pneumothorax, the lung recoils inward toward the hilum.

DIAPHRAGM RUPTURE

Acute diaphragmatic rupture occurs in 1% to 7% of patients following major blunt trauma (36–38), and the diagnosis is missed on initial presentation in up to 66% of patients (39–45). Seventy-five percent to 95% of patients with acute diaphragm rupture have abnormal chest radiographs, but only

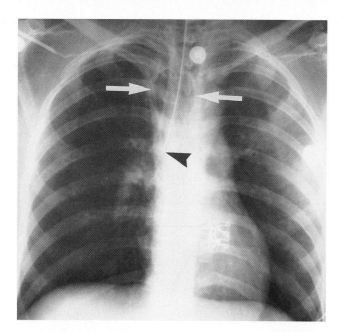

FIGURE 8-16. Tracheal tear. AP supine chest radiograph of a young woman involved in a motor vehicle crash shows an overdistended endotracheal tube balloon (*arrows*) at the site where the balloon herniates through a tracheal tear. Note malpositioning of the tube tip within the right bronchus (*arrowhead*).

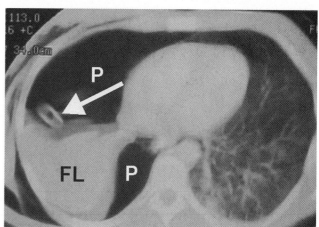

FIGURE 8-18. Fallen lung sign. CT of a patient with an acute traumatic fracture of the right main bronchus shows a large right pneumothorax (*P*), a right chest tube (*arrow*), and collapsed "fallen right lung" (*FL*) positioned in the posterior and lateral right hemithorax. Normally with pneumothorax, the collapsed lung recoils inward toward the hilum.

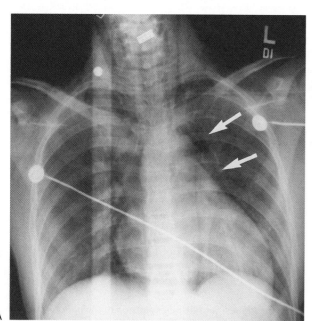

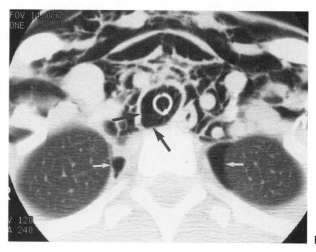

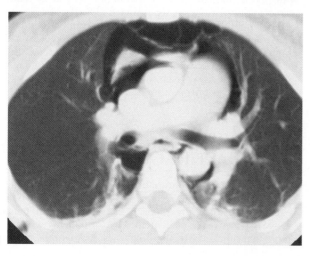

FIGURE 8-17. Tracheal tear. A: AP supine chest radiograph of an 11-year-old girl who impaled her neck on a dumpster bar while riding her bicycle shows a pneumomediastinum with streaks of air in the chest and neck and lateral displacement of the mediastinal pleura (*arrows*). B: CT image shows an overdistended endotracheal tube balloon herniating through a posterolateral tracheal tear (*black arrows*). The endotracheal tube is seen as a white ring within the trachea. Note extensive air within the soft tissues of the neck and bilateral pneumothoraces (*white arrows*). C: CT at a level inferior to (B) shows pneumomediastinum, with air outlining the aorta, superior vena cava, pulmonary artery, and thymus.

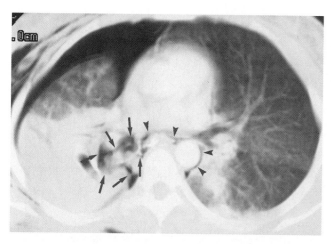

FIGURE 8-19. Fractured bronchus intermedius. CT of a young woman involved in a motor vehicle crash shows leakage of air from a fractured bronchus intermedius to the pleural space (*arrows*) and mediastinum (*arrowheads*), resulting in pneumothorax and pneumo-mediastinum, respectively. (Reprinted with permission from Collins J. Chest trauma imaging in the intensive care unit. *Respir Care.* 1999;14(9):1044–1063).

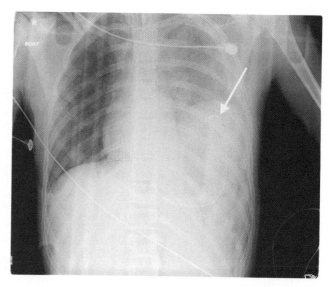

FIGURE 8-21. Diaphragm rupture. AP supine chest radiograph of a patient involved in a motor vehicle crash shows a mass in the left lower hemithorax representing herniated non–air-filled stomach, superior displacement of an intragastric nasogastric tube (*arrow*), and rightward shift of the mediastinum.

17% to 40% have highly suggestive radiographic findings (46–48). Chest radiographic findings of rupture include a normal appearing diaphragm, pneumothorax, displacement of stomach, liver, spleen, colon, or small bowel into the thorax (Fig. 8-20), superior displacement of an intragastric nasogastric tube (Fig. 8-21), pleural effusion, basilar opacity causing inability to visualize the diaphragm, apparent elevation of the diaphragm, an irregular or lumpy diaphragm contour, fractures of the lower ribs, and contralateral shift of the mediastinum

in the absence of a large pleural effusion or pneumothorax (Table 8-2) (49). Rupture of the right hemidiaphragm probably occurs with almost the same frequency as rupture of the left hemidiaphragm, although most clinically recognized diaphragm injuries occur on the left. If diaphragm rupture is not promptly diagnosed, the patient may remain asymptomatic or develop incarceration of herniated abdominal viscera, which can occur at a time remote from the incidence of trauma (Fig. 8-22).

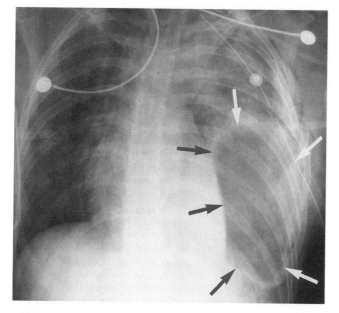

FIGURE 8-20. Diaphragm rupture. AP supine chest radiograph of a 24-year-old woman involved in a motor vehicle crash shows herniation of gas-distended stomach through a left diaphragmatic tear into the left hemithorax (*black and white arrows*). Note the shift of the mediastinum to the right, left rib fractures, and opacification of the left lung from parenchymal injury.

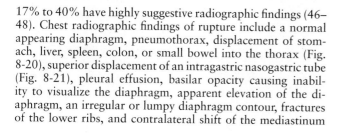

TABLE 8-2

RADIOLOGIC FINDINGS OF DIAPHRAGM RUPTURE

Findings on chest radiography
 Displacement of stomach, liver, spleen, colon, or small bowel into the thorax
 Superior displacement of an intragastric nasogastric tube
 Ipsilateral pleural effusion
 Basilar opacity causing inability to visualize the diaphragm
 Irregular or lumpy diaphragm contour
 Fractures of the lower ribs

Findings on CT scanning
 Direct signs:
  Diaphragmatic discontinuity
  Intrathoracic herniation of abdominal contents
  Waistlike constriction of bowel ("collar sign")
  Dependent viscera sign
 Indirect signs:
  Liver laceration
  Hemoperitoneum
  Hemothorax
  Splenic laceration
  Renal contusion
  Lower lobe atelectasis
  Lower rib fractures

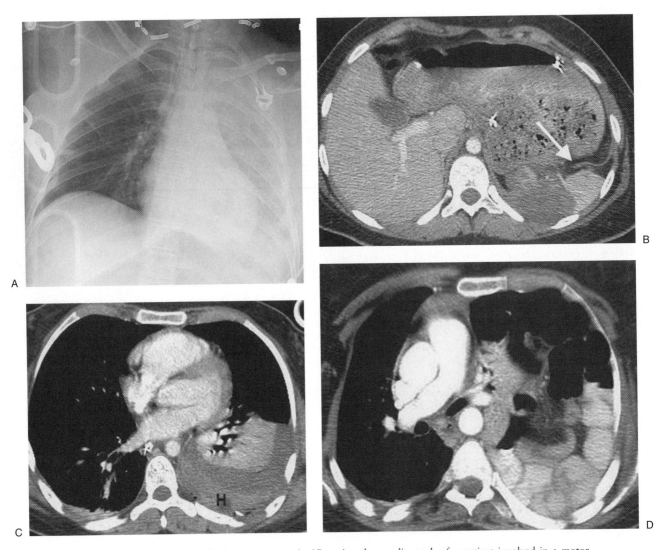

FIGURE 8-22. Unrepaired diaphragm rupture. A: AP supine chest radiograph of a patient involved in a motor vehicle crash shows an opacified left hemithorax. The left hemidiaphragm is not visualized. **B:** CT image shows a discontinuous left hemidiaphragm (*arrow*) and splenic laceration. **C:** CT at a level superior to (**B**) shows a left hemothorax with the "hematocrit sign" (*H*). **D:** CT scan obtained several weeks later shows bowel herniated into the left hemithorax, which has caused rightward shift of the mediastinum.

Multidetector CT has been shown to be useful in making the diagnosis of acute diaphragm rupture, and it is superior to conventional CT because volumetric data acquisition provides high-quality sagittal and coronal reconstructions. Acquisition of data during a single breath-hold decreases slice misregistration (50). Individual diagnostic sensitivity for detecting diaphragmatic rupture on CT scanning is 54% to 73%, and specificity is 86% to 90% (51). Most injuries involve the posterolateral aspect of the diaphragm. Direct CT findings associated with acute rupture include diaphragmatic discontinuity (Fig. 8-23), intrathoracic herniation of abdominal contents, and waistlike constriction of bowel ("collar sign") (Fig. 8-24). In addition, Bergin et al (52) have described the "dependent viscera" sign in CT diagnosis of blunt traumatic diaphragmatic rupture. This sign refers to the upper one third of the liver abutting the posterior right ribs or the bowel or stomach lying in contact with the posterior left ribs. Associated CT findings of diaphragm rupture include liver laceration, hemoperitoneum, hemothorax, splenic laceration, renal contusion, lower lobe atelectasis, and lower rib fractures. Although focal discontinuity of the diaphragm is a direct sign of diaphragmatic rupture, it should be noted that there is a normal increase in di-

aphragmatic defects with age that is not related to trauma (53) (Fig. 8-25).

INJURIES TO THE BONY THORAX

Injury to ribs, clavicles, scapulae, sternum, and spine can occur as a result of blunt chest trauma. Thoracic spine fractures account for 16% to 30% of all spine fractures and result in complete neurologic deficits in approximately 60% of patients (54,55). A supine chest radiograph provides an opportunity to evaluate the thoracic spine, but optimal evaluation requires dedicated frontal and lateral collimated radiographs or CT. Seventy percent to 90% of spine fractures can be seen on conventional radiographs. Findings include cortical disruption and abnormal vertebral body size, shape, opacity and location. CT and magnetic resonance (MR) imaging may show otherwise occult fractures and are the only ways to directly evaluate the integrity of the spinal cord and the intervertebral ligaments (3). CT and MR are more helpful in distinguishing unstable burst fractures from stable, simple, anterior wedge compression fractures (56).

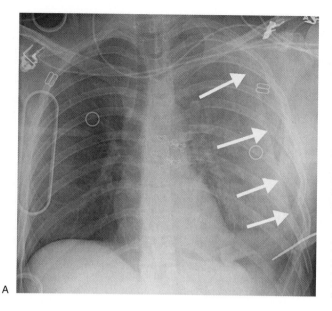

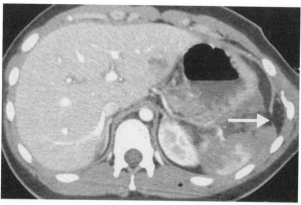

FIGURE 8-23. **Diaphragm rupture. A:** AP supine chest radiograph of a patient involved in a motor vehicle crash shows an opacified left hemithorax and a left pneumothorax (*arrows*). The left hemidiaphragm is not visualized. **B:** CT scan shows discontinuity of the left hemidiaphragm (*arrow*).

Fractures to the upper ribs, clavicle, and upper sternum are important in that they may be accompanied by brachial plexus or vascular injury in 3% to 15% of patients (57). Fractures of the lower ribs should increase suspicion of splenic, hepatic, or renal injury, which can be confirmed with CT. Fractured rib ends may lacerate the pleura or lung, with resultant pulmonary hematoma, hemothorax, or pneumothorax. Fracture of five contiguous ribs or segmental fractures of three or more adjacent ribs (a single rib fractured in two or more locations) can result in paradoxic motion of a "flail" segment during the respiratory cycle, which can impair respiratory mechanics and result in atelectasis and pulmonary infection (Fig. 8-26).

Sternal fractures, which occur in 8% of major thoracic trauma admissions (12), may be associated with myocardial contusion and are often clinically silent. These fractures can-

not be visualized on frontal chest radiographs and may be relatively inconspicuous on lateral chest radiographs, but they are usually readily identified on CT. Most (58% to 80%) sternal fractures occur in the upper or midbody of the sternum (4) and are often associated with retrosternal hematoma (Figs. 8-27 and 8-28). The presence of a fat plane between the hematoma and the aorta implies that the hematoma is not aortic in origin.

Posterior dislocation of the clavicle can result in injury to the great vessels, superior mediastinal nerves, trachea, and esophagus. Although sternoclavicular dislocations can be demonstrated using angled chest radiographs, they are more easily detected with CT (14) (Fig. 8-29).

Scapular fractures are diagnosed on the initial chest radiograph in only a little more than half of patients (58). When scapular fractures are not seen on the initial chest radiograph,

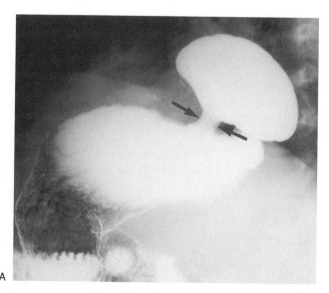

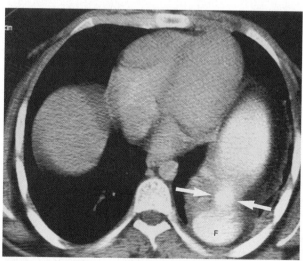

FIGURE 8-24. **Diaphragm rupture. A:** Lateral view of a fluoroscopic upper gastrointestinal tract contrast study shows a waistlike constriction of the stomach ("collar sign"; *arrows*), where the fundus of the stomach herniates through a small diaphragmatic tear into the left hemithorax. **B:** CT scan shows the collar sign (*arrows*). The fundus (*F*) is positioned posteriorly.

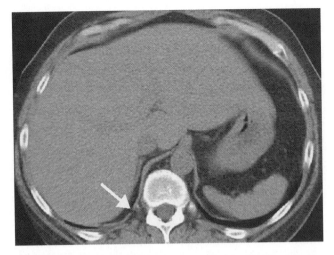

FIGURE 8-25. **Normal diaphragm discontinuity.** CT of a 70-year-old man shows an incidental small discontinuity of the right hemidiaphragm (*arrow*).

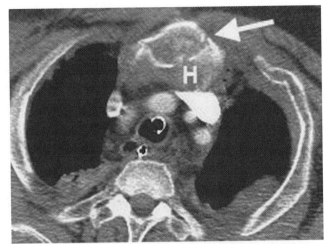

FIGURE 8-27. **Sternal fracture.** CT shows a comminuted fracture of the sternum (*arrow*) and retrosternal hematoma (*H*). Note preservation of the fat plane between the hematoma and the great vessels.

they are visible in retrospect in 72% of cases, not included on the examination in 19%, and obscured by superimposed structures or artifacts in 9% (58) (Fig. 8-30). CT of the chest, especially if used in combination with conventional radiographs, should demonstrate most scapular fractures. Clavicle fractures are common in injured patients and are usually of minimal clinical consequence.

PLEURAL MANIFESTATIONS OF CHEST TRAUMA

Pneumothorax is seen on chest radiography in almost 40% of patients with blunt chest trauma and in up to 20% of patients with penetrating chest injuries (59,60). The most common cause in blunt trauma is assumed to be a rib fracture that

penetrates the visceral pleura; however, pneumothorax in the absence of rib fractures is occasionally seen in adults and is commonly seen in children. Pleural air will rise to the most nondependent portion of the thorax: at the apex in the upright patient and at the anterior, caudal aspect of the pleural space in the supine patient. Radiographic signs of pneumothorax in the supine patient include (a) the deep sulcus sign, which is a deep, lucent costophrenic sulcus (Figs. 8-31 to 8-33); (b) a relative increase in lucency at the affected lung base; and (c) the double diaphragm sign, which is created by the interfaces between the ventral and dorsal portions of the pneumothorax with the anterior and posterior aspects of the hemidiaphragm. CT is much more sensitive for diagnosing pneumothorax in the supine patient than is chest radiography (61,62) and identifies pneumothoraces that cannot be seen on conventional supine radiographs in 10% to 50% of patients who have sustained blunt trauma to the chest (61–63).

Pneumomediastinum may occur in association with pneumothorax. It can be diagnosed on chest radiographs by the

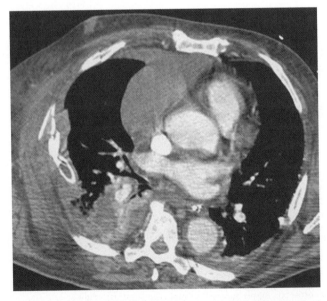

FIGURE 8-26. **Rib fractures and flail chest.** CT of a patient involved in a motor vehicle crash shows a loculated right hemothorax, right chest wall hematoma, and numerous fractured right ribs.

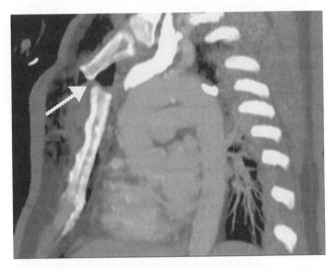

FIGURE 8-28. **Sternal fracture.** Sagittal reformatted CT shows a fracture of the sternum (*arrow*) and posterior displacement of the inferior fracture fragment from the manubrium.

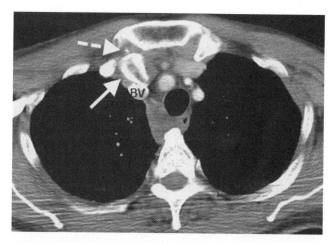

FIGURE 8-29. Sternoclavicular dislocation. CT scan shows posterior displacement of the right clavicular head (*solid arrow*), which impinges upon the right brachiocephalic vein (*BV*). Note a small fracture fragment posterior to the sternum (*dashed arrow*).

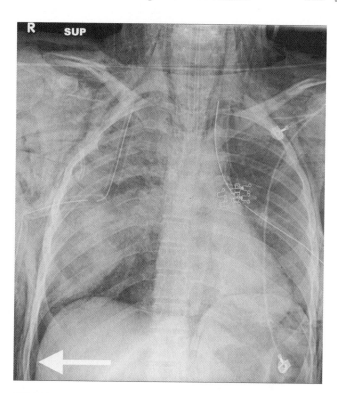

FIGURE 8-31. Deep sulcus sign. AP supine chest radiograph shows a right basilar pneumothorax (*arrow*), which creates a deep, "tongue-like" costophrenic sulcus.

presence of abnormal lucencies in the mediastinum that highlight the contours of the aorta and pulmonary artery and displace the mediastinal pleura laterally, and by the "continuous diaphragm sign," which is produced by the presence of air between the pericardium and the diaphragm. Pneumomediastinum can be easily identified on chest CT and may signal the presence of an underlying laceration of the pharynx, esophagus, or tracheobronchial airway.

Pleural effusions that develop in the acute posttraumatic setting usually represent hemothorax, and a rapidly expanding pleural effusion is most likely to be caused by arterial bleeding. CT can be helpful in distinguishing hematoma from other pleural collections by showing the high CT attenuation of blood (64) (Fig. 8-34). Rupture of the thoracic duct, which is uncommon, produces chylothorax, with milky fluid recovered through thoracentesis. Rupture of the thoracic duct in the lower thorax produces right-sided chylothorax, whereas rup-

ture above the level where the thoracic duct crosses the midline in the midthorax produces left-sided chylothorax. CT is superior to chest radiography in distinguishing pleural fluid from other causes of radiographic density, such as atelectasis, parenchymal injury, or pneumonia, and it can show loculation of pleural fluid and delineate complex pleuroparenchymal opacities.

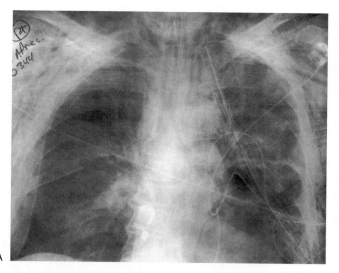

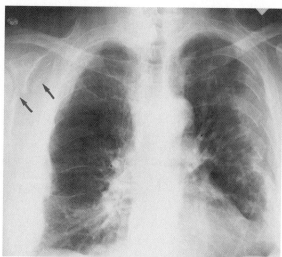

FIGURE 8-30. Scapular fracture. A: AP supine chest radiograph of a 62-year-old man involved in a motor vehicle crash shows massive bilateral chest wall subcutaneous emphysema, obscuring bony and lung parenchymal detail. B: PA upright chest radiograph obtained 10 days later shows a comminuted right scapular fracture (*arrows*), previously obscured by subcutaneous emphysema and film labeling, and multiple rib fractures resulting in bilateral flail chest. (Reprinted with permission from Collins J. Chest trauma imaging in the intensive care unit. *Respir Care.* 1999;14(9):1044–1063.)

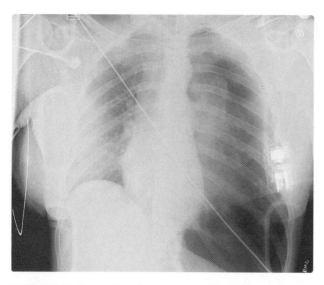

FIGURE 8-32. Deep sulcus sign. AP supine chest radiograph shows a large left apical, lateral, and basilar pneumothorax and associated rightward shift of the mediastinum.

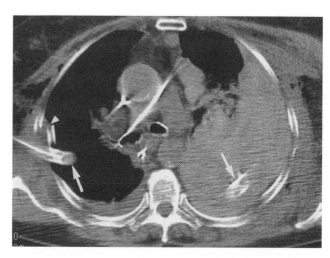

FIGURE 8-34. Traumatic hemothorax. CT of a 78-year-old woman involved in a motor vehicle crash shows a large, high-attenuation, left pleural collection causing shift of the mediastinum to the right; bilateral chest tubes (arrows); and a right rib fracture (arrowhead). Note bilateral chest wall hematomas.

CARDIAC TRAUMA

The heart and pericardium are fairly well protected from non-penetrating injury, and documented traumatic injury is uncommon. The chest radiograph plays a relatively minor role in the evaluation of myocardial injury. Its greatest value is in detecting associated injuries, such as rib fractures, sternal fractures, and pulmonary contusion.

Rapid accumulation of blood in the pericardial space can cause cardiac tamponade and severe hemodynamic compromise. Bedside sonographic evaluation of the heart is the method of choice to quickly and noninvasively detect pericardial fluid. CT is also very sensitive for detecting pericardial fluid and may indicate pericardial hemorrhage, as determined by the high CT attenuation of the fluid (Fig. 8-35). A CT density exceeding 35 Hounsfield units differentiates hemopericardium from transudative pericardial effusions. Cardiac tamponade is suggested by CT findings of distension of the vena cavae, hepatic veins, and renal veins and by development of periportal edema within the liver (14).

Interventricular septal rupture and damage to the mitral valve apparatus can result in congestive heart failure. Mitral regurgitation from the latter may cause asymmetric pulmonary edema, classically of the right upper lobe as a result of the direction of the regurgitant jet. Pneumopericardium can occur when air enters through a pericardial disruption in the presence of pneumothorax (Fig. 8-36).

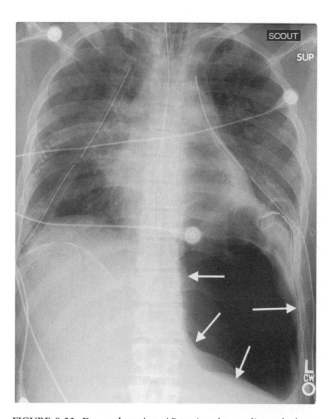

FIGURE 8-33. Deep sulcus sign. AP supine chest radiograph shows a large left basilar pneumothorax (arrows) despite a left chest tube. This case illustrates the importance of including the entire lung base on supine chest radiographs. Otherwise, the presence or size of a large basilar pneumothorax may not be appreciated.

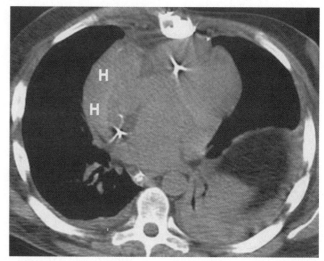

FIGURE 8-35. Hemopericardium. CT shows a crescentic collection of blood (H) compressing the right heart.

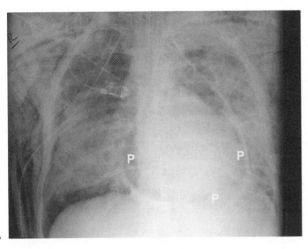
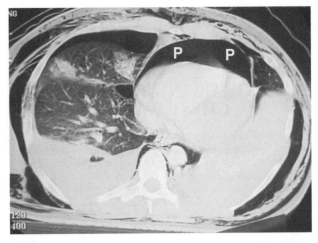

FIGURE 8-36. Pneumopericardium. A: AP supine chest radiograph of a patient involved in a motor vehicle crash shows air surrounding the heart (P). Note right pneumothorax, bilateral parenchymal opacification, and bilateral subcutaneous emphysema. B: CT shows pneumopericardium (P), bilateral pneumothoraces, pneumomediastinum, pleural effusion, and subcutaneous emphysema.

Cardiac contusion may result from blunt chest trauma in 8% to 76% of patients (65,66). The diagnosis is usually made from electrocardiography, nuclear cardiac imaging, or echocardiography. The right ventricle is the most frequently injured, as it comprises almost three times more exposed anterior surface of the heart than does the left ventricle (14). Chest radiography and CT can show sequelae of cardiac contusion, such as congestive heart failure, ventricular aneurysm, or massive cardiac enlargement.

ESOPHAGEAL INJURY

Esophageal tears are more common in patients with penetrating trauma and occur in fewer than 1% of blunt trauma cases (67). Thoracic esophageal tears from trauma are caused almost exclusively by gunshot wounds (16). Esophageal disruption can occur from crushing of the esophagus between the spine and trachea, traction from hyperextension, and direct penetration by cervical spine fracture fragments (68). Most tears occur in the cervical and upper thoracic esophagus, but they also may occur just above the gastroesophageal junction. The thoracic esophagus lies to the left of the trachea at the thoracic inlet but moves to the right as it passes posterior to the aortic arch at the level of the carina. The esophagus crosses back to the left as it enters the stomach. Accordingly, ruptures of the mid- to distal esophagus usually present with a right-sided pleural effusion, and effusions caused by rupture at the gastroesophageal junction occur more commonly on the left.

Chest radiography in patients with esophageal rupture can show persistent severe pneumomediastinum or pneumothorax, pleural effusion, a widened paraspinal line, and retrocardiac lung opacification. CT scans can show similar findings, in addition to leakage of oral contrast from the disrupted esophagus into the mediastinum or pleural space and changes of mediastinitis. The areas of greatest esophageal thickening on CT often

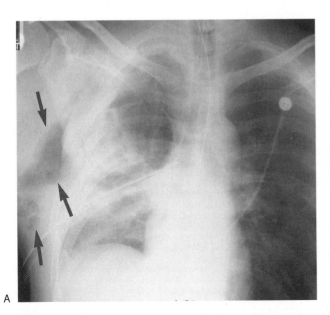
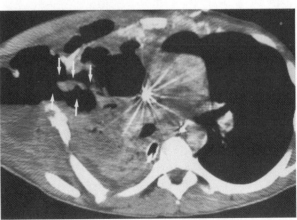

FIGURE 8-37. Broncho-pleural-cutaneous fistula. A: AP upright chest radiograph of a 29-year-old man involved in a motor vehicle crash shows multiple right rib fractures creating a "flail chest," pleural opacification consistent with hemothorax, opacification of the right lung from parenchymal injury, and numerous collections of air within the soft tissues of the right chest wall (arrows). B: CT shows communication between the airways and chest wall hematoma (arrows). (Reprinted with permission from Collins J. Chest trauma imaging in the intensive care unit. Respir Care. 1999; 14(9):1044–1063.)

represent the level of perforation. The perforation itself, however, may be obscured by edema and hemorrhage, and is usually not visualized. The diagnosis is confirmed at fluoroscopy using water-soluble contrast material or with endoscopy.

SOFT TISSUE INJURIES OF THE CHEST WALL

The chest wall has a rich vascular network established by the intercostal and internal mammary arteries. Rib fractures can lacerate intercostal arteries or veins, tear intercostal muscles, or result in bleeding from the raw surface of the bone. In addition, branches of the lateral thoracic artery that supply the pectoral muscles and anastomose with chest wall vessels can be lacerated and bleed. A large amount of blood can collect in the subcutaneous or extrapleural spaces of the chest, especially in the elderly because of skin and subcutaneous tissue laxity. CT scanning can easily distinguish chest wall from parenchymal or mediastinal injury, whereas this differentiation may not be possible with chest radiography. On CT, soft tissue hematomas of the chest wall are readily distinguished from parenchymal injury, and subcutaneous air is distinguished from pneumothorax. CT scanning shows broncho-pleural-cutaneous fistulae, which may not be appreciated on the chest radiograph (Fig. 8-37). Trauma to the breast, which often results in bleeding and hematoma formation, can be produced by a combination of compression and shearing stress produced by a seat belt (Fig. 8-38).

ROLE OF CT IN CHEST TRAUMA

CT scanning is superior to chest radiography in demonstrating pneumothoraces, hemothoraces, pulmonary contusions, and fractures. CT obviates the need for conventional aortography in many patients, and in many institutions CT aortography has become the new gold standard for the diagnosis of acute aortic injury. CT provides a look at the entire chest in addition to the aorta, which is a distinct advantage over conventional aortography. In addition to showing fractures, CT also shows related soft tissue injuries, such as great vessel injury from fracture-dislocation of the clavicle and splenic/liver laceration from ad-

jacent rib fractures. In some cases, CT shows direct signs of tracheobronchial, esophageal, or diaphragmatic injury. Chest CT can be performed quickly on all trauma patients who are referred for abdominal CT as a means of detecting serious chest injuries early.

References

1. Kshettry VR, Bolman RM. Chest trauma. Assessment, diagnosis, and management. *Clin Chest Med.* 1994;15:137–146.
2. Blair E, Topuzlu Z, Davis JH. Delayed or missed diagnosis in blunt chest trauma. *J Trauma.* 1971;11:129–145.
3. Groskin SA. Selected topics in chest trauma. *Semin Ultrasound CT MR.* 1996;17:119–141.
4. Mayberry JC. Imaging in thoracic trauma: the trauma surgeon's perspective. *J Thoracic Imaging.* 2000;15:76–86.
5. Haramati LB, Hochsztein JG, Marciano N, Nathanson N. Evaluation of the role of chest computed tomography in the management of trauma patients. *Emerg Med.* 1996;3:225–230.
6. Stark P. Traumatic rupture of the aorta: a review. *CRC Crit Rev Diagn Imaging.* 1984;21:229–255.
7. Clark DE, Zeiger MA, Wallace KL, et al. Blunt aortic trauma: signs of high risk. *J Trauma.* 1990;30:701–705.
8. Cowley RA, Turney SZ, Hankins JR, et al. Rupture of thoracic aorta caused by blunt trauma: a fifteen year experience. *J Thorac Cardiovasc Surg.* 1990;100:652–660.
9. Kirsh M, Behrendt D, Orringer M, et al. The treatment of acute traumatic rupture of the aorta: a 10-year experience. *Ann Surg.* 1976;184:308–315.
10. Lundevall J. The mechanism of traumatic rupture of the aorta. *Acta Pathol Microbiol Scand.* 1964;62:34–46.
11. Mirvis SE, Bidwell JK, Buddemeyer EU, et al. Value of chest radiography in excluding traumatic aortic rupture. *Radiology.* 1987;163:487–493.
12. Harley DP, Mena I. Cardiac and vascular sequelae of sternal fractures. *J Trauma.* 1986;26:553–555.
13. Parmley CF, Mattingly TW, Manion WC, et al. Nonpenetrating traumatic injury of the aorta. *Circulation.* 1958;17:1086–1101.
14. Mirvis SE, Templeton P. Imaging in acute thoracic trauma. *Semin Roentgenol.* 1992;27:184–210.
15. Marts B, Durham R, Shapiro M, et al. Computed tomography in the diagnosis of blunt thoracic injury. *Am J Surg.* 1994;168:688–692.
16. Poole GV, Morgan DB, Cranston PE, et al. Computed tomography in the management of blunt thoracic trauma. *J Trauma.* 1993;35:296–302.
17. Reginald R. Lung alterations in thoracic trauma. *J Thorac Imaging.* 1987;2:1–11.
18. Schild HH, Strunk H, Weber W, et al. Pulmonary contusion: CT vs plain radiograms. *J Comput Assist Tomogr.* 1989;13:417–420.
19. Smejkal R, O'Malley KF, David E, et al. Routine initial computed tomography of the chest in blunt torso trauma. *Chest.* 1991;100:667–669.
20. Tocino I, Miller MH. Computed tomography in blunt chest trauma. *J Thorac Imaging.* 1987;2:45–59.
21. Toombs BD, Sandler CM, Lester RG. Computed tomography of chest trauma. *Radiology.* 1981;140:733–738.
22. Wagner RB, Crawford WO Jr, Schimpf PP. Classification of parenchymal injuries of the lung. *Radiology.* 1988;167:77–82.
23. Hoff SJ, Shotts SD, Eddy VA, Morris JA Jr. Outcome of isolated pulmonary contusion in blunt trauma patients. *Am Surg.* 1994;60:138–142.
24. Feldman F, Ellis K, Gren WM. The fat embolism syndrome. *Radiology.* 1975;114:535–542.
25. Halttunen PE, Kostianinen SA, Meurala HG. Bronchial rupture caused by blunt chest trauma. *Scand J Cardiovasc Surg.* 1984;18:141–144.
26. Mason AC, Mirvis SE, Templeton PA. Imaging of acute tracheobronchial injury: review of the literature. *Emerg Radiol.* 1994;1:250–260.
27. Guest JL, Anderson JN. Major airway injury in closed chest trauma. *Chest.* 1977;72:63–66.
28. Kirsch MM, Orringer MB, Behrendt DM, Sloan H. Management of tracheobronchial disruption secondary to nonpenetrating trauma. *Ann Thorac Surg.* 1976;22:93–101.
29. Spencer JA, Rogers CE, Westaby S. Clinico-radiological correlates in rupture of the major airways. *Clin Radiol.* 1991;43:371–376.
30. Hood RM, Sloan HE. Injuries of the trachea and major bronchi. *J Thorac Cardiovasc Surg.* 1959;38:458–480.
31. Chesterman JT, Satsangi PN. Rupture of the trachea and bronchi by closed injury. *Thorax.* 1966;21:21–27.
32. Kelly JP, Webb WR, Moulder PV, et al. Management of airway trauma. I. Tracheobronchial injuries. *Ann Thorac Surg.* 1985;40:551–555.
33. Polansky A, Resnick D, Sofferman RA, Davidson TM. Hyoid bone elevation: a sign of tracheal transection. *Radiology.* 1984;150:117–120.
34. Rollins RJ, Tocino I. Early radiographic signs of tracheal rupture. *AJR Am J Roentgenol.* 1989;148:695–698.
35. Oh KS, Fleischner FG, Wyman SM. Characteristic pulmonary finding in traumatic complete transection of a main-stem bronchus. *Radiology.* 1969;92:371–372.

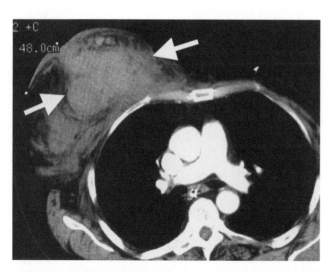

FIGURE 8-38. Breast hematoma. CT of a woman involved in a motor vehicle crash shows a high-attenuation collection of blood in the right breast (*arrows*), a result of shearing stress produced by a seat belt.

36. Estrera A, Platt M, Mills L. Traumatic injuries of the diaphragm. *Chest.* 1979;75:306–313.
37. Meyers BF, McCabe CJ. Traumatic diaphragmatic hernia: occult marker of serious injury. *Ann Surg.* 1993;218:783–790.
38. Voeller GR, Reisser JR, Fabian TC, et al. Blunt diaphragm injuries: a five-year experience. *Am Surg.* 1990;56:28–31.
39. Ball T, McCrory R, Smith JO, Clements JL Jr. Traumatic diaphragmatic hernia: errors in diagnosis. *AJR Am J Roentgenol.* 1982;138:633–637.
40. Estrera AS, Landay MJ, McClelland RN. Blunt traumatic rupture of the right hemidiaphragm: experience in 12 patients. *Ann Thorac Surg.* 1985;39:525–530.
41. Gourin A, Garzon AA. Diagnostic problems in traumatic diaphragmatic hernia. *J Trauma.* 1974;14:20–31.
42. Hood RM. Traumatic diaphragmatic hernia. *Ann Thorac Surg.* 1971;12:311–324.
43. Kearney PA, Rouhana SW, Burney RE. Blunt rupture of the diaphragm: mechanism, diagnosis and treatment. *Ann Emerg Med.* 1989;18:1326–1330.
44. Wienceck RG, Wilson RF, Steiger Z. Acute injuries of the diaphragm: an analysis of 165 cases. *J Thorac Cardiovasc Surg.* 1986;92:989–993.
45. Wise L, Connors J, Hwang YH, Anderson C. Traumatic injuries to the diaphragm. *J Trauma.* 1973;13:946–950.
46. Gelman R, Mirvis SE, Gens D. Diaphragmatic rupture due to blunt trauma: sensitivity of plain chest radiographs. *AJR Am J Roentgenol.* 1991;156:51–57.
47. Minagi H, Brody W, Laing F. The variable roentgen appearance of traumatic diaphragmatic hernia. *J Can Assoc Radiol.* 1977;28:124–128.
48. Payne J, Yellin A. Traumatic diaphragmatic hernia. *Arch Surg.* 1982;117:18–24.
49. Groskin SA. Selected topics in chest trauma. *Radiology.* 1992;183:605–617.
50. Israel RS, Mayberry JC, Primack SL. Diaphragmatic rupture: use of helical CT scanning with multiplanar reformations. *AJR Am J Roentgenol.* 1996;167:1201–1203.
51. Murray JG, Caoili E, Gruden JF, et al. Acute rupture of the diaphragm due to blunt trauma: diagnostic sensitivity and specificity of CT. *AJR Am J Roentgenol.* 1996;166:1035–1039.
52. Bergin D, Ennis R, Keogh C, et al. The "dependent viscera" sign in CT diagnosis of blunt traumatic diaphragmatic rupture. *AJR Am J Roentgenol.* 2001;177:1137–1140.
53. Caskey CI, Zerhouni EA, Fishman EK, et al. Aging of the diaphragm: a CT study. *Radiology.* 1989;171:385–389.
54. Meyer S. Thoracic spine trauma. *Semin Roentgenol.* 1992;27:254–261.
55. Pal J, Mulder D, Brown R, et al. Assessing multiple trauma: is the cervical spine enough? *J Trauma.* 1988;28:1282–1284.
56. Ballock RT, Mackersie R, Abitbol JJ, et al. Can burst fractures be predicted from plain radiographs? *J Bone Joint Surg Br.* 1992;74:147–150.
57. Greene R. Lung alterations in thoracic trauma. *J Thorac Imaging.* 1987;2:1–11.
58. Harris RD, Harris JH Jr. The prevalence and significance of missed scapular fractures in blunt chest trauma. *AJR Am J Roentgenol.* 1988;151:747–750.
59. Ashbaugh DG, Peters GN, Halgrimson FG, et al. Chest trauma: analysis of 685 patients. *Arch Surg.* 1967;95:546–554.
60. Con JH, Hardy JD, Fain WR, et al. Thoracic trauma: analysis of 1022 cases. *J Trauma.* 1963;3:22–40.
61. Tocino IM, Miller MH, Frederick PR, et al. CT detection of occult pneumothorax in head trauma. *AJR Am J Roentgenol.* 1984;143:987–990.
62. Wall SD, Federle MP, Jeffrey RB, et al. CT diagnosis of unsuspected pneumothorax after blunt abdominal trauma. *AJR Am J Roentgenol.* 1983;141:919–921.
63. Wolfman NT, Gilpin JW, Bechtold RE, et al. Occult pneumothorax in patients with abdominal trauma: CT studies. *J Comput Assist Tomogr.* 1993;17:56–59.
64. Mirvis SE, Tobin KD, Kostrubiak I, et al. Thoracic CT in detecting occult disease in critically ill patients. *AJR Am J Roentgenol.* 1987;148:685–689.
65. Hossack KF, Moreno CA, Vanway CW, et al. Frequency of cardiac contusion in non-penetrating chest injury. *Am J Cardiol.* 1988;61:391–394.
66. Rosenbaum RC, Johnston GS. Posttraumatic cardiac dysfunction: assessment with radionuclide ventriculography. *Radiology.* 1986;61:391–394.
67. Biquet JF, Dondelinger RF, Roland D. Computed tomography of thoracic aortic trauma. *Eur Radiol.* 1996;6:25–29.
68. Mirvis SE. Imaging of thoracic trauma. In: Turney SZ, Rodriguez A, Cowley RA, eds. *Management of Cardiothoracic Trauma.* Baltimore: Williams & Wilkins; 1990.

CHAPTER 9

PLEURA, CHEST WALL, AND DIAPHRAGM

LEARNING OBJECTIVES

1. Recognize and name four causes of a large unilateral pleural effusion on a chest radiograph or computed tomograph (CT).
2. Describe the difference in appearance of a pulmonary abscess and an empyema on chest radiograph or CT.
3. Recognize diffuse pleural thickening, as seen in fibrothorax, malignant mesothelioma, and pleural metastases.
4. Recognize a pneumothorax on an upright and supine chest radiograph.
5. Recognize imaging findings suggesting a tension pneumothorax or hydrothorax and describe the acute clinical implications.
6. Recognize a pleural-based mass with bone destruction or infiltration of the chest wall on a chest radiograph or CT; name four likely causes.
7. Recognize pleural calcification on a chest radiograph or CT and suggest the likely diagnosis of asbestos exposure (bilateral involvement) or old tuberculosis or trauma (unilateral involvement).
8. Recognize the typical chest radiographic appearances of pleural effusion, given differences in patient positioning, and describe the role of the lateral decubitus view to evaluate pleural effusion.
9. Recognize apparent unilateral elevation of the diaphragm on a chest radiograph and suggest a specific etiology with supportive history and associated chest radiograph findings.

The chest wall, pleura, and diaphragm enclose the outer lung. All are intimately associated with each other, which occasionally makes it difficult to determine the origin of a mass involving one or more of these compartments (Fig. 9-1). Disorders involving the chest wall, pleura, or diaphragm—resulting in a "pleural-based" mass—can arise from one of these compartments, an adjacent compartment, or another part of the body (as with metastatic neoplasms). Certain radiologic features can help determine the origin of an apparent pleural-based mass and narrow the list of diagnostic possibilities.

PLEURA

The pleura is composed of visceral and parietal serous membranes. The lungs and interlobar fissures are invested in the visceral pleura, whereas the parietal pleura lines the ribs, diaphragm, and mediastinum. The visceral and parietal pleura are continuous with one another as they are reflected around the hilum and the inferior pulmonary ligament. Inferiorly, the parietal pleura is situated within the costophrenic sulcus. The area between the two pleural layers forms a "potential space," which can be enlarged when filled with fluid, cells, or air. Normally, there is approximately 1 to 5 mL of pleural fluid within this space (1). Because the total thickness of the pleural space and the normal visceral and parietal pleura is only 0.2 to 0.4 mm, the pleural layers are not usually identified on radiographs or computed tomographic (CT) scans of the chest except (a) when outlined by air or extrapleural fat, (b) where the visceral pleura invaginates into the lung to form the fissures, or (c) where the two lungs contact each other at junctional lines (2). The parietal pleura is separated from the ribs and intercostal muscles by a layer of fatty areolar connective tissue and a layer of endothoracic fascia. The parietal pleura receives vascular supply from and is drained by the systemic circulation, whereas the visceral pleura is supplied and drained mainly by the pulmonary circulation. Lymphatic drainage of the visceral pleura is by way of a lymphatic plexus that covers the surface of the lung just beneath the visceral pleura (3). These lymphatics do not connect with the pleural space. The parietal pleura is the primary drainage route for fluid in the pleural space,

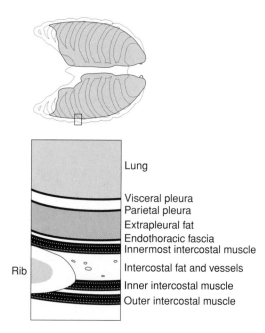

FIGURE 9-1. Association between the lung, pleura, and chest wall. The lungs are invested in the visceral pleura, whereas the parietal pleura lines the ribs and soft tissues of the chest wall, diaphragm, and mediastinum. The parietal pleura is separated from the ribs and intercostal muscles by fat and endothoracic fascia. The total thickness of the pleura and "potential" pleural space is only 0.2 to 0.4 mm.

Labels in figure:
Lung
Visceral pleura
Parietal pleura
Extrapleural fat
Endothoracic fascia
Innermost intercostal muscle
Intercostal fat and vessels
Inner intercostal muscle
Outer intercostal muscle
Rib

as it contains lymphatics that connect to the intercostal, internal mammary, and mediastinal lymph node chains (3). Except in rare circumstances (e.g., in some cases after cardiothoracic surgery or trauma), the right and left pleural spaces do not communicate with each other.

A pleural-based density is one that, in some projection, presents a more or less sharp border indicative of a pleural surface, with a projected center lying outside the parenchyma of the lung. It may be in one of five locations: (i) extrapleural, (ii) parietal pleural, (iii) interpleural, (iv) visceral pleural, or (v) subpleural (Fig. 9-2). When associated with a rib le-

sion, an extrapleural lesion is most likely a hematoma (as from a rib fracture) or a tumor (with rib metastasis); when there is no rib lesion, it is likely a lipoma or lymphoma (when a patient is known to have lymphoma). Lesions involving the parietal pleura are usually calcified and represent plaques from prior asbestos exposure. Interpleural density is common and can represent loculated pleural effusion or metastatic tumor. Visceral pleural lesions are uncommon but usually represent pleural thickening from asbestos exposure (whereas calcified asbestos-related plaques more frequently involve the parietal pleura). Subpleural densities are parenchymal and generally do

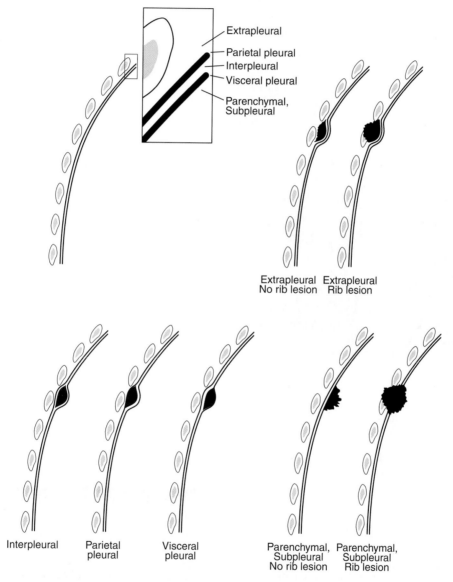

FIGURE 9-2. Radiologic pleural-based densities. A pleural-based density has margins that are partially or completely well circumscribed, indicating contiguity with a pleural surface. There are five types of pleural-based densities, depending on the location of origin. An *extrapleural density* originates in the chest wall, and when it does not extend into the pleura and lung, it has a sharp medial margin where it contacts the parietal pleura. When the adjacent rib is involved, rib fracture with hematoma or neoplasm should be considered. *Parietal* and *visceral pleural densities* are usually asbestos-related pleural plaques, which may or may not be calcified. *Interpleural densities* most commonly represent loculated pleural effusions; when intrafissural in location they may be recognized on chest radiography by characteristic "beaking" at the ends of the fluid collection where the pleural layers of a fissure meet (producing a "pseudotumor"). *Subpleural densities* are parenchymal and usually have an indistinct lung parenchymal margin. If the lesion extends into the pleura and chest wall, all the margins of the lesion may be indistinct. Etiologies to consider when a subpleural density involves the pleura or chest wall are neoplasm and infection (especially fungal, mycobacterial, and actinomycotic).

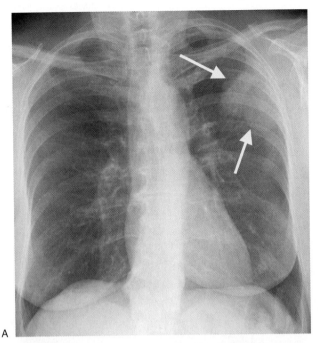

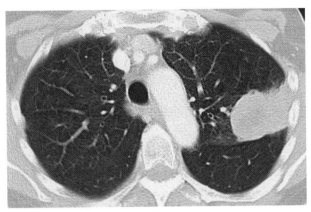

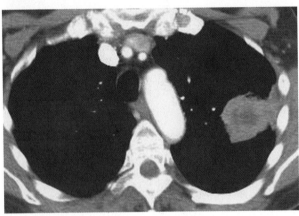

A

B

C

FIGURE 9-3. Subpleural squamous cell bronchogenic carcinoma. A: Posteroanterior (PA) chest radiograph of a 67-year-old woman shows a mass in the left upper hemithorax (*arrows*) that is contiguous with the pleural surface. **B:** CT with lung windowing shows the mass abutting the lateral pleural surface and major fissure. **C:** CT with mediastinal windowing shows that the mass is contiguous with the pleural surface. Centrally, the mass contains areas of low attenuation, consistent with necrosis.

not have a sharp margin with the lung (Fig. 9-3), but on occasion tumors in the apex of the lung (so-called Pancoast tumors) can appear fairly well circumscribed (Fig. 9-4). The etiology of many soft tissue masses, regardless of their origin, cannot be distinguished on radiography or CT of the chest, except in the case of lipoma, which has a characteristic low attenuation value on CT.

Pleural Effusions

Pleural effusions develop when there is excess pleural fluid produced, diminished resorption of fluid from the pleural space, or both. The fluid can originate from the pleura or be extrapleural in origin (Fig. 9-5). Pleural effusions are categorized as either transudates or exudates. The distinction is based on the specific gravity, protein, and lactate dehydrogenase (LDH) content of the fluid, with transudates having a specific gravity of 1.016 or less, a protein content of 3 g/dL or less, a ratio of pleural fluid protein to serum protein of <0.5, an LDH ratio (pleural fluid to serum) of <0.6, and an absolute pleural LDH level of <200 IU/L (4). Transudates develop primarily as a result of changes in microvascular pressure and plasma oncotic pressure, whereas exudates are caused by an altered pleural surface, with an increase in permeability or a decrease in lymph flow. The list

of causes of pleural effusions is lengthy (Table 9-1), but more than 90% of effusions result from heart failure, ascites, pleuropulmonary infection, malignancy, or pulmonary embolism (5).

TABLE 9-1

COMMON CAUSES OF PLEURAL EFFUSION

Infection
Neoplasm
Cardiovascular disease (congestive heart failure)
Cirrhosis
Hypoproteinemia
Pancreatitis
Uremia
Subdiaphragmatic abscess
Trauma (hemothorax, chylothorax)
Occupational (asbestos)
Collagen vascular disease (systemic lupus erythematosus)
Hypothyroidism (often with pericardial effusion)
Pulmonary embolism

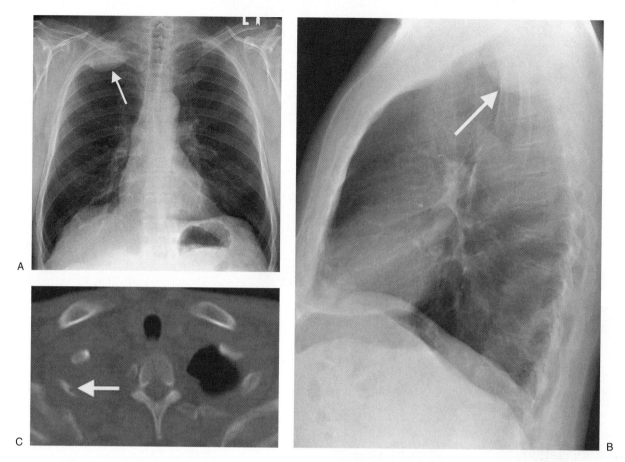

FIGURE 9-4. Pancoast tumor. PA (**A**) and lateral (**B**) chest radiographs of a 61-year-old man with right shoulder pain and a 40–pack-year history of cigarette smoking shows a circumscribed mass (*arrow*) in the right apex. **C:** CT with bone windowing shows the mass filling the right lung apex and destruction of the right second rib (*arrow*).

The appearance of an effusion depends on the patient's position at the time of the radiologic examination and on the mobility of the effusion. In an upright person, fluid collects mainly in the lower pleural space, as long as it is freely mobile, creating a homogeneous opacity with a curvilinear upper border that is sharply marginated and concave to the lung (Fig. 9-6). Fluid can collect in the fissures, creating a "pseudotumor" that conforms to the edges of the fissures and resolves with clearing of lung edema (Figs. 9-7 and 9-8). Occasionally, large quantities of pleural fluid accumulate in a "subpulmonic location"

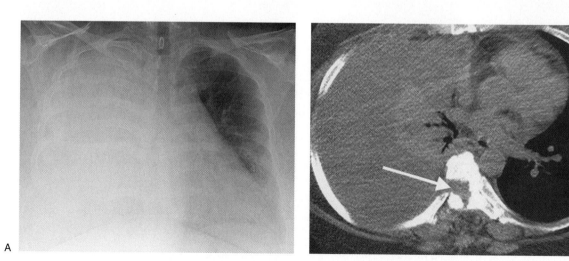

FIGURE 9-5. Cerebrospinal fluid leak into pleural space. A: PA chest radiograph of a 42-year-old man who recently underwent partial corpectomy of the thoracic spine at several levels shows complete opacification of the right hemithorax and shift of the mediastinum to the left. **B:** Non–contrast-enhanced CT shows a large right pleural effusion, collapse of the right lung, mediastinal shift to the left, findings of corpectomy, and continuity of fluid from the spine into the pleural space (*arrow*).

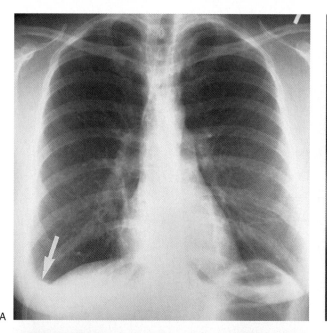

A

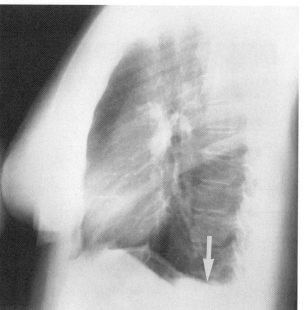

B

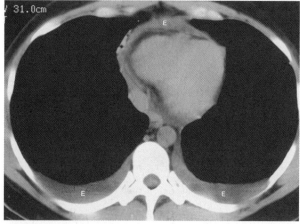

C

FIGURE 9-6. Pleural and pericardial effusions. A: PA chest radiograph of a woman with hypothyroidism shows blunting of the right costophrenic angle, producing a "meniscus" (*arrow*). **B:** Lateral chest radiograph shows blunting of both costophrenic angles posteriorly (*arrow*). **C:** CT shows bilateral pleural and pericardial effusions (*E*).

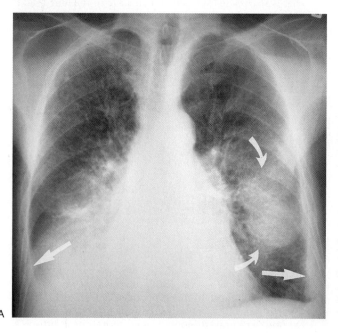

A

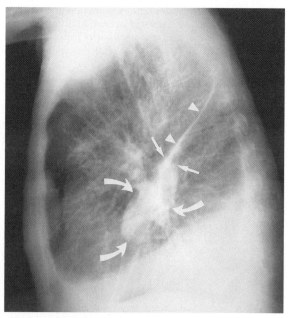

B

FIGURE 9-7. Pulmonary edema and pleural fluid pseudotumor. A: PA chest radiograph shows enlargement of the cardiac silhouette, interstitial pulmonary edema, and displacement of the inferolateral lungs from the chest wall and diaphragm by pleural effusion (*straight arrows*). There is a hazy "mass" in the left middle and lower hemithorax (*curved arrows*). **B:** Lateral chest radiograph shows that the "mass" or "pseudotumor" (*curved arrows*) blends in with the left major fissure (*straight arrows*); this is characteristic of pleural fluid within the fissure. The superior aspect of the left major fissure is thickened as a result of pleural fluid and subpleural edema (*arrowheads*).

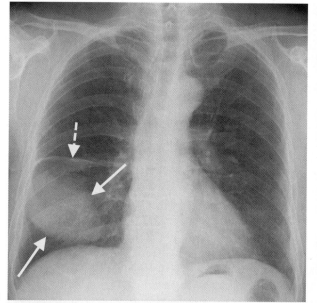

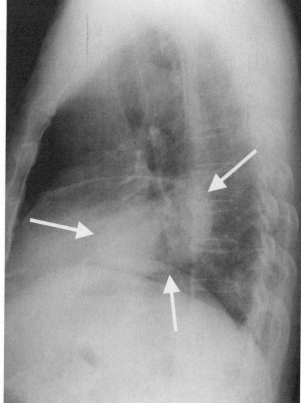

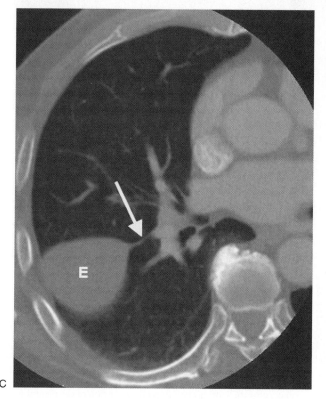

FIGURE 9-8. Pleural fluid pseudotumor. A: PA chest radiograph shows a circumscribed ovoid mass in the right lower hemithorax (*solid arrows*) and thickening of the minor fissure (*dashed arrow*). B: Lateral view shows that the mass (*arrows*) is oriented in the direction of and superimposed on the major fissure. C: CT (bone windowing) shows that the mass is of fluid attenuation, representing pleural effusion (*E*), and is contiguous with the thickened major fissure (*arrow*).

rather than in the general pleural cavity. In this case, the upper edge of the fluid mimics the contour of the diaphragm on the chest radiograph, creating the appearance of an "elevated diaphragm," which usually peaks more laterally than normal. When this occurs on the left, the gastric air bubble and upper surface of the "hemidiaphragm" are separated more than usual. In supine patients, freely mobile fluid layers posteriorly, creating hazy, veillike opacification of the affected hemithorax with preserved vascular shadows. Depending on the size of the effusion, this can be a subtle finding; when bilateral, it may not be detected at all, especially when small, or it may be confused with pulmonary edema. Other findings of pleural effusions in supine patients include blunting of the costophrenic

angle (although this is often a false-positive finding) (6), capping of the lung apex, thickening of the minor fissure, and widening of the paraspinal soft tissues. Lateral decubitus views can be useful in verifying pleural effusions when the supine examination is equivocal, and they can allow determination of whether pleural fluid is mobile or not. The lateral decubitus view is much more sensitive than the upright view for the detection of pleural effusions; it can demonstrate as little as 5 mL of pleural fluid (Fig. 9-9) (7).

CT can detect smaller amounts of pleural fluid than can chest radiography (8). In addition, CT enables determination of whether fluid is loculated, the extent and localization of loculated fluid for purposes of drainage, assessment of pleural

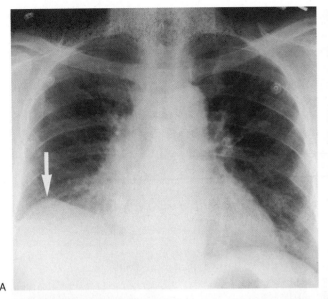

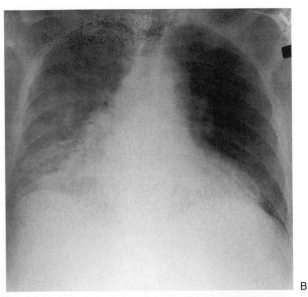

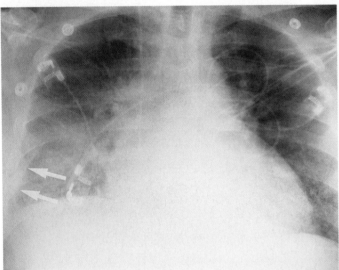

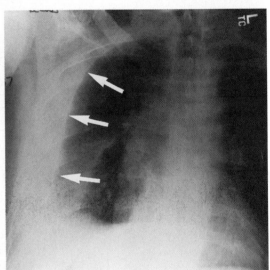

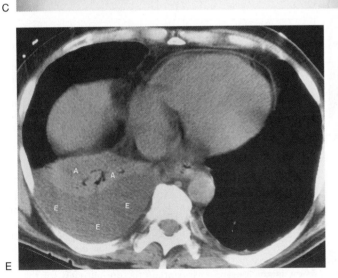

FIGURE 9-9. Positional appearances of pleural fluid on chest radiography and CT. **A:** PA upright chest radiograph shows apparent elevation of the right hemidiaphragm. The dome of the right hemidiaphragm appears to be displaced laterally (*arrow*), a clue to the diagnosis of pleural fluid collecting in a "subpulmonic" location. **B:** Anteroposterior (AP) supine chest radiograph of the same patient, 3 days later, shows hazy increased opacification of the right hemithorax secondary to pleural fluid layering posteriorly within the pleural space, now the most gravity-dependent portion of the pleural space. **C:** AP semi-upright chest radiograph of the same patient, 2 days after (**B**), shows a combination of pleural fluid layering posteriorly, which produces a hazy opacity in the mid and lower right hemithorax and laterally (*arrows*). **D:** Right lateral decubitus chest radiograph of the same patient, taken on the same day as (**A**), shows pleural fluid freely layering against the now gravity-dependent lateral chest wall, from the costophrenic angle to the lung apex (*arrows*). **E:** CT of the same patient, performed on the same day as (**B**), shows a moderate- to large-sized right pleural fluid collection (*E*), with associated "passive" atelectasis of the right lower lobe (*A*).

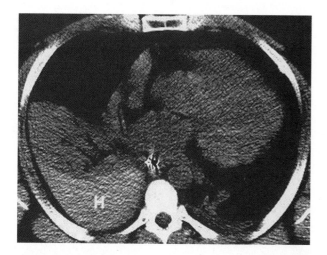

FIGURE 9-10. Hemothorax. CT shows high-attenuation blood (*H*) in the right pleural space.

morphology (irregular thickening and focal masses suggest malignancy), evaluation of underlying parenchymal disease, and differentiation between pleural and parenchymal disease (aided by the use of intravenous contrast material). The attenuation value of pleural fluid on CT enables detection of a hemothorax (Fig. 9-10), which has a higher attenuation value than simple fluid; occasionally, a fluid–fluid or hematocrit level can be seen (see Fig. 8-22).

When a large unilateral effusion is present (Fig. 9-11), four causes should be considered: (i) infection (empyema); (ii) tumor (primary bronchogenic carcinoma, mesothelioma, metastases, and lymphoma); (iii) chylothorax (secondary to tumor, most notably lymphoma, or ruptured thoracic duct); and (iv) hemorrhage (usually from trauma, whether iatrogenic or otherwise) (Table 9-2). Following drainage of a pneumothorax or pleural effusion, the re-expanded lung may become acutely edematous. The edema usually develops within 2 hours of re-expansion, can progress for 1 or 2 days, and resolves within 5 to 7 days. Large pleural collections with complete collapse

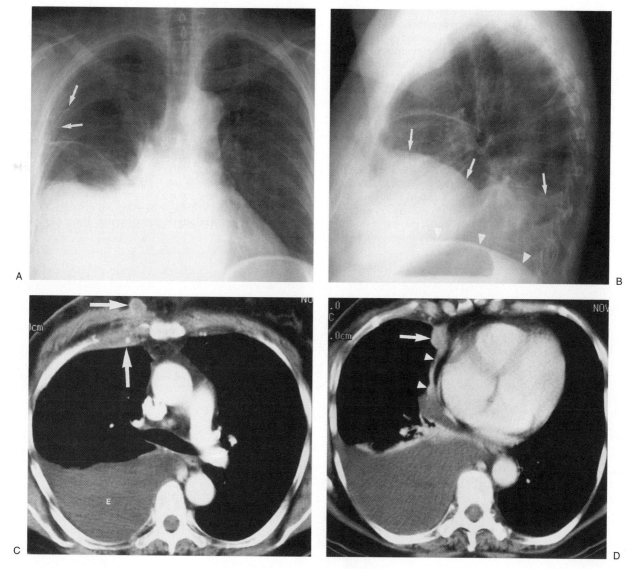

FIGURE 9-11. Malignant pleural effusion. A: PA chest radiograph of a 62-year-old woman with metastatic breast cancer who has had a right mastectomy and axillary node dissection (note surgical clips in right axilla; *arrows*) shows apparent elevation of the right hemidiaphragm. **B:** Lateral chest radiograph also shows apparent elevation of the right hemidiaphragm (*arrows*). The left hemidiaphragm is easily identified (*arrowheads*), as it is just superior to the stomach bubble. **C:** CT shows a large right pleural effusion (*E*) and metastatic breast cancer infiltrating the right chest wall (*arrows*). **D:** CT at a level inferior to (C) shows a metastatic soft tissue mass to the mediastinal pleura (*arrow*) and thickening of the mediastinal pleura (*arrowheads*).

TABLE 9-2

CAUSES OF A LARGE UNILATERAL PLEURAL EFFUSION

"ITCH"
Infection (empyema)
Tumor (primary bronchogenic cancer, metastasis, mesothelioma, lymphoma)
Chylous (ruptured thoracic duct, lymphoma)
Hemorrhage (trauma, either iatrogenic or otherwise)

of the underlying lung, especially when long-standing, predispose to the development of re-expansion pulmonary edema (Fig. 9-12).

Empyema is defined as pus in the pleural cavity. The diagnosis is made when the pleural fluid is obviously purulent, when organisms are identified in the fluid, or when the fluid has an elevated white blood cell count. An empyema is assumed to be present and drainage is indicated when there is associated pneumonia and the fluid pH is below 7.0 or the fluid glucose level is less than 40 mg/dL (9). The radiographic appearance of empyema is that of pleural fluid, which is usually unilateral but when bilateral is substantially greater in volume on the infected side (Fig. 9-13). In contrast to transudative pleural fluid collections, which typically have a smooth margin that is concave to the lung, an empyema will often have a smooth margin that is convex to the lung. Certain CT findings are suggestive of empyema and other exudative effusions, including thickening and enhancement of the parietal and visceral pleura (creating the "split pleura sign") after administration of intravenous contrast material (Figs. 9-14 and 9-15), thickening of the extrapleural subcostal tissues, and increased attenuation of the extrapleural fat. In some cases, empyema can be difficult to distinguish from lung abscess. In general, there is a sharply defined border between an empyema and the lung with dis-

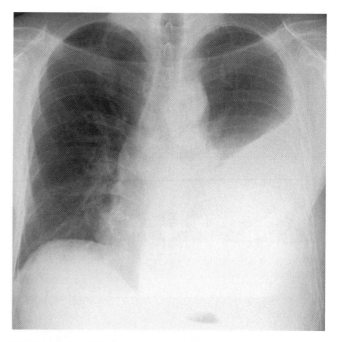

FIGURE 9-13. Tuberculous empyema. PA chest radiograph shows a large left pleural effusion. A large unilateral pleural effusion is worrisome for empyema, hemothorax, malignancy, or chylothorax.

placement and bowing of vessels and bronchi away from the empyema, whereas abscesses lack a discrete boundary between the lesion and the lung parenchyma. Empyemas are often elliptic and have a smooth inner surface, whereas abscesses are more often round and have a relatively thick wall. These features are not always reliable, however, and occasionally it may be impossible to distinguish parenchymal from pleural fluid collections (10).

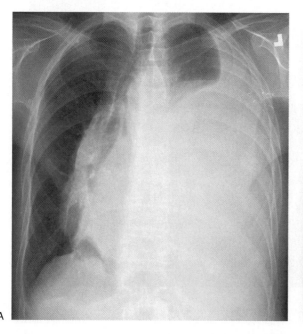
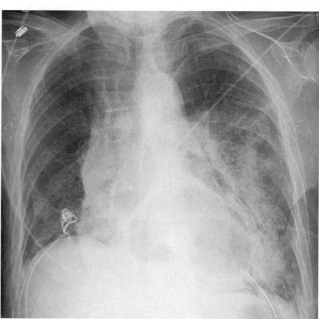

FIGURE 9-12. Re-expansion pulmonary edema. A: PA chest radiograph of a 78-year-old woman with metastatic breast cancer shows a large left pleural effusion associated with collapse of the left lung and shift of the mediastinum to the right. These findings suggest tension hydrothorax. **B:** PA chest radiograph after placement of a left chest tube and adequate drainage of pleural fluid shows re-expansion pulmonary edema on the left.

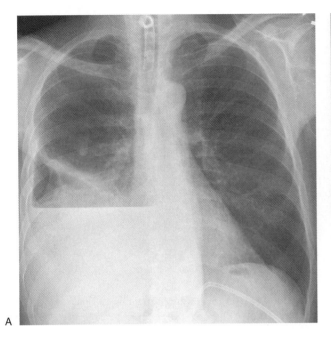

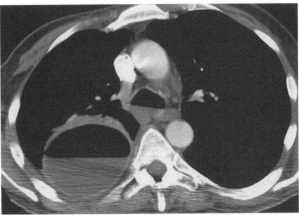

FIGURE 9-14. **Empyema. A:** PA chest radiograph of a 60-year-old man with right lower lobe pneumonia shows a large right hydropneumothorax with air–fluid level. There is an incidental calcified granuloma in the right mid lung. **B:** CT shows a round collection of air and fluid in the right pleural space. The thickened and enhancing separated pleural layers create the "split pleura" sign. Air within an empyema can be secondary to thoracentesis, bronchopleural fistula, or, rarely, a gas-forming organism.

A *chylothorax* contains fluid that is largely chyle (lymph of intestinal origin). Because chyle usually contains suspended fat in the form of chylomicrons, chylothorax fluid may be milky. Three main mechanisms account for chyle collections in the pleural space: (i) leakage from a discrete rupture of the thoracic duct or a large lymphatic vessel, (ii) a general oozing from pleural lymphatics, and (iii) passage of chylous ascites through the diaphragm (11). Approximately 50% of chylothoraces are of neoplastic origin, 25% are traumatic, and 15% are idiopathic (12). Lymphomas make up about 75% of the neoplastic lesions (13), and chylothorax can be the initial feature of lymphomas. The CT attenuation of chyle, despite its fat content, is usually indistinguishable from that of other effusions because chyle is protein rich.

Hemothorax usually results from trauma, either blunt or penetrating trauma to the chest or iatrogenic trauma (such as with central venous catheter placement) (14). A rapidly accumulating pleural fluid collection following trauma is likely of arterial origin. High-pressure bleeding from systemic vessels may be rapid and persistent, with the formation of a ten-sion hemothorax. CT of hemothorax may show areas of hyperdensity (15). With clotting of the blood, loculation occurs; if undrained, a hemothorax may eventually organize and cause pleural thickening (fibrothorax).

Malignant pleural effusions are usually the result of metastases (95% of cases) (16), with bronchogenic cancer accounting for 36% of cases, breast cancer for 25% (Fig. 9-16), lymphoma for 10%, and ovarian and gastric carcinoma for 5% or fewer (Fig. 9-17) (17). Although pleural effusion is often the major component of metastatic disease to the pleura, other findings include pleural nodules or extensive pleural thickening similar to that of mesothelioma. When the pleural metastases are unilateral, the CT findings may be indistinguishable from those of mesothelioma (18).

Malignant mesothelioma is a relatively rare primary tumor of the pleura. Approximately 80% of these lesions occur in individuals who have been exposed to asbestos (19). The lifetime risk for the development of mesothelioma in asbestos workers approaches 10%, and the average latency period is 35 years (20). Radiographic and CT findings include

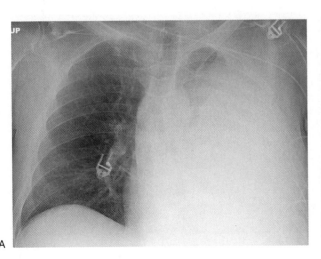

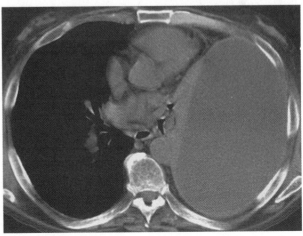

FIGURE 9-15. **Empyema. A:** PA chest radiograph of a 55-year-old man shows a large left pleural effusion, compression of the upper lung, and collapse of the lower lung. **B:** CT shows an elongated ovoid collection of fluid in the left pleural space and collapse of the adjacent lung.

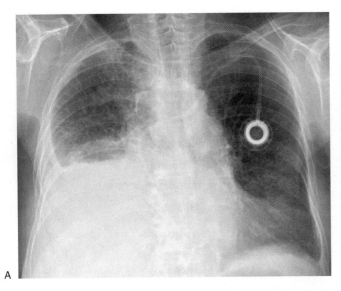
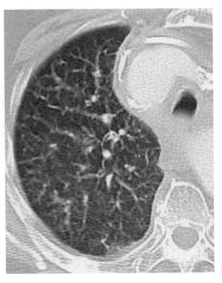

FIGURE 9-16. **Malignant pleural effusion. A:** PA chest radiograph of an 83-year-old woman with metastatic right breast cancer shows a large right pleural effusion and interstitial lung disease. **B:** CT after drainage of right pleural fluid shows nodular thickening of the vascular structures and pulmonary septae on the right, characteristic of lymphangitic carcinomatosis.

nodular or irregular thickening of the visceral and parietal pleura, variable ipsilateral volume loss in the hemithorax, ipsilateral pleural effusion, involvement of the interlobar fissures and mediastinal pleural surfaces, and often fixation of the mediastinum (Figs. 9-18 to 9-20) (21). Approximately 18% of cases are associated with invasion of the chest wall (21).

Pneumothorax

Pneumothorax is defined as a collection of air in the pleural cavity and is divided into spontaneous and traumatic types (Table 9-3). A pneumothorax occurring without an obvious precipitating traumatic event or in a healthy individual is a *pri-*

mary spontaneous pneumothorax. This type of pneumothorax is strongly associated with smoking and tall asthenic men (22). Most patients are between 20 and 40 years of age, and the male-to-female ratio is approximately 5 to 1 (23). The cause is nearly always the rupture of an apical pleural bulla. Without treatment, the likelihood of another pneumothorax is about 40%, and the chance of recurrence rises with each episode (23).

A pneumothorax developing without a precipitating traumatic event in a patient with predisposing lung disease is said to be a *spontaneous secondary pneumothorax* (Figs. 9-21 and 9-22). Chronic obstructive pulmonary disease is the most common cause of secondary spontaneous pneumothorax. About 0.5% of pneumothoraces are associated with lung metastases, of which 89% are caused by sarcomas, with osteogenic

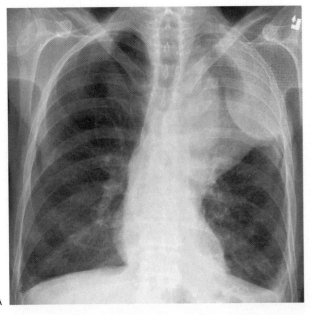
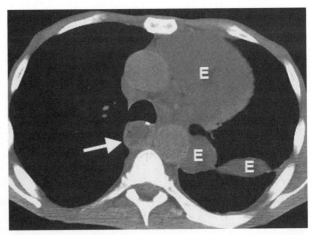

FIGURE 9-17. **Malignant pleural effusion. A:** PA chest radiograph of a 57-year-old man with metastatic esophageal carcinoma who had undergone esophagectomy and gastric pull-through shows a lobulated opacity in the left upper hemithorax. **B:** CT shows loculated pleural fluid (*E*) extending into the fissure. There is fluid in the intrathoracic stomach (*arrow*).

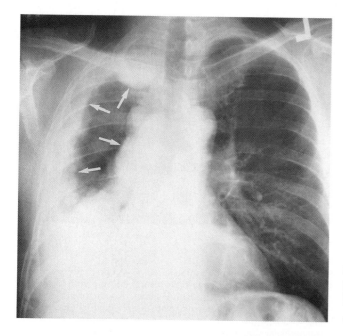

FIGURE 9-18. Malignant mesothelioma. PA chest radiograph of a 53-year-old man shows right pleural opacification with a lobulated contour that involves the entire pleural surface (*arrows*) and is associated with a "fixed mediastinum," meaning no shift right or left, and ipsilateral loss of lung volume, characteristic of malignant mesothelioma.

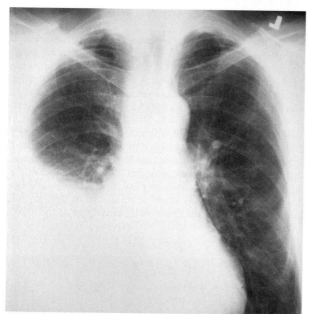

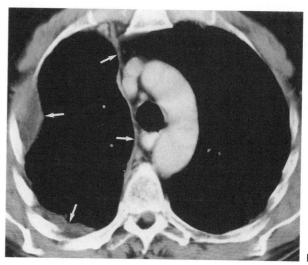

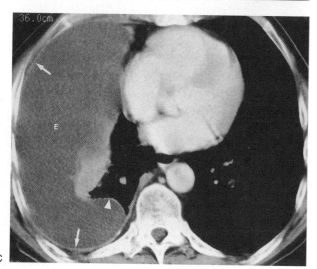

FIGURE 9-19. Malignant mesothelioma. A: PA chest radiograph of a 69-year-old man who worked at a manufacturing plant making brake linings and asbestos shingles shows a large unilateral right pleural effusion. **B:** CT shows thickening of the entire pleural surface (*arrows*). **C:** CT scan at a level inferior to (**B**) shows a large right pleural effusion (*E*) and thickening and enhancement of the parietal (*arrows*) and visceral (*arrowhead*) pleura.

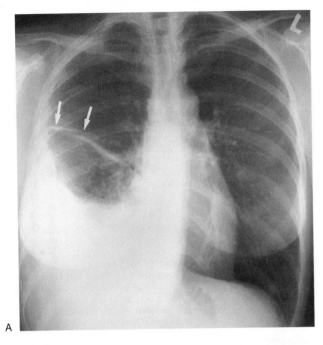

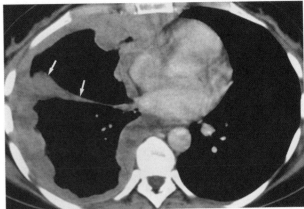

FIGURE 9-20. **Malignant mesothelioma. A:** PA chest radiograph of a 43-year-old man shows a large right pleural effusion with thickening of the minor fissure (*arrows*). **B:** CT shows that the pleural effusion is of higher attenuation compared with simple fluid (consistent with tumor within the pleural space); wraps around the entire pleural surface, including the fissure (*arrows*); and has a lobulated contour.

sarcoma being the most common (24,25). Catamenial pneumothorax is an uncommon disorder that occurs in women, probably caused by air entering the peritoneal cavity by way of the genital tract during menses and proceeding to the pleural cavity through diaphragmatic fenestrations. Catamenial pneumothorax occurs only in relation to the menses, appearing 1 day before or up to 3 days after menses. The pneumothorax is usually small and most often right sided (87%) (26). Recurrence is a characteristic feature of catamenial pneumothorax, and it may be prevented by pregnancy or drugs that suppress ovulation.

As with pleural effusion, the radiographic appearance of pneumothorax depends on the radiographic projection, the patient's position, and the presence or absence of pleural adhesion and subsequent loculation. In the upright patient, air rises in the pleural space and separates the lung from the chest wall, allowing the visceral–pleural line to become visible as a thin curvilinear opacity between vessel-containing lung and the avascular pneumothorax space. The pleural line remains fairly parallel to the chest wall. Curvilinear shadows projected over the lung apex that may mimic the visible visceral–pleural line of a pneumothorax include vascular lines, tubes, clothing, bedding, hair, scapulae, skin folds (Fig. 9-23), and the walls of bullae and cavities. Cysts, bullae, and cavities usually have inner margins that are concave to the chest wall rather than convex. In the supine patient, the highest part of the chest cavity lies anteriorly or anteromedially at the base near the diaphragm, and free pleural air rises to this region (Fig. 9-24). If the pneumothorax is small or moderate in size, the lung is not separated from the chest wall laterally or at the apex and

TABLE 9-3

CAUSES OF PNEUMOTHORAX IN ADULTS

Spontaneous
Primary spontaneous pneumothorax (young healthy smokers)
Chronic obstructive pulmonary disease
Asthma
Cystic fibrosis
Cavitary pneumonia
Pleural metastases (especially osteosarcoma)
Langerhan cell histiocytosis
Lymphangioleiomyomatosis/tuberous sclerosis
Sarcoidosis
Catamenial pneumothorax (related to female menses)

Traumatic
Thoracotomy
Thoracentesis
Percutaneous lung biopsy
Central venous catheter placement
Mechanical ventilation and barotrauma
Blunt or penetrating trauma to chest

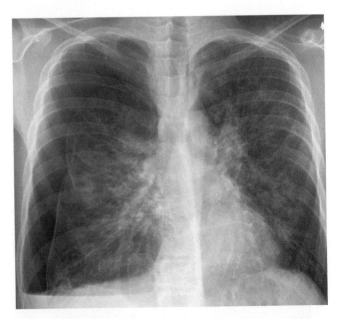

FIGURE 9-21. **Spontaneous secondary pneumothorax.** PA chest radiograph of an 18-year-old man with cystic fibrosis shows a large right hydropneumothorax and severe bilateral cystic bronchiectasis.

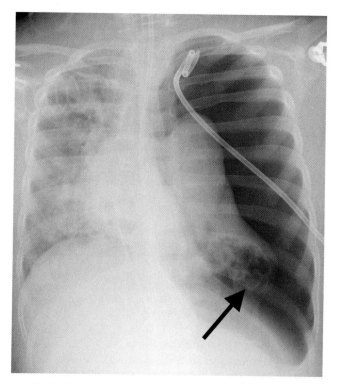

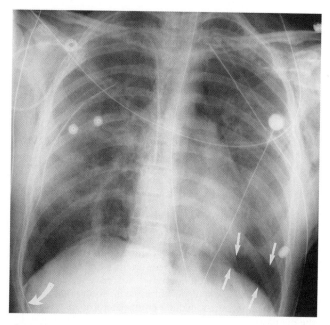

FIGURE 9-22. **Spontaneous secondary pneumothorax.** AP chest radiograph of a 3-year-old boy with respiratory syncytial virus pneumonia shows a large left pneumothorax with shift of the mediastinum to the right. The findings suggest a tension pneumothorax. Numerous cystic lesions, consistent with pneumatoceles, are seen in the collapsed left lung (*arrow*).

FIGURE 9-24. **Pneumothorax in a supine patient.** AP supine chest radiograph shows the "deep sulcus" sign of pneumothorax on the right (*curved arrow*) and a basilar pneumothorax on the left (*straight arrows*).

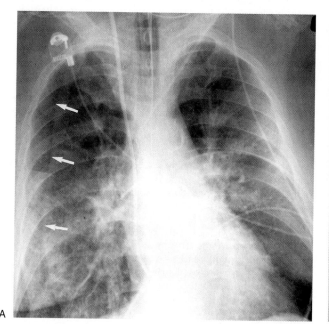

A

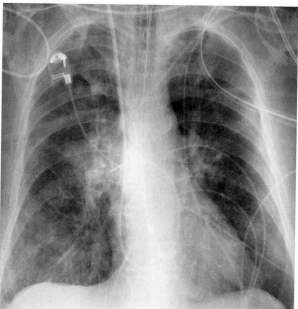

B

FIGURE 9-23. **Skin fold mimicking pneumothorax. A:** AP supine chest radiograph shows opacification of the right medial lung outlined by a sharp edge (skin fold; *arrows*). Note that the lung peripheral to this edge is not hyperlucent, a clue that there is no pneumothorax. **B:** AP upright chest radiograph obtained 1 hour later no longer shows the skin fold. Redundant skin can result in skin folds on the chest radiograph, especially when the patient is supine. Changing patient positioning is often useful in differentiating a skin fold from a pneumothorax.

TABLE 9-4

RADIOGRAPHIC SIGNS OF PNEUMOTHORAX IN THE SUPINE PATIENT

Relative increased lucency of the involved hemithorax
Increased sharpness of the adjacent mediastinal margin and diaphragm
Deep, sometimes "tonguelike" costophrenic sulcus
Visualization of the anterior costophrenic sulcus
Increased sharpness of the cardiac borders
Visualization of the inferior edge of the collapsed lung above the diaphragm
Depression of the ipsilateral hemidiaphragm

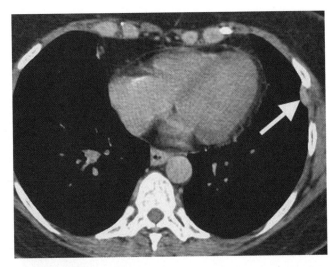

FIGURE 9-26. Malignant mesothelioma. CT scan of a 59-year-old man shows a solitary focal enhancing left pleural soft tissue lesion (*arrow*). At surgery, multiple additional lesions were seen studding the pleural surface.

therefore the pneumothorax may not be appreciated. Signs of pneumothorax in a supine patient are listed in Table 9-4 (27).

A large tension pneumothorax can be a life-threatening situation requiring rapid decompression. Radiologic signs of tension pneumothorax include contralateral displacement of the mediastinum, inferior displacement of the diaphragm, hyperlucent hemithorax, and ipsilateral collapse of the lung (Fig. 9-25).

Localized Pleural Tumors

Focal pleural tumors include localized fibrous tumors of pleura, lipomas, liposarcomas, and invasion of the pleura by adjacent bronchogenic carcinoma. Malignant mesothelioma and metastases may cause focal abnormalities (Fig. 9-26) but are most commonly associated with extensive involvement of the pleura, as previously discussed. Localized fibrous tumor of the pleura is either benign (60%) or malignant (40%) and has a relatively good prognosis when surgically excised (28). It occurs in all age groups, most commonly in patients older than 50, and it is not related to asbestos exposure. Forty percent of these tumors are attached to the pleura by a pedicle, and they may range from 1 to 39 cm in diameter. Calcification is present in 5% of cases.

The radiographic appearance is a mass with a smooth, sharply delineated contour with tapering margins that forms obtuse angles with the chest wall or mediastinum and displaces the adjacent lung parenchyma (Fig. 9-27). Pedunculated tumors may be mobile and change their position with respiration or posture.

Pleural lipomas are rare tumors usually found incidentally on the chest radiograph. On CT, a pleural lipoma appears as a well-defined mass of homogeneous fat attenuation having obtuse angles with the chest wall and displacing the adjacent pulmonary parenchyma (Fig. 9-28) (29). When the tumor is heterogeneous and has attenuation values greater than about 50 Hounsfield units, a liposarcoma should be suspected (Fig. 9-29) (30).

Diffuse Pleural Fibrosis (Fibrothorax)

Fibrothorax (fibrous obliteration of the pleural space) may develop as a result of organized hemorrhagic effusions, tuberculous effusions, other types of empyema, and extensive benign asbestos-related pleural disease. Asbestos-related diffuse pleural thickening is much less common than discrete pleural plaques and involves the visceral rather than the parietal pleura (31). Evidence of underlying parenchymal disease is usually seen in patients with prior tuberculosis or other empyema. Extensive calcification of the fibrothorax favors previous tuberculosis, empyema, hemothorax or trauma (Fig. 9-30) and is seldom seen with asbestos-related diffuse pleural thickening (32). Hemorrhagic effusion, tuberculosis, and other causes of empyema usually lead to unilateral pleural abnormalities, whereas benign asbestos pleurisy usually leads to bilateral pleural abnormalities, whether diffuse pleural thickening or pleural plaques. Involvement of the mediastinal pleura is more common with mesothelioma or other malignancies than with benign fibrothorax (18).

Pleural Plaques

Pleural plaques are circumscribed collections of dense collagenous connective tissue, which may or may not be calcified, and represent the most common manifestation of asbestos exposure (31). The latency period between exposure to asbestos and development of pleural plaques is approximately

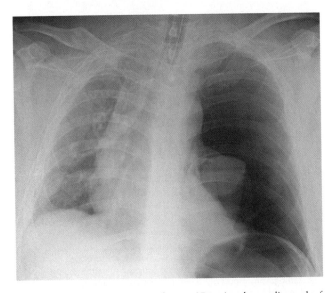

FIGURE 9-25. Tension pneumothorax. AP supine chest radiograph of a 35-year-old man involved in a motor vehicle crash shows a large left pneumothorax, collapse of the left lung, and shift of the mediastinum to the right. The findings suggest a tension pneumothorax, which requires immediate decompression.

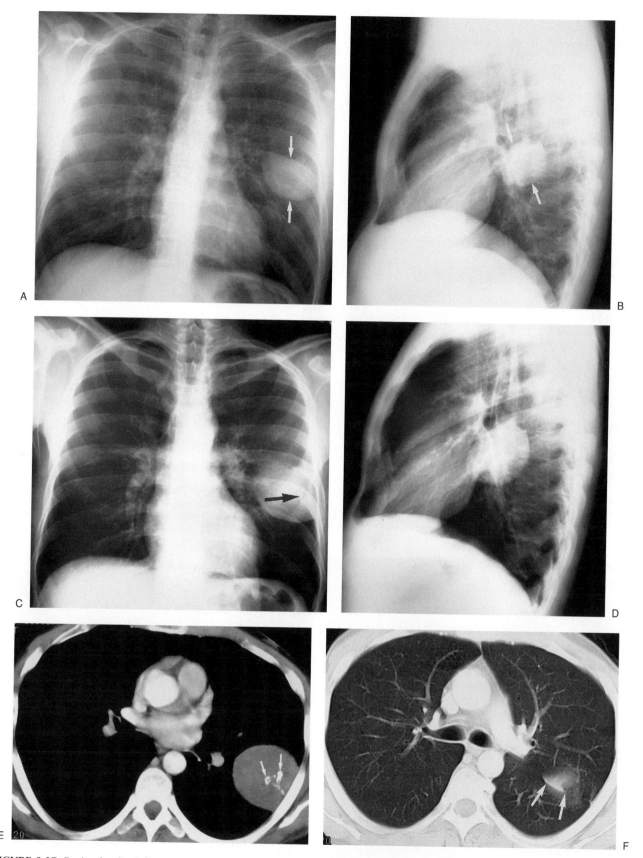

FIGURE 9-27. Benign localized fibrous tumor of the pleura. A: PA chest radiograph of a 32-year-old asymptomatic woman shows a well-circumscribed round mass in the left middle lung (*arrows*). **B:** Lateral view shows that the mass is positioned adjacent to the left major fissure (*arrows*). **C:** PA chest radiograph obtained 4 years later shows that the mass has increased in size. Faint calcification is now visible within the mass (*arrow*). **D:** Lateral view obtained at the same time as (C). **E:** CT shows that the mass is homogeneous, abuts the lateral pleural surface, and has coarse calcifications (*arrows*). **F:** CT with lung windowing shows that the top of the tumor abuts the major fissure (*arrows*).

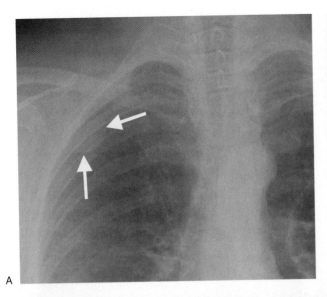

A

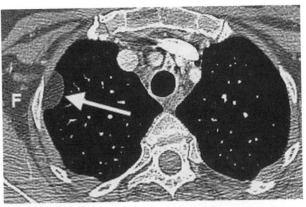

B

FIGURE 9-28. Pleural lipoma. A: PA chest radiograph coned to the right upper lobe shows a circumscribed mass (*arrows*) contiguous with the right lateral chest wall. **B:** CT shows that the mass (*arrow*) is of homogeneous fat attenuation (*F*).

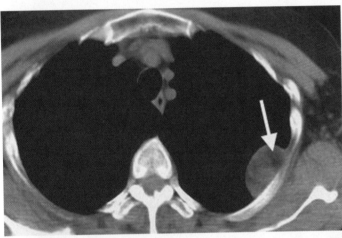

FIGURE 9-29. Benign pleural myelolipoma. CT of a 66-year-old woman shows a circumscribed mass abutting the left lateral chest wall. Although the mass contains central fat (*arrow*), the attenuation of the mass is heterogeneous, and a malignancy, such as liposarcoma, cannot be excluded. The mass was excised and found to be benign.

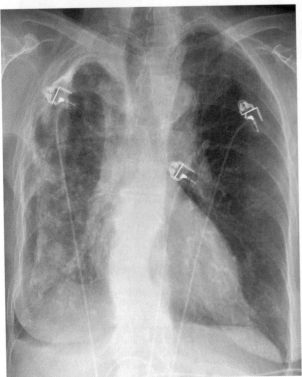

A

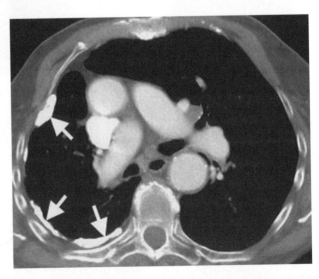

B

FIGURE 9-30. Old tuberculous empyema. A: PA chest radiograph shows dense calcification throughout the right hemithorax. **B:** CT shows dense pleural calcifications (*arrows*) involving only the right hemithorax, associated with loss of lung volume.

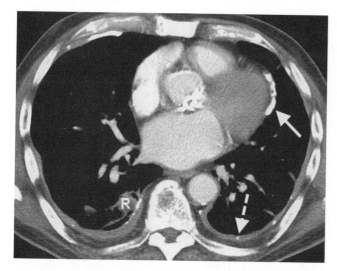

FIGURE 9-31. Calcified pleural and pericardial plaques. CT of an 82-year-old man with prior asbestos exposure shows calcified pericardial (*solid arrow*) and pleural (*dashed arrow*) plaques, in addition to diffuse pleural thickening and rounded atelectasis (*R*).

15 years. The plaques involve mainly the posterior and anterolateral aspects of the pleura, following the contours of the posterolateral seventh to 10th ribs, and the domes of the hemidiaphragms, and spare the lung apices and costophrenic angles. They almost always involve only the parietal pleura but occasionally may be seen in the visceral pleura in the interlobar fissures and sometimes involve the pericardium (Fig. 9-31). On chest radiographs, pleural plaques are unilateral in approximately 25% of cases (33), although more plaques are detected on CT than chest radiography. Pleural plaques are not premalignant, but detection of them is important for three main reasons: (i) in patients with associated interstitial lung disease, the presence of pleural plaques, in the appropriate clinical setting, strongly suggests the diagnosis of asbestosis; (ii) they are virtually pathognomonic of asbestos exposure and should prompt

an occupational history; and (iii) they may encourage a patient to stop smoking, because there is a synergistic interaction between asbestos exposure and smoking in the development of lung cancer. Asbestos-related pleural disease has five manifestations: (i) pleural plaque with or without calcification, (ii) asbestos-related pleural effusion, (iii) diffuse pleural thickening, (iv) rounded atelectasis, and (v) mesothelioma.

CHEST WALL

The thoracic contents are bounded by the chest wall, which consists of skin, subcutaneous tissues, muscles, clavicles, scapulae, ribs, sternum, and spine. Deformities and normal variants of chest wall anatomy are relatively common. Accessory cervical ribs, arising from the seventh cervical vertebra as enlarged costal elements, occur in approximately 0.5% to 1.5% of the population and may lead to thoracic outlet syndrome (34). The most common sternal deformity is pectus excavatum, which is easily appreciated on a lateral chest radiograph as posterior depression of the sternum. On a frontal radiograph, it may cause blurring of the right heart border and displacement of the heart to the left, mimicking a right middle lobe process (Fig. 9-32).

En face, chest wall lesions characteristically appear as homogeneous, often partly rounded opacities with a sharp medial edge and an ill-defined lateral margin. Tangentially, chest wall and localized pleural lesions are convex to the lung and sharply marginated, since they are covered on the lung aspect by pleura (Fig. 9-33). Chest wall masses usually have an obtuse angle of contact with the chest wall. On chest radiographs, localized lesions of the chest wall frequently cannot be distinguished from localized pleural lesions unless there is rib remodeling or destruction. Rib involvement is characteristic of a chest wall lesion and, except for the occasional invasive neoplastic or infective lesion (actinomycosis, tuberculosis), is rarely seen with pleural or lung processes. Masses involving the chest wall include infectious and benign and malignant neoplastic causes (Figs. 9-34 to 9-40) (Table 9-5).

(Text continues on page 160)

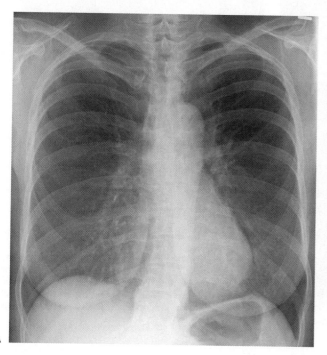
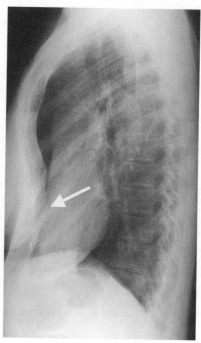

FIGURE 9-32. Pectus excavatum. A: PA chest radiograph of a 60-year-old man shows blurring of the right heart border and displacement of the mediastinum to the left. **B:** Lateral view shows posterior depression of the sternum (*arrow*).

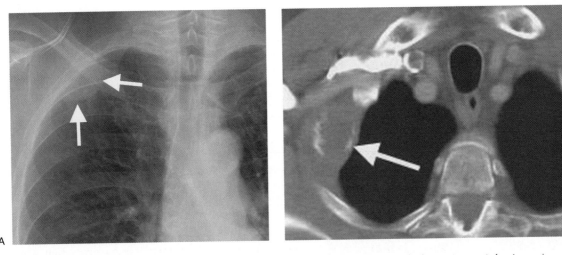

FIGURE 9-33. Lymphoma with rib involvement. A: PA chest radiograph shows a circumscribed mass (*arrows*) that is contiguous with the upper right lateral chest wall. B: CT shows the mass (*arrow*) and destruction of the right second rib.

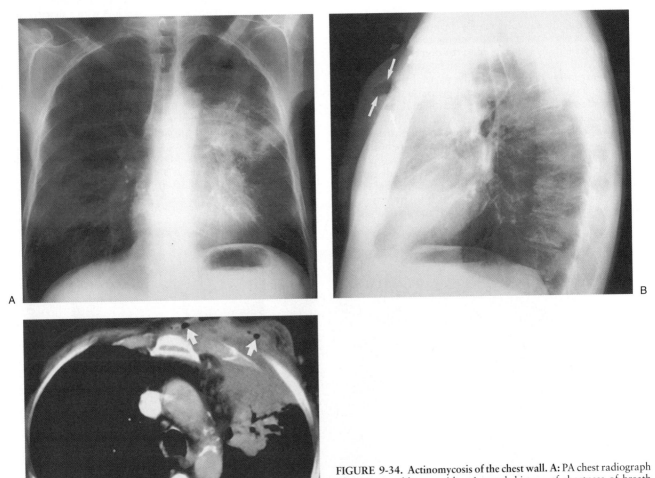

FIGURE 9-34. Actinomycosis of the chest wall. A: PA chest radiograph of a 58-year-old man with a 1-month history of shortness of breath and poor oral hygiene shows airspace disease in the left upper lobe. B: Lateral view shows extension of the left upper lobe pneumonia into the anterior chest wall. There is air within the swollen soft tissues of the chest wall (*arrows*). C: CT shows extension of the left upper lobe pneumonia into the anterior chest wall, along with numerous bubbles of air within the chest wall (*arrows*).

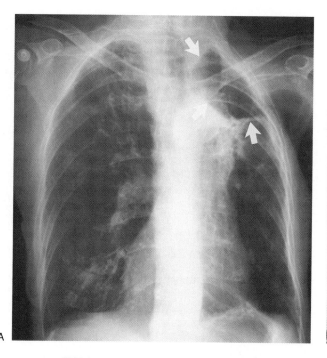

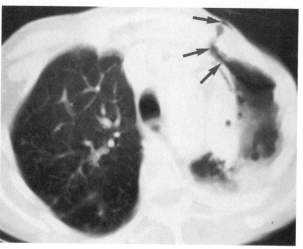

A   B

FIGURE 9-35. Tuberculous pneumonia with broncho-pleural-cutaneous fistula. A: AP upright chest radiograph of an 83-year-old woman with a history of left mastectomy and cobalt radiotherapy 30 years prior, along with a remote history of positive skin test for tuberculosis that was treated with appropriate drug therapy. Now, with a draining left chest wall wound at the surgical scar site, the patient's chest radiograph shows a cavitary mass in the left upper lobe (*arrows*) and scarring in the right upper lobe (unchanged compared with prior chest radiographs). **B:** CT shows air from the cavity communicating with the pleura and skin of the anterior chest wall (*arrows*), so-called empyema necessitatis. Analysis of the fluid draining from the chest wall revealed *Mycobacterium tuberculosis*. The patient was predisposed to the development of reactivation tuberculosis because she had recently been taking high doses of steroids to treat polymyalgia rheumatica.

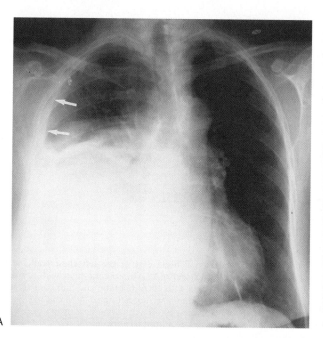

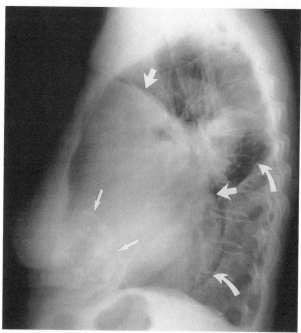

A   B

FIGURE 9-36. Chondrosarcoma of the sternum. A: PA chest radiograph of a 67-year-old woman shows a large area of opacification in the right lower hemithorax, a right pleural effusion (*arrows*), and shift of the mediastinum to the left. **B:** Lateral view shows amorphous calcifications overlying the anterior heart (*smaller arrows*), a large mass within the anterior mediastinum (*larger arrows*), and a pleural effusion (*curved arrows*). (*Continued*)

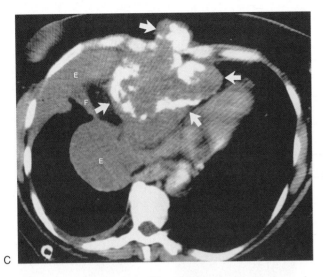

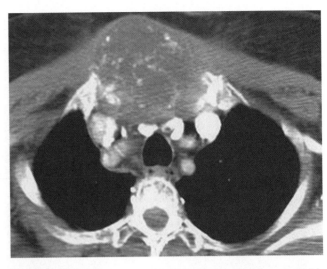

FIGURE 9-36. (*Continued*) **C:** CT, with patient prone, shows a calcified mass arising from the sternum (*arrows*) and a loculated right malignant pleural effusion (*E*) extending into the major fissure (*F*). Differential diagnosis included malignant teratoma, malignant thymoma, and osteogenic sarcoma.

FIGURE 9-37. Sternal metastases. CT of a 64-year-old woman with metastatic endometrial carcinoma shows complete destruction of the sternum by a large soft tissue mass with punctate and curvilinear calcifications.

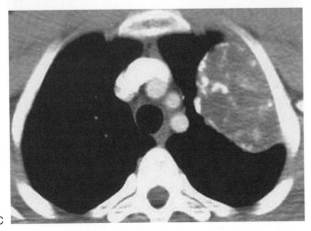

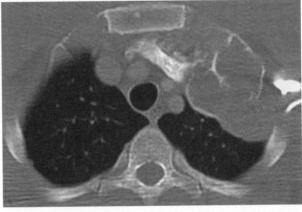

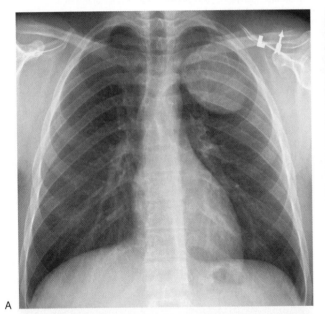

FIGURE 9-38. Aneurysmal bone cyst of the left chest wall. A: PA chest radiograph of a 19-year-old asymptomatic man with a history of Hodgkin disease treated with chemotherapy and radiation shows a circumscribed mass projecting over the left upper lobe and contiguous with the left upper chest wall. **B:** CT with bone windowing shows that the destructive mass arises from the left upper ribs. **C:** CT at a level inferior to (**B**) shows that the mass contains areas of dense calcification. The appearance of this new mass on routine chest radiography was suspicious for a radiation-induced sarcoma.

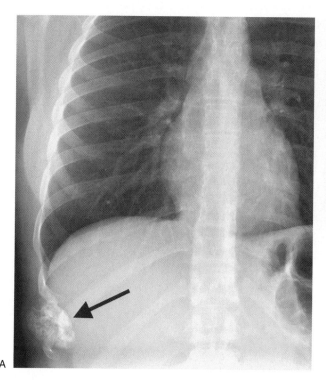

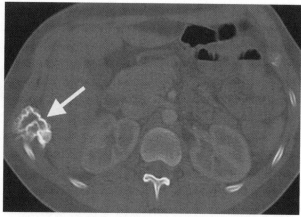

FIGURE 9-39. Benign rib osteochondroma. A: PA chest radiograph of a 20-year-old man shows a calcified mass arising form a lower right lateral rib (*arrow*). B: CT shows continuity of the cortex and marrow of the osteochondroma with that of the host rib, as well as characteristic extension of the osteochondroma on a stalk with a cauliflowerlike head.

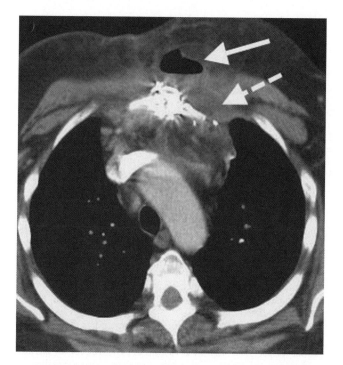

FIGURE 9-40. Sternal wound infection. CT scan of a 47-year-old man several weeks after coronary artery bypass grafting shows an air–fluid level (*solid arrow*) and a focal fluid collection (*dashed arrow*) in the presternal soft tissues and abnormal areas of high attenuation in the retrosternal area. Bacterial infection was confirmed during surgical debridement.

TABLE 9-5

MASSES INVOLVING THE CHEST WALL

Infections
  Mycobacteria
  Fungus
  Nocardia sp.
  Actinomycosis (associated with poor oral hygiene)

Neoplasms
  Bronchogenic carcinoma
  Metastases
  Lymphoma
  Malignant mesothelioma
  Malignant primary bone tumors (multiple myeloma, Ewing sarcoma)
  Benign primary bone tumors (osteochondroma, aneurysmal bone cyst)
  Kaposi sarcoma (in patients with AIDS)
  Bacillary angiomatosis (very vascular; seen in patients with AIDS)
  Neurogenic tumor
  Vascular malformation
  Lipoma/liposarcoma

AIDS, acquired immunodeficiency syndrome.

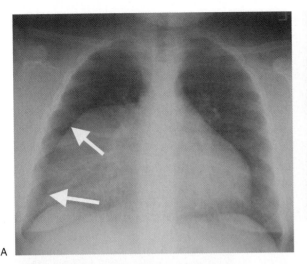

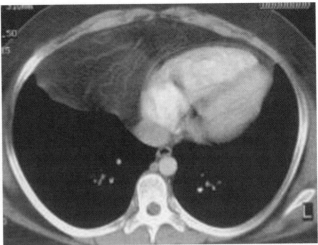

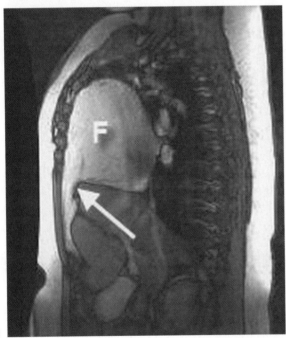

FIGURE 9-41. Foramen of Morgagni hernia. **A:** PA chest radiograph of an 11-year-old girl shows an abnormal right mediastinal contour (*arrows*) and loss of the normal right heart border. **B:** CT shows fat and prominent omental vascular structures anterior to the heart. **C:** Sagittal T1-weighted magnetic resonance image shows a defect in the anterior diaphragm (*arrow*) and herniation of high-signal fat (*F*) into the anterior chest.

DIAPHRAGM

The diaphragm consists of a large, dome-shaped central tendon with a sheet of striated muscle radiating from the central tendon to attach to the seventh through 12th ribs and to the xiphisternum (35). The two crura arise from the upper three lumbar vertebrae and arch upward and forward to form the margins of the aortic hiatus and esophageal hiatus. The diaphragm has a smooth dome shape in most individuals, but a scalloped outline is also common. Radiographically, in most people, the right hemidiaphragm is 1.5 to 2.5 cm higher than the left, but the two hemidiaphragms are at the same level in about 9% of the population, and the left hemidiaphragm is higher than the right (by less than 1 cm) in about 3% of the population (36). Incomplete muscularization, known as *eventration*, is common and frequently involves the anteromedial portion of the hemidiaphragm (usually the right, but occasionally affecting the left), producing a smooth hump on the contour of the diaphragm.

Congenital hernias of the diaphragm are common. Ninety percent of these are Bochdalek hernias, which arise postero-laterally because of failure of the costal and vertebral portions of the diaphragm to fuse. They are more common on the left than the right. Small incidental Bochdalek hernias are seen frequently on CT, often with no more than a small amount of retroperitoneal fat herniating through the defect. Morgagni hernias, most commonly seen on the right, arise anteromedially from failure of the sternal and costal portions of the diaphragm to fuse (Fig. 9-41).

When unilateral elevation of the diaphragm is seen on chest radiography, five diagnostic possibilities should be considered (Table 9-6) (Figs. 9-42 and 9-43). First, however, it is important to determine the chronicity of the elevation, since stability for 2 or more years on chest radiography makes a malignant cause highly unlikely and makes acute processes such as lung collapse and subdiaphragmatic abscess less likely. Subpulmonic effusion was discussed earlier in this chapter. Diaphragmatic rupture was discussed in Chapter 8, and atelectasis is discussed in Chapter 11.

The phrenic nerves, which arise from the third through fifth cervical nerves, supply the diaphragm ("C3, 4, 5 keep the diaphragm alive"). The right phrenic nerve descends at the right side of the superior vena cava and right atrium, in front of the

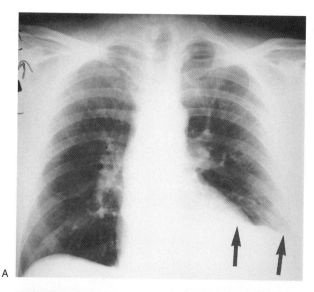

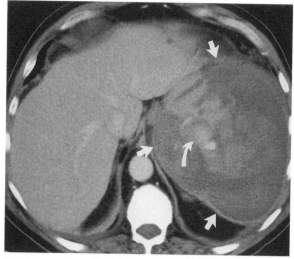

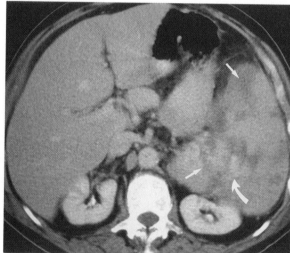

FIGURE 9-42. Elevated diaphragm secondary to subdiaphragmatic splenic hematoma. A: AP upright chest radiograph of a 68-year-old man with left flank pain and chronic lymphocytic lymphoma shows elevation of the left hemidiaphragm (*arrows*). B: CT shows a large subcapsular splenic hematoma (*straight arrows*). The high-attenuation material within the hematoma represents acute bleeding (*curved arrow*). C: CT at a level inferior to (B) shows multiple low-attenuation areas within the spleen from spontaneous splenic rupture (*straight arrows*) and high-attenuation material from acute bleeding (*curved arrow*).

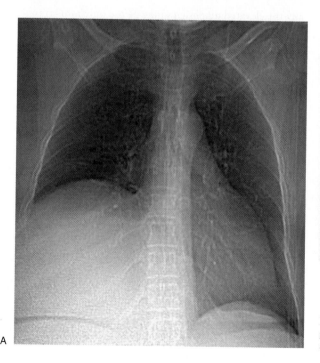

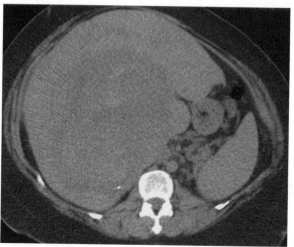

FIGURE 9-43. Elevated diaphragm secondary to hepatic hemangioma. A: CT scout image shows elevation of the right hemidiaphragm. B: Axial CT shows a large hepatic mass.

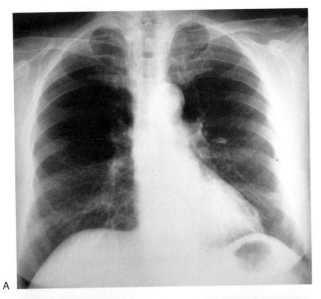

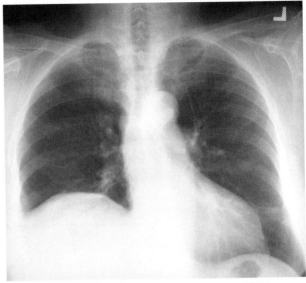

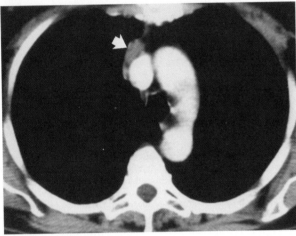

FIGURE 9-44. **Bronchogenic carcinoma invading the phrenic nerve. A:** PA chest radiograph of a 74-year-old woman shows normal positioning of the hemidiaphragms. **B:** PA chest radiograph obtained 1 year later shows elevation of the right hemidiaphragm and no evidence of mediastinal mass. **C:** CT shows a homogeneous soft tissue mass adjacent to the superior vena cava (*arrows*), which proved to be a bronchogenic adenocarcinoma invading the right phrenic nerve. This case illustrates the significance of new diaphragmatic elevation in an adult, even when no mediastinal mass is seen on the chest radiograph.

root of the right lung, between the pericardium and mediastinal pleura. The left phrenic nerve descends between the left subclavian and left common carotid arteries, lateral to the vagus nerve and the arch of the aorta. It passes in front of the root of the left lung between the mediastinal pleura and the pericardium, and its branches pierce the diaphragm immediately to the left of the pericardium. Tumor invading the phrenic nerve on either side can result in elevation of the ipsilateral diaphragm and should always be considered as the cause of an abnormally elevated diaphragm in patients over age 35 unless proven to be stable for 2 years or more on prior chest radiographs (Fig. 9-44). The chest radiograph may not show the tumor itself, and occasion-

ally the elevated diaphragm may be the only radiographic clue to an underlying neoplasm.

References

1. Black LF. The pleural space and pleural fluid. *Mayo Clin Proc.* 1972;47:493–506.
2. Im JG, Webb WR, Rosen A, Gamsu G. Costal pleura: appearances at high-resolution CT. *Radiology.* 1989;171:125–131.
3. Groskin SA. Radiologic–pathologic correlations. In: Groskin SA, ed. *Heitzman's The Lung.* St. Louis, MO: Mosby; 1993:575–609.
4. Light RW. *Pleural Diseases.* Philadelphia: Lea & Febiger; 1983.
5. Jay SJ. Diagnostic procedures for pleural disease. *Clin Chest Med.* 1985;6:33–48.
6. Ruskin JA, Gurney JW, Thorsen MK, et al. Detection of pleural effusions on supine chest radiographs. *AJR Am J Roentgenol.* 1987;148:681–683.
7. Moskowitz H, Platt RT, Schacher R, Mellins H. Roentgen visualization of minute pleural effusion. *Radiology.* 1973;109:33–35.
8. McLoud TC, Flower CDR. Imaging the pleura: sonography, CT, and MR imaging. *AJR Am J Roentgenol.* 1991;156:1145–1153.
9. Light RW. Diseases of the pleura, mediastinum, chest wall, and diaphragm. In: George RB, Light RW, Matthay MA, et al, eds. *Chest Medicine.* Baltimore: Williams & Wilkins; 1990:318–412.
10. Naidich DP, Zerhouni EA, Siegelman SS. Pleura and chest wall. In: Naidich DP, Zerhouni EA, Siegelman SS, eds. *Computed Tomography and Magnetic Resonance of the Thorax.* 2nd ed. New York: Raven Press; 1991:407–471.
11. Nix JT, Albert M, Dugas JE, et al. Chylothorax and chylous ascites: a study of 302 selected cases. *Am J Gastroenterol.* 1957;28:40–53.

TABLE 9-6

UNILATERAL ELEVATED DIAPHRAGM

"PAPER"

Phrenic nerve paralysis (malignant involvement, surgical trauma)

Atelectasis/Abdominal mass

Postsurgical abdominal abscess

Effusion (subpulmonic; creates appearance of elevated diaphragm)

Rupture (trauma)

12. Sassoon CS, Light RW. Chylothorax and pseudochylothorax. *Clin Chest Med.* 1985;6:163–171.
13. MacFarlane JR, Holman CW. Chylothorax. *Am Rev Respir Dis.* 1972;105:287–291.
14. Groskin SA. Selected topics in chest trauma. *Radiology.* 1992;183:605–617.
15. Wolverson MK, Crepps LF, Sundaram M, et al. Hyperdensity of recurrent hemorrhage at body computed tomography: incidence and morphologic variation. *Radiology.* 1983;148:779–784.
16. Godwin JD, ed. *Computed Tomography of the Chest.* Philadelphia: Lippincott; 1984:130–137.
17. Sahn SA. Malignant pleural effusion. In: Fishman AP, ed. *Pulmonary Diseases and Disorders.* 2nd ed. New York: McGraw-Hill; 1988:2159–2169.
18. Leung AN, Müller NL, Miller RR. CT in differential diagnosis of diffuse pleural disease. *AJR Am J Roentgenol.* 1990;154:487–492.
19. Mossman BT, Gee JBL. Asbestos-related diseases. *N Engl J Med.* 1989;320:1721–1730.
20. Antman KH. Clinical presentation and natural history of benign and malignant mesothelioma. *Semin Oncol.* 1981;8:313–320.
21. Kawashima A, Libshitz HI. Malignant pleural mesothelioma: CT manifestations in 50 cases. *AJR Am J Roentgenol.* 1990;155:965–969.
22. Jansveld CAF, Dijkman JH. Primary spontaneous pneumothorax and smoking. *Br Med J.* 1975;4:559–560.
23. Killen DA, Gobbel WG. *Spontaneous Pneumothorax.* Boston: Little, Brown; 1968.
24. Dines DE, Cortese DA, Brennan MD, et al. Malignant pulmonary neoplasms predisposing to spontaneous pneumothorax. *Mayo Clin Proc.* 1973;48:541–544.
25. Janetos GP, Ochsner SF. Bilateral pneumothorax in metastatic osteogenic sarcoma. *Am Rev Respir Dis.* 1963;88:73–76.
26. Carter EJ, Ettensohn DB. Catamenial pneumothorax. *Chest.* 1990;98:713–716.
27. Tocino IM, Miller MH, Fairfax WR. Distribution of pneumothorax in the supine and semirecumbent critically ill adult. *AJR Am J Roentgenol.* 1985;144:901–905.
28. England DM, Hochholzer L, McCarthy MJ. Localized benign and malignant fibrous tumors of the pleura: a clinicopathologic review of 223 cases. *Am J Surg Pathol.* 1989;13:640–658.
29. Buxton RC, Tan CS, Khine NM, et al. Atypical transmural thoracic lipoma: CT diagnosis. *J Comput Assist Tomogr.* 1988;12:196–198.
30. Munk PL, Müller NL. Pleural liposarcoma: CT diagnosis. *J Comput Assist Tomogr.* 1988;12:709–710.
31. Schwartz DA. New developments in asbestos-related pleural disease. *Chest.* 1991;99:191–198.
32. Friedman AC, Fiel SB, Radecki PD, et al. Computed tomography of benign pleural and pulmonary parenchymal abnormalities related to asbestos exposure. *Semin Ultrasound CT MR.* 1990;11:393–408.
33. Withers BF, Ducatman AM, Yang WN. Roentgenographic evidence for predominant left-sided location of unilateral pleural plaques. *Chest.* 1984;95:1262–1264.
34. Kurihara Y, Yakushiji YK, Matsumoto J, et al. The ribs: anatomic and radiologic considerations. *RadioGraphics.* 1999;19:105–119, 151–152.
35. Heitzman ER. The diaphragm: radiologic correlations with anatomy and pathology. *Clin Radiol.* 1990;42:15–19.
36. Felson B. *Chest Roentgenology.* Philadelphia: WB Saunders; 1973.

CHAPTER 10

UPPER LUNG DISEASE, INFECTION, AND IMMUNITY

LEARNING OBJECTIVES

1. List an appropriate differential diagnosis for upper lung disease seen on chest radiography or computed tomography (CT).
2. Describe the radiographic classification of sarcoidosis.
3. State the three most common locations (Garland triad) for adenopathy to occur in the chest of patients with sarcoidosis.
4. List four common etiologies of "eggshell" calcified lymph nodes in the chest.
5. Recognize progressive massive fibrosis secondary to silicosis on chest radiography and CT.
6. Recognize and describe the typical appearance of cystic fibrosis on chest radiography and CT.
7. Describe the radiologic manifestations of primary pulmonary tuberculosis.
8. Name the most common segmental sites of involvement for reactivation tuberculosis in the lung.
9. Define a Ghon lesion (calcified pulmonary parenchymal granuloma) and Ranke complex (calcified node and Ghon lesion); recognize both on a chest radiograph and CT and describe their significance.
10. Suggest the possibility of radiation as a cause of new upper lung opacification on a chest radiograph of a patient with evidence of mastectomy and/or axillary node dissection or known head and neck cancer.
11. Describe the acute and chronic phases of radiation-caused changes in the lungs, including the time course and typical chest radiograph and CT appearances.
12. Recognize the typical appearance of irregular lung cysts

13. on chest CT of a patient with Langerhan cell histiocytosis.
13. Name the major categories of disease that cause chest radiographic or CT abnormalities in the immunocompromised patient.
14. Other than typical bacterial infection, name two important infections and two important neoplasms to consider in patients with acquired immunodeficiency syndrome (AIDS) and chest radiographic or CT abnormalities.
15. Describe the typical chest radiographic and CT appearances of Kaposi sarcoma.
16. Describe the chest radiograph and CT appearances of *Pneumocystis jiroveci* pneumonia.
17. Name four important etiologies of hilar and mediastinal lymphadenopathy in patients with AIDS.
18. Describe the time course and chest radiographic appearance of a blood transfusion reaction.
19. Describe the chest radiographic and CT appearances of a miliary pattern and provide a differential diagnosis.
20. Name and describe the types of pulmonary *Aspergillus* disease.
21. Identify an intracavitary fungus ball on chest radiography and CT.
22. Name the most common pulmonary infections that occur after solid organ (e.g., liver, renal, lung, cardiac) and bone marrow transplantation.
23. Describe the chest radiographic and CT findings of posttransplant lymphoproliferative disorders.

Pulmonary infections are a major cause of morbidity and mortality, especially in immunocompromised patients. Immunocompromised patients have altered immune mechanisms and are predisposed to opportunistic infections. Numerous factors are associated with an immunocompromised state, including but not limited to diabetes; renal or liver failure; advanced age; bone marrow or solid organ transplantation; acquired immunodeficiency syndrome (AIDS); presence of access lines (e.g., intravenous lines, endotracheal tubes, chest tubes); splenectomy, hospital environment (predisposing to nosocomial pneumonia); underlying malignancy; drug therapy (e.g., steroids, chemotherapy); and immune deficiencies (e.g., hypogammaglobulinemia). Some of the clinically important infections and other diseases seen in immunocompetent and immunocompromised patients tend to have an upper lung–predominant distribution (e.g., mycobacterial and fungal dis-

ease). Recognition of an upper lung distribution of disease helps the clinician to form an appropriate differential diagnosis. This chapter begins with a discussion of upper lung disease, including infectious and noninfectious causes, and continues with a review of the disorders that occur in immunocompromised individuals and their radiographic appearances.

UPPER LUNG DISEASE

Upper lung refers to the upper one third of the lung, which includes the majority of the upper lobes and the uppermost portion of the superior segments of the lower lobes. In the normal upright lung, blood flow and ventilation predominate in the lung base; in many lung disorders, however, the greatest degree of abnormality occurs in the upper lung. Alterations in

TABLE 10-1

UPPER LUNG DISEASE

"SHRIMP"
Sarcoidosis
Histiocytosis, Langerhan cell
Radiation pneumonitis (cancers of head/neck and breast)
Infection (tuberculous, fungal)
Metastases[a]
Pneumoconioses[b] (silicosis, coal miner's)

"CASSET"
Cystic fibrosis
Ankylosing spondylitis
Silicosis
Sarcoidosis
Eosinophilic granulomatosis (Langerhan cell histiocytosis)
Tuberculous, fungal infection

[a] See Chapter 7.
[b] See Chapter 3.

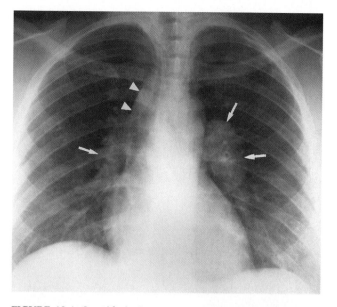

FIGURE 10-1. Sarcoidosis. Posteroanterior (PA) chest radiograph of a 31-year-old woman with class I sarcoidosis shows right paratracheal (*arrowheads*) and bilateral hilar (*arrows*) lymphadenopathy. This pattern of lymphadenopathy is classic for sarcoidosis and is referred to as the 1-2-3 sign or Garland triad.

ventilation–perfusion, lymphatic flow, metabolism, and mechanics are proposed as pathogenic factors in upper lung localization of lung disease (1). Two mnemonics, "SHRIMP" and "CASSET," can be used to recall common and uncommon disorders occurring in the upper lungs (Table 10-1). Because it may be difficult to appreciate a predominantly upper lung distribution of disease on chest radiography, it is useful to consider the differential diagnoses given in Table 10-1, even if the disease appears diffuse, any time the upper lungs are as affected as much or more than the middle and lower lungs.

SARCOIDOSIS

Sarcoidosis is a common systemic disease of unknown etiology characterized by widespread development of noncaseating granulomas. These granulomas are nonspecific and resemble those in many other granulomatous processes, except for tuberculosis, a disease in which caseous necrosis of granulomas is usually seen. Sarcoidosis is ten times more common in African-Americans than in Caucasians (2). Most patients who present with sarcoidosis are between the ages of 20 and 40, but the disease occurs as early as 1 year and as late as 80 years of age (3). The disease is two to three times more common in African-American women than in African-American men (3). The lung is the most commonly involved organ in patients with sarcoidosis and accounts for most of the morbidity and mortality, with an overall mortality rate between 2.2% and 7.6% (3).

Sarcoidosis can be classified according to its appearance on the chest radiograph (Table 10-2) (4). Patients commonly, but not necessarily, progress through each class, and the class at presentation can, but does not always, correlate with prognosis (5). Forty-five percent to 65% of patients are class I at the time of presentation. Lymphadenopathy is the most common intrathoracic manifestation of sarcoidosis and occurs in 75% to 80% of patients at some point in their illness (6). The classic pattern of lymphadenopathy is bilateral hilar and right paratracheal nodal enlargement, the so-called Garland triad or 1-2-3 sign (Figs. 10-1 and 10-2), although any mediastinal nodes can be and frequently are involved. The hilar lymph nodes are usually symmetric in appearance and can be massively enlarged ("potato nodes") but are usually clear of the cardiac borders, a feature that helps distinguish sarcoidosis from lymphomatous lymphadenopathy, as the latter usually abuts the cardiac margins. Of patients with class I disease at initial examination, about 60% go on to complete resolution (7), with parenchymal disease occurring in the remaining patients. Nodal calcification is seen in up to 20% of cases (8), and in some of these cases (approximately 5%), the calcification is of a peripheral "eggshell" pattern (Figs. 10-3 and 10-4). Eggshell calcification is largely limited to sarcoidosis and silicosis, but it can be seen in other disorders (Table 10-3) (9).

Parenchymal disease is seen on chest radiography at the time of presentation in approximately half of patients with sarcoidosis. Radiographic patterns of parenchymal disease include reticulonodular opacities, ill-defined opacities that have an appearance of alveolar filling, large nodules, and lung fibrosis. Reticulonodular opacities are the most common pattern, seen in 75% to 90% of patients with parenchymal disease; the opacities are usually bilaterally symmetric with a distribution predominantly in the middle and upper lungs (10) (Fig. 10-5). In 10% to 20% of patients, opacities with airspace features develop, which can be ill defined or focal, nodular, and well defined. The term *alveolar sarcoid* refers to this pattern, although the "airspace" disease represents an interstitial process that compresses and obliterates alveoli. Alveolar sarcoid generally consists of bilateral, multifocal, poorly defined opacities showing a predilection for the peripheral lungs (11) (Fig. 10-6). The peripheral distribution is particularly well seen with computed tomography (CT).

TABLE 10-2

CLASSIFICATION OF SARCOIDOSIS ON CHEST RADIOGRAPHY

0	Normal chest radiograph
I	Hilar or mediastinal nodal enlargement only
II	Nodal enlargement and parenchymal disease
III	Parenchymal disease only
IV	End-stage lung (pulmonary fibrosis)

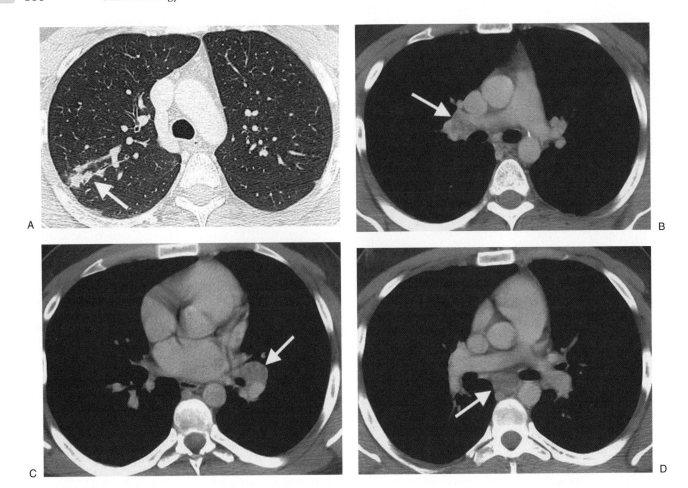

FIGURE 10-2. Sarcoidosis. A: CT of a 23-year-old woman shows ill-defined nodules in a bronchovascular distribution (*arrow*) in the right upper lobe. B: CT with mediastinal windowing shows right hilar lymphadenopathy (*arrow*). C: CT at the level of the inferior pulmonary veins shows left hilar lymphadenopathy (*arrow*). D: CT at the level of the lower lobe pulmonary arteries shows subcarinal lymphadenopathy (*arrow*).

Sarcoid granulomas may resolve completely or heal by fibrosis. Pulmonary fibrosis occurs in approximately 20% of patients with sarcoidosis, and the radiologic features are considered by some authors to be almost pathognomonic. The findings consist of permanent, coarse, linear opacities radiating laterally from the hilum into adjacent upper and middle

lungs. Bullae can form in the upper lungs. The hila are pulled upward and outward, and vessels and fissures are distorted. The fibrosis is occasionally so severe that massive parahilar opacities in the middle and upper lungs, resembling those of progressive massive fibrosis of silicosis, are seen.

CT can define the anatomic location of parenchymal sarcoid granulomas much more accurately (12–14). The most common finding of sarcoidosis on CT is multiple, 1- to 5-mm nodules, usually with irregular margins, in a lymphatic distribution (bronchovascular margins, along interlobular septa, subpleurally, and in the center of secondary pulmonary lobules) (Fig. 10-7). Septal thickening from sarcoidosis has a beaded appearance, a feature that helps distinguish it from pulmonary edema, in which the septal thickening is typically smooth. Patchy ground-glass opacities are seen in about 50% of

FIGURE 10-3. Sarcoidosis. CT shows precarinal lymphadenopathy with rim calcification (*arrow*). This pattern of calcification is referred to as "eggshell" calcification and is commonly seen with sarcoidosis.

TABLE 10-3

COMMON CAUSES OF "EGGSHELL" CALCIFICATION OF NODES IN THE CHEST

"SIT"
Sarcoidosis
Silicosis
Infection (tuberculous, fungal)
Treated lymphoma

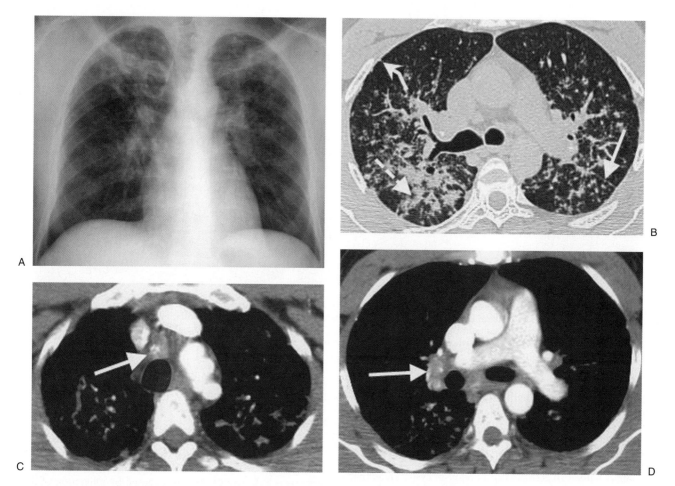

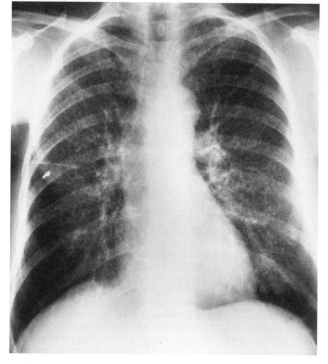

FIGURE 10-4. Sarcoidosis. A: PA chest radiograph of a 37-year-old man shows bilateral upper lobe nodular disease and hilar enlargement (class II). **B:** CT shows nodules of varying size along the fissures (*straight solid arrow*) and bronchovascular bundles (*dashed arrow*) and in a subpleural location (*curved solid arrow*). **C:** CT with mediastinal windowing shows central calcification of right paratracheal lymph nodes (*arrow*). **D:** CT at a lower level shows calcification of right hilar nodes (*arrow*).

FIGURE 10-5. Sarcoidosis. PA chest radiograph shows reticulonodular opacities scattered diffusely throughout the upper and middle lungs. Parenchymal disease without lymphadenopathy indicates class III sarcoidosis.

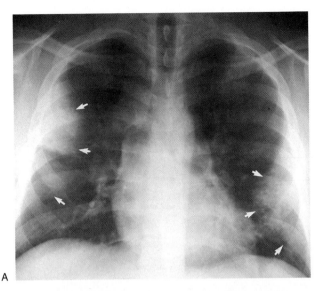
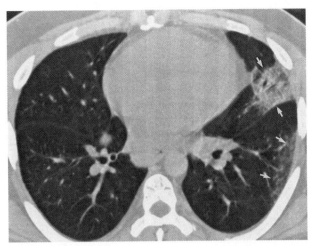

FIGURE 10-6. Sarcoidosis. A: PA chest radiograph of a 28-year-old man with mild shortness of breath shows right paratracheal and bilateral hilar lymphadenopathy and bilateral peripheral areas of consolidation (*arrows*). B: CT shows multifocal opacities in the periphery of the left lung (*arrows*). This pattern of sarcoidosis is referred to as alveolar sarcoid, although pathologically it is seen to be an interstitial process.

patients with sarcoidosis and rarely may be the only CT abnormality (Fig. 10-8). Fibrosis is better characterized on CT than on chest radiography. CT can show findings of sarcoidosis when the chest radiograph is normal, and patients can have a normal CT study yet have sarcoidosis proved by lung biopsy (13).

Fungus balls (mycetomas) can develop in cystic areas that develop from sarcoidosis, and sarcoidosis is the second most common predisposing condition (after tuberculosis) leading to the development of mycetoma (15). Hemoptysis resulting from mycetoma formation can be life threatening. Mycetomas occur in the upper lobes and should be suspected when new opacities are seen in an area of chronic cystic or bullous disease, especially when they are accompanied by new apical pleural or extrapleural opacity on chest radiography. There are myriad other atypical features of sarcoidosis, including pleural effusions, pleural thickening, cavitary nodules, bronchostenosis,

pulmonary artery hypertension from periarterial granulomatosis (Fig. 10-9), cor pulmonale, and pneumothorax from chronic fibrosis.

SILICOSIS

Silicosis is a disease of the lungs caused by inhalation of dust containing silicon dioxide, or silica, the predominant constituent of the earth's crust. Silica dust is prevalent in mining, quarrying, and tunneling operations. Occupations associated with the development of silicosis include mining of heavy metals, the pottery industry, sandblasting, foundry work, and stonemasonry. When silica particles are inhaled, they are deposited in the alveoli and engulfed by alveolar macrophages,

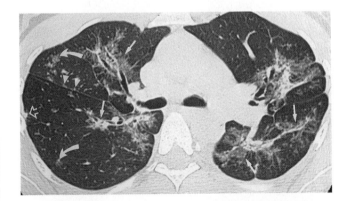

FIGURE 10-8. Sarcoidosis. CT image of a 46-year-old woman with mild shortness of breath shows bilateral areas of abnormal opacification distributed along the central and peripheral bronchovascular bundles (*straight arrows*). Some of the opacities are of ground-glass attenuation, allowing visualization of underlying bronchial and vascular markings. Note small nodules along the right major fissure (*arrowheads*), in the center of secondary pulmonary lobules (*curved arrows*), and in a peripheral subpleural location (*open arrow*). All of these findings illustrate a perilymphatic distribution, which is typical of sarcoidosis.

FIGURE 10-7. Sarcoidosis. CT of a 40-year-old man shows ill-defined nodules in a bronchovascular distribution (*arrows*).

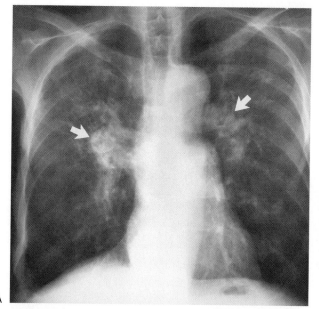

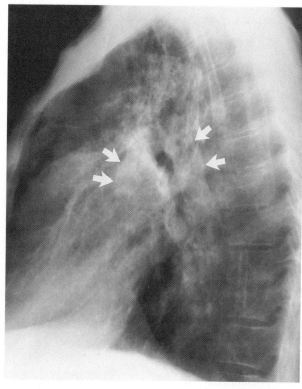

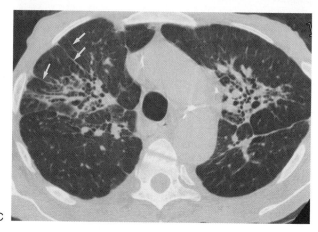

FIGURE 10-9. Sarcoidosis. PA (**A**) and lateral (**B**) chest radiographs of a 69-year-old man with class IV sarcoidosis show enlarged pulmonary arteries (*arrows*) secondary to pulmonary arterial hypertension. Note diffuse upper and middle lung reticulonodular opacities, and note also the upward retraction of the hila. **C:** CT shows bilateral central areas of pulmonary fibrosis with thickening of bronchovascular bundles and traction bronchiectasis. Note parenchymal bands on right (*arrows*).

where they are acted on by lysosomal enzymes. The affected macrophage dies and liberates mediators (leading to stimulation of collagen production) and the silica particles. The silica particles are then free to be taken up by other macrophages, and the cycle continues, leading to progressive lung disease even without continued occupational exposure to silica. Silicosis can be classified as simple silicosis, complicated silicosis, acute silicosis, or Caplan syndrome. Coal worker's pneumoconiosis, caused by inhalation of coal dust, is different pathologically from silicosis, but it produces chest radiographic findings similar to and often indistinguishable from those of silicosis.

Patients with *simple silicosis* are usually asymptomatic. Between 10 and 20 years' exposure is usually necessary before the chest radiograph becomes abnormal (16). The chest radiograph shows multiple nodules, 1 to 10 mm in diameter, with a diffuse but upper lung–predominant distribution (Fig. 10-10). Occasionally, the nodules may calcify. Enlargement of mediastinal and hilar nodes is common and is occasionally associated with eggshell calcification similar to that seen with sarcoidosis.

Complicated silicosis refers to progression of simple silicosis, where the nodules become confluent and larger than 1 cm. On chest radiography, these opacities are seen predominantly in the periphery of the upper lungs, which, over time, tend to migrate toward the hilum as the fibrotic process progresses.

These conglomerate masses, which can reach several centimeters in size and contain obliterated blood vessels and bronchi, are referred to as *progressive massive fibrosis* (Fig. 10-11). The conglomerate masses are often surrounded by paracicatricial emphysema, which is best appreciated on chest CT. As conglomeration of the nodules occurs, the lungs gradually lose volume, and cavitation of the masses can occur. Patients who have advanced to this stage are at increased risk of active tuberculosis, and this diagnosis should be suspected when a new area of cavitation is seen on chest radiography.

Acute silicosis is a rare condition related to heavy acute exposure to silica in enclosed spaces with minimal or no protection. Histologically, the appearance is identical to that of pulmonary alveolar proteinosis; hence the term *silicoproteinosis* is used. The disease is rapidly progressive, often leading to death as a result of respiratory failure. The chest radiographic pattern is that of nonspecific diffuse airspace disease or ground-glass opacities, with a perihilar distribution and air bronchograms identical to the radiographic findings of pulmonary edema.

Caplan syndrome consists of the presence of large necrobiotic rheumatoid nodules superimposed on a background of simple silicosis. The syndrome is a manifestation of rheumatoid lung disease and is seen in both coal worker's pneumoconiosis and silicosis.

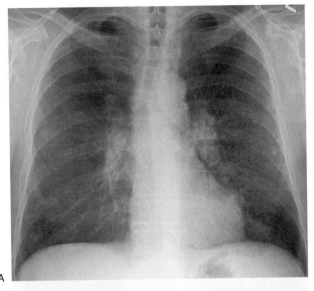

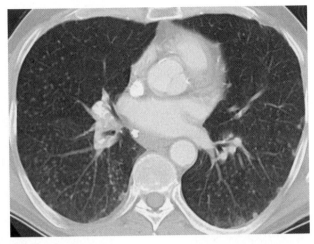

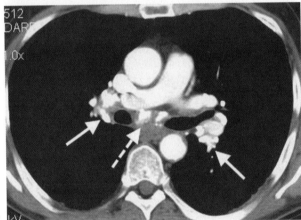

FIGURE 10-10. Simple silicosis. A: PA chest radiograph of a foundry worker shows numerous bilateral ill-defined tiny nodules, creating an overall increase in lung opacity. B: On CT, the nodules are much better appreciated. C: CT with mediastinal windowing shows densely calcified hilar (*solid arrows*) and subcarinal (*dashed arrow*) lymph nodes.

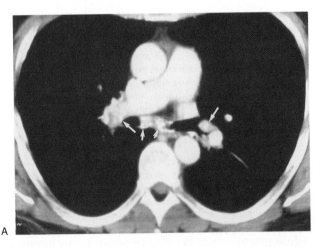

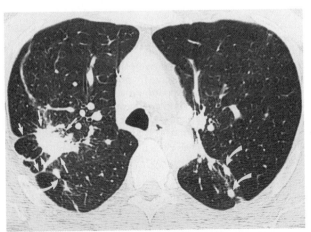

FIGURE 10-11. Complicated silicosis. A: CT of a 52-year-old man who had spent many years working in a sand pit shows calcification of hilar (*long arrows*) and subcarinal (*short arrows*) nodes. B: CT with lung windowing shows "progressive massive fibrosis" in the right upper lobe (*long straight arrows*) and early conglomeration of nodules in the superior segments of the lower lobes (*curved arrows*). Multiple parenchymal bands are seen on the right (*short straight arrows*).

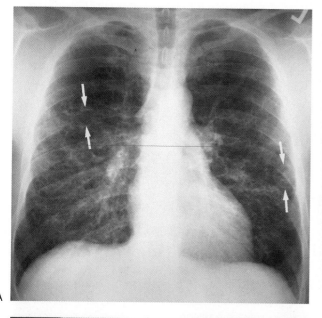

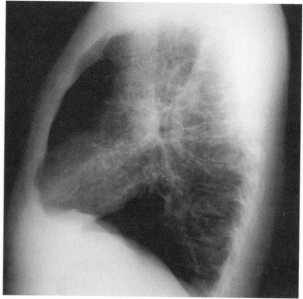

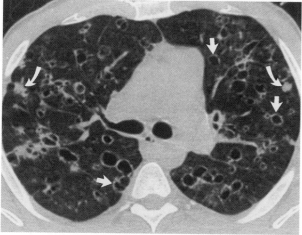

FIGURE 10-12. Langerhan cell histiocytosis. PA (A) and lateral (B) chest radiographs of a 32-year-old male cigarette smoker show bilateral reticular interstitial opacities and thin-walled cysts (*arrows*). Note increased lung volumes. C: CT shows bilateral thin-walled cysts, with rounded and irregular shapes (*straight arrows*), and ill-defined nodules (*curved arrows*).

LANGERHAN CELL HISTIOCYTOSIS

Langerhan cell histiocytosis (LCH), also referred to as *histiocytosis X* or *eosinophilic granuloma*, is a granulomatous disorder of unknown cause characterized by the presence within the granulomas of a histiocyte, the Langerhan cell. The disease is equally prevalent in male and female patients, it is unusual in African-Americans (17), and 95% of adult patients are cigarette smokers (17). In most patients, symptoms appear in the third or fourth decades, but the disease can occur in teenagers and those over age 60. The diagnosis can be made in asymptomatic patients with abnormal chest radiographs. Pneumothorax is a classic manifestation of LCH, and the frequency of pneumothorax as the initial manifestation is as high as 14% (18). The pneumothoraces are commonly recurrent and may be bilateral. Approximately one third of patients with LCH improve, one third remain stable, and one third deteriorate (18).

The chest radiograph of patients with LCH shows a diffuse, symmetric, reticulonodular pattern or, less commonly, a solely nodular pattern. Both patterns have a predominantly middle and upper lung distribution. The nodules are usually ill defined, vary in size from 1 to 15 mm, and are often innumerable but can be few in number. Large nodules can mimic metas-

tases. With time, small cystic airspaces develop, and larger airspaces up to 5 cm in diameter will form only rarely. Because of the development of these abnormal airspaces, lung volume does not decrease with time but often increases. Pleural effusion and hilar or mediastinal nodal enlargement are uncommon.

CT of the lungs shows cysts and nodules, often in combination (19,20) (Fig. 10-12). Cysts range in diameter from 1 to 30 mm or more and, unlike centrilobular emphysema, usually have very thin discrete walls and no centrilobular core structure. Some cysts have bizarre shapes, which can help to distinguish them from the uniformly round cysts that are typical of lymphangioleiomyomatosis. Nodules are typically 1 to 5 mm in diameter, have irregular margins, and may be cavitary. The disease is thought to progress from solid nodules to cavitary nodules to cysts, although this is controversial. End-stage disease can resemble that of generalized centrilobular pulmonary emphysema.

RADIATION PNEUMONITIS

Radiation injury to the lung is most commonly seen after radiation therapy for breast cancer, lung cancer, and Hodgkin disease. On the chest radiograph, the changes of radiation

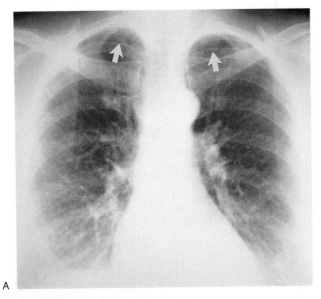

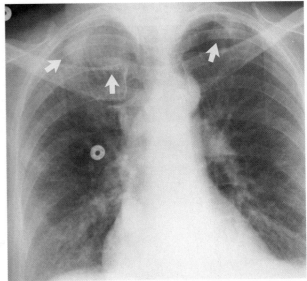

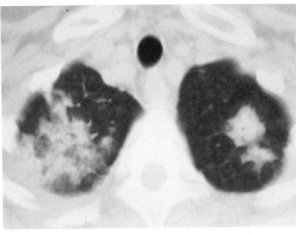

FIGURE 10-13. Radiation pneumonitis. A: PA chest radiograph of a 60-year-old woman 3 months after radiation treatment to the neck for a piriform sinus carcinoma. Subtle areas of abnormal opacification are seen at both apices (*arrows*). **B:** PA chest radiograph obtained 2 months later shows progression of apical opacities (*arrows*). **C:** CT shows bilateral apical airspace disease without anatomic or geographic distribution. Bronchoscopic biopsy of the right apex was negative for organisms, and the opacities gradually resolved without treatment on follow-up chest radiographs.

pneumonitis are almost always confined to the field of irradiation. The first change is a diffuse haze in the irradiated region, with obscuration of the normal vascular markings. Patchy opacities appear, which may coalesce into a nonanatomic but geometric area of pulmonary opacification. These radiographic changes usually appear about 8 weeks after treatment, depending on the radiation dose and dosing interval (21); peak reaction occurs at 3 to 4 months. With time, the opacities become more linear or reticular, and fibrous contraction and distortion of lung architecture occurs. The fibrosis and contraction continue over a 12- to 18-month period. When only the apices of the lung are affected by radiation, such as with treatment for head and neck neoplasms, the radiographic changes do not appear geometric but ill defined and patchy (Fig. 10-13). When bilateral apical airspace opacities are seen on chest radiography, radiation pneumonitis should be considered in the appropriate patient population. Radiation of the axilla, an adjuvant treatment for patients with breast cancer who have undergone lumpectomy or mastectomy, can result in ipsilateral peripheral upper lung patchy airspace opacities (Fig. 10-14).

TUBERCULOSIS

Once a disease of childhood, more than half of cases of initial infection with *Mycobacterium tuberculosis*, or primary tuberculosis (TB), are now seen in the adult population (22). In

primary tuberculous infections, the pulmonary focus and lymphadenopathy may resolve without a trace, or they may leave a focus of caseous necrosis, scarring, or calcification. Several terms are used to describe the form of tuberculosis that develops after a primary infection under the influence of established hypersensitivity including *reactivation TB*, *postprimary TB*, and *secondary TB*.

The predominant radiographic feature of *primary TB* is the presence of hilar lymphadenopathy (usually unilateral) and mediastinal lymphadenopathy contiguous to the affected hilum. Lymphadenopathy is less common and milder in adults than in children, with the exception of immunocompromised adults, especially those with AIDS. On CT, the enlarged nodes typically have a low-density center with rim enhancement (Fig. 10-15) (23). The pulmonary foci of primary TB are randomly distributed throughout the lungs, and they range from small, occasionally imperceptible, ill-defined parenchymal opacities to segmental or lobar consolidation, often with an appearance similar to that of other bacterial pneumonias (Figs. 10-16 and 10-17). The incidence of cavitation varies between 10% and 30% (22). Hilar or mediastinal lymph node calcification is observed in 35% of cases (24). Pleural effusions are not uncommon, are generally unilateral, and are usually, but not always, associated with some identifiable pulmonary parenchymal disease (Fig. 10-18). Bronchial stenosis, bronchial occlusions, and polypoid endobronchial tuberculous lesions may be seen on CT.

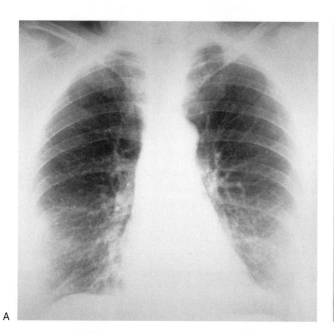
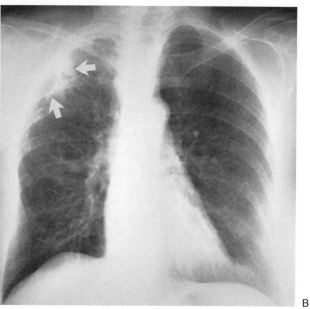

FIGURE 10-14. Radiation pneumonitis. A: Normal baseline PA chest radiograph of a 71-year-old woman. B: PA chest radiograph obtained 11 months later shows interval right mastectomy for treatment of breast cancer (note hyperlucent right lower hemithorax) and surgical clips in the right axilla. Note new abnormal areas of nonsegmental opacification in the periphery of the right upper lobe (arrows) from recent radiation to the axilla.

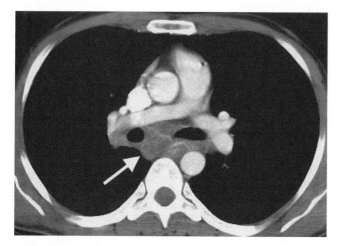

FIGURE 10-15. Primary tuberculosis. CT shows low-density subcarinal nodes with partial rim enhancement (arrow).

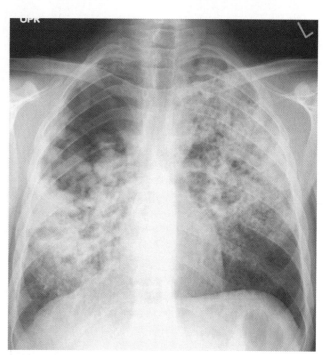

FIGURE 10-16. Primary tuberculosis. PA chest radiograph shows diffuse nodular airspace disease.

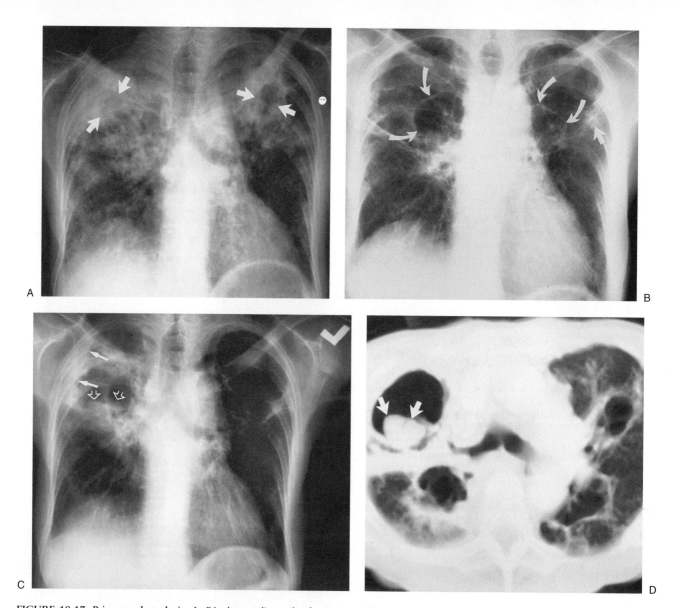

FIGURE 10-17. Primary tuberculosis. A: PA chest radiograph of a 71-year-old man with fever, hemoptysis, and weight loss shows bilateral patchy airspace opacities, with areas of cavitation in the upper lobes (*arrows*). Sputum contained numerous *M. tuberculosis* organisms. **B:** PA chest radiograph taken 9 months later shows changes of healing in upper lobes consisting of linear opacities (*straight arrow*) and thin-walled cavities (*curved arrows*). **C:** PA chest radiograph 2 months after (**B**) shows new right apical pleural thickening (*solid arrows*) and increased opacification of the right upper lobe. A fungus ball (aspergilloma) is seen within a right upper lobe cavity (*open arrows*). **D:** CT shows fungus ball in right upper lobe cavity (*arrows*). Note the cystic changes of healed TB in left upper lobe.

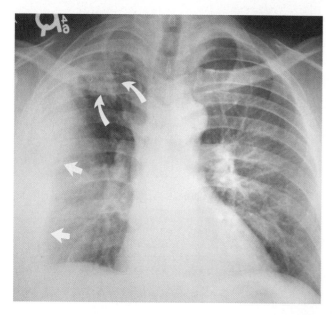

FIGURE 10-18. Primary tuberculosis. PA chest radiograph of a 39-year-old man shows abnormal right upper lobe opacification (*curved arrows*) and a large loculated right pleural effusion (*straight arrows*). Freely layering pleural fluid collects inferiorly, within the most gravity-dependent portion of the pleural space, in upright positioning, and the pleural fluid in this case tracks superiorly along the chest wall.

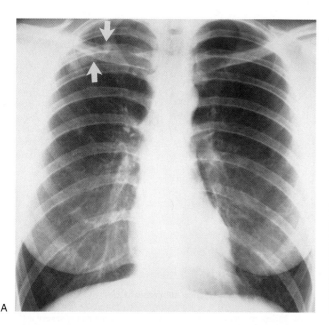
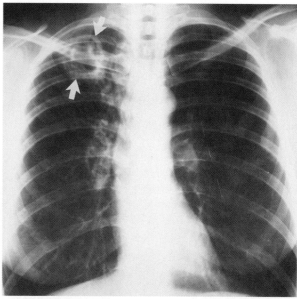

FIGURE 10-19. Reactivation tuberculosis. A: PA chest radiograph of a 44-year-old man shows a partially calcified opacity in the right upper lobe (*arrows*), which was unchanged in comparison with multiple prior chest radiographs and thus consistent with prior TB infection of indeterminate activity. B: PA chest radiograph obtained 6 years later shows a new cavity in the right upper lobe (*arrows*). Sputum contained *M. tuberculosis* organisms.

The earliest chest radiographic findings of *reactivation TB* consist of one or more ill-defined patchy opacities, with or without small satellite foci in the adjacent lung, occurring in the posterior segments of the upper lobes in the majority of patients and in the superior segment of the lower lobes in most of the remainder of patients. This distribution of disease is very helpful in suggesting the diagnosis of reactivation TB. Cavitation with or without the presence of air–fluid levels is a distinct feature of reactivation TB and indicates a high likelihood of active infection (Figs. 10-19 to 10-21). The presence of cavitation implies that the disease is highly contagious, and patients with cavitary disease should be placed under immediate infective precautions (respiratory isolation) on the basis of radiographic findings alone. With healing, the chest radiograph shows gradually increasing definition of the lung opacities, development of fibrosis in the surrounding lung, contraction and volume loss of the affected segment or lobe with fissural displacement or distortion of the vascular structures in the hilum, bronchiectasis, and calcification (Fig. 10-22). Fluid levels in cavities disappear, and the cavities either disappear or persist with a smooth inner wall.

Other patterns of reactivation TB include lobar pneumonia, diffuse bronchopneumonia, endobronchial TB, tuberculoma formation, miliary TB, and tuberculous pleuritis. A

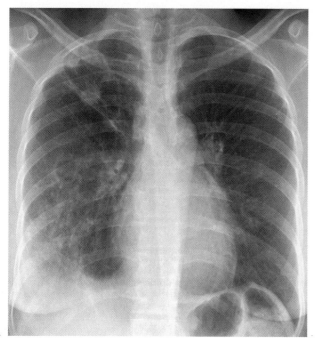
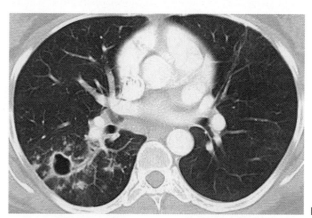

FIGURE 10-20. Reactivation tuberculosis. A: PA chest radiograph of a 30-year-old man from Africa who had been treated for tuberculosis 10 years earlier shows elevation of the minor fissure, right apical pleural opacity, and ill-defined opacities throughout the right lung. B: CT shows a thin-walled cavity, thickening of the bronchovascular bundles, and ill-defined nodules in the superior segment of the right lower lobe.

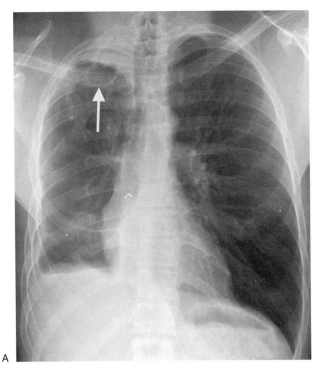

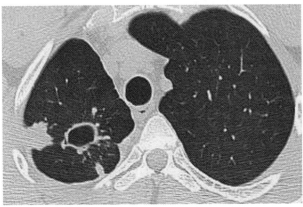

FIGURE 10-21. Reactivation tuberculosis. PA chest radiograph of a 28-year-old man with a prior history of right middle and lower lobectomy and right pleurodesis, currently taking steroids for severe asthma, shows right apical pleural opacity and a thin-walled cyst (*arrow*) in the right upper lung. Both were new findings compared with prior chest radiographs. **B:** CT shows the cyst and surrounding ill-defined nodules in the posterior right upper lobe.

calcified lymph node may erode into an adjacent airway, becoming a broncholith, and be associated with hemoptysis or postobstructive atelectasis or pneumonia. Broncholiths can be suggested when a previously documented nodal calcification on chest radiography has disappeared or changed position. On rare occasion, a patient can cough up pieces of a calcified broncholith, a phenomenon referred to as lithoptysis. Tuberculomas are discrete tumorlike foci of TB in which there is a fine balance between inflammation and healing. The margins of a tuberculoma are usually well circumscribed. Tuberculomas may be

single or multiple, are occasionally as large as 5 cm in diameter, and may grow slowly over an extended period of time. Calcification develops in the central caseous core with time and may be seen radiographically, but it is better characterized with CT. When the calcification is dense and assumes the majority of the volume of the tuberculoma as seen on chest radiography, the diagnosis of a benign inactive granuloma can be assumed. Such a parenchymal tuberculoma, known as a Ghon lesion, in combination with calcified nodes, is referred to as a Ranke complex. Miliary TB, which results from hematogenous dissemination

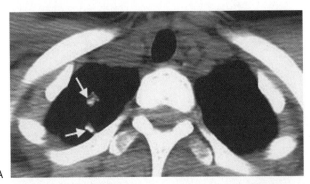

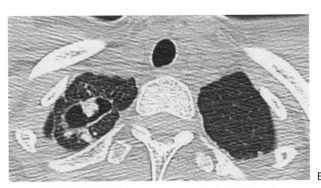

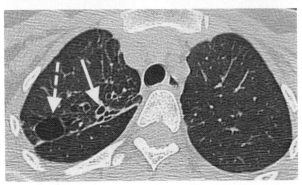

FIGURE 10-22. Healed tuberculosis. **A:** CT shows calcified nodules in the right upper lobe (*arrows*). **B:** CT with lung windowing shows a thin-walled cyst. The mural nodule along the anterior cyst wall and the nodule posterior to the cyst represent the calcified nodules seen in (**A**). **C:** CT at a more inferior level shows bronchiectasis (*solid arrow*) and a second thin-walled cyst (*dashed arrow*). The findings were unchanged in comparison with multiple CT scans obtained during the prior 3 years.

of disease, is an uncommon but serious complication of both primary and reactivation TB. The chest radiograph shows innumerable 2- to 3-mm nodules likened to millet seeds in size and appearance. The nodules are uniformly distributed and equal in size. Because there is a threshold below which the nodules are imperceptible, miliary TB can be present in patients with a "normal" chest radiograph. Miliary TB does not leave residual calcifications.

A number of mycobacteria other than *M. tuberculosis* can cause pulmonary infection. These atypical mycobacteria are common in the natural environment, and numerous species exist, including *M. kansasii* and *M. avium-intracellulare*; the latter is a very important pathogen in human immunodeficiency virus (HIV)–infected individuals. The classic features of atypical mycobacterial infections of the lung are those of a chronic indolent fibrocavitary process, usually involving one or both apical regions of the lungs in a middle-aged or older individual with underlying chronic obstructive pulmonary disease (25), or in chronic lower lung bronchiectasis. In many cases, the radiographic features are indistinguishable from those of reactivation TB. The lesions have the same predilection for the posterior aspects of the upper lobes or the superior segments of the lower lobes as reactivation TB. Cavitation occurs in up to 96% of patients with atypical mycobacterial infection (26).

ASPERGILLUS LUNG DISEASE

Fungi of the genus *Aspergillus* are ubiquitous saprophytes that are commonly laboratory contaminants but on occasion can become human pathogens. Infection is acquired primarily through the respiratory tract. Exposure to *Aspergillus* is almost universal, yet the nonimmunocompromised patient usually does not develop *Aspergillus* infection (27).

Aspergillosis represents a spectrum of diseases based on the degree of immune impairment at one end of the spectrum and hypersensitivity at the other end of the spectrum (28). Four basic types of pulmonary aspergillosis are (i) noninvasive (saprophytic), (ii) semi-invasive, (iii) invasive, and (iv) allergic.

Noninvasive pulmonary aspergillosis refers to colonization of a pre-existing cavity or cystic area in the lung with *Aspergillus* organisms, creating a "fungus ball" or mycetoma. Prior tuberculous infection, emphysematous bullae, sarcoidosis (Fig. 10-23), or other processes, such as ankylosing spondylitis, that result in cavities, cysts, or cystic bronchiectasis, can lead to mycetoma formation (29,30). In noninvasive aspergillosis, the fungus causes the development of vascular granulation tissue within the cavity wall, which can lead to hemoptysis. With peripheral cavities, there is also a pleural response to the

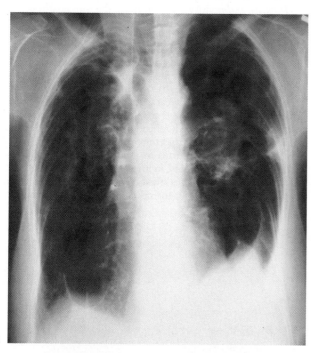

A

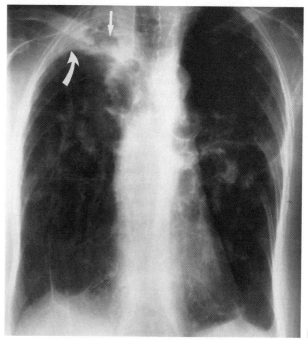

B

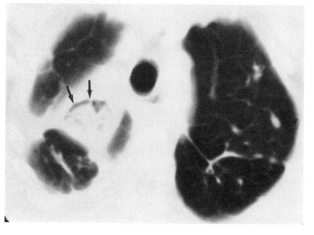

C

FIGURE 10-23. Noninvasive pulmonary aspergillosis. A: Baseline PA chest radiograph of a 79-year-old woman with class IV sarcoidosis shows retraction of the hila bilaterally, bilateral upper lobe fibrosis, and tenting of the hemidiaphragms from upper lobe volume loss. **B:** PA chest radiograph taken 2 years later shows increased right apical pleural thickening (*curved arrow*) and a fungus ball (aspergilloma) in the right upper lobe cavity (*straight arrow*). **C:** CT shows opacity within the right upper lobe cavity, representing vascular granulation tissue and fungal organisms. A small amount of air is seen within the cavity (*arrows*).

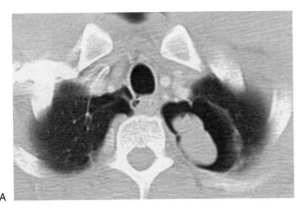
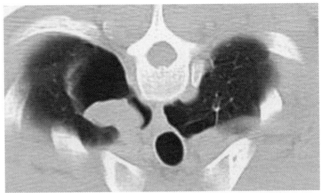

FIGURE 10-24. Noninvasive pulmonary aspergillosis. A: Supine CT image of a 41-year-old man with hemoptysis shows a thin-walled cavity in the left upper lobe containing an ovoid mass of soft tissue attenuation. B: Prone CT image shows movement of the mass to the dependent aspect of the cavity. Movement of an intracavitary fungus ball with change in patient positioning is typical of noninvasive aspergillosis.

presence of the organism, leading to marked pleural thickening and extrapleural fatty hypertrophy as clues to the chronic inflammation. Chest radiography and CT typically show a mobile, intracavitary mass, usually in an upper lobe (Figs. 10-24 and 10-25). Specific therapy is not required for patients with an asymptomatic aspergilloma; however, this type of aspergillosis can cause massive hemoptysis that can sometimes lead to death. Bronchial artery embolization, surgery, or instillation of amphotericin B into the aspergilloma cavity can be used to treat patients with an aspergilloma and hemoptysis.

Semi-invasive pulmonary aspergillosis refers to a chronic, indolent form of *Aspergillus* infection that leads to cavity formation and then a classic aspergilloma. This form of aspergillosis tends to occur in patients with depressed immune systems (e.g., those with a neoplasm, those who have undergone radiation, those who are of advanced age or debilitated, those with diabetes or chronic obstructive lung disease, or those on chronic corticosteroid therapy) (31). The disease typically begins as an upper lung opacity on chest radiography, which, over a period of weeks to months, gradually develops cavi-

tation with formation of an "air crescent sign." As the disease progresses, extensive apical pleural thickening develops. As cavitation progresses, a thick-walled cavity often becomes thin walled, containing a mycetoma (Fig. 10-26). Therapy is the same as for noninvasive aspergillosis.

Invasive pulmonary aspergillosis is the most pathologically aggressive form of aspergillosis and occurs in severely immunocompromised patients (Fig. 10-27). Chest radiographs show a solitary pulmonary nodule or mass, or multifocal opacities. In some cases, multiple poorly defined nodules (likely representing infarcts) are seen and extend to the periphery of the lungs. In patients with leukemia, cavitation of the nodules develops as the neutrophil count recovers from the chemotherapy-induced nadir (32). Cavitation leads to the air crescent sign, which is seen as a crescent-shaped collection of air between the cavity wall and the intracavitary contents. In contrast to noninvasive and semi-invasive forms of aspergillosis, in which a fungus ball occupies the cavity, in invasive aspergillosis the central mass within the cavity is almost always necrotic lung and not an aspergilloma. Early in the course of infection during bone

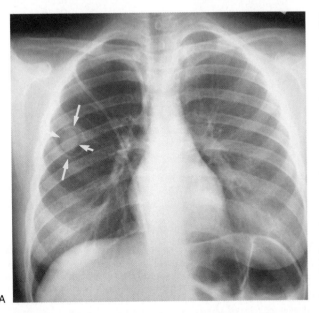
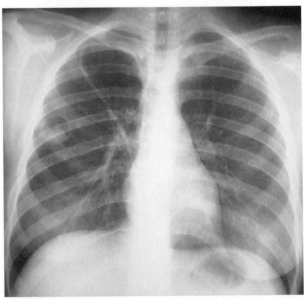

FIGURE 10-25. Noninvasive pulmonary aspergillosis. A: PA chest radiograph of a 14-year-old girl with a thin-walled cavity in the right upper lobe (*long arrows*) containing a fungus ball (*short arrows*). B: PA chest radiograph after change in patient position shows movement of the mobile fungus ball.

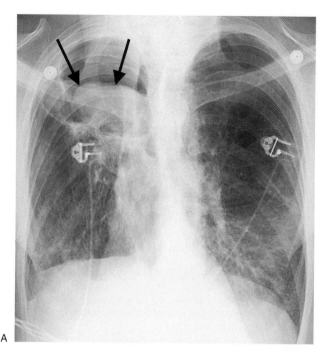

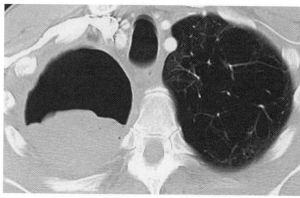

FIGURE 10-26. Semi-invasive pulmonary aspergillosis. A: PA chest radiograph of a 49-year-old woman with hemoptysis shows a rounded opacity (*arrows*) within a right upper lobe cavity. There is retraction of the right hilum along with elevation of the right hemidiaphragm. B: CT shows a fungus ball within the right upper lobe cavity. Note severe changes of emphysema in the left lung.

marrow aplasia, before air crescent formation or cavitation, CT often shows the CT "halo sign," a zone of ground-glass opacification surrounding the pulmonary nodule or mass. In patients with acute leukemia, the presence of the CT halo sign (representing a zone of hemorrhage) strongly suggests the diagnosis of invasive aspergillosis (Fig. 10-28) (33). Intravenous amphotericin B remains the frontline therapy for invasive aspergillosis. Patients who do not respond to therapy usually die of the disease.

Allergic bronchopulmonary aspergillosis (ABPA) is a form of hypersensitivity reaction to inhaled *Aspergillus* organisms. It is seen most commonly in patients with underlying asthma, it is seen in approximately 10% of patients with cystic fibrosis, and it is seen occasionally in patients with no known underlying pulmonary disease (34). The fungus grows noninvasively within the bronchi, releasing an antigen that causes host sensitization and a subsequent immunologic reaction. Mucus traps the organisms in the bronchi. Bronchiectasis either results from or is a predisposing factor to development of ABPA. Patients with ABPA typically present with symptoms of asthma.

Typical radiographic findings consist of central bronchiectasis with mucoid material filling the bronchi. The appearance of mucus-filled bronchi on chest radiography has been variously described as finger in glove, rabbit ears, Mickey Mouse, toothpaste-shaped, and Y- or V-shaped opacities. The diagnosis of ABPA is based on major and minor criteria (35). Major criteria include asthma, blood eosinophilia, immediate skin reactivity to *Aspergillus* antigen, increased serum immunoglobulin E, transient or fixed pulmonary opacities on chest radiography, and central bronchiectasis. Minor criteria include fungal organisms in the sputum, history of expectoration of brown plugs or flecks, and delayed skin reactivity to fungal antigens. Because ABPA is an allergic disease, the primary treatment consists of corticosteroids.

Bronchocentric granulomatosis, characterized histologically by necrotizing granulomas that may obstruct and destroy bronchioles, is a histopathologic pattern that is generally believed to represent a nonspecific response to a variety of forms of airway injury. Approximately half of all cases are associated with asthma and ABPA, and among these patients,

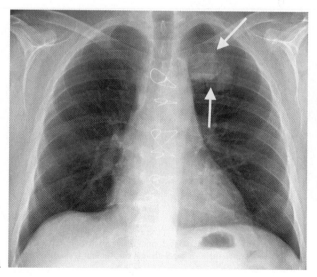

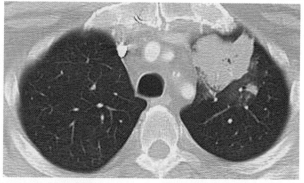

FIGURE 10-27. Invasive pulmonary aspergillosis. A: PA chest radiograph of a 57-year-old woman with a transplanted heart shows focal airspace opacity in the left upper lobe (*arrows*). B: CT shows dense airspace opacity and surrounding halo of ground-glass opacity in the left upper lobe.

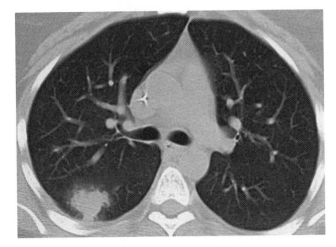

FIGURE 10-28. Invasive pulmonary aspergillosis. CT of a 30-year-old woman with leukemia and fever shows an ill-defined nodule with a halo of ground-glass opacity in the right lung.

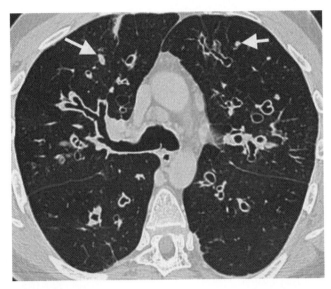

FIGURE 10-30. Cystic fibrosis. CT of a 37-year-old woman shows bilateral bronchiectasis and mucoid-impacted airways (*arrows*).

bronchocentric granulomatosis may represent a histopathologic manifestation of fungal hypersensitivity. *Aspergillus* hyphae can be identified within the granulomas in up to 50% of patients. Although the imaging features may be similar to those of conventional ABPA, the lung involvement in bronchocentric granulomatosis is more commonly focal and peripheral (36).

CYSTIC FIBROSIS

Cystic fibrosis is an autosomal recessive disease involving chromosome 7 and characterized by dysfunction of exocrine glands, which form a thick, tenacious material. The incidence is 1 in 1,600 live births, with Caucasians affected most frequently. Organs involved include the lung, upper respiratory tract, pancreas, liver, gallbladder, and reproductive tract. The earliest chest radiographic findings include peribronchial inflammatory changes (peribronchial cuffing) and both atelectasis and hyperinflation. With progression of the disease, ring shadows and tram tracking are seen as signs of bronchiectasis, usually with an upper lobe predominance (Fig. 10-29). Not uncommonly, air–fluid levels can be seen in areas of cystic bronchiectasis. Small, ill-defined or tubular opacities occur as a result of mucus plugging in dilated airways (Figs. 10-30 and 10-31). Larger

opacities usually represent pneumonia, most commonly caused by *Staphylococcus aureus* or *Pseudomonas* species. Bilateral hilar lymphadenopathy is common. Severe disease can lead to pulmonary arterial hypertension and cor pulmonale, which may be suggested when enlargement of the central pulmonary arteries and enlargement of the right heart, respectively, are seen on the chest radiograph. ABPA occurs in 10% of patients with cystic fibrosis, as discussed earlier in this chapter. Hypertrophic pulmonary osteoarthropathy, a disorder involving the long bones and joints, occurs in approximately 15% of patients with cystic fibrosis.

RADIOLOGIC ABNORMALITIES IN IMMUNOCOMPROMISED PATIENTS

Infection is the leading cause of chest radiographic abnormalities in immunocompromised patients and is a direct result of a deficiency in immune defenses (e.g., immunoglobulin abnormalities, cell-mediated dysfunction, and phagocytic defense disorders) or a nonspecific reduction in host resistance

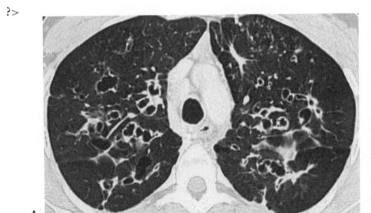

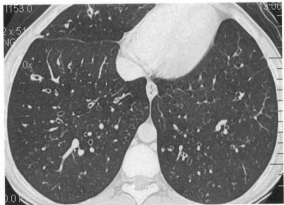

FIGURE 10-29. Cystic fibrosis. A: CT of a 29-year-old woman shows bilateral cystic bronchiectasis and thickening of bronchial walls. Small nodules in the left upper lobe likely represent mucoid-impacted bronchioles. B: CT at a more inferior level shows similar but less severe findings. Cystic fibrosis typically involves the upper lungs to a greater degree than the lower lungs.

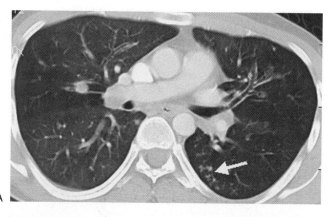 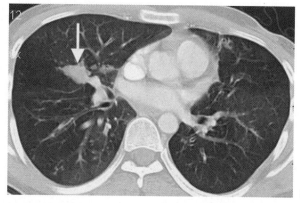

FIGURE 10-31. Cystic fibrosis and *Mycobacterium avium* infection. A: CT shows small nodular and linear branching opacities (*arrow*) in the left lower lobe, consistent with bronchiolar spread of mycobacterial disease. Note bronchiectasis in both upper lobes. **B:** CT at a more inferior level shows a markedly distended, mucoid-impacted bronchus in the right middle lobe (*arrow*). This finding is suggestive of ABPA, which patients with cystic fibrosis are predisposed to develop.

(e.g., advanced age, alcoholism, diabetes, starvation or malnutrition, and cancer). In addition to infection, radiographic abnormalities in immunocompromised patients can result from many other causes, as listed in Table 10-4.

Infection

Bacterial agents are the most frequent causes of pneumonia in immunocompromised patients. Patients receiving steroids and patients with renal transplants are particularly susceptible to infection with *Legionella* organisms. *L. pneumophila* manifests as progressive parenchymal consolidation, sometimes with cavitation and pleural effusion. *L. micdadei* pneumonia results in well-circumscribed nodular densities with central cavitation (37). *Nocardia asteroides* infection occurs most commonly in immunosuppressed patients, including those with AIDS and solid organ transplants. Chest radiographs show lobar or mul-

tilobar areas of consolidation, or they show solitary or multiple ill-defined pulmonary nodules with a tendency to cavitate and invade surrounding structures such as the chest wall (38,39).

TB in immunocompromised patients occurs most commonly in the AIDS population. In non-AIDS immunocompromised patients, TB is usually caused by reactivation of a dormant lesion. The radiographic features typically consist of apical and posterior segmental fibronodular disease in the upper lobes with or without cavitation (40). Infection with atypical mycobacteria can have a similar appearance, but there is a tendency toward increased cavitation relative to total lung involvement, thin-walled cavities with less dense surrounding parenchymal opacification, less bronchogenic and more contiguous spread, more involvement of the apical and anterior segments of the upper lobes, and marked pleural thickening over the involved areas of the lung (40).

A. fumigatus is an important fungal pathogen in immunocompromised patients, especially those with lymphoma or leukemia. The different types of *Aspergillus* lung disease were discussed earlier in this chapter.

Candida albicans is another fungal agent that causes pneumonia in a substantial number of patients with leukemia or lymphoma. Chest radiographs most commonly show diffuse bilateral nonsegmental patchy alveolar or mixed alveolar–interstitial opacities. A pattern of miliary opacities can also be seen (41).

Mucormycosis results from infection with one of the phycomycetes and has a 100% mortality rate in the absence of treatment. Patients susceptible to mucormycosis include those with leukemia or lymphoma and those with diabetes mellitus. Pathologically, mucormycosis is fungal vascular invasion resulting in infarction (42). The most common radiographic abnormality is a single pulmonary nodule, mass, or focus of consolidation, frequently with cavitation. This is usually accompanied by infection of the paranasal sinuses, brain, and meninges.

Cryptococcosis, discussed later in this chapter, is the most common fungal pulmonary infection in patients with AIDS. Widespread dissemination of the organisms causing blastomycosis, coccidiomycosis, and histoplasmosis can occur in immunocompromised patients, but radiodiagnostic features are lacking; attention is usually given to excluding more common opportunistic fungi.

The most common virus to cause pneumonia in immunocompromised patients is Cytomegalovirus (CMV). The radiographic appearances include diffuse interstitial opacities, often with a nodular pattern. Other important viruses, especially in

TABLE 10-4

CAUSES OF RADIOGRAPHIC ABNORMALITIES IN IMMUNOCOMPROMISED PATIENTS

Infection
  Bacterial (typical)
  Mycobacterial
  Fungal
  Viral (Cytomegalovirus pneumonia)

Neoplasm
  Lymphoma and other lymphoproliferative disorders
  Leukemia
  Metastases/recurrence of primary tumor

Transfusion reaction

Graft-versus-host disease (after bone marrow transplantation)

Radiation pneumonitis
  Acute
  Chronic

Adverse drug reaction
  Early (noncytotoxic)
  Late (cytotoxic)

Hemorrhage

patients with lymphoma, are the varicella-zoster virus and the herpes simplex virus.

Neoplasm

Patients with lymphoma or leukemia can have pulmonary involvement of their disease. Leukemic infiltration of the lungs, pleura, or mediastinum, although common pathologically, does not appear to be a cause of pulmonary symptoms and is rarely a cause of radiographic abnormalities. Radiographs and CT scans of the chest are often normal in pathologically proven cases. Diffuse pulmonary disease is more likely to represent pneumonia or hemorrhage than leukemic infiltration (43). Radiographically visible leukemic infiltrates are virtually confined to patients with high peripheral blast counts (44). Leukostasis—the accumulation of leukemic cells in small pulmonary blood vessels in patients with leukemia—can result in diffuse airspace opacities on chest radiography, which is felt to be caused by pulmonary edema rather than the accumulation of leukemic cells (45). Distinguishing pneumonia from pulmonary lymphoma can be difficult or impossible radiographically.

In patients with an underlying nonpulmonary primary malignancy, the development of multiple, well-circumscribed pulmonary nodules of varying sizes is highly suspicious for metastatic disease. Infection, especially from fungal agents, and septic emboli should be considered in the differential diagnosis.

Certain populations of patients are predisposed to developing lymphoproliferative disorders, which can range from benign lymphoid hyperplasia to frank malignancy. This topic is discussed in the later sections on AIDS and lung transplantation.

Transfusion Reaction

Transfusion reactions are leukoagglutinin reactions that occur approximately 4 hours after blood transfusion. Acute reactions can be difficult to distinguish radiographically from volume overload with pulmonary edema (Fig. 10-32). True reactions are caused by an excess of antibodies in the donor serum directed against the recipient's white blood cells, leading to the abrupt onset of fever, chills, tachypnea, and tachycardia, coincident with the development of varying radiographic patterns of noncardiac pulmonary edema (46). The edema can persist for 24 to 48 hours, and it does not respond to diuresis but can respond to steroids.

Drug Reaction

Drug reactions can be categorized as *cytotoxic* (late) or *noncytotoxic* (early). The most common are cytotoxic reactions, which are well known in patients receiving a variety of chemotherapeutic agents (especially azathioprine, bleomycin, busulfan, cyclophosphamide, cytosine arabinoside, and methotrexate) (47). Between 2 and 6 months after completion of chemotherapy, the patient develops a cough, fever, and dyspnea. The chest radiograph shows either diffuse interstitial or hazy alveolar opacities (Fig. 10-33). Pleural effusions are uncommon. The resulting lung injury is compounded by chest radiation, oxygen therapy, and concurrent administration of other cytotoxic drugs. Two types of noncytotoxic drug reactions are *hypersensitivity reactions* and *noncardiac pulmonary edema* (47). Hypersensitivity reactions occur within hours or days of the initial administration of the drug. The patient develops an acute cough, fever, and dyspnea. Peripheral eosinophilia is often present. The chest radiograph typically shows nonspecific diffuse interstitial opacities that can progress to airspace disease.

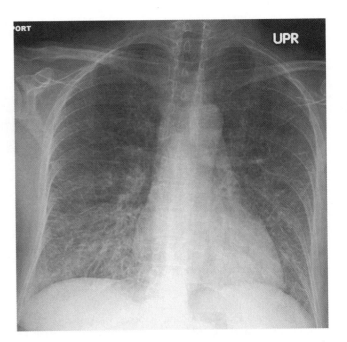

FIGURE 10-32. Transfusion-related lung injury. PA chest radiograph of a woman with abrupt onset of fever, chills, tachypnea, and tachycardia 4 hours after blood transfusion shows bilateral interstitial lung disease with prominent Kerley lines.

Hemorrhage

Pulmonary hemorrhage can occur in patients who develop thrombocytopenia after treatment of leukemia or after bone marrow transplantation, and it can be associated with an underlying bleeding tendency, infection, or diffuse alveolar damage. Pulmonary hemorrhage is seen in approximately 75% of patients with leukemia at autopsy (48), and alveolar lung disease from pulmonary hemorrhage alone occurs in up to 40% of patients with leukemia (49). The chest radiograph initially shows focal or, more commonly, multifocal airspace opacities that are gradually replaced by interstitial opacities as the by-products of blood breakdown are cleared by alveolar macrophages and transported through the lymphatic system in the interstitial spaces of the lungs.

AIDS

The majority of patients with AIDS eventually suffer from one or more forms of pulmonary disease. The chest radiograph has an important function in detecting the presence of disease, and in some cases it strongly suggests a specific diagnosis. The distinct radiographic features of disorders seen in patients with AIDS are outlined in Tables 10-5 and 10-6.

The bacterial agents that most commonly cause pneumonia in AIDS patients are the same organisms that cause pneumonia in the population at large (*Streptococcus pneumoniae* and *Haemophilus influenzae*). Septic emboli, usually owing to *S. aureus*, occur most commonly in AIDS patients who are intravenous drug abusers or who have central venous catheters in place (Fig. 10-34). Other bacterial agents associated with AIDS include the *Legionella* organisms (Fig. 10-35), *Mycoplasma* species, and *Rhodococcus equi* (50). The radiographic findings of single or multiple segmental or lobar areas of consolidation are the same as those in non-AIDS patients. The diagnosis, however, can be confounded by the presence of coexistent infections or other disease processes.

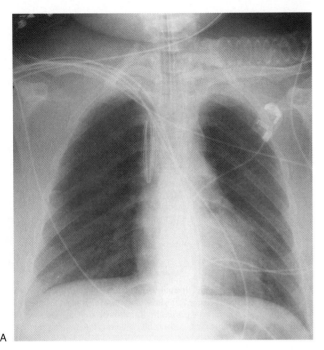
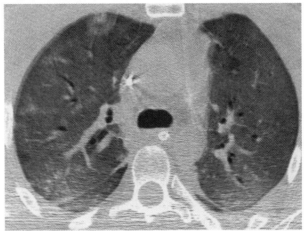

A   B

FIGURE 10-33. Bleomycin toxicity. **A:** Anteroposterior (AP) supine chest radiograph of a 30-year-old woman with Hodgkin disease shows subtle bilateral hazy opacification of the lungs. **B:** CT shows bilateral diffuse ground-glass opacification. The underlying bronchovascular markings remain visible. Motion artifact is present because of the inability to suspend respiration during scanning.

TABLE 10-5

RADIOGRAPHIC FEATURES OF COMMON DISORDERS IN PATIENTS WITH AIDS

Pneumocystis jiroveci *pneumonia*
  Typically, NO effusions or lymphadenopathy
  Bilateral perihilar or diffuse alveolar or reticulonodular
    opacities
  Lung cysts, often multiseptated, with associated
    spontaneous pneumothorax
  Upper lung predominance in some cases
Mycobacterial disease
  Tuberculosis
    Can manifest as primary or reactivation disease
    Responds rapidly to therapy unless the strain is drug
      resistant
    Can be spread to normal healthy people
  Mycobacterium avium-intracellulare complex
    Newly acquired, not reactivation
    Not transmitted to normal, healthy people
    Does not respond rapidly to treatment
Kaposi sarcoma
  Most common malignancy in AIDS
  Nearly all patients have mucocutaneous lesions
  Bilateral perihilar opacities with bronchovascular
    distribution
  Poorly defined, "flame-shaped" parenchymal nodules
  Pleural effusions common
  Kerley B lines common
AIDS-related lymphoma
  Occurs with severe immunocompromise
  Solitary or multiple lung nodules or masses
  Pleural or pericardial effusions common
  Lymphadenopathy common
  Can be rapidly progressive

AIDS, acquired immunodeficiency syndrome.

Other than typical community-acquired bacterial disease, the two most important infections to consider in AIDS patients are mycobacterial disease and *Pneumocystis jiroveci* pneumonia (PCP). There has been an increase in incidence of TB as a result of the AIDS epidemic. TB in patients with AIDS usually represents a reactivation of a previously acquired disease (51), and it occurs with less severe degrees of immunocompromise than other opportunistic infections in HIV-infected patients. With lesser degrees of immunocompromise, TB usually manifests as cavitary disease involving the apicoposterior segments of the upper lobes and superior segments of the lower lobes, without lymphadenopathy. As the immunocompromise worsens, a form of TB resembling primary TB develops—even though the disease is usually reactivation TB—with prominent lymphadenopathy and dissemination of disease throughout the lungs, pleura, and other parts of the body (Figs. 10-36 and 10-37). Intrathoracic lymphadenopathy is not a feature of the diffuse lymphadenopathy syndrome found in HIV infection, and it signifies an active complication of HIV infection such as TB (52).

TABLE 10-6

HILAR AND MEDIASTINAL LYMPHADENOPATHY AND AIDS

Tuberculosis[a]
Mycobacterium avium-intracellulare complex[a]
Fungal (especially *Cryptococcus*)
Lymphoma[a]
Kaposi sarcoma
Bronchogenic carcinoma (? increased incidence in AIDS
  patients)

Lymphadenopathy is NOT a feature of Pneumocystis jiroveci pneumonia.
AIDS, acquired immunodeficiency syndrome.
[a] Bulky nodes are a common feature.

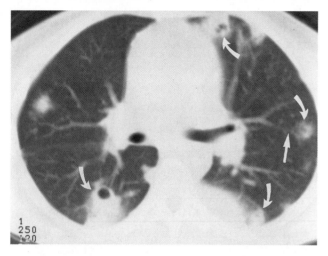

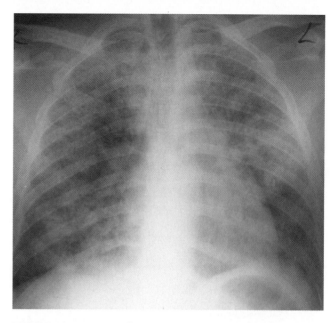

FIGURE 10-34. Septic emboli. CT of a 3-year-old girl with AIDS shows multiple ill-defined nodules with cavitation in a predominantly peripheral distribution (*curved arrows*). A "feeding vessel" leads to one of the nodules in the left upper lobe (*straight arrow*), indicating a hematogenous process. (Reprinted with permission from Kuhlman JE. Pulmonary manifestations of acquired immunodeficiency syndrome. *Semin Roentgenol.* 1994;29:242–274.)

FIGURE 10-35. *Legionella* pneumonia. AP upright chest radiograph of a 27-year-old man with AIDS shows bilateral diffuse airspace opacity, a nonspecific pattern of parenchymal disease that can be seen with many types of pneumonias, pulmonary edema, and pulmonary hemorrhage.

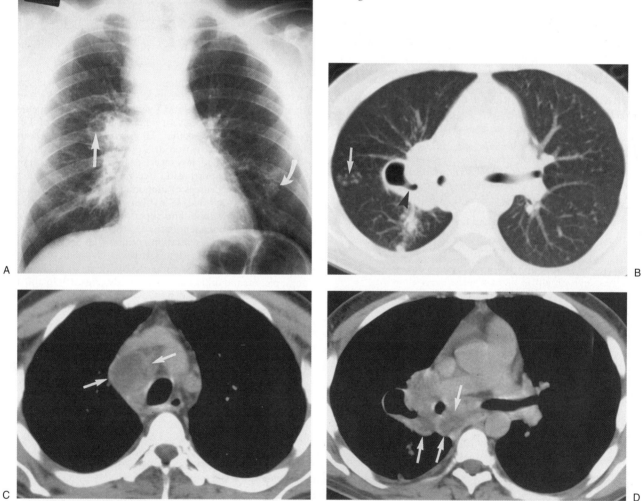

FIGURE 10-36. Tuberculosis. A: PA chest radiograph of a 27-year-old man with AIDS shows an air–fluid level adjacent to the right hilum (*straight arrow*), fullness to the right infrahilar area, and abnormal opacity in the left lower lung (*curved arrow*). **B:** CT shows cavitation of a right hilar mass that communicates with a central bronchus (*arrowhead*). Small nodules in the periphery of the posterior segment of the right upper lobe (*arrow*) and larger nodules in the superior segment of the right lower lobe are consistent with endobronchial spread of TB. **C:** CT with mediastinal windowing shows low-attenuation paratracheal lymphadenopathy (*arrows*). **D:** CT at a level inferior to (**C**) shows low-attenuation right hilar and subcarinal lymphadenopathy (*arrows*). (Courtesy of Janet E. Kuhlman, MD, University of Wisconsin Hospital and Clinics, Madison.)

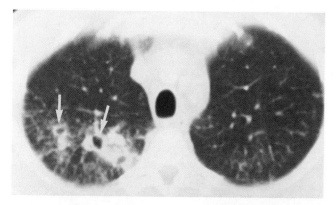

FIGURE 10-37. **Tuberculosis.** CT scan of a 49-year-old man with AIDS shows cavitary, ill-defined nodules (*arrows*) in the posterior segment of the right upper lobe and superior segment of the right lower lobe, along with peripheral small linear and nodular opacities bilaterally. (Courtesy of Janet E. Kuhlman, MD, University of Wisconsin Hospital and Clinics, Madison.)

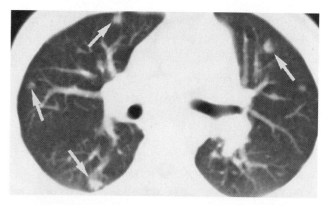

FIGURE 10-39. *Mycobacterium avium* **pneumonia.** CT of a man with AIDS shows bilateral small ill-defined nodules (*arrows*) in a predominantly peripheral distribution. (Reprinted with permission from Kuhlman JE. Pulmonary manifestations of acquired immunodeficiency syndrome. *Semin Roentgenol.* 1994;29:242–274.)

Numerous nontuberculous mycobacterial agents affect patients with AIDS, but *M. avium-intracellulare* predominates. Radiographs or CT scans of the chest show hilar and mediastinal lymphadenopathy with or without diffuse nodular or patchy alveolar parenchymal opacities (Figs. 10-38 and 10-39). Cavitation in pulmonary opacities is uncommon. The infection is extremely resistant to treatment.

The microbe that causes PCP in humans is a distinct phylogenetic fungal species called *P. jiroveci* (pronounced "yee-row-vet-zee") (53). PCP has long been the most common serious AIDS-defining opportunistic infection in the United States. The introduction of highly active antiretroviral therapy (HAART) for the treatment of HIV infection has been accompanied by substantial reductions in mortality and the incidence of opportunistic infections, including PCP (53). Despite these advances, *P. jiroveci* remains a major pathogen in HIV-infected persons who either are not receiving or are not responding to HAART and among those who are unaware of their HIV status. PCP is also of clinical importance in people who are immunocompromised for reasons other than HIV, such as organ or bone marrow transplantation (Fig. 10-40) or after receiving chemotherapy for malignant diseases (Fig. 10-41) (53).

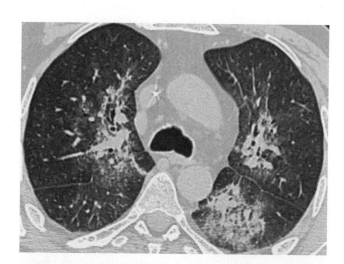

FIGURE 10-40. *Pneumocystis jiroveci* **pneumonia.** CT of a 53-year-old man with a bone marrow transplant shows bilateral dense airspace and ground-glass opacities associated with airway dilatation. The distribution is predominantly central and upper lung.

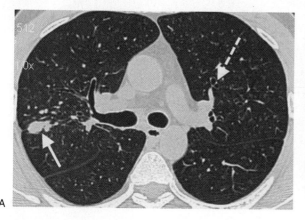

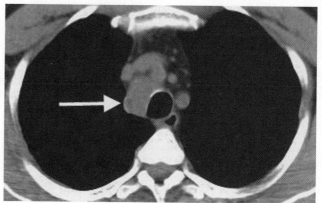

FIGURE 10-38. *Mycobacterium avium* **pneumonia. A:** CT of a 56-year-old man with AIDS shows an impacted bronchus in the right upper lobe (*solid arrow*), which is surrounded by small nodules, and bronchiectasis (*dashed arrow*). **B:** CT with mediastinal windowing shows bulky right paratracheal lymphadenopathy (*arrow*).

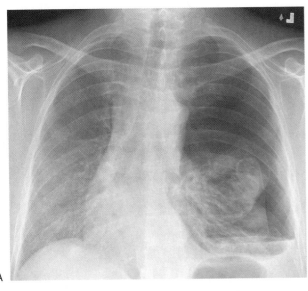

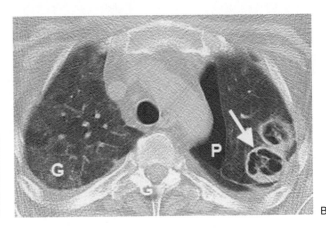

A

B

FIGURE 10-41. *Pneumocystis jiroveci* pneumonia. A: PA chest radiograph of a 46-year-old man undergoing treatment for a brain tumor and acute shortness of breath shows a large left pneumothorax and shift of the mediastinum to the right. B: CT shows multiseptated cysts (*arrow*), left pneumothorax (*P*) after chest tube placement, and patchy ground-glass opacity (*G*). This constellation of findings is very suggestive of PCP.

The chest radiograph is abnormal in more than 90% of patients with PCP; it most commonly shows diffuse opacity of the lung parenchyma, which is finely reticular in early stages but progresses to confluent airspace disease (54). Patients receiving aerosolized pentamidine show an increased tendency to develop focal parenchymal opacity, particularly in the upper lungs (55) (Fig. 10-42), although an apical predominance of disease can be seen even in patients not receiving pentamidine prophylaxis (56). Pneumatoceles can develop in patients with AIDS and PCP (Figs. 10-41 and 10-43), which can lead to pneumothorax. When the chest radiograph is normal, CT may show diffuse ground-glass opacities. Pleural effusions and lymphadenopathy are rare with PCP. As the disease evolves,

CT can show calcification in hilar, mediastinal, and abdominal lymph nodes.

Viruses, especially CMV, are an infrequent cause of clinical pneumonia in HIV-infected patients, even though CMV is often isolated from the lungs in patients with AIDS. To be able to name CMV as the cause of pneumonia in AIDS patients, CMV must be recovered by culture, CMV inclusion bodies must be identified in lavage or biopsy samples, and progressive pneumonia responding to an antiviral agent must be present. Viral pneumonias result in diffuse parenchymal opacities on chest radiography, similar in appearance to pulmonary edema of noncardiac origin, without substantial pleural effusions or lymphadenopathy (Fig. 10-44).

Numerous fungal agents can cause pneumonia in patients with AIDS. Cryptococcosis is the most common fungal pulmonary infection, and it usually coexists with cryptococcal meningitis. Chest radiographs show focal or diffuse reticular or reticulonodular opacities, a miliary nodular pattern (Fig. 10-45), or focal airspace opacities. Lymphadenopathy, pleural effusions, and cavitation are frequent findings (57).

FIGURE 10-42. *Pneumocystis jiroveci* pneumonia. PA chest radiograph of a 41-year-old man with AIDS, who had been treated with inhaled pentamidine, shows bilateral interstitial and alveolar opacities with an upper lung–predominant distribution.

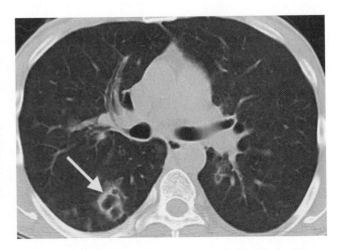

FIGURE 10-43. *Pneumocystis jiroveci* pneumonia. CT of a 37-year-old man with AIDS shows a multiseptated cyst in the right lower lobe (*arrow*) and scattered ground-glass opacities.

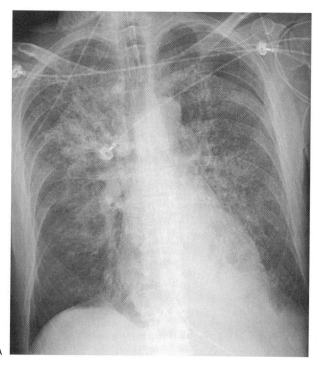

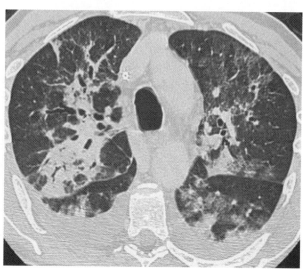

FIGURE 10-44. *Pneumocystis jiroveci* pneumonia and Cytomegalovirus pneumonia. A: PA chest radiograph of a 60-year-old man with AIDS shows nonspecific diffuse bilateral interstitial and airspace opacities. B: CT shows nonspecific findings of bilateral dense airspace and ground-glass opacities associated with airway dilatation. Imaging of immunocompromised patients is often confounded by the presence of multiple ongoing disease processes.

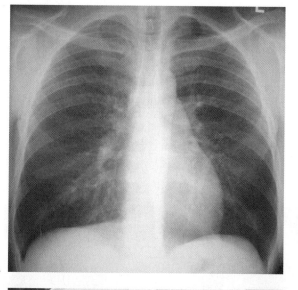

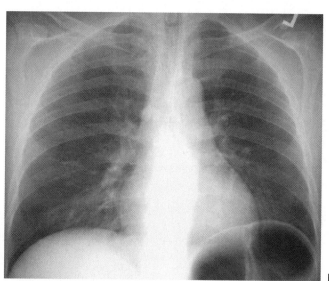

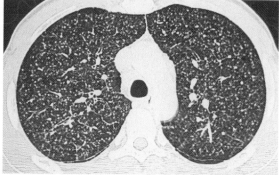

FIGURE 10-45. Cryptococcal pneumonia. A: PA chest radiograph of a 43-year-old man with AIDS, fever, night sweats, and weight loss shows diffuse bilateral hazy opacity. B: Prior chest radiograph is normal. C: CT shows numerous randomly distributed miliary nodules.

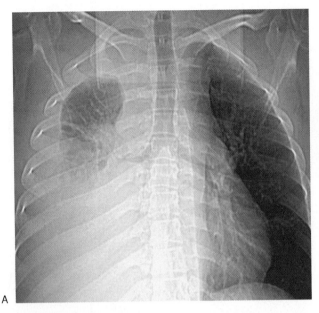

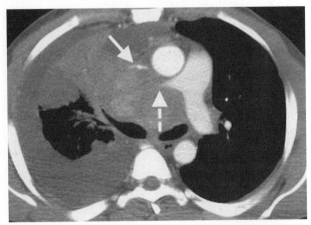

FIGURE 10-46. Large-cell lung cancer. A: CT scout image of a 37-year-old man with AIDS and multiple distended neck and anterior chest wall veins shows a large right pleural effusion and collapse of most of the right lung. **B:** Axial CT shows extensive tumor infiltrating the mediastinum, resulting in slitlike narrowing of the superior vena cava (*solid arrow*), encasement of the right pulmonary artery (*dashed arrow*), and a large right pleural effusion.

Pulmonary aspergillosis occurs in the terminal stages of AIDS, usually when other opportunistic infections or AIDS-related malignancies are present.

The two most important malignancies to consider in patients with AIDS are Kaposi sarcoma and lymphoproliferative disease. There is also a possible increased incidence of bronchogenic cancer in patients with AIDS, which is highly aggressive and occurs in patients who are younger than those who have bronchogenic cancer without AIDS (Fig. 10-46). Kaposi sarcoma is the most common malignancy (58). Pulmonary Kaposi sarcoma is rare in the absence of cutaneous involvement, providing a helpful clue to the diagnosis. Chest radiographic findings are nonspecific, and Kaposi sarcoma, like other disor-

ders in patients with AIDS, often coexists with opportunistic infections. Two patterns can be seen: (i) diffuse linear and reticular interstitial opacities (including Kerley B lines) or (ii) diffuse nodular opacities. A perihilar distribution predominates with both patterns, reflecting a bronchovascular distribution (59) (Fig. 10-47). The bronchovascular nodules can have a flame-shaped appearance. Pleural effusions are common and can be large. Hilar and mediastinal lymphadenopathy is common, although not bulky; the CT attenuation of these nodes can be relatively high after injection of intravenous contrast material because of the hypervascularity of Kaposi sarcoma.

Pulmonary lymphoma is the second most common intrathoracic malignancy associated with HIV infection (58). Most are

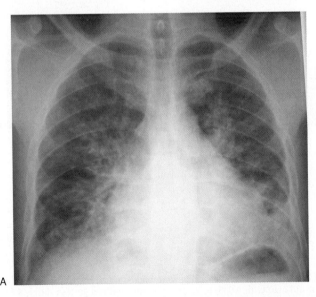

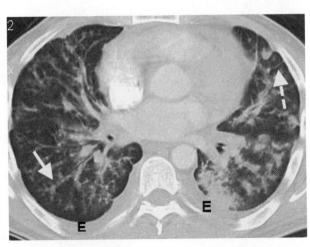

FIGURE 10-47. Kaposi sarcoma. A: PA chest radiograph of a 49-year-old man with AIDS, cutaneous lesions, nonproductive cough, and shortness of breath shows bilateral ill-defined nodular thickening of the bronchovascular bundles. **B:** CT shows nodular bronchovascular thickening (*solid arrow*), septal thickening (Kerley lines; *dashed arrow*), and bilateral pleural effusions (*E*). The findings are very suggestive of Kaposi sarcoma.

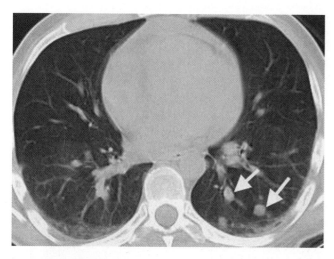

FIGURE 10-48. Large-cell lymphoma. CT of a man with AIDS and profound immunosuppression shows multiple circumscribed pulmonary nodules (*arrows*).

of the B-cell Hodgkin type. These lymphomas are usually aggressive, widely disseminated, and almost always associated with extranodal disease. It is a later feature of AIDS that occurs in severely immunocompromised patients. The chest radiographic and CT appearances are similar to those of non–AIDS-related lymphomas, including pulmonary masses or nodules (Fig. 10-48), lymphadenopathy (Fig. 10-49), and pleural effusions (60). There is a strong association between the presence of the Epstein-Barr virus and lymphoproliferative disorders of many kinds in immunocompromised patients, including those with AIDS. The most common CT appearance in these patients is multiple nodules with a bronchovascular and subpleural distribution affecting predominantly the middle and lower lungs (61).

Lymphocytic interstitial pneumonia (LIP) is characterized by infiltration of the peribronchial interstitial tissues of the lung by mature polyclonal lymphocytes, plasma cells, and im-munoblasts. Although LIP is usually a diffuse interstitial process with a basilar predominance, one or more nodular masses frequently develop (62). The diffuse interstitial pattern can be miliary in appearance, an appearance similar to that of miliary TB. LIP is more common in children than in adults and is an AIDS-defining illness in children. Other lymphoproliferative disorders seen in patients with AIDS include lymphocytic bronchiolitis and pulmonary lymphoid hyperplasia.

BONE MARROW TRANSPLANTATION

Pulmonary infections occur in at least half of all patients after bone marrow transplantation and are the most significant cause of death in this patient population (63) (Fig. 10-50). Infections occurring in immunocompromised patients were discussed earlier in this chapter.

Graft-versus-host disease (GVHD) results from the transplantation of immunocompetent donor lymphocytes that attack the recipient's tissues, especially the skin, liver, and gastrointestinal tract. Acute GVHD occurs 20 to 100 days after transplantation and involves primarily extrapulmonary organs. Chronic GVHD occurs at least 100 days after transplantation in approximately one third of patients surviving this long (64), and it results in lymphocytic infiltration of the airways and obliterative bronchiolitis. Chest radiograph and CT findings include diffuse patchy perihilar opacities, reflecting the airway distribution of disease. In severe cases, a diffuse interstitial pattern is seen. CT may be normal on inhalational images but may show air trapping on exhalational images, reflecting obliterative bronchiolitis.

Pulmonary veno-occlusive disease rarely occurs in patients after bone marrow transplantation but can lead to patient death. The pulmonary veins thrombose and develop intimal fibrosis, possibly as a result of pulmonary infection. Occlusion of the pulmonary veins leads to pulmonary venous and capillary congestion, pulmonary edema, alveolar hemosiderin deposits, pulmonary arterial hypertension, and right heart failure. Chest radiographs, when abnormal, show signs of pulmonary arterial hypertension (enlarged central pulmonary arteries) and, in some cases, interstitial and alveolar pulmonary edema (65). The left atrium is not enlarged, differentiating this entity from mitral valve disease and left atrial myxoma.

Pulmonary hemorrhage can occur in the absence of any evidence of a coagulopathy and in the absence of hemoptysis. It usually develops within 20 days of transplantation and is a fulminant condition with a 75% mortality rate. Chest radiographs most commonly show diffuse alveolar lung disease, although in some cases a pattern of reticular interstitial disease predominates (66).

LUNG TRANSPLANTATION

The first successful lung transplantation was performed in 1983. As of June 2004, 3,154 heart–lung and 19,296 lung transplantations had been performed according to data from an international registry (67). Single lung transplantation is the preferred procedure for lung replacement because fewer donor organs are required compared with heart–lung or bilateral lung transplantation. Cystic fibrosis is the most common indication for bilateral lung transplantation because of the incidence of recurrent infections in the native lung after single lung transplantation and institution of immunosuppression.

In single lung transplantation, the chest is entered through the bed of the fifth rib. This avoids complications of a sternotomy, which is performed for heart–lung and double lung transplantation. The surgery involves pulmonary artery,

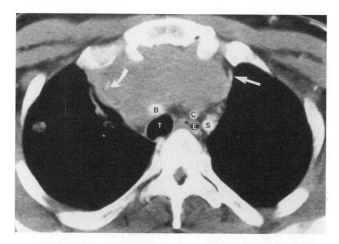

FIGURE 10-49. AIDS-related lymphoma. CT shows a large anterior mediastinal mass encasing the right brachiocephalic vein (*curved arrow*), displacing the left brachiocephalic vein laterally (*straight arrow*), and displacing the brachiocephalic artery (*B*), left common carotid artery (*C*), left subclavian artery (*S*), trachea (*T*), and esophagus (*E*) posteriorly. (Reprinted with permission from Kuhlman JE. AIDS-related tumors of the chest. In: Husband JES, Reznele RH, eds. *Imaging in Oncology.* Oxford, UK: ISIS Medical Media; 1998:1003–1018.)

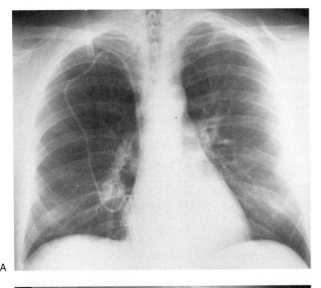

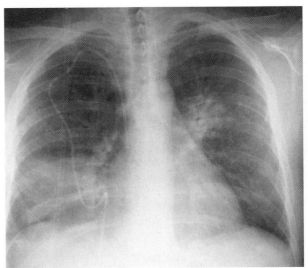

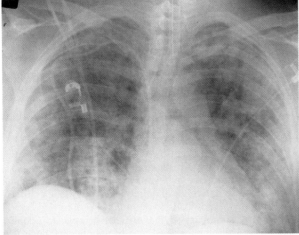

FIGURE 10-50. **Respiratory syncytial virus pneumonia. A:** Baseline PA chest radiograph of a 23-year-old man 21 days after bone marrow transplantation. **B:** PA chest radiograph taken 9 days later shows new bilateral interstitial and alveolar opacities. **C:** AP supine chest radiograph taken 4 days after (**B**) shows progression of diffuse parenchymal disease, correlating with the clinical onset of acute respiratory distress syndrome (ARDS). Note new endotracheal tube. The patient died from fulminant viral pneumonia and ARDS.

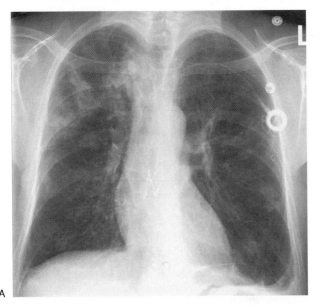

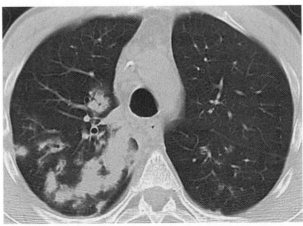

FIGURE 10-51. **Streptococcal pneumonia. A:** PA chest radiograph of a 40-year-old man with bilateral lung transplants shows bilateral patchy airspace opacities. **B:** CT shows airspace opacities that are not specific for any infectious organism. The findings can also be seen with acute rejection.

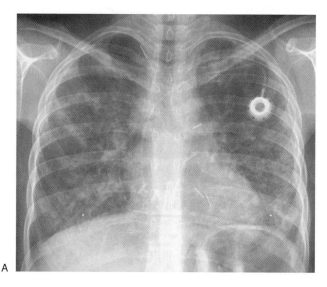
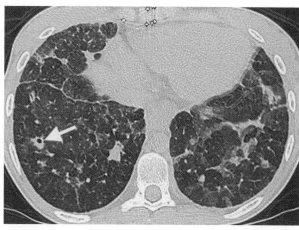

FIGURE 10-52. Staphylococcal pneumonia. A: PA chest radiograph of an 18-year-old woman with bilateral lung transplants shows diffuse bilateral interstitial and airspace opacities. B: CT shows multifocal dense airspace and ground-glass opacities and small cavitary nodules (*arrow*).

bronchial, and donor–recipient left atrial cuff anastomoses (68). Bilateral lung transplantation involves sequential single lung transplants and is commonly performed via a "clamshell" approach through a lower sternotomy.

Infection is the leading cause of death in the lung transplant population, accounting for 48% of early postoperative mortality (69). Factors that increase the susceptibility to infection include immunosuppression, reduced mucociliary clearance, interruption of lymphatic drainage, and direct and constant contact of the transplant with the outside environment via the airways (70). Bacterial agents predominate in the first month after transplantation (Figs. 10-51 and 10-52), CMV infections occur mainly in the second and third months (Fig. 10-53), and fungal infections (Fig. 10-54) occur both early and later after transplantation (70–73). PCP is uncommon secondary to an-

tibiotic prophylaxis. If CMV pneumonia develops, a fulminant course proceeding to respiratory failure and death within a few days can develop (74).

Acute rejection may be observed at any point after transplantation, with the first episode occurring as early as 48 hours and most occurring in the first 100 days after surgery. Most recipients experience at least one episode (75). CT of the chest shows ground-glass opacification as the only significant finding (76). Chest radiograph and CT findings overlap with those of infection (77).

Reperfusion edema is seen within 24 hours after transplantation and resolves over a period of days to months, usually within 1 to 2 weeks. The radiographic appearance ranges from mild perihilar haze to dense consolidation, and it results from surgical trauma, ischemia, organ preservation, denervation,

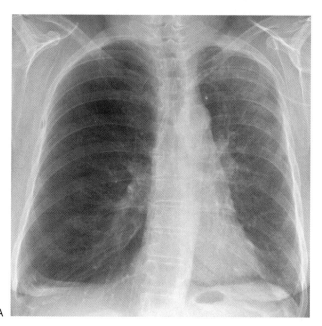
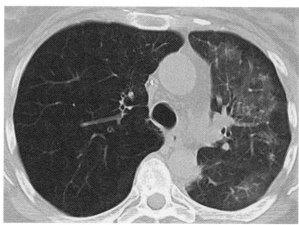

FIGURE 10-53. Cytomegalovirus pneumonia. A: PA chest radiograph of a 55-year-old man with a left lung transplant shows abnormal opacity in the left upper lobe. Note the hyperlucent and hyperexpanded native right emphysematous lung. B: CT shows ground-glass opacity involving only the left transplant lung and severe changes of emphysema in the native right lung.

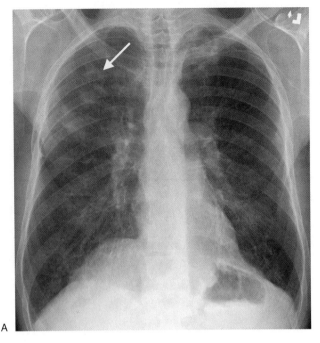

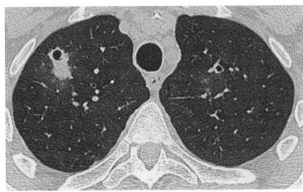

FIGURE 10-54. Invasive pulmonary aspergillosis. A: PA chest radiograph of a 35-year-old man with bilateral lung transplants shows multiple nodules, some with evidence of cavitation (*arrow*), in the right upper lung. B: CT shows a cavitary nodule in the right upper lobe with a halo of ground-glass opacity. There is a smaller thin-walled cavity in the left upper lobe.

and lymphatic interruption (70). The diagnosis is one of exclusion and is characterized by all radiographic changes beginning soon after surgery that are not the result of left ventricular failure, rejection, fluid overload, infection, or atelectasis (75).

Pleural effusions are common after lung transplantation, secondary to impaired fluid clearance through the lymphatics of the visceral pleura. Most effusions develop immediately following surgery and continue for up to 9 days, with output declining steadily during the first week (78). Pneumothoraces are evident on postoperative radiographs in 60% of patients; they are generally small and apical in location (79).

Chronic rejection is a major problem in patients surviving longer than 3 months, and it occurs in more than 50% of patients. Obliterative bronchiolitis represents the patho-

logic finding in chronic rejection. CT findings of bronchiectasis/bronchiolectasis, decreased vascular markings, and air trapping on exhalational scans are findings associated with obliterative bronchiolitis (71,72,80).

Posttransplantation lymphoproliferative disease, thought to be induced by the Epstein-Barr virus, manifests as a spectrum of lymphoproliferation that ranges from a mild, polyclonal lymphoid hyperplasia to frank lymphoma. Of all transplantation procedures, this disorder occurs most often after lung transplantation, with a prevalence of 5% to 20%, occurring most often within the first year after surgery (81). Intrathoracic involvement is most commonly characterized by the presence of discrete nodules, either solitary or multiple, with or without mediastinal lymphadenopathy (Fig. 10-55)

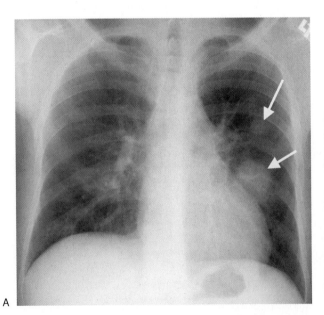

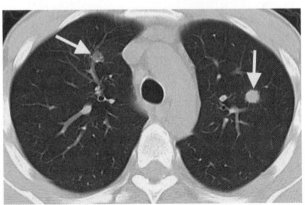

FIGURE 10-55. Posttransplant lymphoproliferative disorder. A: PA chest radiograph of a 32-year-old woman with bilateral lung transplants shows multiple pulmonary nodules (*arrows*). B: CT confirms multiple circumscribed pulmonary nodules (*arrows*). The nodule in the right lung is related to a bronchovascular bundle, a common pattern of distribution of nodules in patients with this disorder.

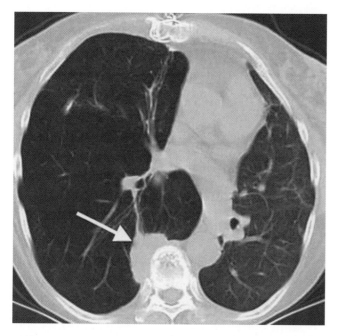

FIGURE 10-56. Squamous cell bronchogenic carcinoma. CT of a 65-year-old woman with a left lung transplant and a 35–pack-year history of cigarette smoking shows a right paravertebral mass (*arrow*). Note the severe changes of emphysema in the native right lung and normal perfusion to the left transplant lung.

(61,81,82). Bronchogenic carcinoma occurs after lung transplantation, most commonly in the native lung in patients with single lung transplantation for emphysema (Fig. 10-56) or idiopathic pulmonary fibrosis (83).

Recurrence of disease has occurred in patients transplanted for sarcoidosis (most common), LCH, lymphangiomyomatosis, bronchioloalveolar carcinoma, desquamative interstitial pneumonitis, pulmonary alveolar proteinosis, giant cell interstitial pneumonitis, diffuse panbronchiolitis, talc granulomatosis, and bronchiectasis from aspiration (84). It is important to consider recurrence of native disease when new abnormalities are seen on chest radiography or CT in the appropriate clinical situation.

References

1. Gurney JW, Schroeder BA. Upper lobe lung disease: physiologic correlates. *Radiology.* 1988;167:359–366.
2. Benatar SR. A comparative study of sarcoidosis in white, black and coloured South Africans. In: Williams WJ, Davies BH, eds. *Eighth International Conference on Sarcoidosis and Other Granulomatous Diseases.* Cardiff, Wales: Alpha Omega; 1980:508–513.
3. Mayock RL, Bertrand P, Morrison CE, et al. Manifestations of sarcoidosis: analysis of 145 patients, with a review of nine series selected from the literature. *Am J Med.* 1963;35:67–89.
4. DeRemee RA. The roentgenographic staging of sarcoidosis. *Chest.* 1983;83:128–133.
5. Siltzbach LE. The Kveim test in sarcoidosis: a study of 750 patients. *JAMA.* 1961;178:476–482.
6. Kirks DR, Greenspan RH. Sarcoid. *Radiol Clin North Am.* 1973;11:279–294.
7. Ellis K, Renthal G. Pulmonary sarcoidosis: roentgenographic observations on course of disease. *AJR Am J Roentgenol.* 1962;88:1070–1083.
8. Israel HL, Lenchner G, Steiner RM. Late development of mediastinal calcification in sarcoidosis. *Am Rev Respir Dis.* 1981;124:302–305.
9. Gross BH, Schneider HJ, Proto AV. Eggshell calcification of lymph nodes: an update. *AJR Am J Roentgenol.* 1980;135:1265–1268.
10. Smellie H, Hoyle C. The natural history of pulmonary sarcoidosis. *Q J Med.* 1960;29:539–559.
11. Battesti JP, Saumon G, Valeyre D, et al. Pulmonary sarcoidosis with an alveolar radiographic pattern. *Thorax.* 1982;37:448–452.
12. Brauner MW, Grenier P, Mompoint D, et al. Pulmonary sarcoidosis: evaluation with high-resolution CT. *Radiology.* 1989;172:467–471.
13. Lynch DA, Webb WR, Gamsu G, et al. Computed tomography in pulmonary sarcoidosis. *J Comput Assist Tomogr.* 1989;13:405–410.
14. Müller NL, Kullnig P, Miller RR. The CT findings of pulmonary sarcoidosis: analysis of 25 patients. *AJR Am J Roentgenol.* 1989;152:1179–1182.
15. Rockoff SD, Rohatgi PK. Unusual manifestations of thoracic sarcoidosis. *AJR Am J Roentgenol.* 1985;144:513–528.
16. Ziskind M, Jones RN, Weill H. Silicosis: state of the art. *Am Rev Respir Dis.* 1976;113:647–665.
17. Marcy TW, Reynolds HY. Pulmonary histiocytosis X. *Lung.* 1985;163:129–150.
18. Lacronique J, Roth C, Battesti JP, et al. Chest radiological features of pulmonary histiocytosis X: a report based on 50 adult cases. *Thorax.* 1982;37:104–109.
19. Brauner MW, Grenier P, Mouelhi MM, et al. Pulmonary histiocytosis X: evaluation with high-resolution CT. *Radiology.* 1989;172:255–258.
20. Moore ADA, Godwin JD, Müller NL, et al. Pulmonary histiocytosis X: comparison of radiographic and CT findings. *Radiology.* 1989;172:249–254.
21. Libshitz HI, Shuman LS. Radiation-induced pulmonary change: CT findings. *J Comput Assist Tomogr.* 1984;8:15–19.
22. Woodring JH, Vandiviere JH, Fried AM, et al. Update: the radiographic features of pulmonary tuberculosis. *AJR Am J Roentgenol.* 1986;146:497–506.
23. Im J-G, Song KS, Kang HS, et al. Mediastinal tuberculous lymphadenitis: CT manifestations. *Radiology.* 1987;164:115–119.
24. Weber AL, Bird KT, Janower ML. Primary tuberculosis in childhood with particular emphasis on changes affecting the tracheobronchial tree. *AJR Am J Roentgenol.* 1968;103:123–132.
25. Woodring JH, Vandiviere HM. Pulmonary disease caused by nontuberculous mycobacteria. *J Thorac Imag.* 1990;5:64–76.
26. Christensen EE, Dietz GW, Ahn CH, et al. Radiographic manifestations of pulmonary *Mycobacterium kansasii* infections. *AJR Am J Roentgenol.* 1978;131:985–993.
27. Miller WT. Aspergillosis: a disease with many faces. *Sem Roentgenol.* 1996;31:52–66.
28. Gefter W. The spectrum of pulmonary aspergillosis. *Thorac Imaging.* 1992;7:56–74.
29. Bardana EJ Jr. The clinical spectrum of aspergillosis. Part 2. Classification and description of saprophytic, allergic, and invasive variants of human disease. *CRC Crit Rev Clin Lab Sci.* 1980;13:85–96.
30. Wolfschlager C, Khan F. Aspergillomas complicating sarcoidosis: a prospective study in 100 patients. *Chest.* 1980;86:585–591.
31. Gefter WB, Weingrad TR, Epstein DM, et al. Semi-invasive pulmonary aspergillosis. *Radiology.* 1981;140:313–321.
32. Albelda SM, Talbot GH, Gerson SL, et al. Pulmonary cavitation and massive hemoptysis in invasive pulmonary aspergillosis: influence on bone marrow recovery in patients with acute leukemia. *Am Rev Respir Dis.* 1985;131:115–121.
33. Kuhlman JE, Fishman EK, Siegelman SS. Invasive pulmonary aspergillosis in acute leukemia: characteristic findings on CT, the CT halo sign, and the role of CT in early diagnosis. *Radiology.* 1985;157:611–614.
34. Sauter B, Speich R, Russi EW, et al. Cavernous destruction of an upper lung lobe in a healthy young man: an unusual roentgenographic presentation of allergic bronchopulmonary aspergillosis. *Chest.* 1994;105:1871–1872.
35. Rosenberg M, Patterson R, Mintzer R, et al. Clinical and immunologic criteria for the diagnosis of allergic bronchopulmonary aspergillosis. *Ann Intern Med.* 1977;86:405–414.
36. Katzenstein AL, Liebow AA, Friedman PJ. Bronchocentric granulomatosis, mucoid impaction and hypersensitivity reactions to fungi. *Am Rev Respir Dis.* 1975;111:497–537.
37. Pope TL, Armstrong P, Thomas R, et al. Pittsburgh pneumonia agent: chest film manifestations. *AJR Am J Roentgenol.* 1983;138:237–241.
38. Feigin DS. Nocardiosis of the lung: chest radiographic findings in 21 cases. *Radiology.* 1986;159:9–14.
39. Kramer MR, Uttamchandani RB. The radiographic appearance of pulmonary nocardiosis associated with AIDS. *Chest.* 1990;98:382–385.
40. McLoud TC. Pulmonary infections in the immunocompromised host. *Radiol Clin North Am.* 1989;27:1059–1066.
41. Pagani JJ, Libshitz HI. Opportunistic fungal pneumonias in cancer patients. *AJR Am J Roentgenol.* 1981;137:1033–1039.
42. Meyer RD, Rosen P, Armstrong D. Phycomycosis complicating leukemia and lymphoma. *Ann Intern Med.* 1972;77:871–879.
43. Lee WA, Hruban RH, Kuhlman JE, et al. High-resolution computed tomography of inflation-fixed lungs: pathologic-radiologic correlation of pulmonary lesions in patients with leukemia, lymphoma or other hematopoietic proliferative disorders. *Clin Imaging.* 1992;16:15–24.
44. Kovalski R, Hansen-Flaschen J, Lodato R, et al. Localized leukemic pulmonary infiltrates. *Chest.* 1990;97:674–678.
45. van Buchem MA, Wondergem JH, Kool LJS, et al. Pulmonary leukostasis: radiologic-pathologic study. *Radiology.* 1987;165:739–741.
46. Ward HN. Pulmonary infiltrates associated with leukoagglutinin transfusion reactions. *Ann Intern Med.* 1970;73:689–694.

47. Dee P. Drug- and radiation-induced lung disease. In: Armstrong P, Wilson AG, Dee P, et al, eds. *Imaging of Diseases of the Chest*. 2nd ed. St. Louis: Mosby–Year Book; 1995:464–466.

48. Maile CW, Moore AV, Ulreich S, et al. Chest radiographic-pathologic correlation in adult leukemia patients. *Invest Radiol*. 1983;18:495–499.

49. Tenholder MF, Hooper RG. Pulmonary infiltrates in leukemia. *Chest*. 1980;78:468–473.

50. Polsky B, Gold JWM, Whimbey E, et al. Bacterial pneumonia in patients with the acquired immunodeficiency syndrome. *Ann Intern Med*. 1986;104: 38–41.

51. Pitchenik AE, Rubinson HA. The radiographic appearance of tuberculosis in patients with the acquired immunodeficiency syndrome (AIDS) and pre-AIDS. *Am Rev Respir Dis*. 1985;131:393–396.

52. Stern RG, Gamsu G, Golden JA, et al. Intrathoracic adenopathy: differential feature of AIDS and diffuse lymphadenopathy syndrome. *AJR Am J Roentgenol*. 1984;142:689–692.

53. Stringer JR, Beard CB, Miller RF, Wakefield AE. A new name (*Pneumocystis jiroveci*) for pneumocystis from humans. *Emerg Infect Dis*. 2002 Sep;8:891–896. Available online at: http://www.cdc.gov/ncidod/EID/vol8no9/02-0096.htm. Accessed February 28, 2006.

54. Goodman PC, Gamsu G. Pulmonary radiographic findings in the acquired immunodeficiency syndrome. *Postgrad Radiol*. 1987;7:3–15.

55. Abd AG, Nierman DM, Ilowite JS, et al. Bilateral upper lobe *Pneumocystis carinii* pneumonia in a patient receiving inhaled pentamidine prophylaxis. *Chest*. 1988;94:329–331.

56. Baughman RP, Dohn MN, Shipley R, et al. Increased *Pneumocystis carinii* recovery from the upper lobes in *Pneumocystis* pneumonia: the effect of aerosol pentamidine prophylaxis. *Chest*. 1993;103:426–432.

57. Chechani V, Kamholz SL. Pulmonary manifestations of disseminated cryptococcosis in patients with AIDS. *Chest*. 1990;98:1060–1066.

58. Kaplan MH, Susin M, Pahwa SG, et al. Neoplastic complications of HTLV-III infection: lymphomas and solid tumors. *Am J Med*. 1987;82:389–396.

59. Naidich DP, Tarras M, Garay SM, et al. Kaposi's sarcoma: CT-radiographic correlation. *Chest*. 1989;96:723–728.

60. Sider L, Weiss AJ, Smith MD, et al. Varied appearance of AIDS-related lymphoma in the chest. *Radiology*. 1989;171:629–632.

61. Collins J, Müller NL, Leung AN, et al. Epstein-Barr virus associated lymphoproliferative disease of the lung: CT and histologic findings. *Radiology*. 1998;208:749–759.

62. Oldman SAA, Castillo M, Jacobson FL, et al. HIV-associated lymphocytic interstitial pneumonia: radiologic manifestations and pathologic correlation. *Radiology*. 1989;170:83–87.

63. Krowka MJ, Rosenow EC, Hoagland HC. Pulmonary complications of bone marrow transplantation. *Chest*. 1985;87:237–246.

64. Lum LG, Storb R. Bone marrow transplantation. In: Flye M, ed. *Principles of Organ Transplantation*. Philadelphia: WB Saunders; 1989:478–499.

65. Shackleford GD, Sacks EJ, Mullins JD, et al. Pulmonary veno-occlusive disease: case report and review of the literature. *AJR Am J Roentgenol*. 1977;128:643–648.

66. Witte RJ, Gurney JW, Robbins RA, et al. Diffuse pulmonary alveolar hemorrhage after bone marrow transplantation: radiographic findings in 39 patients. *AJR Am J Roentgenol*. 1991;157:461–464.

67. The International Society for Heart and Lung Transplantation. International Registry for Heart and Lung Transplantation: Twenty-Second Annual Report. Available at: http://www.ishlt.org/registries/slides.asp?slides=heartLungRegistry. Accessed July 5, 2006.

68. Kshettry VR, Shumway SJ, Gauthier RL, et al. Technique of single-lung transplantation. *Ann Thorac Surg*. 1993;55:1019–1021.

69. Ettinger NA, Trulock EP. Pulmonary considerations of organ transplantation: part 3. *Am Rev Respir Dis*. 1991;144:443–451.

70. Engeler CE. Heart-lung and lung transplantation. *Radiol Clin North Am*. 1995;33:559–580.

71. Medina LS, Siegel MJ. CT of complications in pediatric lung transplantation. *RadioGraphics*. 1994;14:1341–1349.

72. Murray JG, McAdams HP, Erasmus JJ, et al. Complications of lung transplantation: radiologic findings. *AJR Am J Roentgenol*. 1996;166:1405–1411.

73. Patel SR, Kirby TJ, McCarthy PM, et al. Lung transplantation: the Cleveland Clinic experience. *Cleve Clin J Med*. 1993;60:303–319.

74. Bonser RS, Fragomeni LS, Jamieson SW. Heart-lung transplantation. *Invest Radiol*. 1989;24:310–322.

75. Garg K, Zamora MR, Tuder R, et al. Lung transplantation: indications, donor and recipient selection, and imaging of complications. *RadioGraphics*. 1996;16:355–367.

76. Loubeyre P, Revel D, Delignette A, et al. High-resolution computed tomographic findings associated with histologically diagnosed acute lung rejection in heart-lung transplant recipients. *Chest*. 1995;107:132–138.

77. Bergin CJ, Castellino RA, Blank N, et al. Acute lung rejection after heart-lung transplantation: correlation of findings on chest radiographs with lung biopsy results. *AJR Am J Roentgenol*. 1990;155:23–27.

78. Judson MA, Handy JR, Sahn SA. Pleural effusions following lung transplantation: time course, characteristics, and clinical implications. *Chest*. 1996;109:1190–1194.

79. Chiles C, Guthaner DF, Jamieson SW, et al. Heart-lung transplantation: the postoperative chest radiograph. *Radiology*. 1985;154:299–304.

80. Leung AN, Fisher K, Valentine V, et al. Bronchiolitis obliterans after lung transplantation: detection using expiratory HRCT. *Chest*. 1998;113:365–370.

81. Armitage JM, Kormos RL, Stuart RS, et al. Post-transplant lymphoproliferative disease in thoracic organ transplant patients: ten years of cyclosporine-based immunosuppression. *J Heart Lung Transplant*. 1991;10:877–887.

82. Dodd GD III, Ledesma-Medina J, Baron RL, et al. Post-transplant lymphoproliferative disorder: intrathoracic manifestations. *Radiology*. 1992;184:65–69.

83. Collins J, Kazerooni EA, Lacomis J, et al. Bronchogenic carcinoma after lung transplantation: frequency, clinical characteristics, and imaging findings. *Radiology*. 2002;224:131–138.

84. Collins J, Hartman MJ, Warner TF, et al. Frequency and CT findings of recurrent disease after lung transplantation. *Radiology*. 2001;219:503–509.

CHAPTER 11

ATELECTASIS

LEARNING OBJECTIVES

1. Recognize partial or complete atelectasis of the following on a chest radiograph or computed tomography:

   - Right upper lobe
   - Right middle lobe
   - Right lower lobe
   - Right upper and middle lobe
   - Right middle and lower lobe

   - Left upper lobe
   - Left lower lobe

2. Recognize complete collapse of the right or left lung on a chest radiograph or computed tomography and list an appropriate differential diagnosis for the etiology of the collapse.

3. Recognize lung collapse related to massive pleural effusion on a frontal chest radiograph.

Atelectasis is defined as "diminished volume affecting all or part of a lung, which may or may not include loss of normal lucency in the affected part of lung (this finding is not to be confused with diminished volume produced by resection of pulmonary tissue)" (1). The term *atelectasis* is derived from the Greek words *ateles* and *ektasis* and means "incomplete expansion" (2–4). The term *collapse* is used when a whole lobe or lung is involved. Pulmonary atelectasis is one of the most commonly encountered abnormalities in chest radiology. Recognizing an abnormality on chest radiography as being caused by atelectasis can be crucial in understanding the underlying pathology, such as a case of left upper lobe collapse in an adult with endobronchial carcinoma obstructing the left upper lobe bronchus. In this chapter, *atelectasis* will be used to describe pulmonary loss of volume without substantial filling of alveolar spaces. The term *alveolar lung disease* implies filling of alveolar spaces with fluid or other material. This chapter will review the types of atelectasis based on mechanism, the signs of atelectasis, and the radiologic manifestations of lobar and nonlobar atelectasis.

TYPES OF ATELECTASIS

Pulmonary atelectasis can be divided into six types, based on mechanism: resorptive, adhesive, compressive, passive, cicatrization, and gravity-dependent. Whereas atelectasis can be divided into types based on these different mechanisms, in any given patient several mechanisms can occur simultaneously.

Resorptive atelectasis, the most common type, results from resorption of gas from the alveoli when communications between the alveoli and the trachea are obstructed. Resorptive atelectasis is therefore also referred to as *obstructive atelectasis*. The obstruction can occur at the bronchial or bronchiolar level. The most important condition producing intrinsic bronchial obstruction is bronchogenic carcinoma. Other causes of bronchial obstruction include other primary lung and metastatic neoplasms, inflammatory etiologies (especially tuberculous or fungal infection), aspirated foreign bodies, mucous plugging, a malpositioned endotracheal tube (Fig. 11-1), and extrinsic compression of an airway by neoplasm, lymphadenopathy, aortic aneurysm, or cardiac enlargement. Resorptive atelectasis is most commonly caused by obstruction of the small peripheral bronchioles, from impairment of mucociliary transport and pooling of retained secretions in the smaller airways. The larger airways are often patent and filled with air, resulting in air bronchograms within the atelectatic lung (Fig. 11-2). The presence of air bronchograms within the atelectatic lung usually, but not always, indicates the absence of a central obstructing neoplasm. Some of the conditions known to impair mucociliary clearance include thoracic and abdominal pain, central nervous system depression, respiratory depressant medication, general anesthesia, endotracheal intubation, and inhalation of toxic fumes or smoke (5). Resorptive

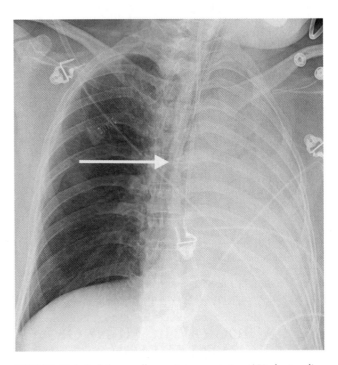

FIGURE 11-1. Left lung collapse. Anteroposterior (AP) chest radiograph shows the tip of the endotracheal tube (*arrow*) in the right main bronchus, resulting in collapse of the left lung. The left hemithorax is completely opaque and the mediastinum is shifted to the left.

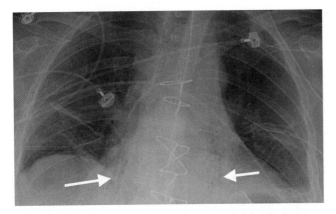

FIGURE 11-2. Bibasilar resorptive atelectasis. AP chest radiograph shows abnormal opacity associated with air bronchograms (*arrows*) in the lower lobes. There are other areas of linear subsegmental atelectasis more superiorly in the lower lungs.

TABLE 11-1

RADIOGRAPHIC SIGNS OF ATELECTASIS

Crowding of pulmonary vessels
Crowded air bronchograms
Displacement of interlobar fissures
Abnormal pulmonary opacification
Obscured heart or diaphragm borders
Diaphragm elevation
Displacement of mediastinal structures
Hilar displacement
Compensatory hyperexpansion of surrounding lung
Approximation of ribs

atelectasis can also be associated with certain chronic obstructive airway diseases (e.g., asthma, chronic bronchitis, and emphysema), and it can be seen in acute bronchitis, bronchiolitis, and aspiration and other types of pneumonia from obstruction of small airways by inflammatory exudate.

Atelectasis resulting from surfactant deficiency is termed *adhesive atelectasis*. Insufficient surfactant leads to alveolar collapse; once collapsed, the alveolar walls tend to adhere, making re-expansion difficult. Diffuse surfactant deficiency can result from hyaline membrane disease, acute respiratory distress syndrome, smoke inhalation, cardiac bypass surgery, uremia, and prolonged shallow breathing (5).

Compressive atelectasis is caused by any space-occupying lesion of the thorax compressing the lung and forcing air out of the alveoli. Such space-occupying lesions include pleural effusion (including empyema), pneumothorax, pleural tumors, large pulmonary parenchymal masses, large emphysematous bullae, and lobar emphysema (6). Diaphragmatic hernias and abdominal distension from a variety of causes can also compress the lung.

The distinction between compressive and *passive atelectasis* is not clear cut. Any space-occupying mass within the thorax can either compress the lung or allow the lung to retract, passively, from the lung's normal elastic recoil mechanism.

Volume loss resulting from decreased pulmonary compliance as the result of pulmonary fibrosis is termed *cicatrization atelectasis*. This type of atelectasis is often associated with bronchiectasis in the affected lung. A number of conditions can result in pulmonary fibrosis and cicatrization atelectasis—for example, idiopathic pulmonary fibrosis, sarcoidosis, pneumoconioses, collagen vascular diseases, chronic tuberculous and fungal infections, and radiation fibrosis.

Normally, the most gravity-dependent portions of lung receive greater perfusion and have less alveolar expansion than non–gravity-dependent portions of lung. These gravity-dependent alterations in alveolar volume are normal but can exacerbate atelectasis in the dependent portions of the lungs, particularly in bedridden hospitalized patients with prolonged shallow breathing. Atelectasis occurring from these forces is termed *gravity-dependent atelectasis*.

RADIOGRAPHIC SIGNS OF ATELECTASIS

Radiographic signs of atelectasis are outlined in Table 11-1 (5). Opacification of atelectatic lung may not be seen until a considerable loss of volume has occurred. When edema fluid

is drawn into the collapsing lung, pneumonia has resulted in atelectasis, or postobstructive pneumonitis is present, there can be abnormal opacification of lung without substantial evidence of volume loss. Elevation of the diaphragm as a sign of volume loss is most easily appreciated when comparison is made to a normal baseline radiograph. A key radiographic feature of upper lobe atelectasis is superior displacement of the hilus. Conversely, in lower lobe atelectasis, the hilus is displaced inferiorly. There is usually no hilar displacement with right middle lobe or lingula atelectasis. Displacement of a fissure follows the movement of the atelectatic lung and is most apparent with atelectasis of an entire lobe. Lung surrounding atelectatic lung often hyperexpands in an attempt to fill in the missing volume of lung; this is referred to as compensatory hyperexpansion or sometimes confusingly referred to as compensatory emphysema. Emphysema is a pathologic condition involving destruction of alveolar walls. Although emphysematous lungs are invariably hyperinflated, hyperexpanded lungs are not invariably emphysematous. If atelectasis affects only one lung, the ribs on that side may come to lie closer together than the ribs on the contralateral normal side. This should be distinguished from the approximation of ribs caused by poor patient positioning at the time the radiograph was obtained.

One of the pitfalls in diagnosing left lower lobe atelectasis is artifactual loss of the medial margin of the left hemidiaphragm and abnormal opacity in the left lower lung as a result of incorrect angulation of the x-ray beam. Lordotic angulation of the beam by as little as 10 degrees results in the beam no longer being tangential to the apex of the hemidiaphragm, creating illusory opacity in the left retrocardiac region that may be interpreted as atelectasis or airspace disease in the left lower lobe. Normal appearing diaphragms and lungs on a lateral view are helpful in making the distinction.

LOBAR ATELECTASIS

In an adult with lobar atelectasis, a central obstructing neoplasm should always be considered as the underlying cause. Bronchogenic carcinoma is relatively uncommon in adults under the age of 40, when bronchial carcinoid tumor is more likely. In children with lobar collapse, an aspirated foreign body or asthma is the usual cause. In postoperative patients, the most common cause is a mucous plug.

With right upper lobe atelectasis, the major and minor fissures move upward (Figs. 11-3 to 11-6); with severe atelectasis, the lung can approximate the mediastinum and lung apex. With complete atelectasis, or collapse of the right upper lobe, the minor fissure parallels the mediastinum and resembles pleural thickening or mediastinal widening. Compensatory hyperexpansion of the middle and right lower lobes leads to outward and upward displacement of the right lower lobe pulmonary

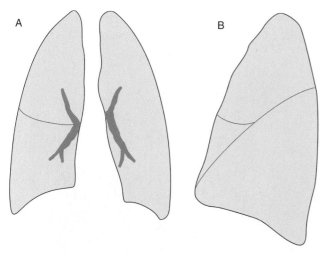

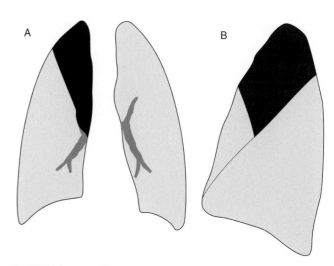

FIGURE 11-3. Normal lung volumes and fissures. Frontal (**A**) and lateral (**B**) views of the chest show normal positions of the minor (horizontal, right-sided) and major (oblique, bilateral) fissures. The major fissures are often superimposed on the lateral chest radiograph and are usually not seen on the frontal view.

FIGURE 11-4. Right upper lobe atelectasis. A: Frontal view of the chest shows elevation of the minor fissure and increased opacification of the right upper medial lung (*black area*). **B:** Lateral view shows elevation of the minor fissure and superior portion of the right major fissure, as well as opacification of the upper lung.

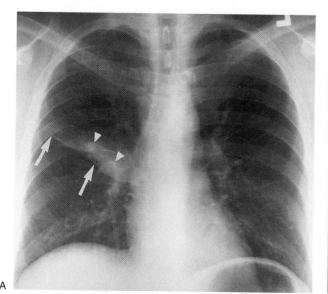

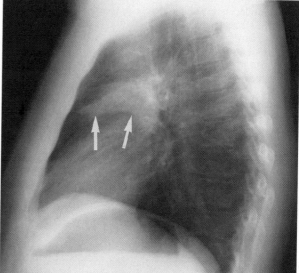

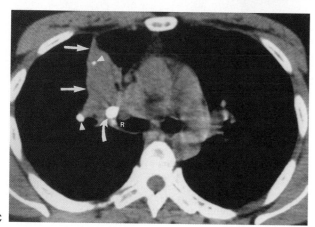

FIGURE 11-5. Right upper lobe segmental atelectasis. A: Posteroanterior (PA) chest radiograph of a 35-year-old man with lithoptysis (literally "coughing up stones," but representing calcified lymph nodes that have eroded into the airway, usually secondary to tuberculosis or histoplasmosis) shows partial collapse of the right upper lobe. The minor fissure is elevated (*arrows*), outlining the inferior margin of the opacified, atelectatic lung. Note calcified densities (*arrowheads*) overlying the opacified lung centrally and peripherally. **B:** Lateral view shows elevation of the minor fissure (*arrows*) outlining the inferior margin of the opacified, atelectatic right upper lobe. **C:** CT shows the smooth and fairly straight fissural margin of the atelectatic right upper lobe (*straight arrows*), calcified granulomas within the atelectatic right upper lobe (*arrowheads*), and an obstructing broncholith (*curved arrow*) within the right upper lobe bronchus (*R*).

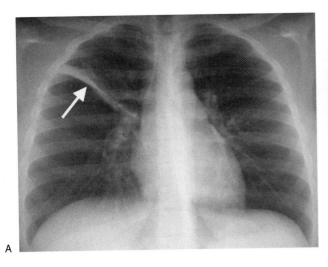

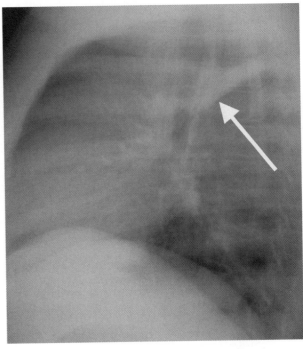

FIGURE 11-6. Right upper lobe segmental atelectasis. A: PA chest radiograph of a 15-year-old girl with asthma shows elevation of the minor fissure (*arrow*). **B:** Lateral view shows elevation of the superior portion of the right major fissure (*arrow*) outlining a linear band of atelectatic lung.

artery. Upward angulation of the right mainstem and lower lobe bronchi may be difficult to appreciate on chest radiography. Two radiologic signs are associated with right upper lobe atelectasis. The Golden S sign, or S sign of Golden (see Fig. 2-11), refers to right upper lobe collapse around a central obstructing mass. The juxtaphrenic peak sign (see Fig. 2-14) refers to a small triangular shadow based on the apex of the dome of the right hemidiaphragm with loss of silhouette of the adjacent hemidiaphragm. On computed tomography (CT), a collapsed right upper lobe appears as a triangular soft tissue density lying against the mediastinum and the anterior chest wall. The border formed by the major fissure posteriorly and the minor fissure laterally is sharp.

Atelectasis of the right middle lobe can be easily overlooked on the frontal chest radiograph. Loss of silhouette of the right border of the heart is often seen, but not always. The atelectatic lobe is more readily recognized on the lateral chest radiograph as a well-defined linear or triangular band of density lying between the major and minor fissures (with approximation of these fissures) and extending downward and forward from the hilum (Fig. 11-7). The collapsed lobe can be very thin and misinterpreted as a thickened fissure. On CT scans, right middle lobe collapse appears as a triangular density bounded posteriorly by the major fissure, medially by the mediastinum at the level of the right atrium, and anteriorly by the minor fissure (Figs. 11-8 and 11-9). The posterior boundary should be well defined. Chronic atelectasis of the right middle lobe is referred to as *middle lobe syndrome*, a term that was coined in 1948 to describe the presence of right middle lobe atelectasis and chronic inflammation secondary to enlarged lymph nodes impinging on the middle lobe bronchus (7). The middle lobe bronchus is long and narrow, and it is more easily obstructed at its origin by lymph nodes than are other bronchi. The syndrome was initially described with tuberculosis, but it may also be seen in other infections and endobronchial tumors; it may even be seen in the absence of obstruction.

Combined atelectasis of the right upper and middle lobes is unusual because there is no single bronchus to the right upper and middle lobes that does not also supply the right lower lobe. The cause is almost always cancer beginning in the upper lobe bronchus and growing down one side of the bronchus inter-

medius to involve the middle lobe bronchus. The appearance of combined right upper and middle lobe atelectasis is similar to that seen with left upper lobe atelectasis.

Combined right lower and middle lobe atelectasis is a fairly common combination, is seen with obstruction to the bronchus intermedius, and is similar in appearance to right lower lobe atelectasis on both posteroanterior (PA) and lateral chest radiographs (Fig. 11-10). With combined right lower and middle lobe atelectasis, however, the abnormal parenchymal opacity extends all the way to the lateral costophrenic angle on the PA view and from the front to the back of the thorax on the

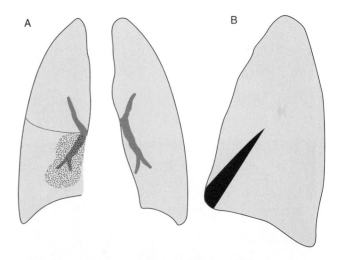

FIGURE 11-7. Right middle lobe atelectasis. A: Frontal view of the chest shows loss of the right heart border and an ill-defined area of increased opacification in the right medial lung (*stippled area*). **B:** Lateral view shows triangular area of opacification (*black area*) overlying the heart, with approximation of the minor and major fissures. (Reprinted with permission from Collins J. 1996 Joseph E. Whitley, MD, Award. Evaluation of an introductory course in chest radiology. *Acad Radiol.* 1996;3:994–999.)

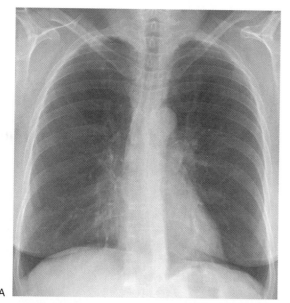

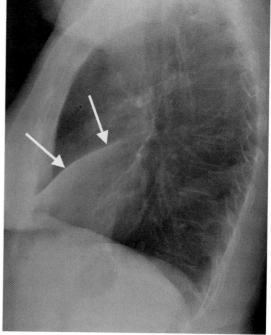

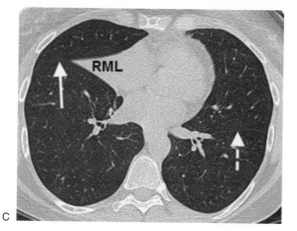

FIGURE 11-8. Right middle lobe atelectasis. A: PA chest radiograph of a 52-year-old woman with shortness of breath and cough shows hazy opacity in the right medial lung and loss of the right heart border. B: Lateral view shows a linear opacity overlying the heart (*arrows*), representing the collapsed right middle lobe. C: CT shows a triangular opacity adjacent to the right heart border representing right middle lobe collapse (*RML*). The right major fissure (*solid arrow*) is displaced anteriorly compared with the normally positioned left major fissure (*dashed arrow*). At bronchoscopy, thick secretions were seen in the right middle lobe bronchus.

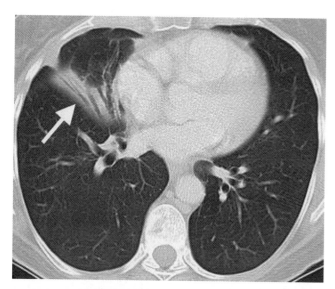

FIGURE 11-9. Right middle lobe atelectasis. CT of a 53-year-old man with asthma shows anterior displacement of the major fissure (*arrow*) and crowding of bronchi in the opacified segment of right middle lobe.

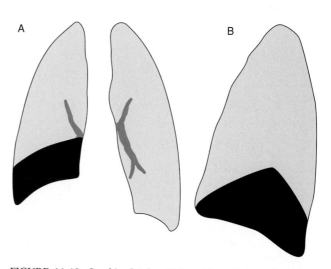

FIGURE 11-10. Combined right middle and lower lobe atelectasis. A: Frontal view of the chest shows elevation of the right hemidiaphragm, depression of the minor fissure, and increased opacification in the right lower lung that extends to the lateral costophrenic angle (*black area*). B: Lateral view shows depression of the minor and major fissures and increased opacification of the inferior lung, extending from anterior to posterior (*black area*).

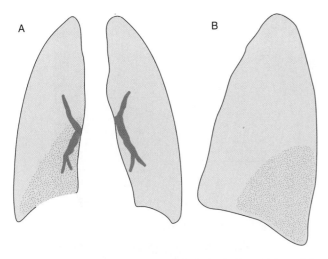

FIGURE 11-11. **Right lower lobe atelectasis. A:** Frontal view of the chest shows loss of the medial right hemidiaphragm border, elevation of the right hemidiaphragm, and increased opacification of the right medial lower lung (*stippled area*). **B:** Lateral view shows increased opacification of the posterior inferior lung (*stippled area*).

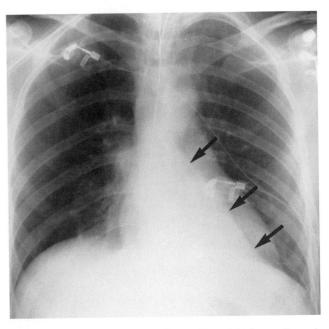

FIGURE 11-13. **Left lower lobe collapse.** AP upright chest radiograph of a 17-year-old boy shows downward and medial displacement of the left major fissure (*arrows*), a triangular area of increased opacification over the left heart, and loss of the left medial diaphragmatic contour.

lateral view. On the frontal radiograph, there is a superficial resemblance to an elevated diaphragm, but the lung above it (right upper lobe) is unusually clear instead of appearing "expiratory." The diagnosis is made much more easily with CT because the bronchi can be identified individually.

Atelectasis of either lower lobe results in backward and medial rotation of the major fissure, as well as downward displacement of the upper half of the fissure. With right lower lobe atelectasis, the minor fissure can be displaced inferiorly (Figs. 11-11 and 11-12). The atelectatic lobe lies posteromedially in the lower thoracic cavity, with a resulting triangular

opacity based on the diaphragm and mediastinum, and with the fissure running obliquely through the thorax (Figs. 11-13 and 11-14). When a lower lobe collapses completely, it becomes very thin and appears on the PA chest radiograph as a sliver lying against the mediastinum. On the lateral radiograph, lower lobe atelectasis results in loss of the outline of the posterior half of the hemidiaphragm shadow. Also, with lower lobe atelectasis, the lower vertebrae appear more opaque than the vertebrae higher up; this results in a situation that is the opposite of

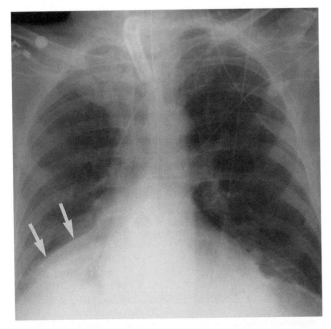

FIGURE 11-12. **Bilateral lower lobe atelectasis.** AP supine chest radiograph of a 61-year-old man shows partial loss of the contours of the hemidiaphragms bilaterally, abnormal opacification of the lung bases, and inferior displacement of the minor fissure (*arrows*).

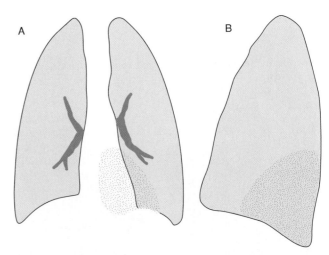

FIGURE 11-14. **Left lower lobe atelectasis. A:** Frontal view of the chest shows loss of the medial left hemidiaphragm border, elevation of the left hemidiaphragm, and increased opacification of the left medial lower lung (*stippled area*). **B:** Lateral view shows increased opacification of the posterior inferior lung (*stippled area*).

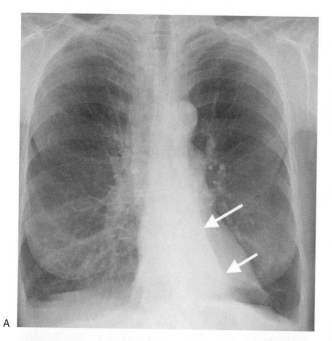

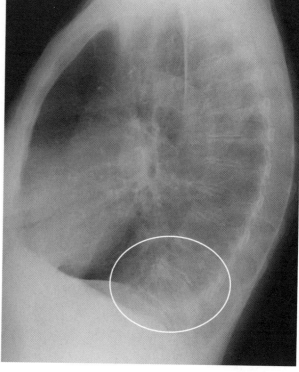

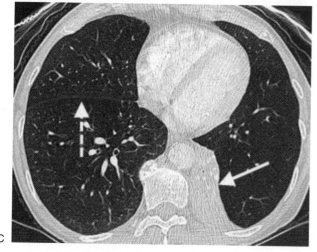

FIGURE 11-15. Left lower lobe collapse. A: PA chest radiograph of a 65-year-old woman shows inferior displacement of the left major fissure (*arrows*) and a triangular area of abnormal opacity projected over the left heart. **B:** Lateral view shows abnormal opacity overlying the lower spine (*circle*), the so-called spine sign. **C:** CT shows the collapsed left lower lobe hugging the spine, outlined laterally by the inferiorly displaced major fissure (*solid arrow*). Note the normal position of the right major fissure (*dashed arrow*).

normal, where the opacity gradually decreases in moving from superior to inferior along the thoracic spine and has been called the spine sign (Fig. 11-15). On CT scans, a collapsed lower lobe produces a triangular opacity in the posterior chest against the spine.

The radiologic appearance of left upper lobe atelectasis is markedly different from that of right upper lobe atelectasis because there is no minor fissure on the left. In left upper lobe atelectasis, the lobe collapses forward, pulling the expanding lower lobe behind it (Fig. 11-16). On the frontal radiograph, the atelectatic lobe is seen as hazy opacification extending out from the left hilum, often reaching the lung apex, fading laterally and inferiorly (Figs. 11-17 and 11-18). It is important not to mistake the abnormal parenchymal opacity as representing pneumonia, and this mistake will not be made if the other signs of volume loss are appreciated. These signs include loss of the left cardiomediastinal silhouette, elevation of the left hemidiaphragm, and shift of the mediastinal structures to the left. With complete collapse, the upper margin of the aortic arch is visible because the superior segment of the lower lobe hyperexpands to take the place of the posterior segment of the

upper lobe. This crescentic lucency, which represents the hyperexpanded superior segment of the left lower lobe invaginating between the aortic arch and collapsed left upper lobe, is referred to as the luftsichel sign (see Chapter 2). This sign can be seen on the frontal chest radiograph and on CT. The hyperexpansion of the left lower lobe also results in elevation of the left hilum and outward angulation of the left lower lobe pulmonary artery. The left main bronchus assumes a near horizontal course and the lower lobe bronchus runs more vertically than normal. On the lateral radiograph, the major fissure is displaced anteriorly, paralleling the anterior chest wall; the atelectatic left upper lobe is seen as an abnormal band of retrosternal opacification. Left upper lobe atelectasis in an adult patient is especially important to recognize because of the frequency with which it is caused by endobronchial carcinoma.

Complete collapse of either lung results in opacification of the hemithorax and shift of the mediastinal structures to the side of collapse (Fig. 11-19). There is usually hyperexpansion of the opposite lung into the involved hemithorax. The differential diagnosis of an opaque hemithorax with volume loss includes congenital absence of a lung (the bony thorax on

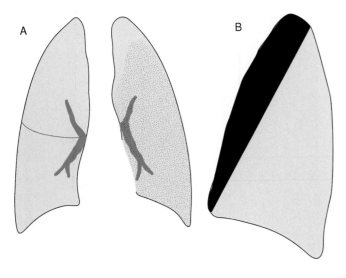

FIGURE 11-16. Left upper lobe atelectasis. A: Frontal view of the chest shows loss of the left heart border, elevation of the left hemidiaphragm, and increased opacification of the left lung (*stippled area*). B: Lateral view shows anterior displacement of the major fissure and increased retrosternal opacification (*black area*). (Reprinted with permission from Collins J. Joseph E. Whitley, MD, Award. Evaluation of an introductory course in chest radiology. *Acad Radiol.* 1996;3:994–999.)

the affected side is usually underdeveloped), remote traumatic injury to the bronchus on the affected side (Fig. 11-20), and pneumonectomy (hilar surgical clips provide a clue to the underlying cause of mediastinal shift). Intubated patients are at increased risk of mucous plugging of the airways, and whenever acute lobar or complete lung collapse is seen in this patient population, mucous plugging should be suspected (Fig. 11-21). It is important to recognize lung collapse related to massive pleural effusion, which can (but does not always) result in opacity of the ipsilateral hemithorax and shift of the mediastinum to the *opposite* side (Fig. 11-22). Parenchymal masses may be obscured on chest radiography when accompanied by lung collapse secondary to central obstruction or massive pleural effusion. In some cases, an opaque hemithorax may represent a combination of a parenchymal mass, lung collapse, and pleural effusion. The overall balance of volume loss and mass effect will determine the position of the mediastinum.

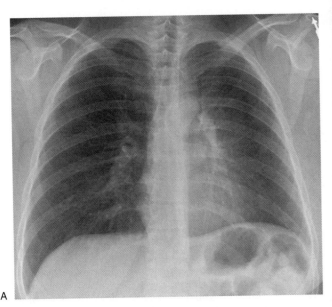

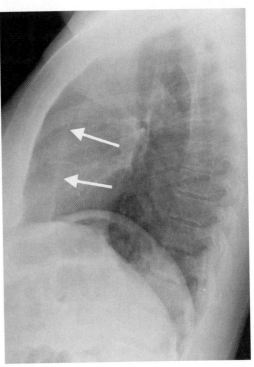

FIGURE 11-17. Left upper lobe collapse. A: PA chest radiograph of a 44-year-old man with a 6-month history of recurrent pneumonia shows elevation of the left hemidiaphragm, hazy opacity of the left hemithorax, and loss of the left heart border. B: Lateral view shows anterior displacement of the left major fissure (*arrows*) and increased retrosternal opacity. Bronchoscopic biopsy of a left upper lobe endobronchial mass confirmed the diagnosis of a bronchial carcinoid tumor as the cause of the left upper lobe collapse.

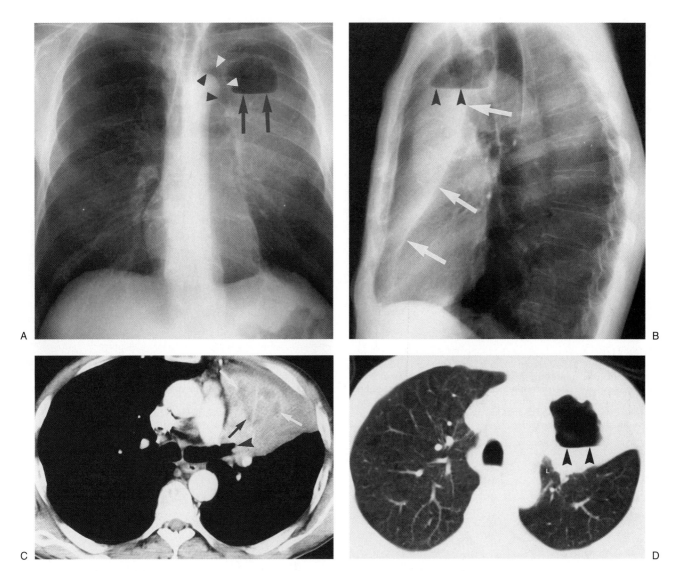

FIGURE 11-18. Left upper lobe collapse. A: PA chest radiograph of a 54-year-old man with a cavitary left upper lobe squamous cell bronchogenic carcinoma shows hazy opacification of the left upper and middle lung, elevation of the left hemidiaphragm, and loss of a portion of the left upper heart border. Note air–fluid level within the left upper lobe (*arrows*). There is a crescentic lucency between the aortic arch and the collapsed left upper lobe (*black and white arrowheads*) representing hyperexpansion of the superior segment of the left lower lobe (the luftsichel sign). **B:** Lateral view shows anterior displacement of the major fissure (*arrows*), abnormal retrosternal opacification representing the collapsed left upper lobe, and air–fluid level within the left upper lobe (*arrowheads*). **C:** CT shows abrupt cutoff of the left upper lobe bronchus (*arrowhead*) from an obstructing endobronchial carcinoma and distal collapse of the left upper lobe. Note areas of low attenuation (*arrows*) within the collapsed left upper lobe, representing trapped mucus, pneumonia, or both. **D:** CT with lung windowing shows the cavitary cancer in the left upper lobe, with an air–fluid level (*arrowheads*). Note hyperexpansion of the superior segment of the left lower lobe between the aortic arch and collapsed left upper lobe, accounting for the radiographic luftsichel sign (*L*).

NONLOBAR ATELECTASIS

For descriptive purposes, atelectasis can be divided into several types other than lobar atelectasis, depending on the anatomic location of the atelectatic lung. *Round atelectasis* is a form of chronic atelectasis associated with pleural disease, often benign asbestos-related pleural disease, and is discussed in Chapter 3.

Discoid atelectasis, also referred to as *platelike* or *linear atelectasis*, is a form of peripheral pulmonary volume loss that is not secondary to bronchial obstruction. First described in 1936

by Fleischner (8) and, therefore, also referred to as Fleischner lines, the atelectasis is disc or plate shaped. Discoid atelectasis usually abuts the pleura and is perpendicular to the pleural surface; the thickness ranges from a few millimeters to a centimeter or more, and the lesions are therefore usually seen as linear or bandlike opacities. The mechanism of discoid atelectasis is hypoventilation, which leads to alveolar collapse. Although often of little clinical significance, multiple areas of discoid atelectasis can be physiologically significant in certain conditions, such as after general anesthesia.

The radiographic identification of *subsegmental atelectasis* can be difficult. When atelectasis is present at the subsegmental

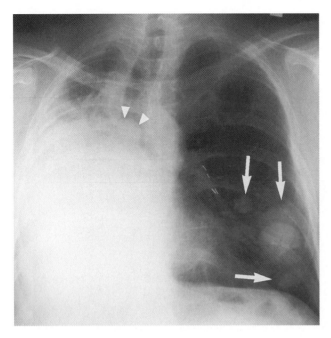

FIGURE 11-19. Atelectasis of the right lung. PA chest radiograph of a 40-year-old man with metastatic frontal sinus fibrosarcoma shows nearly complete collapse of the right lung, with only partial aeration of the right upper lobe. The mediastinal structures are shifted to the right. A large, rounded endobronchial metastasis is obstructing the right main bronchus (*arrowheads*), and numerous parenchymal metastases are seen within the left lung (*arrows*).

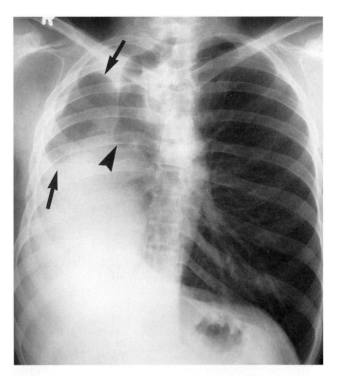

FIGURE 11-20. Collapse of the right lung. PA chest radiograph of a 30-year-old man with a history of a "punctured lung" during a motor vehicle crash 11 years previously. There is complete collapse of the right lung and compensatory hyperexpansion of the left lung into the right hemithorax (*arrows*). Note the bronchial cutoff sign on the right (*arrowhead*), where the bronchus was fractured and healed with granulation tissue.

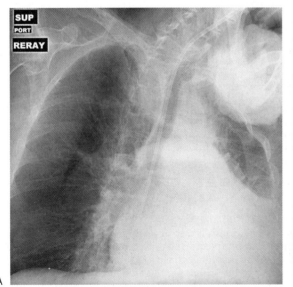

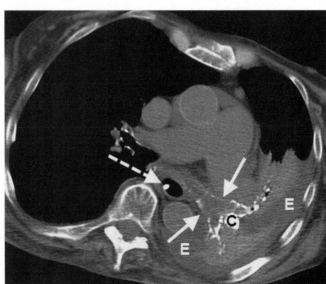

FIGURE 11-21. Left lung atelectasis. A: AP supine chest radiograph of an 82-year-old woman with dementia and respiratory distress shows nearly complete collapse of the left lung. Note mediastinal shift to the left. B: CT shows that the left main bronchus (*solid arrows*), lingular bronchus, and left lower lobe superior segment bronchus (all outlined by calcified walls) are airless and filled with low-attenuation material (mucus). There is a densely calcified left hilar lymph node (C). Pleural effusion (E) outlines the collapsed left lung. A feeding tube is present within the esophagus (*dashed arrow*).

pulmonary lobules collapse within the affected segment or lobe, crowded vessels and bronchi, hilar displacement, or fissural displacement will become apparent.

Generalized or *diffuse atelectasis* is a term used to describe widespread volume loss in the lungs in the absence of specific signs of linear, segmental, or lobar atelectasis (5). There can be marked arteriovenous shunting, but the opacification of the lungs may be mild or unapparent; high positioning of the diaphragm may be the only radiographic clue to the presence of volume loss. Most of these cases are interpreted as "poor inspiratory effort." When generalized atelectasis is associated with diffuse pulmonary opacification, the interpretation is often diffuse pneumonia or pulmonary edema. The abnormally high diaphragm provides a clue to the correct diagnosis, but in practice it is often impossible to distinguish diffuse atelectasis from poor inspiratory effort or pulmonary edema.

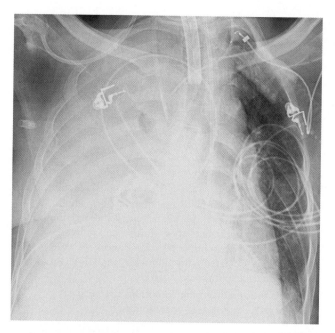

FIGURE 11-22. Massive right pleural effusion. AP supine chest radiograph of a 55-year-old man with end-stage liver disease and shortness of breath shows opacification of the right hemithorax and shift of the mediastinum to the left, away from the opaque hemithorax.

level, many secondary pulmonary lobules within the affected segment or lobe may remain aerated, whereas others collapse. In such cases, and when multifocal, the degree of volume loss can be minimal, and the radiograph may show only patchy opacities resembling bronchopneumonia. As more secondary

References

1. Fleischner Society. Glossary of terms for thoracic radiology: recommendation of the nomenclature committee of the Fleischner Society. *AJR Am J Roentgenol.* 1984;143:509–517.
2. Fraser RG, Paré JAP, Paré PD, et al. *Diagnosis of Diseases of the Chest.* 3rd ed. Philadelphia: WB Saunders; 1988:472–545.
3. Heitzman ER. *The Lung: Radiologic Pathologic Correlations.* 2nd ed. St. Louis: Mosby; 1984:457–501.
4. Felson B. *Chest Roentgenology.* Philadelphia: WB Saunders; 1973:92–133.
5. Woodring JH, Reed JC. Types and mechanisms of pulmonary atelectasis. *J Thorac Imaging.* 1996;11:92–108.
6. Naidich DP, McCauley DI, Khouri NF, et al. Computed tomography of lobar collapse. II. Collapse in the absence of endobronchial obstruction. *J Comput Assist Tomogr.* 1983;7:758–767.
7. Graham EA, Burford TH, Mayer JH. Middle lobe syndrome. *Postgrad Med.* 1948;4:29–43.
8. Fleischner F. Uber das Wesen der basalen horizontalen Schattenstreifen im Lungenfeld. *Wein Arch Intern Med.* 1936;28:461.

CHAPTER 12

PERIPHERAL LUNG DISEASE

LEARNING OBJECTIVES

1. Recognize a pattern of peripheral lung disease on chest radiography or computed tomography and give an appropriate differential diagnosis, including a single most likely diagnosis when supported by associated radiologic findings or clinical information (e.g., peripheral lung disease associated with paratracheal and bilateral hilar lymphadenopathy in an asymptomatic patient with alveolar sarcoidosis; peripheral lung disease associated with a markedly elevated blood eosinophil count in a patient with eosinophilic pneumonia; peripheral opacities associated with multiple rib fractures and pneumothorax in a patient with acute chest trauma and pulmonary contusions; and multiple peripheral wedge-shaped opacities associated with pulmonary emboli in a patient with multiple pulmonary infarcts).

2. Name four predisposing conditions that lead to cryptogenic organizing pneumonitis.

The diseases in this chapter are not ordinarily discussed together. Alveolar sarcoidosis, usual interstitial pneumonitis, and contusions are, in fact, discussed in chapters 10, 3, and 8, respectively. Cryptogenic organizing pneumonitis (COP) (previously referred to as *bronchiolitis obliterans organizing pneumonia*) and eosinophilic pneumonia (EP) could be discussed in a chapter on diffuse interstitial lung disease. Pulmonary infarcts are discussed with pulmonary emboli in Chapter 17. However, these disorders have been categorized together here because of their propensity for producing a predominantly peripheral distribution of disease on chest radiography and computed tomography (CT). A simple mnemonic, "AEIOU," can be used to remember those disorders that have a peripheral distribution of disease (Table 12-1 and Fig. 12-1). It needs to be mentioned, however, that these disorders frequently do not manifest as recognizable peripheral opacities on chest radiography or CT, so a lack of peripheral opacities does not exclude these disorders. If there is any hint of a peripheral distribution of disease on the chest radiograph, CT can be very helpful in better defining the morphology and distribution of disease (Fig. 12-2).

ALVEOLAR SARCOIDOSIS

Sarcoidosis is a systemic disease of unknown etiology that is characterized by widespread development of noncaseating granulomas. More complete discussions of this disorder are found in chapters 3, 6, and 10. This section will be limited to a discussion of those patients with sarcoidosis who have so-called "alveolar" opacities on chest radiography or CT.

Although the term *alveolar sarcoidosis* is used, the process is predominantly interstitial, with compression and obliteration of alveoli creating the appearance of alveolar filling on radiologic imaging. Histologically, these lesions are seen to represent confluent interstitial granulomas. The radiographic appearance of airspace (alveolar) opacities develops in 10% to 20% of patients with sarcoidosis. The radiologic appearance is that of bilateral, multifocal, poorly defined opacities that range in size from 1 to 10 cm and show a predilection for the peripheral middle lung, sparing the costophrenic angles (1–3) (Fig. 12-3). The peripheral distribution is better seen and on occasion appreciated only on CT. Air bronchograms are common. Associated CT findings of reticulonodular opacities, especially in a lym-

phatic distribution, and mediastinal and hilar lymphadenopathy provide clues to the correct diagnosis. Most patients with alveolar sarcoidosis have accompanying lymphadenopathy (4) (Fig. 12-4). When only peripheral opacities are seen, the appearance can be indistinguishable from those of COP or EP. Although all three disorders can present with blood eosinophilia, the degree of eosinophilia is most pronounced with EP. The peripheral opacities of alveolar sarcoidosis can clear rapidly with or without steroid treatment (1).

EOSINOPHILIC PNEUMONIA

The term *pulmonary eosinophilia*, synonymous with *pulmonary infiltration with eosinophilia*, describes a group of diseases in which blood and/or tissue eosinophilia affects major airways and lung parenchyma (5). Blood eosinophilia, however, is not necessary to make a diagnosis of eosinophilic lung disease. The number of diseases included under the umbrella term *pulmonary eosinophilia* are numerous. A simple mnemonic, "NAACP," and the term *idiopathic* can be used to remember the major classifications of disorders that constitute pulmonary eosinophilia (Table 12–2). This section will focus on parasitic infections and idiopathic pulmonary eosinophilia.

TABLE 12-1

DISORDERS FREQUENTLY MANIFESTING AS PERIPHERAL OPACITIES ON CHEST RADIOGRAPHY OR COMPUTED TOMOGRAPHY

"AEIOU"
Alveolar sarcoidosis
Eosinophilic pneumonia
Infarcts
COP (cryptogenic organizing pneumonia)
UIP ([usual interstitial pneumonitis] and DIP [desquamative interstitial pneumonitis])
ContUsions

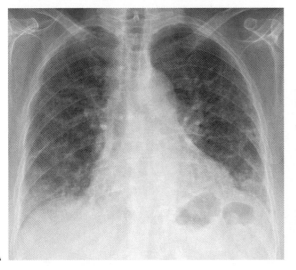
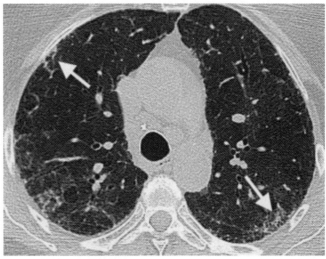

FIGURE 12-1. **Usual interstitial pneumonitis. A:** Posteroanterior (PA) chest radiograph of a 72-year-old woman with scleroderma shows low lung volumes and bilateral reticular interstitial lung disease. **B:** CT shows that the reticular opacities have a subpleural, peripheral distribution (*arrows*).

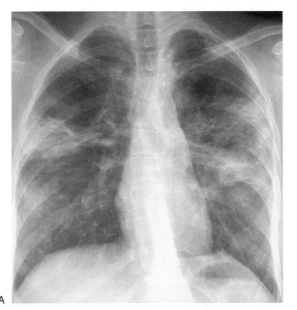

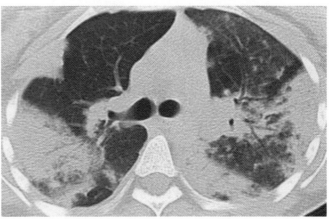

FIGURE 12-2. **Eosinophilic pneumonia. A:** PA chest radiograph of a 21-year-old woman shows bilateral airspace opacities that extend to the lung periphery. **B:** CT better shows the peripheral distribution of disease. Note prominent air bronchograms.

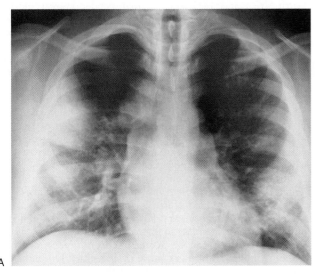

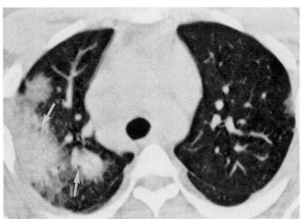

FIGURE 12-3. **Alveolar sarcoidosis. A:** PA chest radiograph of a 28-year-old asymptomatic man shows nonsegmental peripheral airspace disease and bilateral hilar and mediastinal lymphadenopathy. **B:** CT shows bilateral peripheral airspace disease. Note air bronchograms (*arrows*), a common feature of alveolar sarcoidosis.

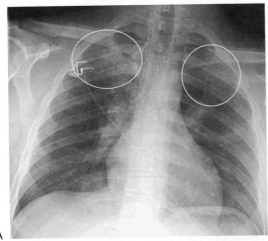

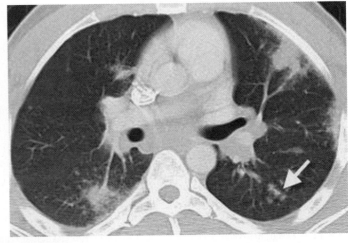

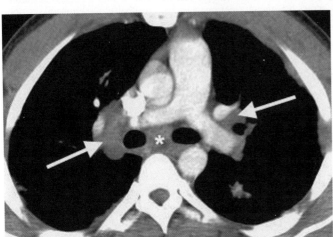

FIGURE 12-4. Alveolar sarcoidosis. A: PA chest radiograph of a 29-year-old man shows ill-defined opacities in the upper lungs (*circles*). B: CT image shows a peripheral distribution of airspace disease. Note nodular beading of a left lower lobe bronchovascular bundle (*arrow*), a characteristic feature of sarcoidosis. C: CT with mediastinal windowing shows bilateral hilar (*arrows*) and subcarinal (*asterisk*) lymphadenopathy. Most patients with alveolar sarcoidosis have accompanying lymphadenopathy.

TABLE 12-2

CLASSIFICATION OF EOSINOPHILIC LUNG DISEASE

"NAACP" and Idiopathic

Neoplasms
  Bronchogenic carcinoma
  Metastases
  Lymphoma

Asthma

Allergic disorders
  Allergic bronchopulmonary aspergillosis
  Drug-induced disease
  Extrinsic allergic alveolitis (hypersensitivity pneumonitis)

Collagen vascular and granulomatous disorders
  Rheumatoid lung disease
  Churg-Strauss syndrome
  Wegener granulomatosis
  Sarcoidosis

Parasitic disorders and other infections
  Tropical pulmonary eosinophilia
  Helminth infections (worm infestation)
  Fungal infections
  Other bacterial, viral, and protozoal infections

Idiopathic
  Acute eosinophilic pneumonia (Löffler syndrome)
  Chronic eosinophilic pneumonia

Tropical pulmonary eosinophilia is a systemic disease caused by hypersensitivity to microfilariae, which are the early larval forms of various filarial nematodes, most notably *Brugia malayi* and *Wuchereria bancrofti* (6). The disease is endemic in the Indian subcontinent, Southeast Asia, the South Pacific, North Africa, and South America. In nonendemic areas, the disease is seen in immigrants. The predominant respiratory symptom is chronic cough, which is often worse at night. Patients have marked blood eosinophilia, elevated immunoglobulin E (IgE) levels, and a high titer of antifilarial antibody. The chest radiograph is abnormal in the majority of patients, with the most common abnormality being fine linear opacities that are distributed diffusely and symmetrically. Small nodules, ranging in size from 1 to 5 mm, are seen in about half of cases. Hilar lymphadenopathy is uncommon and, when present, is mild (7). An important diagnostic criterion is rapid response to treatment with diethylcarbamazine. Chronic interstitial fibrosis can develop in some patients (8).

The larval stages of a number of worms other than filarial nematodes can pass through the lung and cause EP. These include *Ascaris lumbricoides, Strongyloides stercoralis, Toxocara canis, Trichuris trichiura,* and *Schistosoma* sp. The radiologic pattern is usually identical to that of acute EP.

Cryptogenic EP can be acute or chronic, depending on whether the condition lasts more or less than 1 month (9). The 1-month criterion is arbitrary, and the distinction between acute and chronic EP is not always clear. Acute EP, also referred to as Löffler syndrome, is characterized by blood eosinophilia; mild or absent symptoms and signs (cough, fever, dyspnea);

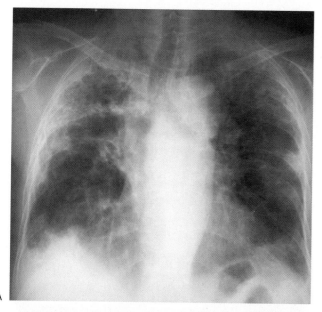

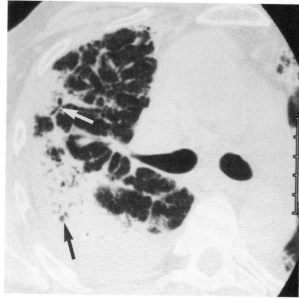

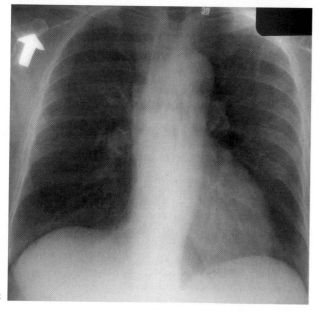

FIGURE 12-5. Chronic eosinophilic pneumonia. A: PA chest radiograph of a 62-year-old woman shows bilateral interstitial and airspace opacities, which are worse in the peripheral lungs, and elevation of the right hemidiaphragm related to right upper lobe volume loss. Based on the findings on this single exam, with no prior chest radiograph for comparison, both acute and chronic processes must be considered. B: CT of the right lung better shows the peripheral distribution of airspace disease. Note air bronchograms (*arrows*), which are a common feature of EP. No honeycombing is seen. C: PA chest radiograph obtained 2 months later, after treatment with steroids, shows complete clearing of bilateral peripheral lung disease.

one or more nonsegmental mixed interstitial and alveolar pulmonary opacities that are transitory or migratory; and spontaneous clearing of opacities (within 1 month). The pulmonary opacities have a tendency to be predominantly peripheral in distribution. One way of remembering this peripheral distribution is to think of EP as being the opposite of PE (pulmonary edema). The classic distribution of pulmonary edema is a *central* batwing or butterfly pattern of alveolar lung disease, which is just the opposite of the *peripheral* alveolar opacities seen with EP. Pleural effusions and lymphadenopathy are not features of acute EP.

Chronic EP is most prevalent in the third to seventh decades of life, with women outnumbering men by 2 to 1 (10). Symptoms of dyspnea, cough, wheeze, malaise, weight loss, fever, and night sweats can be mild or severe. Blood eosinophilia occurs in the majority of patients. Serum IgE is normal or only mildly elevated, which is helpful in distinguishing the condition from allergic bronchopulmonary aspergillosis and tropical and parasitic pulmonary eosinophilias, in which serum

IgE levels are markedly elevated. The classic findings on chest radiograph and CT are nonspecific peripheral, nonsegmental, homogeneous alveolar opacities, often with air bronchograms (10,11) (Figs. 12-5 and 12-6). In a minority of patients, the opacities are central in distribution or both central and peripheral (Fig. 12-7). Chronic EP is sensitive to steroid therapy; rapid clearing of radiologic abnormalities is usually seen within a few days, with complete clearing by 1 month. Relapse is common, and the majority of patients need long-term low-dose steroids, distinguishing this disease from acute EP (12). The radiologic manifestations can be migratory, occurring in new locations with relapse.

PULMONARY INFARCTION

Only 15% or fewer of thromboemboli cause pulmonary infarction (13). It is unknown why some emboli cause infarction

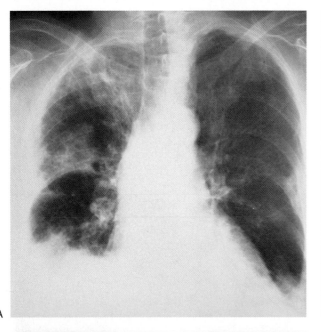

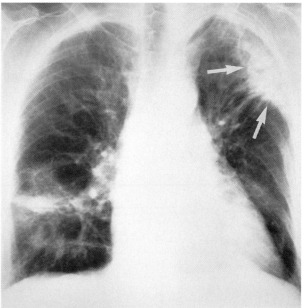

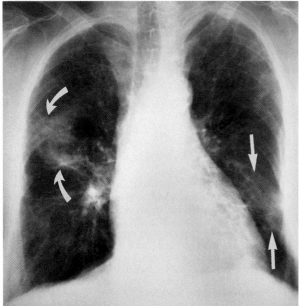

FIGURE 12-6. Chronic eosinophilic pneumonia, recurrent. A: PA chest radiograph of an 85-year-old woman shows bilateral, ill-defined parenchymal opacities in a predominantly peripheral distribution. The right lung is more involved than the left. **B:** PA chest radiograph taken 5 months later shows clearing of much of the right lung and worsening disease in the periphery of the left lung (*arrows*). **C:** PA chest radiograph obtained 1 month after (**B**) shows partial clearing of the left upper lung, worsening disease in the left mid peripheral lung (*straight arrows*), and worsening disease in the right middle lung (*curved arrows*). Migratory lung disease is a characteristic feature of EP.

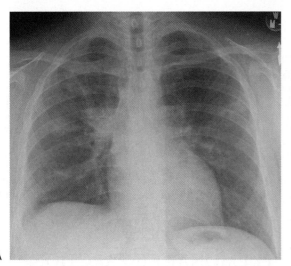

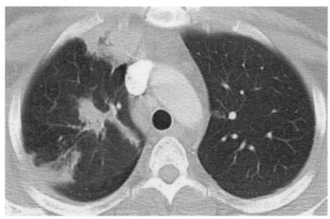

FIGURE 12-7. Chronic eosinophilic pneumonia. A: PA chest radiograph of a 30-year-old woman with several months' history of productive cough, fever, fatigue, chills, and dyspnea on exertion, treated unsuccessfully with several courses of antibiotics, shows bilateral ill-defined opacities, predominantly in the mid lungs. **B:** CT shows peripheral and central airspace disease. (*Continued*)

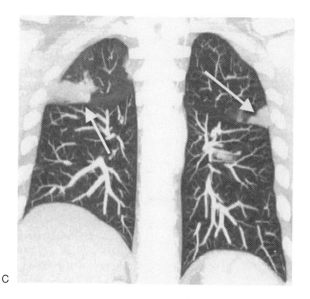

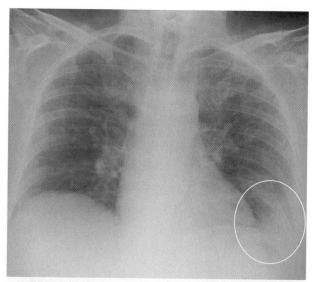

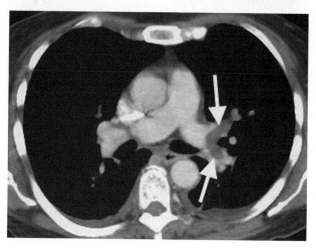

C

FIGURE 12-7. (*Continued*) **C:** CT coronal reformatted image clearly shows the subpleural, peripheral distribution of disease (*arrows*). The patient improved rapidly with steroid treatment.

and others do not, but it is likely a result of compromise of both the pulmonary and bronchial arterial circulation. This is most likely to occur with peripheral emboli and in patients with left heart failure or circulatory shock (14). It is known that bronchial circulation alone can sustain the lung parenchyma without infarction occurring (15).

No chest radiographic sign is specific for pulmonary embolism or infarction, and the sensitivity of chest radiography for these conditions is poor. Even with large pulmonary artery clot burden, the chest radiograph can be normal (16). The main role of the chest radiograph, therefore, is to exclude other diagnoses that might mimic pulmonary embolism clinically, such as pneumonia or pneumothorax.

Pulmonary infarction results in airspace opacities that are usually multifocal and predominantly in the lower lungs. They usually appear within 12 to 24 hours after the embolic event. The opacities are classically peripheral, with a triangular or rounded shape (thus the term "Hampton hump"), and they are always in contact with the pleural surfaces (Fig. 12-8). The apex or hump of the opacity is directed toward the lung hilum. Occasionally, lobar consolidation resembling pneumonia can occur. Air bronchograms are rarely present. It is important to

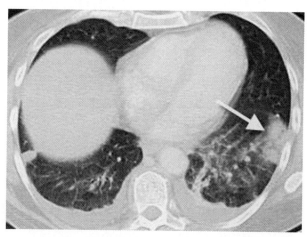

FIGURE 12-8. Pulmonary infarct. A: PA chest radiograph of a 52-year-old woman with acute pulmonary embolism shows focal airspace disease at the left costophrenic angle (*circle*). **B:** CT shows bilateral subpleural airspace opacities, which are largest in the left lower lobe (*arrow*), and bilateral pleural effusions. **C:** CT with mediastinal windowing confirms the presence of a central filling defect (*arrows*) within otherwise opacified lingular and left lower lobe pulmonary arteries, characteristic features of acute pulmonary emboli.

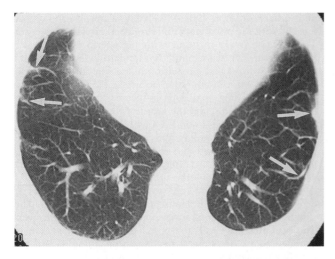

FIGURE 12-9. Pulmonary infarcts. CT of a 69-year-old man 10 weeks after a confirmed acute pulmonary embolic event shows residual subpleural scarring related to bilateral pulmonary infarcts (*arrows*).

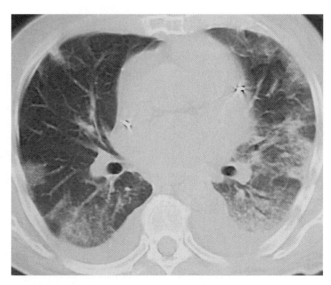

FIGURE 12-11. Cryptogenic organizing pneumonitis. CT shows bilateral dense airspace and ground-glass opacities in a peripheral distribution. The patient had COP related to amiodarone lung toxicity.

note that the opacities can be a result of a combination of atelectasis and pulmonary hemorrhage without infarction, in which case clearing occurs within a week. Infarction takes several months to resolve, often with residual scarring (Fig. 12-9). As infarcts resolve, they melt away "like an ice cube" (giving rise to the melting ice cube sign; see Fig. 2-16). The opacity clears from the periphery first, whereas in pneumonia the opacity clears homogeneously (both centrally and peripherally) at the same time. Cavitation can occur within infarcts but is rare without coexisting infection, either secondary infection of an infarct or a result of septic emboli or vasculitis. Pleural effusions related to pulmonary emboli are usually small, unilateral, and associated with pulmonary infarction.

CRYPTOGENIC ORGANIZING PNEUMONITIS

COP, previously referred to as bronchiolitis obliterans organizing pneumonia, is a clinicopathologic entity of unknown cause characterized by nonspecific clinical symptoms of cough and dyspnea and by equally nonspecific chest radiographic findings of patchy, peripheral airspace opacities. COP should not be confused with bronchiolitis obliterans, also known as obliterative bronchiolitis or constrictive bronchiolitis, a separate entity that is discussed in Chapter 13. Although COP is idiopathic in etiology, several precipitating conditions leading to organizing

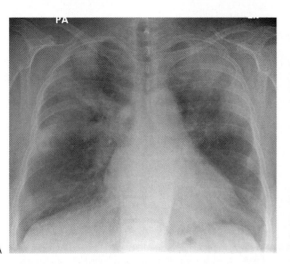

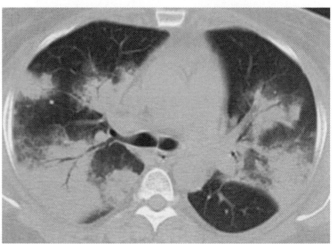

FIGURE 12-10. Cryptogenic organizing pneumonitis. A: PA chest radiograph of a 53-year-old man with rheumatoid arthritis shows bilateral peripheral airspace disease involving predominantly the upper and middle lungs. **B:** CT confirms the peripheral distribution of disease and shows prominent air bronchograms.

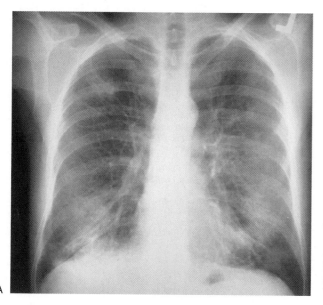

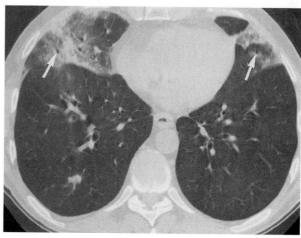

FIGURE 12-12. Cryptogenic organizing pneumonitis. A: PA chest radiograph of a 52-year-old man after bone marrow transplant for leukemia shows bilateral ill-defined parenchymal opacities. B: CT shows that the opacities are peripheral and nonsegmental. Note air bronchograms (*arrows*).

pneumonitis have been identified, including infections (most notably viral), connective tissue disorders (Fig. 12-10), drug toxicity (Fig. 12-11), inhalation of noxious fumes, and lung and bone marrow transplantation (Fig. 12-12). Patients with COP are generally 55 to 60 years of age, and half of them have a history of an influenza-like prodrome followed by an illness of about 3 months characterized by cough, exertional dyspnea, malaise, fever, and weight loss (17).

Radiographs and CT scans of the chest resemble those of many other types of pneumonia and show bilateral, patchy, nonsegmental, airspace opacities with a peripheral and basilar predominance (18). The opacities may contain air bronchograms. On occasion, the opacities are not peripheral in distribution but are central and centered along bronchovascular bundles. Although COP is usually a bilateral process, occasionally only one lung is involved or is much more involved than the other lung (Fig. 12-13). Areas of ground-glass attenuation are common and may be the only finding on CT.

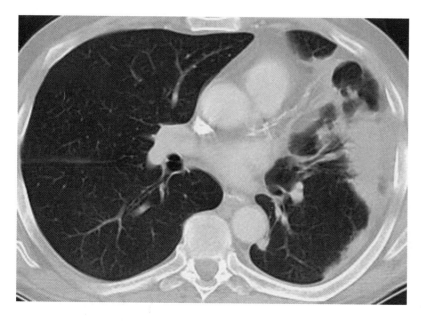

FIGURE 12-13. Cryptogenic organizing pneumonia. CT of a 66-year-old man with rheumatoid arthritis shows peripheral airspace disease involving only the left lung.

References

1. Battesti JP, Saumon G, Valeyre D, et al. Pulmonary sarcoidosis with an alveolar radiographic pattern. *Thorax.* 1982;37:448–452.
2. Rabinowitz JG, Ulreich S, Soriano C. The usual unusual manifestations of sarcoidosis and the "hilar haze"—a new diagnostic aid. *AJR Am J Roentgenol.* 1974;120:821–831.
3. Shigematsu N, Emori K, Matsuba K, et al. Clinicopathologic characteristics of pulmonary acinar sarcoidosis. *Chest.* 1978;73:186–188.
4. Kirks DR, McCormick VD, Greenspan RH. Pulmonary sarcoidosis: roentgenologic analysis of 150 patients. *AJR Am J Roentgenol.* 1973;117:777–786.
5. Fraser RG, Paré JAP, Paré PD. *Diagnosis of Diseases of the Chest.* 3rd ed, vol 2. Philadelphia: WB Saunders; 1989.
6. Otteson EA, Nutman TB. Tropical pulmonary eosinophilia. *Ann Rev Med.* 1992;43:417–424.
7. Webb JKG, Job CK, Gault EW. Tropical eosinophilia: demonstration of microfilariae in lung, liver, and lymph nodes. *Lancet.* 1960;1:835–842.
8. Udwadia FE. Tropical eosinophilia: a review. *Respir Med.* 1993;87:17–21.
9. Crofton JW, Livingstone JL, Oswald NC, et al. Pulmonary eosinophilia. *Thorax.* 1952;7:1–35.
10. Jederlinic PJ, Sicilian L, Gaensler EA. Chronic eosinophilic pneumonia: a report of 19 cases and a review of the literature. *Medicine.* 1988;67:154–162.
11. Mayo JR, Müller NL, Road J, et al. Chronic eosinophilic pneumonia: CT findings in six cases. *AJR Am J Roentgenol.* 1989;153:727–730.
12. Naughton M, Fahy J, Fitzgerald MX. Chronic eosinophilic pneumonia: a long-term follow-up of 12 patients. *Chest.* 1993;103:163–165.
13. Moser KM. Pulmonary embolism: state of the art. *Am Rev Respir Dis.* 1977;115:829–852.
14. Tsao MS, Schraufnagel D, Wang NS. Pathogenesis of pulmonary infarction. *Am J Med.* 1982;72:599–606.
15. Dalen JE, Haffajee CI, Alpert JS, et al. Pulmonary embolism, pulmonary hemorrhage and pulmonary infarction. *N Engl J Med.* 1977;296:1431–1435.
16. Wenger NK, Stein PD, Willis PW. Massive acute pulmonary embolism: the deceivingly nonspecific manifestations. *JAMA.* 1972;220:843–844.
17. King TE, Mortenson RL. Cryptogenic organizing pneumonitis: the North American experience. *Chest.* 1992;102(suppl):8S–13S.
18. Izumi T, Kitaichi M, Nishimura K, et al. Bronchiolitis obliterans organizing pneumonia: clinical features and differential diagnosis. *Chest.* 1992;102:715–719.

AIRWAYS

Airway disorders can be categorized into those that involve the trachea, those that involve the bronchi, and those that involve the bronchioles, the smallest branching airways leading to alveoli. Many disorders can, and frequently do, involve more than one airway compartment. Tracheal disorders will be discussed first, and disorders involving both the bronchi and bronchioles will be discussed together. The reader is referred to Chapter 1 for a discussion of normal anatomy of the airways.

TRACHEAL DISORDERS

Tracheal shape varies, depending on the phase of the respiratory cycle. The intrathoracic trachea is round or elliptic on inspiration images and flat or horseshoe shaped during and at the end of a forced exhalation as a result of anterior bowing of the posterior noncartilaginous tracheal membrane during exhalation (1). Upper limits of normal for coronal and sagittal tracheal dimensions, respectively, as determined by chest radiographs, are 25 mm and 27 mm for men and 21 mm and 23 mm for women. The lower limit of normal for both dimensions is 13 mm in men and 10 mm in women (2). Mean measurements on computed tomography (CT) of anteroposterior (AP) and transverse diameters of the extrathoracic trachea, respectively, are 20.1 mm and 18.4 mm (3); these can increase by as much as 15% in men with aging (4).

CT is superior to chest radiography for detection of abnormalities of the trachea and main bronchi; sensitivities in detecting disease on chest radiographs and CT are 66% and 97%, respectively (5). Spiral multidetector CT, which allows for the acquisition of a whole thoracic volume during a single breath-hold, eliminating respiratory motion, is the technique of choice for noninvasive imaging of the airways. Volume acquisition with multidetector CT has fostered a renewed interest in two-dimensional and three-dimensional (3D) reconstructions applied to the tracheobronchial tree. Potential clinical applications of 3D reconstructions, such as shaded surface display and volume rendering, include assisting with diagnoses, replacing bronchoscopy in some instances, and helping in surgical plan-

ning and endobronchial treatments (6). In the case of a lesion that completely obstructs an airway, CT allows visualization of the airway beyond the obstruction. However, CT's virtual bronchoscopy is currently unable to show mucosal detail, and 3D postprocessing methods are time consuming to perform and rarely performed in routine clinical practice.

Patients with tracheal disease can be asymptomatic or may present with cough, dyspnea, wheezing, or stridor. Because of the variety of conditions that can cause wheezing, a misdiagnosis of asthma is common (7). Tracheal disorders are generally organized into those that cause tracheal widening and those that cause narrowing. CT can demonstrate the degree of widening or narrowing, in addition to the location and extent of tracheal abnormality; it can also demonstrate the presence of associated extraluminal disease, postobstructive atelectasis, and pneumonia. Magnetic resonance imaging (MRI) is a valuable method for observing the trachea because of its multiplanar demonstration of the airway, the mediastinal vessels, and the other structures simultaneously, without the need for contrast medium or exposing the patient to radiation. MRI is particularly useful in children and in patients with either vascular rings or tracheal compression by the innominate artery.

Disorders That Cause Tracheal Widening

Congenital or nonacquired diffuse tracheal widening is much less common than tracheal narrowing and has a more limited differential diagnosis. The Mounier-Kuhn syndrome, which affects primarily men in the fourth and fifth decades, accounts for almost all cases of nonacquired tracheal widening (8). Thought to be congenital (9), it is an abnormality of the trachea and main bronchi characterized by atrophy or absence of elastic fibers and thinning of muscle, which allows the trachea and main bronchi to become flaccid and markedly dilated on inspiration, with narrowing or collapse on expiration or cough. The abnormal airway dynamics and pooling of secretions in broad outpouchings, or diverticula, of redundant musculomembranous tissue between the cartilaginous rings predispose patients to the

TABLE 13-1

DISORDERS THAT CAUSE TRACHEOBRONCHOMEGALY

Nonacquired
  Mounier-Kuhn syndrome

Acquired
  Common
    Normal aging
    Chronic airway infection
    Cigarette smoking
    Chronic bronchitis
    Emphysema
    Cystic fibrosis
    Diffuse pulmonary fibrosis
  Uncommon
    Playing wind instruments
    Inhalation of noxious fumes
    Chronic intubation
    Ehlers-Danlos syndrome
    Cutis laxa
    Marfan syndrome
    Ataxia-telangiectasia
    Ankylosing spondylitis
    Kenny-Caffey syndrome
    Brachmann-de Lange syndrome
    Connective tissue diseases
    Bruton-type agammaglobulinemia
    Light-chain deposition disease

TABLE 13-2

DISORDERS THAT CAUSE TRACHEAL NARROWING

Extrinsic
  Masses (e.g., thyroid, aberrant vessels, enlarged nodes)
  Fibrosing mediastinitis

Intrinsic
  Congenital tracheal narrowing
  Infection
  Granulomatous disorders (e.g., Wegener granulomatosis, sarcoidosis)
  Neoplasms
  Trauma, including intubation
  Amyloidosis
  Relapsing polychondritis
  Tracheobronchopathia osteochondroplastica
  Saber-sheath trachea
  Idiopathic

development of chronic pulmonary suppuration, bronchiectasis, emphysema, and pulmonary fibrosis (10). The trachea is involved from the subglottic region to the carina. A tracheal diameter greater than 3 cm is required for diagnosis, and tracheal widths up to 5.5 cm have been recorded (8). The radiographic and CT features of the condition include marked dilatation of the trachea and mainstem bronchi, tracheal diverticulosis, and a variable incidence of bronchiectasis and chronic pulmonary parenchymal disease (11,12).

Several conditions can result in acquired tracheobronchomegaly that may closely resemble that seen in Mounier-Kuhn syndrome (Table 13-1). Some degree of tracheal dilatation may be seen with aging (4,13) and in musicians who play wind instruments (13). Chronic infection, cigarette smoking, chronic bronchitis, emphysema, cystic fibrosis (CF), inhalation of noxious fumes, chronic intubation, and diffuse pulmonary fibrosis can also result in tracheobronchomegaly (10,14,15). Other conditions associated with tracheal widening, which may in fact be related to Mounier-Kuhn syndrome, are Ehlers-Danlos syndrome and cutis laxa (16,17). Although tracheal narrowing is the usual end result in relapsing polychondritis—a disorder of cartilaginous inflammation involving the nose, ear, trachea, and joints—diffuse tracheal widening may develop occasionally (18). In contrast, nasal and ear cartilage abnormalities are absent in Mounier-Kuhn syndrome. Additional causes of secondary tracheobronchomegaly are listed in Table 13-1. Nevertheless, the majority of cases appear to be sporadic, predominantly occurring in men in the third and fourth decades of life (9).

Disorders That Cause Tracheal Narrowing

Tracheal narrowing is seen with a variety of disorders and can be idiopathic (7,19–21) (Table 13-2). Strictures of the trachea are usually caused by damage from a cuffed endotracheal or tracheostomy tube or trauma to the neck (22). Postintubation tracheal injuries remain the most common indication for tracheal resection and reconstruction, despite identification of the causes of these lesions and development of techniques for their avoidance (23). Tracheomalacia, which is diagnosed when the trachea collapses more than 50% on expiration, can also be caused by trauma, and it may be recognized only on dynamic or expiratory CT scanning (1,24).

Saber-sheath trachea is diffuse *intrathoracic* narrowing of the trachea, with the coronal diameter reaching two thirds (or less) of the sagittal diameter when measured 1.0 cm above the top of the aortic arch (25). More than 95% of patients with this deformity have clinical evidence of chronic obstructive pulmonary disease (COPD), and saber-sheath trachea is considered an insensitive but specific sign for COPD on standard chest radiography (Fig. 13-1) (25,26).

Relapsing polychondritis is a systemic autoimmune connective tissue disease in which cartilage is affected diffusely by recurrent episodes of inflammation. The pinnal, nasal, laryngeal, and tracheal cartilages are most commonly involved. The major airways are involved in more than 50% of cases, and recurrent pneumonia is the most common cause of death in these patients (8,27). CT shows diffuse or multifocal fixed narrowing of the tracheobronchial lumen, with associated thickening of the wall (28,29). Dense calcium deposits may be seen in the thickened tracheal cartilage (30).

Amyloidosis of the respiratory tract, both primary and secondary, is a rare condition that produces focal or diffuse irregular narrowing of the airway by submucosal deposits of amyloid (22). Both radiography and CT of the chest can demonstrate diffuse narrowing or show nodular protrusions into the tracheal lumen that can be calcified (Fig. 13-2) (8).

Tracheobronchopathia osteochondroplastica is a benign condition characterized by multiple submucosal osteocartilaginous growths along the inner anterolateral surfaces of the trachea (31,32). Although the etiology is unknown, theories have linked this disorder to chronic inflammation, degenerative processes, amyloidosis, and neoplasia (33–35). Radiography and CT of the chest show multiple sessile nodular tumors, with or without calcification, extending over a long segment of the trachea and into the main bronchi. In contrast, the nodules in amyloidosis may be circumferential and can be distinguished from those of tracheobronchopathia osteochondroplastica, in which there is always sparing of the posterior membranous wall.

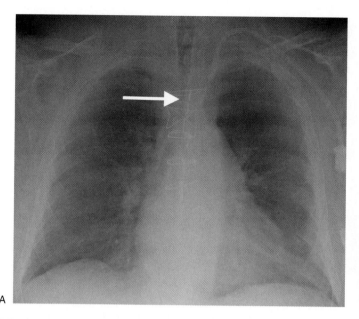
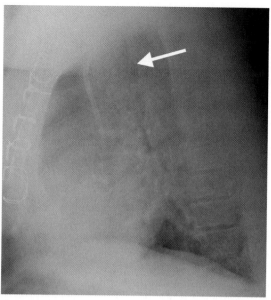

FIGURE 13-1. Saber-sheath trachea. A: Posteroanterior (PA) chest radiograph of a 67-year-old man with emphysema shows narrowing of the coronal diameter of the trachea (*arrow*). **B:** On the lateral view, the tracheal diameter (*arrow*) is normal or slightly enlarged.

Wegener granulomatosis is characterized by granulomatous vasculitis of the upper and lower respiratory tract, usually in conjunction with renal and other organ involvement. The CT appearance of airway involvement includes circumferential narrowing of the airway lumen, abnormal soft tissue within the tracheal rings, and dense irregular calcification of the tracheal cartilages (36). Sarcoidosis is another granulomatous disorder

that may rarely involve the trachea and bronchi. Granulomatous sarcoid lesions may exist intrinsically in the airway, or enlarged hilar nodes may compress the bronchi extrinsically (37,38).

Many viral, bacterial, or fungal diseases can involve the trachea. In North America, most cases of laryngotracheobronchitis are viral in nature; subglottic or laryngeal narrowing is

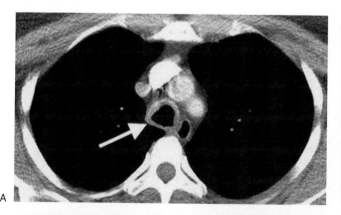
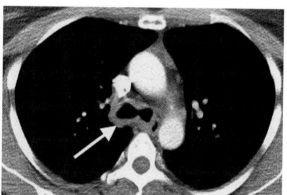
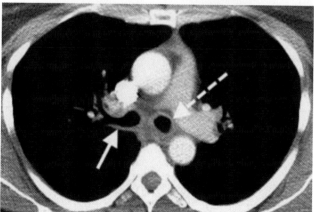

FIGURE 13-2. Tracheobronchial amyloidosis. A: CT of a 44-year-old woman with dysphagia and dyspnea on exertion shows circumferential thickening and calcification of the tracheal wall (*arrow*). **B:** CT at a more inferior level shows thickening of the walls of the main bronchi (*arrow*). **C:** CT at a level inferior to (**B**) shows thickening of the wall of the right upper lobe bronchus (*solid arrow*) and left main bronchus (*dashed arrow*).

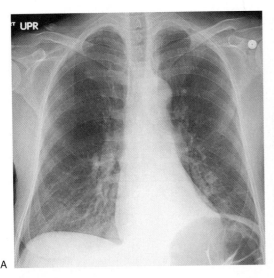

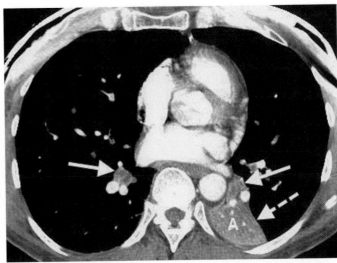

FIGURE 13-3. Mucous plugging. A: PA chest radiograph of a 45-year-old woman with shortness of breath after cervical spine fusion shows abnormal opacities in both lower lobes and volume loss in the left lower lobe. **B:** CT shows low-attenuation material in both lower lobe segmental bronchi (*solid arrows*), postobstructive atelectasis of the left lower lobe (*A*), and posteromedial displacement of the left major fissure (*dashed arrow*).

common, but radiographically demonstrable tracheal narrowing is unusual (7).

it can be helpful to selectively repeat the scan at the region of interest after the patient has coughed.

Tracheobronchial Filling Defects

In adults, tracheobronchial filling defects are usually produced by mucus (Fig. 13-3) or neoplasms (Figs. 13-4 to 13-7). Less common causes include papilloma, infections (Fig. 13-8), foreign bodies (Fig. 13-9), broncholiths (Fig. 13-10), and other miscellaneous disorders. If mucus is suspected on a CT scan,

Tracheoesophageal Fistulas

Tracheoesophageal fistulas in adults are almost exclusively acquired lesions. They occur as a complication of intrathoracic malignancies (accounting for 60% of cases), infection, and

(Text continues on page 221)

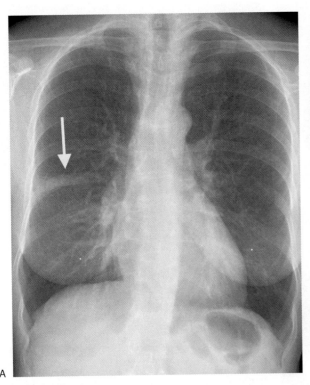

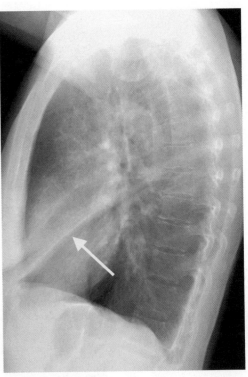

FIGURE 13-4. Tracheal adenoid cystic carcinoma. A: PA chest radiograph of a 59-year-old man with recurrent right middle lobe pneumonia and cough shows a linear band of opacity in the right middle lung (*arrow*). **B:** Lateral view shows an oblique band of opacity paralleling the inferior aspect of the major fissure (*arrow*). (*Continued*)

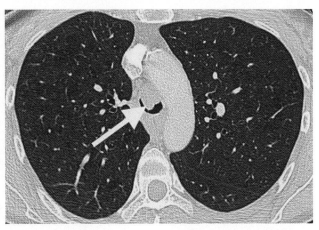

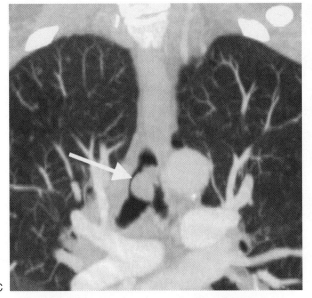

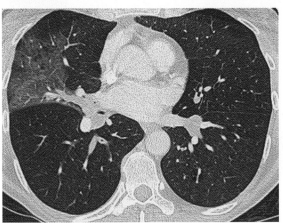

FIGURE 13-4. (*Continued*) C: Coronal reformatted CT shows a lobular soft tissue mass (*arrow*) almost completely obstructing the lumen of the trachea just above the level of the carina. D: Axial CT shows that the mass (*arrow*) almost completely fills the lumen of the trachea. E: CT at the level of the inferior pulmonary veins shows postobstructive atelectasis and pneumonia in the right middle lobe.

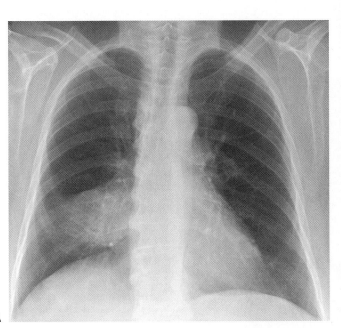

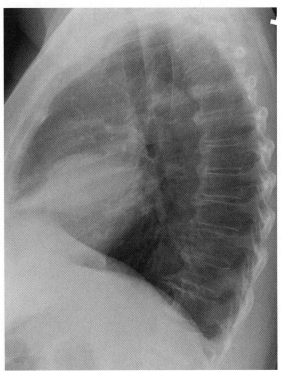

FIGURE 13-5. **Metastatic endometrial carcinoma. A:** PA chest radiograph of a 75-year-old woman shows a mass adjacent to the right hilum. **B:** Lateral view shows the mass projected over the heart. The contours of the mass suggest that it is related to the inferior edge of the major fissure. (*Continued*)

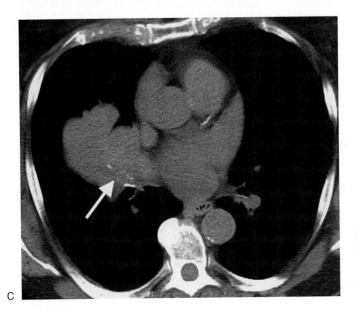

C

FIGURE 13-5. (*Continued*) C: Axial CT shows low-attenuation material obliterating the lumen of the right middle lobe bronchus (*arrow*). Note that the bronchial wall is outlined by calcium. Tumor is growing through the bronchus into the right middle lobe. The opacity seen on the chest radiograph represents tumor and collapsed right middle lobe.

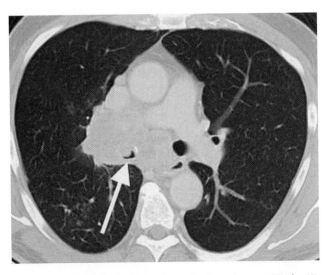

FIGURE 13-6. **Endobronchial non–small cell carcinoma.** CT of a 63-year-old woman with cough shows a soft tissue mass that almost completely obliterates the lumen of the bronchus intermedius (*arrow*).

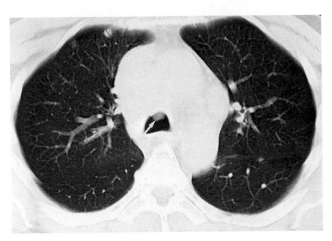

FIGURE 13-7. **Tracheal metastasis.** CT of a 64-year-old woman with renal cell carcinoma shows a soft tissue mass adjacent to the anterior wall of the trachea (*arrow*) representing one of many biopsy-proven metastases to the trachea. Mucus could have a similar appearance, but it will usually clear with a repeated scan after the patient clears the throat.

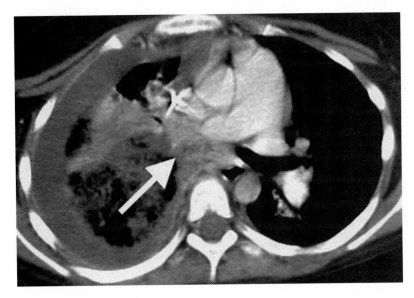

FIGURE 13-8. **Endobronchial blood clot.** CT of a 10-year-old girl with leukemia and *Rhizopus* necrotizing pneumonia shows a filling defect occluding the bronchus intermedius (*arrow*). The right middle and lower lobes were surgically resected; pathology showed pulmonary artery and vein thromboses, diffuse pneumonia and pulmonary hemorrhage, and clotted blood in the bronchus intermedius.

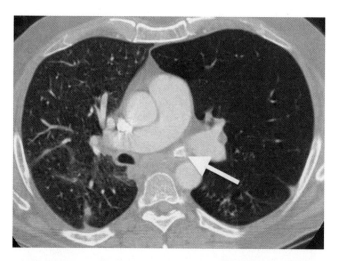

FIGURE 13-9. Endobronchial foreign body. CT shows a radiopaque foreign body (*arrow*) in the left main bronchus. Note the hyperlucency and hyperinflation of the left upper and lower lobes secondary to air trapping. A chicken bone was removed from the airway.

trauma (39,40). The diagnosis is usually made with a fluoroscopic contrast study but can be made, in some cases, with CT. In addition to demonstrating the site of a fistula, CT can suggest the etiology and detect pulmonary and mediastinal complications (41).

Congenital Tracheobronchial Anomalies

Congenital tracheobronchial anomalies can present as life-threatening emergencies at birth, or they may go undiagnosed for years. Clinical symptoms are often nonspecific, and radiographic evaluation is frequently required to localize and characterize the lesion before endoscopy, surgery, or medical management. The radiologist must be on the alert for unsuspected

additional associated anomalies involving airways, lungs, great vessels, and the esophagus, which occur with relative frequency.

Tracheal webs produce localized areas of narrowing with no associated deformity of the underlying cartilage. The thickness of the webs determines the severity of obstruction and the therapeutic approach (42). Congenital tracheal stenosis may occur in any portion of the trachea, usually involving more length and depth of the trachea than webs, and is more likely to require resection rather than dilatation alone. Stenosis secondary to long-term compression by a dilated esophagus, abnormal great vessels, or cervicomediastinal masses results in a focal fibrous and cartilaginous deformity that persists for some time after the mass is removed. Congenital tracheal stenosis is frequently associated with bronchial stenosis; pulmonary hypoplasia or agenesis; tracheal bronchus; tracheoesophageal fistula; tracheomalacia; anomalies of vertebrae, ribs, and thumbs; and cardiac anomalies.

Tracheomalacia is an abnormally flaccid trachea that may involve all or part of the trachea and results in abnormal anteroposterior tracheal collapse during expiration of $\geq 50\%$ of cross-sectional area. The innominate artery compression syndrome can result in secondary tracheomalacia, in which there is persistent narrowing of the anterior tracheal wall at the level of the thoracic inlet. Short trachea, which occurs when there are 15 or fewer tracheal rings, can be diagnosed on CT when the tracheal bifurcation lies above the fourth thoracic vertebral body in children younger than 2 years old or above the fifth thoracic vertebra thereafter (43).

Aberrant tracheal bronchus (so-called "pig bronchus," or bronchus suis), the most common anomalous airway pattern, is reported in 2% of children during bronchoscopy examination (44). It occurs most commonly in boys, arising most often from the right lateral tracheal wall within 2 cm of the carina. It can be asymptomatic, or it may result in right upper lobe infection, atelectasis, or bronchiectasis, usually from a stenotic bronchial segment and poorly cleared secretions. The CT appearance is that of a bronchus arising from the trachea in a section more cephalad than the carina (Fig. 13-11) (45).

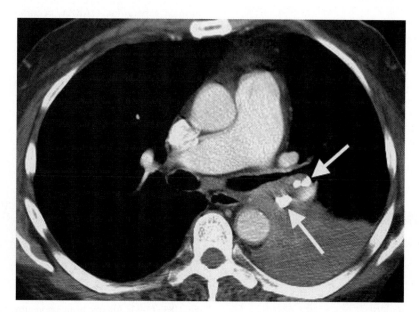

FIGURE 13-10. Broncholithiasis. CT of a 72-year-old man with cough, wheezing, and increasing shortness of breath shows large calcifications in the left hilum and left lower lobe bronchus (*arrows*). Note postobstructive atelectasis of the left lower lobe.

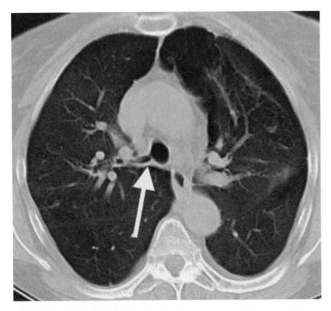

FIGURE 13-11. Aberrant tracheal bronchus. CT of a 58-year-old woman with cough and recurrent pneumonia shows a so-called "pig bronchus" (*arrow*) arising from the right lateral wall of the trachea, above the level of the carina.

CHRONIC OBSTRUCTIVE PULMONARY DISEASE

COPD refers to a group of disorders characterized by chronic or recurrent obstruction to airflow. Five principal disorders fall under this heading (Table 13-3), although the term is commonly used clinically to refer to emphysema. Because these disorders are sometimes difficult to distinguish from one another on chest radiography, the term *COPD* should not be restricted to emphysema.

Asthma

There is no universally accepted definition of asthma; it may be regarded as a diffuse, obstructive lung disease with hyperreactivity of the airways to a variety of stimuli and a high degree of reversibility of the obstructive process, which may occur either spontaneously or as a result of treatment. Asthma is a complex disorder involving biochemical, autonomic, immunologic, infectious, endocrine, and psychologic factors in varying degrees in different individuals. Both large and small airways may be involved, again to varying degrees. The three elements that contribute to airway obstruction in asthma are: (i) spasm of smooth muscle; (ii) edema and inflammation of the mucous membranes lining the airways; and (iii) intraluminal exudation

TABLE 13-3
CHRONIC OBSTRUCTIVE PULMONARY DISEASE
"ABCCE" Asthma Bronchiectasis Chronic bronchitis/bronchiolitis Cystic fibrosis Emphysema

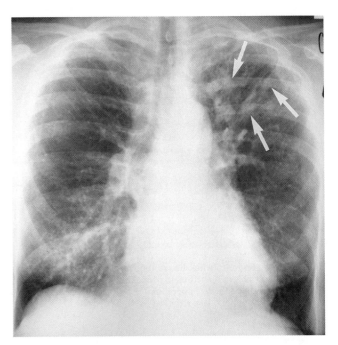

FIGURE 13-12. Allergic bronchopulmonary aspergillosis. PA chest radiograph of a 64-year-old woman with a long history of asthma shows multiple tubular opacities in the left upper lobe (*arrows*) representing dilated bronchi filled with mucus, debris, and fungal hyphae.

of mucus, inflammatory cells, and cellular debris. Asthma can be a benign, self-limiting problem; it can lead to acute respiratory failure; or it can be a chronic, recurrent disease that leads to debilitating, irreversible airflow obstruction and COPD. Emphysema is not a prominent finding in the lungs of nonsmoking patients with asthma, even in those with severe disease (46).

Chest radiographs of patients with asthma can be normal, show increased lung markings and hyperinflation, or show low lung volumes and multifocal atelectasis. CT findings can include bronchiectasis involving mostly subsegmental and distal bronchi, bronchial wall thickening, small centrilobular opacities, and decreased lung attenuation (47). Allergic bronchopulmonary aspergillosis (ABPA) occurs with a greater prevalence in patients with asthma and CF (48) (Figs. 13-12 and 13-13). Central bronchiectasis on CT is the hallmark of ABPA.

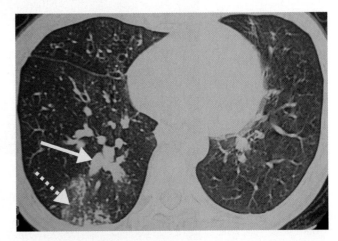

FIGURE 13-13. Allergic bronchopulmonary aspergillosis. CT shows central bronchial dilatation and impaction (*solid arrow*). Peripheral nodular and ground-glass opacities (*dashed arrow*) represent impaction of small airways and peribronchiolar inflammation.

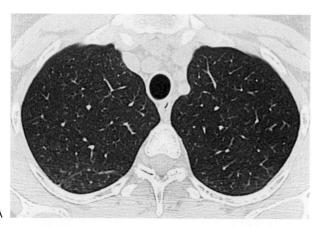
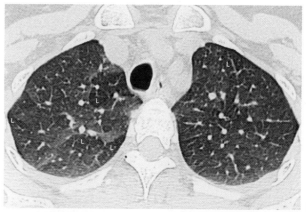

A   B

FIGURE 13-14. Asthma. A: Inspiratory CT of a 34-year-old woman with steroid-dependent asthma is normal. Note the round contour of the trachea. B: Expiratory image at the same level as (A) shows areas of lucency (*L*), representing air trapping. Note the flattened posterior tracheal contour on expiration.

Bronchial wall thickening in asthma (which is assessed subjectively on CT) may reflect bronchial and peribronchial inflammation as well as increased smooth muscle, mucous gland, cartilage, and submucosal area (49,50). Areas of hyperlucency are caused by decreased lung perfusion secondary to reflex vasoconstriction in hypoventilated areas, and by air trapping (51) (Fig. 13-14). Emphysema seen on the CT scans of patients with asthma is attributed to cigarette smoking (52). Small centrilobular opacities may correspond to plugging or to thickening of the bronchiole walls (49). Because central airway lesions and mitral stenosis can produce symptoms attributed to asthma, the airways, cardiac silhouette, and pulmonary vasculature should always be evaluated closely on every chest radiograph when the clinical history is "asthma." The chest radiograph should also be assessed for evidence of pneumonia, which is known to exacerbate asthma, and pneumomediastinum (Fig. 13-15)

and pneumothorax, as evidence of alveolar rupture that can be caused by wheezing and coughing (Table 13-4).

Bronchiectasis

Bronchiectasis, defined as irreversible dilatation of the bronchial tree, can cause chronic sputum production and hemoptysis, and it can be described morphologically as *cylindric, varicose, cystic,* or *traction* in type (53). Cylindric bronchiectasis, the mildest form, is characterized by smooth, uniformly dilated bronchi (Figs. 13-16 and 13-17). Sectioned lengthwise, these bronchi resemble nontapering "tram tracks"; sectioned crosswise, the bronchi appear round or oval. Beaded dilatation of bronchi describes the varicose type (Fig. 13-18); cystic bronchiectasis, the most severe type, is characterized by cysts in clusters, often with air–fluid levels (Figs. 13-19 and 13-20). Traction bronchiectasis refers to irreversible dilatation of bronchi and bronchioles in areas of pulmonary fibrosis. It occurs predominantly in the peripheral portions of lung, where bronchi contain less supporting cartilage (see Fig. 3-3B) (54). There are numerous causes of bronchiectasis; these can be remembered with the mnemonic "BRONCHIECTASIS" (Table 13-5).

Although patients with bronchiectasis rarely have a normal chest radiograph (55), the chest radiographic findings are neither sufficiently sensitive nor specific enough to be of value

FIGURE 13-15. **Pneumomediastinum.** PA chest radiograph of a patient with asthma shows mediastinal air outlining the heart (*dashed arrow*) and extending into the neck bilaterally (*solid arrows*).

TABLE 13-4

THINGS TO LOOK FOR ON THE CHEST RADIOGRAPH WHEN THE PATIENT HISTORY IS "ASTHMA"

"PHAME"
Pneumothorax
Pneumomediastinum
Hyperinflation
Atelectasis
Mucous plugging (ABPA)
Mitral stenosis (patients can present with symptoms of "asthma")
Endotracheal lesion (e.g., patients with carcinoid tumor can present with symptoms of "asthma")

ABPA, allergic bronchopulmonary aspergillosis.

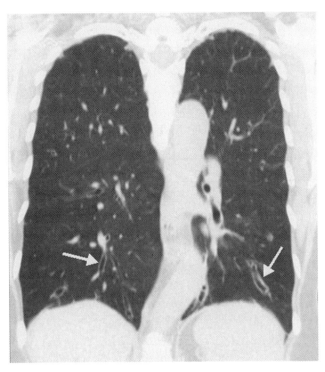

FIGURE 13-16. Cylindric bronchiectasis. Coronal reformatted CT shows smooth, uniformly dilated bronchi (*arrows*), predominantly in the lower lungs.

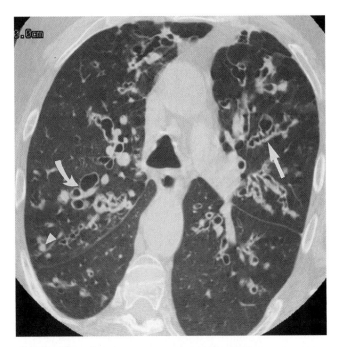

FIGURE 13-18. Varicose and cystic bronchiectasis. CT of a 66-year-old man shows dilated bronchi and bronchioles. In profile, some of the bronchiectatic airways have the "beaded" appearance of varicose bronchiectasis (*straight arrow*); in cross section, some are grouped together like a "cluster of grapes," as is seen with cystic bronchiectasis (*curved arrow*). The bronchial and bronchiolar walls are thickened. Some of the dilated bronchioles are filled with mucus, forming peripheral nodular opacities (*arrowhead*).

in the accurate assessment of bronchiectasis, and they are unreliable in determining the severity and extent of the disease (55–57). The common radiographic findings are loss of definition and increase in number and size of the bronchovascular markings (caused by peribronchial inflammation/fibrosis and the presence of retained secretions), tram tracking, tubular or ring-shaped opacities with central lucency if the airways are air filled, central opacity if there is mucoid impaction, and cystic spaces that can be up to 2 cm in diameter.

Early studies assessing the accuracy of conventional CT in diagnosing bronchiectasis resulted in sensitivities of 60% to 80% and specificities of 86% to 100% (57–60). With the use of 1.5-mm collimation at 10-mm intervals, sensitivity with CT

improved to a range of 96% to 98%, with specificity of 93% to 99% (61,62). Thin-section CT is now the accepted gold standard for diagnosing bronchiectasis. With current state-of-the-art multidetector CT, routine imaging of the lungs with 3-mm collimation and 1.25-mm reformatting will allow for diagnosis of most cases of bronchiectasis, even very mild cases. The most reliable finding for the diagnosis of cylindric bronchiectasis is visualization of bronchi within 1 cm of costal or paravertebral pleura, or visualization of bronchi abutting the mediastinal pleura. Although lack of normal bronchial tapering and increased bronchoarterial ratios are helpful in the diagnosis of

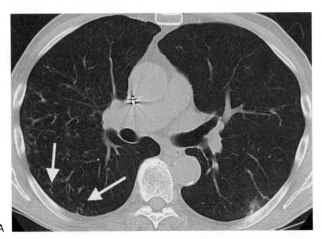

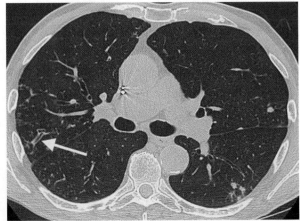

FIGURE 13-17. Atypical mycobacterial bronchiolitis. A: CT shows tree-in-bud opacities in the periphery of the right lower lobe (*arrows*). **B:** Thin-section CT (1.25 mm) shows cylindric bronchiolectasis in the right lower lobe (*arrow*). Note bronchiolar opacities in the left lower lobe as well.

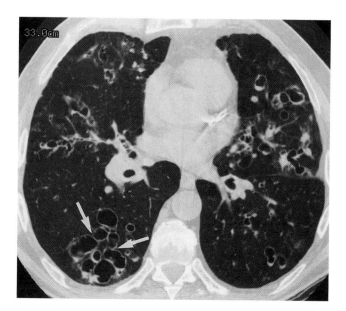

FIGURE 13-19. Cystic bronchiectasis. CT of a 65-year-old woman with a history of *Pasteurella multocida* infection of the lungs shows dilated bronchi and bronchioles, forming a "cluster of grapes" in the right lower lobe (*arrows*).

TABLE 13-5

CAUSES OF BRONCHIECTASIS

"BRONCHIECTASIS"
Broncholith
Retraction of parenchyma (fibrosis)
Obstruction by foreign body
Neoplastic obstruction
Cartilage deficiency (Williams-Campbell syndrome)
Cilia syndrome (Kartagener syndrome)
Host defenses down (agammaglobulinemia)
Infection
Emphysema
Cystic fibrosis
Chronic granulomatous disease
Tuberculosis
Allergic bronchopulmonary aspergillosis
Swyer-James syndrome
Inhalation injury (ammonia, gastric acid)
Sarcoidosis (uncommon)

bronchiectasis, these findings can also be seen in 10% to 20% of healthy subjects.

Despite the ease with which bronchiectasis can be identified on CT in most cases, there are a number of potential pitfalls (63). These include artifacts from both respiratory and cardiac motion, and inappropriate collimation and electronic windowing. A number of diffuse lung diseases can simulate bronchiectasis, especially cystic bronchiectasis; these include Langerhan cell histiocytosis, lymphangioleiomyomatosis, cystic changes related to connective tissue diseases or lymphocytic interstitial pneumonitis or in patients with acquired immunodeficiency syndrome and *Pneumocystis jiroveci* pneumonia, emphysema, and cystic metastases. The characteristic combination of "cyst" paired with the accompanying pulmonary artery is sometimes helpful in confirming bronchiectasis, as is variation in the sizes of bronchiectatic "cysts" with inspiration and expiration, a feature that is not usually seen with other types of cystic lesions. Following cystlike lesions from one CT scan section to another and noting their relationship to central airways and their "tubular" nature also allow for accurate distinction between bronchiectasis and other cystic diseases, in most cases. This can be facilitated by reconstructing multidetector CT data to create maximum-intensity-projection images and coronal reformations.

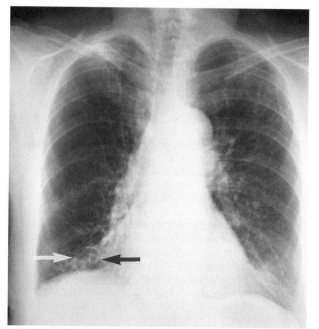

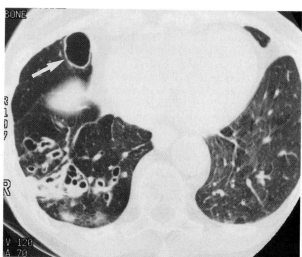

FIGURE 13-20. Cystic bronchiectasis. A: PA chest radiograph of a 78-year-old woman shows increased "interstitial markings" in the lower lungs. There is a prominent thin-walled "ring shadow" in the right middle lobe (*arrows*). B: CT shows thick-walled, dilated bronchioles forming a "cluster of grapes" in the right lower lobe and a large dilated airway in the right middle lobe (*arrow*). Patchy areas of dense airspace opacity in the right lower lobe were thought to represent acute pneumonia.

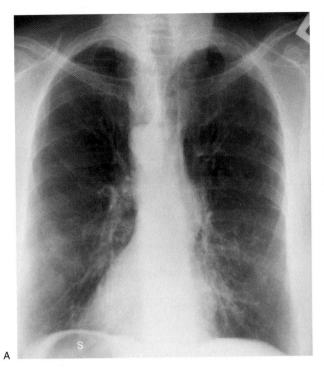

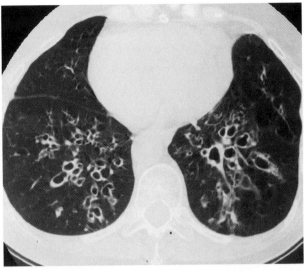

FIGURE 13-21. Kartagener syndrome. A: PA chest radiograph of a woman with sinusitis shows dextrocardia, a right-sided stomach bubble (*S*), and subtle bilateral lower lobe "interstitial" opacities. B: CT shows bilateral lower lobe cystic bronchiectasis.

The dyskinetic cilia syndrome, first described in 1976 (64), represents a spectrum of genetically determined defects in ciliary structure and function that interfere with mucociliary clearance. Although the term *immotile cilia syndrome* has been used, in many cases the cilia demonstrate some motility (although dyskinetic). Described conditions include (a) situs inversus, paranasal sinusitis, and bronchiectasis (the three major components of Kartagener syndrome) (Figs. 13-21 and 13-22); (b) recurrent upper and lower respiratory tract infections; (c) and immotile sperm and infertility.

Cystic Fibrosis

CF is a relatively common genetic disorder that affects the upper and lower respiratory tracts, pancreas, liver and gallbladder, intestines, and genital tract. Approximately one in 1,600 live births is affected by this autosomal recessive disease, which occurs predominantly in Caucasians. In 1985, the CF defect was determined to be located on chromosome 7 (65), and 4 years later the CF gene was identified by positional cloning (66–68). This new knowledge gave rise to new therapies, including in vivo gene therapy (69). The median survival age rose from about 18 years in 1976 to 29 years in the early 1990s (70,71).

Chest radiographic findings in adult patients with CF include hyperinflation and atelectasis as well as bronchiectasis (72). CT shows the presence, severity, and extent of bronchiectasis, peribronchial thickening, mucous plugging (Fig. 13-23), abscesses, bullae, lung collapse, and dense parenchymal opacification (73) (Fig. 13-24). In early stages of the disease, the upper lungs are involved to a greater extent than the lower lungs (Fig. 13-25). As the disease progresses, the process becomes more diffuse and an upper lung–predominant pattern may not be appreciated.

Chronic Bronchitis

Chronic bronchitis is defined clinically as a chronic or recurrent increase in the volume of mucoid bronchial secretions sufficient to cause expectoration, occurring on most days during at least 3 consecutive months for no less than 2 consecutive years (74). It is common among cigarette smokers. The diagnosis is based on the presence of chronic productive cough in the absence of any specific cause, such as bronchiectasis or chronic infection. The radiographic features are nonspecific and include tubular shadows, thickened bronchial walls, hyperinflation of the lungs, and areas of pulmonary oligemia. The term *dirty lung* has been used to describe the increase in bronchovascular markings. Hyperinflation and oligemia are probably a result of associated pulmonary emphysema. Findings of centrilobular emphysema can predominate on CT of patients with chronic bronchitis. Radiographic and CT features are insensitive and nonspecific, and a high degree of interobserver variability further limits the diagnostic capabilities of imaging.

Bronchiolitis

Evaluation of the bronchioles, defined as peripheral airways that do not contain cartilage, requires an understanding of the anatomy of the secondary pulmonary lobule, the smallest portion of lung that is surrounded by connective tissue septa. The lobular bronchioles measure no more than 1 mm in diameter (75), and their walls are less than 0.1 mm thick. Normal bronchioles are generally not seen on thin-section CT. However, bronchiolar abnormalities may be detected when there is thickening of the bronchiolar wall, peribronchiolar inflammation and fibrosis, and bronchiolectasis with or without filling of the dilated bronchiole with secretions (76).

Another CT feature of bronchiolar (small-airway) disease is a mosaic pattern of lung attenuation, which can also be seen with pulmonary vascular and infiltrative lung diseases. In cases of small airway disease, areas of variable lung attenuation that form a mosaic pattern, which is accentuated during forced exhalation, represent air trapping, hypoxic vasoconstriction, and mechanical pressure on blood vessels (77). On CT obtained at end-exhalation, air trapping is recognized as a lack of increase in attenuation or a lack of decrease in volume of areas of abnormally lucent lung. In small airway disease, the size and number of vessels in the abnormally lucent area of lung are decreased relative to areas of higher-attenuation lung. Air trapping can

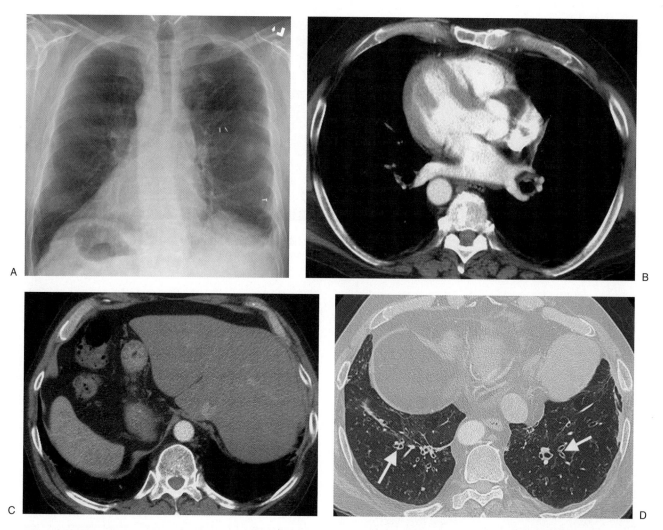

FIGURE 13-22. Kartagener syndrome. A: PA chest radiograph of a 56-year-old man shows dextrocardia and a right-sided stomach bubble. **B:** CT confirms dextrocardia. **C:** CT at a level inferior to (**B**) shows situs inversus, with the liver on the left and the spleen on the right. **D:** CT with lung windowing shows bibasilar bronchiectasis (*arrows*).

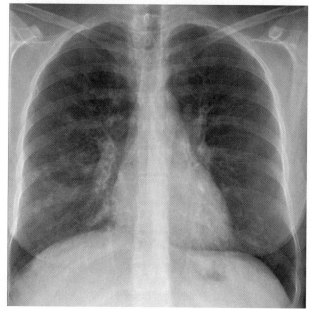

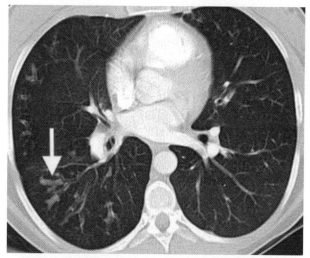

FIGURE 13-23. Cystic fibrosis. A: PA chest radiograph of a 28-year-old woman with cystic fibrosis shows bilateral bronchiectasis, along with tubular and nodular opacities representing mucus-impacted airways. **B:** CT shows mucous plugging of distal airways (*arrow*).

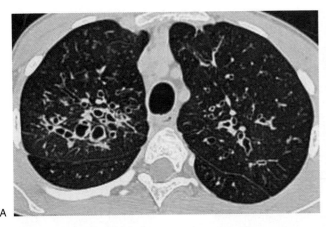
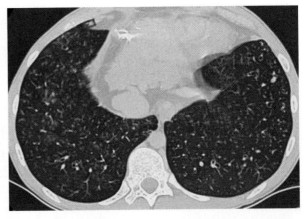

FIGURE 13-24. Cystic fibrosis. A: CT of a 22-year-old man with cystic fibrosis shows extensive bronchiectasis and bronchial wall thickening in the upper lobes. B: CT at a more inferior level shows extensive involvement of the small airways.

also be seen with pulmonary vascular diseases but not with infiltrative diseases.

Obliterative bronchiolitis (OB) is defined pathologically as irreversible fibrosis of small-airway walls that causes the airway lumina to become narrow or obliterated. *Constrictive bronchi-* *olitis*, which emphasizes the fibrotic and extrinsic nature of the lesion, is a synonym for OB and is favored by some authors since it avoids confusion with bronchiolitis obliterans organizing pneumonia, a condition now more commonly referred to as cryptogenic organizing pneumonia (78). The clinical criteria

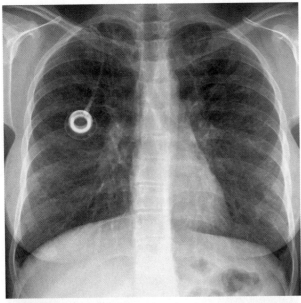
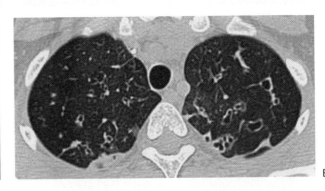
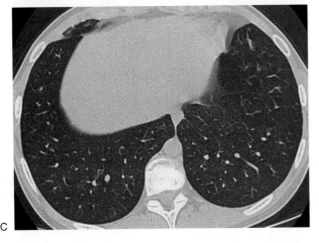

FIGURE 13-25. Cystic fibrosis. A: PA chest radiograph of a 19-year-old man with cystic fibrosis shows diffuse bilateral bronchiectasis, bronchial wall thickening, and areas of mucoid impaction. B: CT of the upper lungs confirms the chest radiographic findings. C: CT at a more inferior level shows normal lung bases. Early in the course of the disease process, it is typical for the upper lungs to be more involved than the lower lungs. As the disease progresses, an upper lung predominance may not be appreciated.

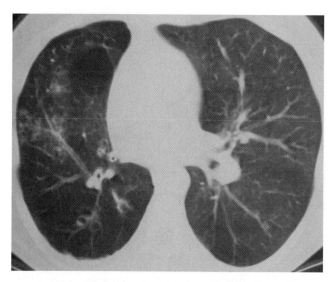

FIGURE 13-26. Swyer-James syndrome. CT shows bronchiectasis, bronchiolectasis, tree-in-bud opacities, and bullae in the right lung. The right lung is hyperlucent as a result of air trapping related to obliterative bronchiolitis. The right pulmonary artery is diminutive, another feature of Swyer-James syndrome.

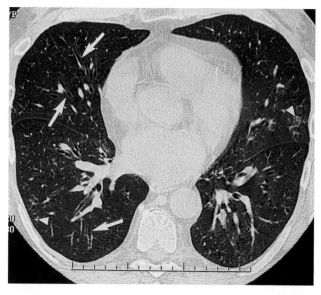

FIGURE 13-28. Diffuse panbronchiolitis. CT of a 61-year-old non-smoking man with chronic sinusitis, cough, fever, shortness of breath, scant sputum production, and mixed restrictive and obstructive pattern on pulmonary function tests shows cylindric bronchiectasis and bronchiolectasis (arrows), along with peripheral nodular and linear branching opacities representing dilated, impacted bronchioles (arrowheads).

used for the diagnosis of OB are irreversible airflow limitation, with a forced expiratory volume in 1 second (FEV_1) that is less than 60% of the predicted value, in the absence of emphysema, chronic bronchitis, asthma, or other cause of airway obstruction (79). OB and cryptogenic organizing pneumonia are not thought to be related, although they can occur as a result of similar etiologic factors. Both are commonly idiopathic. OB is a common sequela of heart or lung transplantation, representing chronic rejection in lung transplantation, and bone marrow transplantation, where OB represents chronic graft-versus-host disease. OB is a component of Swyer-James syndrome related to childhood viral infection (Fig. 13-26).

Chest radiographs are usually normal in OB but can show slowly progressive hyperinflation. The CT findings include bronchiolectasis, centrilobular branching structures and nodules caused by peribronchiolar thickening and bronchiolectasis with secretions (80), and mosaic lung attenuation (80–83) (Fig. 13-27). Interpretation of air trapping must be made with cau-

tion, because occasional isolated areas of lobular air trapping can be seen in healthy individuals (51).

Pathologic changes occur in the small airways of essentially all smokers (84,85). Respiratory bronchiolitis, also referred to as smoker's bronchiolitis (86,87), involves the respiratory bronchioles and is characterized by mild chronic inflammation of the bronchioles associated with accumulation of pigmented macrophages in respiratory bronchioles and adjacent alveoli. The condition may be severe enough to produce clinical symptoms of cough and shortness of breath and to produce CT abnormalities, including areas of ground-glass attenuation, centrilobular micronodules, and air trapping (88,89). The abnormalities usually involve predominantly the upper lungs (a distribution similar to that of smoking-related centrilobular emphysema) but may be diffuse.

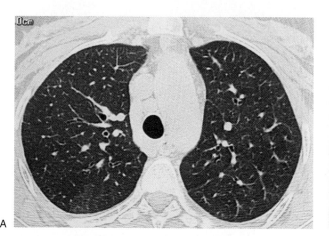
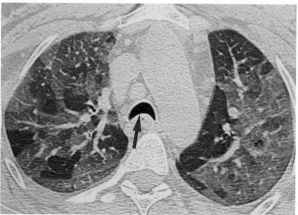

FIGURE 13-27. Obliterative bronchiolitis. A: Inspiratory CT of a 40-year-old woman with a transplanted heart is normal. B: Expiratory CT shows diffuse areas of abnormal parenchymal lucency, representing air trapping. Note anterior bowing of posterior membranous trachea on expiration (arrow).

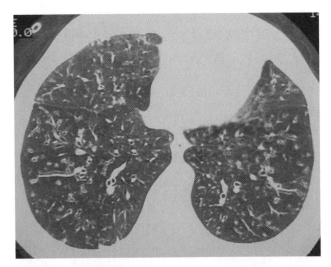

FIGURE 13-29. Diffuse panbronchiolitis. CT shows diffuse bronch-iectasis, bronchiolectasis, airway wall thickening, and tree-in-bud opacities.

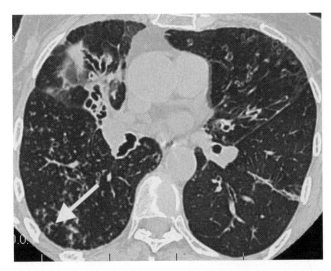

FIGURE 13-31. Atypical mycobacterial bronchiolitis. CT of an 88-year-old woman with chronic cough shows varicose and cystic bronchiectasis in the right middle lobe and tree-in-bud opacities in the right lower lobe (arrow).

Diffuse panbronchiolitis is an inflammatory lung disease of unclear etiology that is prevalent in Asians and rare in Euro-peans and North Americans. Histologically, there is thickening of the walls of respiratory bronchioles and associated peribron-chiolitis, and, in advanced stages, bronchiolectasis (90). The chest radiograph can show disseminated small nodular opaci-ties up to 2 mm in size (91). The findings on CT have been clas-sified into four types: (a) nodules alone, (b) nodules associated with branching linear opacities, (c) nodules with ring-shaped or small tubular opacities (probable bronchiolectasis), and (d) large cystic opacities accompanied by dilated proximal bronchi (90,92) (Figs. 13-28 and 13-29).

Bronchopneumonia, regardless of the type of infectious agent, can result in centrilobular nodules or branching struc-tures on CT, which are related to peribronchiolar consolidation or pus-filled small airways (91), and it is the most common cause of the "tree-in-bud" pattern seen on CT (93,94) (Figs. 13-30 to 13-34). Aspiration of infected or other material into

the small airways is another common cause of the tree-in-bud pattern (Figs. 13-35 and 13-36).

Emphysema

Pulmonary emphysema, as defined by the National Heart, Lung, and Blood Institute, is "an abnormal permanent enlarge-ment of the airspaces distal to the terminal bronchioles, ac-companied by destruction of the alveolar walls, and without obvious fibrosis" (95). Three different morphologic subtypes of emphysema have been described according to their location in the secondary pulmonary lobule: centrilobular, panlobular, and paraseptal (distal lobular) (Table 13–6). A fourth type of emphysema, paracicatricial emphysema, results from and is

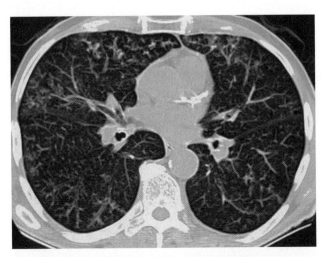

FIGURE 13-30. Infectious bronchiolitis. Maximum-intensity-projec-tion CT of an 81-year-old man with cough and weight loss shows diffuse bronchiolitis, with prominent tree-in-bud opacities in the pe-riphery of the lungs.

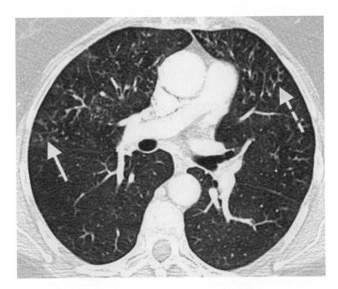

FIGURE 13-32. Atypical mycobacterial bronchiolitis. CT of a 69-year-old woman with fever and cough shows tree-in-bud opacities in the right middle lobe (solid arrow) and cylindric bronchiectasis in the lingula (dashed arrow).

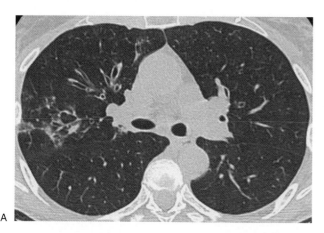
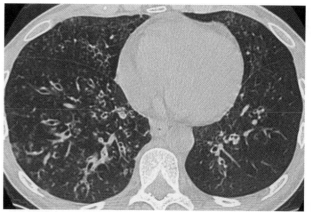

FIGURE 13-33. *Mycobacterium avium* complex infection. **A:** CT of a 58-year-old woman shows cylindric bronchiectasis in the right middle lobe. **B:** Extensive bronchiectasis, bronchiolectasis, airway wall thickening, and tree-in-bud opacities are seen in the lower lobes.

always associated with pulmonary fibrosis and therefore does not meet the strict definition of emphysema.

Emphysema is found at autopsy in up to 66% of adult patients (96,97), but clinical detection of disease during life is difficult unless the condition is advanced. The presence of airflow obstruction alone is a sensitive indicator of the presence of emphysema but is not specific, since asthma, irreversible small-airway disease, and certain forms of interstitial lung disease may also result in decreased FEV_1 (95,98,99). Evidence of impairment in gas transfer, as assessed with carbon monoxide diffusing capacity, is more sensitive than abnormal spirometry for the diagnosis of emphysema; it is also nonspecific, however, and patients may have up to 30% of their lung involved with emphysema but have no evidence of functional impairment (100). The accuracy of diagnosis based on findings from chest radiographs depends on the severity of parenchymal destruction (101,102). CT findings correlate with the presence and severity of morphologic emphysema better than chest radiographic findings or results of pulmonary function tests (103,104), although several studies that assessed CT with 10-mm and 1-mm collimation concluded that CT consistently underestimates the extent of centrilobular and panlobular emphysema and the

severity of emphysema when compared with pathologic assessment (105–108). In spite of these limitations, CT is currently the best way to detect emphysema in living patients.

The most common form of emphysema, centrilobular emphysema, is strongly associated with cigarette smoking, with the severity of emphysema increasing with the number of cigarettes smoked (109,110). Centrilobular emphysema results from destruction of alveoli around the proximal respiratory bronchiole and characteristically has a predominantly upper lung distribution. Although the upper lungs are more severely affected by emphysema, the degree of emphysema in the lower lungs has a stronger correlation with pulmonary function abnormalities. This indicates that the upper lungs are physiologically a relatively silent region, where extensive destruction may occur before functional abnormalities become detectable (111).

Panlobular emphysema has a characteristic lower lobe–predominant distribution; this is the type of emphysema seen in patients with α-1-antitrypsin deficiency (Fig. 13-37). In panlobular emphysema, the alveoli are destroyed throughout the secondary pulmonary lobule. The same findings of basilar

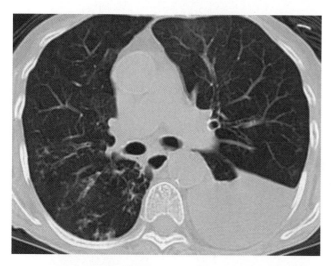

FIGURE 13-34. Infectious bronchiolitis. CT of a 72-year-old man with methicillin-resistant *Staphylococcus aureus* pneumonia shows tree-in-bud opacities in the right lower lobe and dense airspace opacity and volume loss in the left lower lobe.

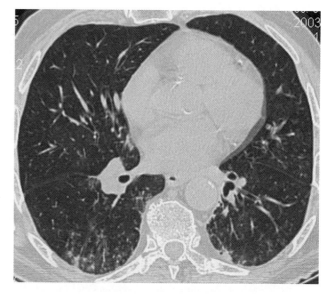

FIGURE 13-35. Aspiration. CT of a 77-year-old man with recurrent aspiration shows bronchiectasis and tree-in-bud opacities in both lower lobes.

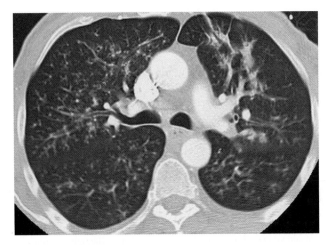

FIGURE 13-36. Aspiration. CT of a 57-year-old man with Parkinson disease and recurrent aspiration shows diffuse tree-in-bud opacities.

TABLE 13-6
FEATURES OF THREE MORPHOLOGIC SUBTYPES OF EMPHYSEMA

Centrilobular
    Involves central portion of secondary pulmonary lobule
    Usually a result of cigarette smoking
    Upper lung–predominant distribution
    "Swiss cheese" appearance on CT (early on)

Panacinar
    Involves entire secondary pulmonary lobule
    Seen in α-1-antitrypsin deficiency
    Lower lung–predominant distribution
    "Lung simplification" appearance on CT

Paraseptal
    Bullae or air cysts in a subpleural location
    Associated with spontaneous pneumothorax
    Most common in lung apices

CT, computed tomography.

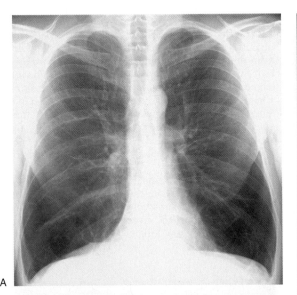

A

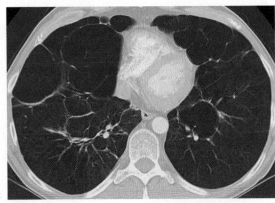

C

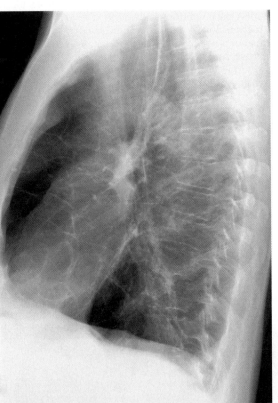

B

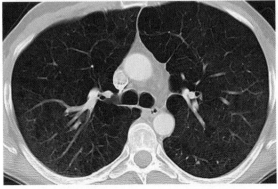

D

FIGURE 13-37. Alpha-1-antitrypsin deficiency. A: PA chest radiograph of a 43-year-old man shows hyperinflation and hyperlucency in the lower lungs. B: Lateral view shows increased retrosternal lucency and flattening of the diaphragm. C: CT shows bullous emphysema in the lower lungs. D: CT at a more superior level shows less severe emphysema. Compared with smoking-related centrilobular emphysema, emphysema caused by α-1-antitrypsin deficiency, although diffuse, is more severe in the lower lungs.

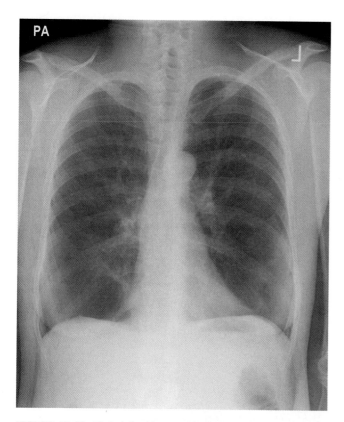

FIGURE 13-38. **Methylphenidate (Ritalin) lung.** PA chest radiograph of a woman who intravenously injected crushed Ritalin tablets shows emphysema in the lower lungs, which is similar in appearance to the findings of α-1-antitrypsin deficiency.

emphysema can be seen in patients who intravenously inject methylphenidate (crushed Ritalin tablets) (Fig. 13-38) (112).

Paraseptal emphysema is a focal or multifocal abnormality involving the periphery of the pulmonary lobule that is almost always seen in the periphery of the lung along the fissures and at sharp pleural reflections. Coalescence of paraseptal emphysema leads to the formation of bullae and is important in the development of spontaneous pneumothorax (113,114). Paraseptal emphysema should not be confused with honeycombing, which has thicker walls and is associated with fibrosis (115).

Criteria for chest radiographic diagnosis of emphysema include two or more of the following:

1. Depression and flattening of the diaphragm on the posteroanterior (PA) chest radiograph and blunting of costophrenic angles, with the actual level of the diaphragm not as significant as the contour (this can be determined from a straight line connecting the costophrenic junction to the vertebrophrenic junction on each side; if the highest level of the diaphragm contour is less than 1.5 cm above this line, the diaphragm can be recorded as flat).
2. Irregular radiolucency of the lung, as a result of irregularity in distribution of the emphysematous tissue destruction.
3. Increased retrosternal radiolucency, as seen on the lateral view, measuring 2.5 cm or more from the sternum to the most anterior margin of the ascending aorta.
4. Flattening or even concavity of the diaphragm contour on the lateral chest radiograph, as determined by the presence of a sternodiaphragmatic angle of 90 degrees or larger (100) (Fig. 13-39).

Other findings include increased AP diameter of the chest, saber-sheath configuration of the trachea, narrow cardiomediastinal silhouette, and enlargement of the central pulmonary arteries and right ventricle when pulmonary artery hypertension and cor pulmonale are present, respectively.

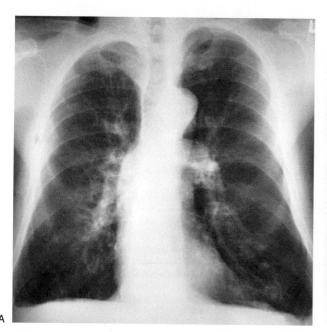
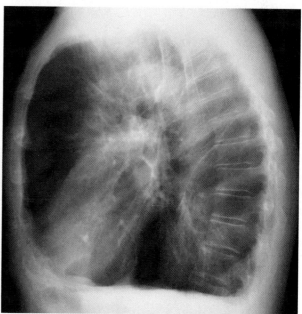

FIGURE 13-39. **Emphysema.** PA (**A**) and lateral (**B**) chest radiographs of a long-time cigarette smoker show flattening of the diaphragm with blunting of the costophrenic angles, increased retrosternal lucency, increased AP diameter of the chest, and prominent central pulmonary arteries. Note that the sternodiaphragmatic angle is greater than 90 degrees, indicative of extreme flattening and even minimal concavity of the diaphragmatic contour, as seen on the lateral view.

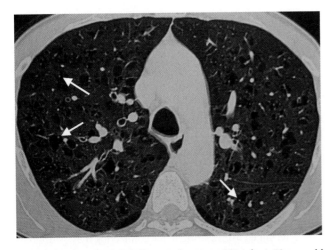

FIGURE 13-40. Centrilobular emphysema. CT of a 50-year-old woman with a long history of cigarette smoking shows focal areas of low attenuation creating a "Swiss cheese" appearance. Note a central nodular opacity within several of the areas of lucency (*arrows*); these opacities represent the lobular arteries. This finding helps to distinguish emphysema from cystic lung diseases.

Thin-section CT shows centrilobular emphysema as focal areas of low attenuation up to 1 cm in diameter within a homogeneous background of lung parenchyma; occasionally, this results in a "Swiss cheese" appearance. These areas of low attenuation are usually round or oval, have no definable wall, and are often associated with a small centrilobular "dot" representing the normal centrilobular core structures (Fig. 13-40). The appearance of panlobular emphysema on CT is large, extensive areas of uniform low attenuation with a lower lobe–predominant distribution associated with a reduction in the size and number of pulmonary vessels. No peripheral preservation of the lobule occurs, and therefore no striking difference in density exists between affected lobules and a homogeneous background of normal pulmonary parenchyma. Because of this, mild to moderate disease can be easily missed and the extent of disease underestimated (116). Paraseptal emphysema appears as multiple small subpleural airspaces ranging from a few millimeters to 1 cm in diameter (117).

Bullae, a term used synonymously with blebs, are described as air-filled structures greater than 1 cm in diameter, with thin walls, occurring in a subpleural or intraparenchymal location. They are usually multiple or associated with paraseptal, centrilobular, or panlobular emphysema (118). Giant bullous emphysema, or vanishing lung syndrome (Fig. 13-41), is

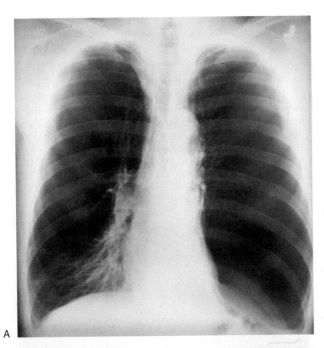

A

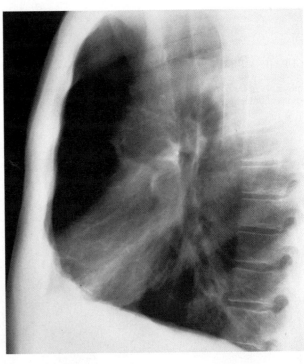

B

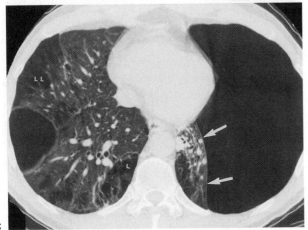

C

FIGURE 13-41. Giant bullous emphysema. PA (A) and lateral (B) chest radiographs of a 47-year-old man with progressive severe shortness of breath shows marked hyperinflation and hyperlucency of the lungs. The vascular markings are sparse (so-called vanishing lung sign), with the majority of residual perfusion going to the right medial base. The crowding of vascular markings at the right lung base, from compressive emphysema, should not be mistaken for focal pneumonia. Pneumothorax can be confused with this appearance; in some cases, CT is the only way to exclude a pneumothorax. C: CT shows a huge bulla in the left upper lobe that displaces the major fissure posteriorly and medially (*arrows*) and a prominent bulla in the right lower lobe. Note abnormal lucent emphysematous spaces within the lungs (L).

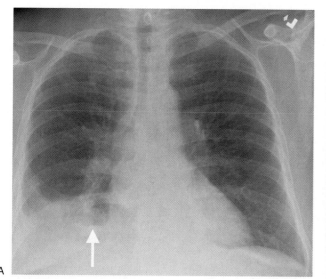

A

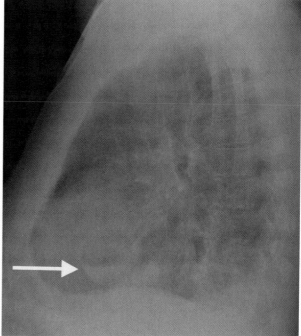

B

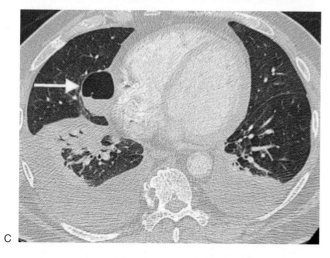

C

FIGURE 13-42. Infected bulla. A: PA chest radiograph of a 68-year-old man shows an air–fluid level in the right medial base (*arrow*). B: Lateral view shows a thin-walled cystic structure with an air–fluid level (*arrow*) in the right middle lobe. C: CT confirms a thin-walled bulla with an air–fluid level in the right middle lobe (*arrow*). Additional bullae were seen at several other levels on CT.

characterized by large bullae that are several centimeters in diameter and in some cases large enough to fill an entire hemithorax. When giant bullae impair pulmonary function and are associated with compressed lung on CT, the usual method of treatment is surgical resection (bullectomy) (119). On occa-

sion, bullae can become infected and present as cystic masses with air–fluid levels (Figs. 13-42 and 13-43).

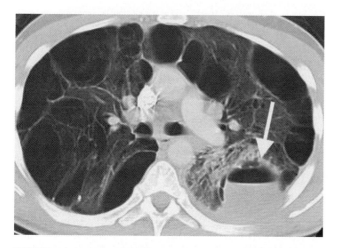

FIGURE 13-43. Infected bulla. CT of a 39-year-old man with α-1-antitrypsin deficiency shows a bulla with an air–fluid level (*arrow*) in the left lower lobe.

References

1. Stern EJ, Graham CM, Webb WR, et al. Normal trachea during forced expiration: dynamic CT measurements. *Radiology.* 1993;187:27–31.
2. Breatnach E, Abbott GC, Fraser RG. Dimensions of the normal human trachea. *AJR Am J Roentgenol.* 1984; 141:903–6.
3. Brown BM, Oshita AK, Castellino RA. CT assessment of the adult extrathoracic trachea. *J Comput Assist Tomogr.* 1983;7(3):415–418.
4. Gibellino F, Osmanliev DP, Watson A, et al. Increase in tracheal size with age—implications for maximal expiratory flow. *Am Rev Respir Dis.* 1985;132:784–787.
5. Kwong JS, Adler BD, Padley SPG, et al. Diagnosis of diseases of the trachea and main bronchi: chest radiography vs CT. *AJR Am J Roentgenol.* 1993;161:519–522.
6. Ferretti GR, Vining DJ, Knoplioch J, et al. Tracheobronchial tree: three-dimensional spiral CT with bronchoscopic perspective. *J Comput Assist Tomogr.* 1996;20:777–781.
7. Kwong JS, Müller NL, Miller RR. Diseases of the trachea and mainstem bronchi: correlation of CT with pathologic findings. *Radiographics.* 1992;12:645–657.
8. Choplin RH, Wehunt WD, Theros EG. Diffuse lesions of the trachea. *Semin Roentgenol.* 1993;28:38–50.
9. Bateson EM, Woo-Ming M. Tracheobronchomegaly. *Clin Radiol.* 1973;24:354–358.
10. Woodring JH, Howard RS II, Rehm SR. Congenital tracheobronchomegaly (Mounier-Kuhn syndrome): a report of 10 cases and review of the literature. *J Thorac Imaging.* 1991;6(2):1–10.

11. Dunne MG, Reiner B. CT features of tracheobronchomegaly. *J Comput Assist Tomogr.* 1988;12:388–391.
12. Shin MS, Jackson RM, Ho KJ. Tracheobronchomegaly (Mounier-Kuhn syndrome): CT diagnosis. *AJR Am J Roentgenol.* 1988;150:777–779.
13. Fiser F, Tomanek A, Rimanova V, et al. Tracheobronchomegaly. *Scand J Respir Dis.* 1969;50:147–155.
14. Bhutani VK, Ritchie WG, Shaffer TH. Acquired tracheomegaly in very preterm neonates. *Am J Dis Child.* 1986;140:449–452.
15. Woodring JH, Barrett PA, Rehm SR, et al. Acquired tracheomegaly in adults as a complication of diffuse pulmonary fibrosis. *AJR Am J Roentgenol.* 1989;152:743–747.
16. Cavanaugh MJ, Cooper DM. Chronic pulmonary disease in a child with the Ehlers-Danlos syndrome. *Acta Paediatr Scand.* 1976;65:679–684.
17. Wanderer AA, Ellis EF, Goltz RW, et al. Tracheobronchiomegaly and acquired cutis laxa in a child: physiologic and immunologic studies. *Pediatrics.* 1969;44:709–715.
18. Feist JH, Johnson TH, Wilson RJ. Acquired tracheomalacia: etiology and differential diagnosis. *Chest.* 1975;68:340–345.
19. Armstrong P, Wilson AG, Dee P, et al. *Imaging of Diseases of the Chest.* St. Louis: Mosby—Year Book; 1995:818.
20. Shepard JO, McLoud TC. Imaging the airways: computed tomography and magnetic resonance imaging. *Clin Chest Med.* 1991;12(1):151–168.
21. Stern EJ, Gamsu G. CT of the trachea and central bronchi. *Radiologist.* 1994;1(6):335.
22. Gamsu G, Webb WR. Computed tomography of the trachea and mainstem bronchi. *Semin Roentgenol.* 1983;18:51–60.
23. Grillo HC, Donahue DM, Mathisen DJ, et al. Postintubation tracheal stenosis: treatment and results. *J Thorac Cardiovasc Surg.* 1995;109:486–492.
24. Quint LE, Whyte RI, Kazerooni EA, et al. Stenosis of the central airways: evaluation by using helical CT with multiplanar reconstructions. *Radiology.* 1995;194:871–877.
25. Greene R, Lechner GL. "Saber-sheath" trachea: a clinical and functional study of marked coronal narrowing of the intrathoracic trachea. *Radiology.* 1975;115:265–268.
26. Greene R. "Saber-sheath" trachea: relation to chronic obstructive pulmonary disease. *AJR Am J Roentgenol.* 1978;130:441–445.
27. Fraser RG, Paré JAP, Paré PD, et al, eds. *Diagnosis of Diseases of the Chest.* 3rd ed. Philadelphia: WB Saunders; 1990:1987–2003.
28. Davis SD, Berkmen YM, King T. Peripheral bronchial involvement in relapsing polychondritis: demonstration by thin-section CT. *AJR Am J Roentgenol.* 1989;153:953–954.
29. Müller NL, Miller RR, Ostrow DN, et al. Clinico-radiologic-pathologic conference: diffuse thickening of the tracheal wall. *Can Assoc Radiol J.* 1989;40:213–215.
30. Im J-G, Chung JW, Han SK. CT manifestations of tracheobronchial involvement in relapsing polychondritis. *J Comput Assist Tomogr.* 1988;12:792–793.
31. Lundgren R, Stjernberg NL. Tracheobronchopathia osteochondroplastica: a clinical bronchoscopic and spirometric study. *Chest.* 1981;80:706–709.
32. Secrest PG, Kendig TA, Beland AJ. Tracheobronchopathia osteochondroplastica. *Am J Med.* 1964;36:815–818.
33. Alroy GG, Lichtig C, Kaftori JK. Tracheobronchopathia osteoplastica: end stage of primary lung amyloidosis?. *Chest.* 1972;61:465–468.
34. Way SP. Tracheopathia osteoplastica. *J Clin Pathol.* 1967;20:814–820.
35. Young RH, Sandstrom RE, Mark GJ. Tracheopathia osteoplastica: clinical, radiologic, and pathologic correlations. *J Thorac Cardiovasc Surg.* 1980;79:537–541.
36. Stein MG, Gamsu G, Webb WR, et al. Computed tomography of diffuse tracheal stenosis in Wegener granulomatosis. *J Comput Assist Tomogr.* 1986;10:868–870.
37. Mendelson DS, Norton K, Cohen BA, et al. Bronchial compression: an unusual manifestation of sarcoidosis. *J Comput Assist Tomogr.* 1983;7:892–894.
38. Westcott JL, Noehren TH. Bronchial stenosis in chronic sarcoidosis. *Chest.* 1973;63:893–897.
39. Coleman FP. Acquired non-malignant esophagorespiratory fistula. *Am J Surg.* 1957;93:321–328.
40. Spalding AR, Burney DP, Richie RE. Acquired benign bronchoesophageal fistulas in adults. *Ann Thorac Surg.* 1979;28:378–383.
41. Vaid YN, Shin MS. Computed tomography evaluation of tracheoesophageal fistula. *J Comput Tomogr.* 1986;10:281–285.
42. Carpenter LM, Merten DF. Radiographic manifestations of congenital anomalies affecting the airway. *Radiol Clin North Am.* 1991;29:219–240.
43. Wells AL, Wells TR, Landing BH, et al. Short trachea, a hazard in tracheal intubation of neonates and infants: syndromal associations. *Anesthesiology.* 1989;71:367–373.
44. McLaughlin FJ, Strieder DJ, Harris GBC, et al. Tracheal bronchus: association with respiratory morbidity in childhood. *J Pediatr.* 1985;106:751–755.
45. Shipley RT, McLoud TC, Dedrick CG, et al. Computed tomography of the tracheal bronchus. *J Comput Assist Tomogr.* 1985;9(1):53–55.
46. Thurlbeck W. Pathology of chronic airflow obstruction. *Chest.* 1990;97(suppl 2):6S–10S.
47. Grenier P, Mourey-Gerosa I, Benali K, et al. Abnormalities of the airways and lung parenchyma in asthmatics: CT observations in 50 patients and inter- and intraobserver variability. *Eur Radiol.* 1996;6:199–206.
48. Neeld DA, Goodman LR, Gurney JW, et al. Computerized tomography in the evaluation of allergic bronchopulmonary aspergillosis. *Am Rev Respir Dis.* 1990;142:1200–1205.
49. Paganin F, Trussard V, Seneterre E, et al. Chest radiography and high resolution computed tomography of the lungs in asthma. *Am Rev Respir Dis.* 1992;146:1084–1087.
50. Carroll N, Elliot J, Morton A, et al. The structure of large and small airways in nonfatal and fatal asthma. *Am Rev Respir Dis.* 1993;147:405–410.
51. Stern EJ, Frank MS. Small airway diseases of the lungs: findings at expiratory CT. *AJR Am J Roentgenol.* 1994;163:37–41.
52. Kondoh Y, Taniguchi H, Yokoyama S, et al. Emphysematous change in chronic asthma in relation to cigarette smoking: assessment by computed tomography. *Chest.* 1990;97:845–849.
53. Reid LM. Reduction in bronchial subdivision in bronchiectasis. *Thorax.* 1950;5:233–247.
54. Westcott JL, Cole SR. Traction bronchiectasis in end-stage pulmonary fibrosis. *Radiology.* 1986;161:665–669.
55. Gudbjerg CE. Roentgenologic diagnosis of bronchiectasis. An analysis of 112 cases. *Acta Radiol.* 1955;43:210–226.
56. Currie DC, Cooke JC, Morgan AD, et al. Interpretation of bronchograms and chest radiographs in patients with chronic sputum production. *Thorax.* 1987;42:278–284.
57. Silverman PM, Godwin JD. CT/bronchographic correlations in bronchiectasis. *J Comput Assist Tomogr.* 1987;11(1):52–56.
58. Cooke JC, Currie DC, Morgan AD, et al. Role of computed tomography in diagnosis of bronchiectasis. *Thorax.* 1987;42:272–277.
59. Müller NL, Bergin CJ, Ostrow DN, et al. Role of computed tomography in the recognition of bronchiectasis. *AJR Am J Roentgenol.* 1984;143:971–976.
60. Phillips MS, Williams MP, Flower CDR. How useful is computed tomography in the diagnosis and assessment of bronchiectasis? *Clin Radiol.* 1986;37:321–325.
61. Grenier P, Maurice F, Musset D, et al. Bronchiectasis: assessment by thin-section CT. *Radiology.* 1986;161:95–99.
62. Young K, Aspestrand F, Kolbenstvedt A. High resolution CT and bronchography in the assessment of bronchiectasis. *Acta Radiol.* 1991;32(6):439–441.
63. McGuinness G, Naidich DP, Leitman BS, et al. Bronchiectasis: CT evaluation. *AJR Am J Roentgenol.* 1993;160:253–259.
64. Afzelius BA. A human syndrome caused by immotile cilia. *Science.* 1976;193:317–319.
65. Tsui LC, Buchwald M, Barker D, et al. Cystic fibrosis locus defined by a genetically linked polymorphic DNA marker. *Science.* 1985;230:1054–1057.
66. Kerem B, Rommens JM, Buchanan JA, et al. Identification of the cystic fibrosis gene: genetic analysis. *Science.* 1989;245:1073–1080.
67. Riordan JR, Rommens JM, Kerem B, et al. Identification of the cystic fibrosis gene: cloning and characterization of complementary DNA. *Science.* 1989;245:1066–1073.
68. Rommens JM, Iannuzzi MC, Kerem B, et al. Identification of the cystic fibrosis gene: chromosome walking and jumping. *Science.* 1989;245:1059–1065.
69. Davis PB, Drumm M, Konstan MW. Cystic fibrosis. *Am J Respir Crit Care Med.* 1996;154:1229–1256.
70. Cystic Fibrosis Foundation. *Patient Registry 1994 Annual Data Report.* Bethesda, MD: Cystic Fibrosis Foundation; 1995.
71. Fitzsimmons SC. The changing epidemiology of cystic fibrosis. *J Pediatr.* 1993;122:1–9.
72. Friedman PJ, Harwood IR, Ellenbogen PH. Pulmonary cystic fibrosis in the adult: early and late radiologic findings with pathologic correlation. *AJR Am J Roentgenol.* 1981;136:1131–1144.
73. Bhalla M, Turcois N, Aponte V, et al. Cystic fibrosis: scoring system with thin-section CT. *Radiology.* 1991;179:783–788.
74. Fletcher CM, Pride NB. Definitions of emphysema, chronic bronchitis, asthma, and airflow obstruction: twenty-five years on from the CIBA Symposium. *Thorax.* 1984;39:81–85.
75. Kuhn C III. Normal anatomy and histology. In: Thurlbeck WM, Churg AM, eds. *Pathology of the Lung.* 2nd ed. New York: Thieme; 1995:1–36.
76. Murata K, Itoh H, Todo G, et al. Centrilobular lesions of the lung: demonstration by high-resolution CT and pathologic correlation. *Radiology.* 1986;161:641–645.
77. Stern EJ, Müller NL, Swensen SJ, et al. CT mosaic pattern of lung attenuation: etiologies and terminology. *J Thorac Imaging.* 1995;10:294–297.
78. Teel GS, Engeler CE, Tashijian JH, et al. Imaging of small airways disease. *Radiographics.* 1996;16:27–41.
79. Turton CW, Williams G, Green M. Cryptogenic obliterative bronchiolitis in adults. *Thorax.* 1981;36:805–810.
80. Padley SPG, Adler BD, Hansell DM, et al. Bronchiolitis obliterans: high-resolution CT findings and correlation with pulmonary function tests. *Clin Radiol.* 1993;47:236–240.
81. Lynch DA, Brasch RC, Hardy KA, et al. Pediatric pulmonary disease: assessment with high-resolution ultrafast CT. *Radiology.* 1990;176:243–248.
82. Morrish WF, Herman SJ, Weisbrod GL, et al. Bronchiolitis obliterans after lung transplantation: findings at chest radiography and high-resolution CT. *Radiology.* 1991;179:487–490.
83. Sweatman MC, Millar AB, Strickland B, et al. Computed tomography in adult obliterative bronchiolitis. *Clin Radiol.* 1990;41:116–119.

84. Finkelstein R, Cosio M. Disease of the small airways in smokers: smokers' bronchiolitis. In: Epler G, ed. *Diseases of the Bronchioles*. New York: Raven Press; 1994:115–137.
85. Remy-Jardin M, Remy J, Gosselin B, et al. Sliding thin slab, minimum intensity projection technique in the diagnosis of emphysema: histopathologic—CT correlation. *Radiology*. 1996;200:665–671.
86. Myers JL, Veal CF, Shin MS, et al. Respiratory bronchiolitis causing interstitial lung disease: a clinicopathologic study of six cases. *Am Rev Respir Dis*. 1987;135:880–884.
87. Wright JL, Cagle P, Churg A, et al. State of the art: diseases of the small airways. *Am Rev Respir Dis*. 1992;146:240–262.
88. Gruden JF, Webb WR. CT findings in a proved case of respiratory bronchiolitis. *AJR Am J Roentgenol*. 1993;161:44–46.
89. Remy-Jardin M, Remy J, Gosselin B, et al. Lung parenchymal changes secondary to cigarette smoking: pathologic—CT correlations. *Radiology*. 1993;186:643–651.
90. Akira M, Kitatani F, Yong-Sik L, et al. Diffuse panbronchiolitis: evaluation with high-resolution CT. *Radiology*. 1988;168:433–438.
91. Gruden JF, Webb WR, Warnock M. Centrilobular opacities in the lung on HRCT: diagnostic considerations and pathologic correlation. *AJR Am J Roentgenol*. 1994;162:569–574.
92. Homma H, Yamanaka A, Tanimoto S, et al. Diffuse panbronchiolitis: a disease of the transitional zone of the lung. *Chest*. 1983;83:63–69.
93. Aquino SL, Gamsu G, Webb WR, et al. Tree-in-bud pattern: frequency and significance on thin section CT. *J Comput Assist Tomogr*. 1996;20:594–599.
94. Collins J, Blankenbaker D, Stern EJ. CT patterns of bronchiolar disease: what is "tree-in-bud"? *AJR Am J Roentgenol*. 1998;171:365–370.
95. Snider GL. Distinguishing among asthma, chronic bronchitis, and emphysema. *Chest*. 1985;87:35S–39S.
96. Sobonya RE, Burrows B. The epidemiology of emphysema. *Clin Chest Med*. 1983;4:351–358.
97. Thurlbeck WM. Overview of the pathology of pulmonary emphysema in the human. *Clin Chest Med*. 1983;4:337–350.
98. Gelb AF, Gold WM, Wright RR, et al. Physiologic diagnosis of subclinical emphysema. *Am Rev Respir Dis*. 1973;107:50–63.
99. Snider GL. Chronic obstructive pulmonary disease—a continuing challenge. *Am Rev Respir Dis*. 1986;133:942–944.
100. Pratt PC. Role of conventional chest radiography in diagnosis and exclusion of emphysema. *Am J Med*. 1987;82:998–1006.
101. Schmidt RA, Glenny RW, Godwin JD, et al. Panlobular emphysema in young intravenous Ritalin abusers. *Am Rev Respir Dis*. 1991;143:649–656.
102. Sherman CB, Hudson LD, Pierson DJ. Severe precocious emphysema in intravenous methylphenidate (Ritalin) abusers. *Chest*. 1987;92:1085–1087.
103. Kinsella M, Müller NL, Abboud RT, et al. Quantitation of emphysema by computed tomography using a "density mask" program and correlation with pulmonary function tests. *Chest*. 1990;97:315–321.
104. Morrison NJ, Abboud RT, Ramadan F, et al. Comparison of single breath carbon monoxide diffusing capacity and pressure-volume curves in detecting emphysema. *Am Rev Respir Dis*. 1989;139:1179–1187.
105. Bergin C, Müller NL, Nochols DM, et al. The diagnosis of emphysema. A computed tomographic-pathologic correlation. *Am Rev Respir Dis*. 1986;133:541–546.
106. Foster WL Jr, Pratt PC, Roggli VL, et al. Centrilobular emphysema: CT-pathologic correlation. *Radiology*. 1986;159:27–32.
107. Hayhurst MD, Flenley DC, McLean A, et al. Diagnosis of pulmonary emphysema by computerized tomography. *Lancet*. 1984;2:320–322.
108. Miller RR, Müller NL, Vidal S, et al. Limitation of computed tomography in the assessment of emphysema. *Am Rev Respir Dis*. 1989;139:980–983.
109. Auerbach O, Hammond EC, Garfinkel L, et al. Relationship of smoking and age to emphysema: whole-lung section study. *N Engl J Med*. 1972;286:853–857.
110. Niewoehner DE. Cigarette smoking, lung inflammation, and the development of emphysema. *J Lab Clin Med*. 1988;111:15–27.
111. Gurney JW, Jones KK, Robbins RA, et al. Regional distribution of emphysema: correlation of high-resolution CT with pulmonary function tests in unselected smokers. *Radiology*. 1992;183:457–463.
112. Stern EJ, Frank MS, Schmutz JF, et al. Panlobular pulmonary emphysema caused by i.v. injection of methylphenidate (Ritalin): findings on chest radiographs and CT scans. *AJR Am J Roentgenol*. 1994;162(3):550–560.
113. Anderson AE Jr, Furlaneto JA, Foraker AG. Bronchopulmonary derangements in non-smokers. *Am Rev Respir Dis*. 1970;101:518–527.
114. Tuddenham WJ. Glossary of terms for thoracic radiology: recommendations of the Nomenclature Committee of the Fleischner Society. *AJR Am J Roentgenol*. 1984;143:509–517.
115. Stern EJ, Frank MS. CT of the lung in patients with pulmonary emphysema: diagnosis, quantification, and correlation with pathologic and physiologic findings. *AJR Am J Roentgenol*. 1994;162:791–798.
116. Spouge D, Mayo JR, Cardoso W, et al. Panacinar emphysema: CT and pathologic findings. *J Comput Assist Tomogr*. 1993;17(5):710–713.
117. Thurlbeck WM. *Morphology of Emphysema and Emphysema-like Conditions*. Philadelphia: WB Saunders; 1976:96–234.
118. Reid L. *The Pathology of Emphysema*. London: Lloyd-Duke (Medical Books); 1967.
119. Martinez F. Surgical therapy for chronic obstructive pulmonary disease: conventional bullectomy and lung volume reduction surgery in the absence of giant bullae. *Semin Respir Crit Care Med*. 1999;20:351–364.

CHAPTER 14

UNILATERAL HYPERLUCENT HEMITHORAX

LEARNING OBJECTIVES

1. Recognize a unilateral hyperlucent hemithorax on a chest radiograph or computed tomography (CT).
2. Describe the common causes of a unilateral hyperlucent hemithorax on a chest radiograph or CT.
3. List an appropriate differential diagnosis when a hyperlucent hemithorax is seen on a chest radiograph or

CT and suggest a specific diagnosis when certain associated findings are seen (e.g., absence of a breast after mastectomy, absence of a pectoralis muscle in Poland syndrome, unilateral or asymmetric bullous disease/emphysema, or air trapping on exhalation imaging in a patient with Swyer-James syndrome or an endobronchial foreign body).

The most common chest radiographic causes of a unilateral hyperlucent hemithorax do not reflect an intrinsic abnormality of the lung itself. Improper patient positioning is the most common cause. A slight degree of patient rotation will result in disparity in overall lung opacity on the posteroanterior (PA) chest radiograph. By the same mechanism, scoliosis, if severe, may cause asymmetry of lung density. Mastectomy results in asymmetry of soft tissues overlying the lungs and relative radiolucency on the side of breast removal (Fig. 14-1). This common cause of unilateral hyperlucent hemithorax is easily overlooked

unless the observer is methodical in always evaluating soft tissues on a chest radiograph. Absence of the sternocleidomastoid muscle results in hyperlucency in the upper hemithorax (Fig. 14-2). Absence of the pectoralis muscle also results in hyperlucency of the ipsilateral hemithorax (Fig. 14-3 and 14-4). When associated with ipsilateral syndactyly, brachydactyly, and rib anomalies, the condition is called Poland syndrome.

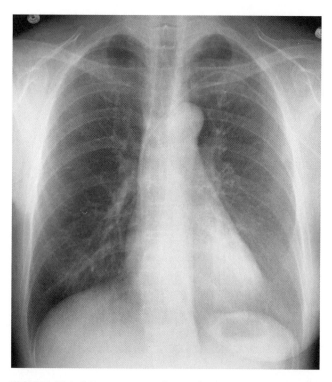

FIGURE 14-1. Mastectomy. PA chest radiograph of a woman after right mastectomy for breast cancer. Note the presence of a breast shadow on the left and the absence on the right; as a result, the right lung appears relatively hyperlucent compared with the left.

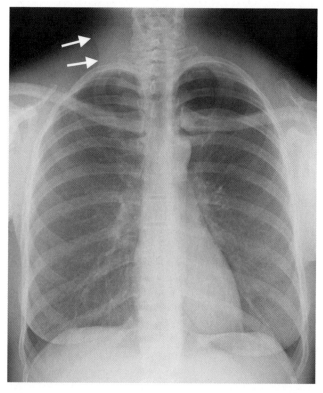

FIGURE 14-2. Absence of sternocleidomastoid muscle. PA chest radiograph of a 47-year-old woman with thyroid carcinoma who underwent left radical neck dissection shows hyperlucency of the left upper hemithorax. Note a normal sternocleidomastoid muscle shadow on the right (*arrows*) and absence of the shadow on the left.

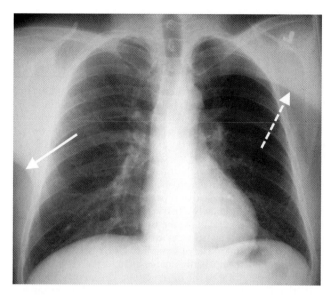

FIGURE 14-3. Absence of pectoralis muscle. PA chest radiograph shows relative hyperlucency of the left hemithorax because of the absence of left pectoralis muscle. Note the normal pectoralis muscle shadow on the right (*solid arrow*) and abnormal elevation of the skin fold on the left (*dashed arrow*).

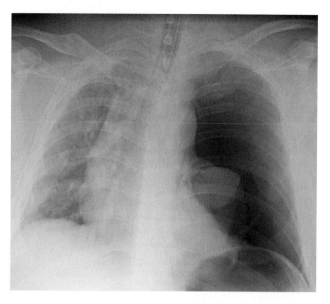

FIGURE 14-5. Tension pneumothorax. Anteroposterior supine chest radiograph of a 35-year-old man involved in a motor vehicle crash shows a large left pneumothorax, collapse of the left lung, and mediastinal shift to the right. The left hemithorax is hyperlucent compared with the right.

A large pneumothorax results in hyperlucency of the ipsilateral hemithorax and can be recognized by observing displacement of the visceral pleural line, absence of lung markings distal to the displaced pleural line, and contralateral shift of the mediastinum (Fig. 14-5). Patients who have had pulmonary resections or who have lobar atelectasis may also show lucency of the residual aerated lung in the involved hemithorax because of compensatory hyperexpansion. A common cause of hyperlucent hemithorax in some hospitals is unilateral lung transplantation for pulmonary emphysema, where the native emphysematous lung is radiolucent relative to the lung transplant, which receives the bulk of the pulmonary perfusion (Fig. 14-6). In some cases of hyperlucent hemithorax, the lucent side is normal and the opposite side is abnormally radiopaque. Dif-

fuse pleural thickening on the more opaque side or pleural fluid layering posteriorly on a supine radiograph are frequent causes.

The origins of true unilateral hyperlucent lung will be the focus of this chapter. After faulty radiologic technique and chest wall defects are excluded as possible sources, the causes of unilateral hyperlucent lung can be categorized into those primarily related to airway obstruction and those primarily related to decreased pulmonary blood flow (Table 14-1).

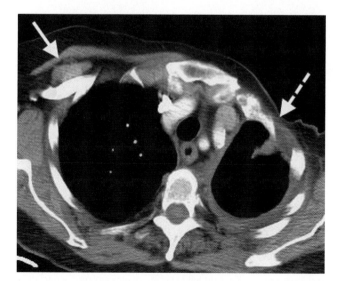

FIGURE 14-4. Absence of pectoralis muscles. Computed tomography (CT) of a woman who underwent left radical mastectomy for breast cancer shows pectoral muscles on the right (*solid arrow*) and absence of pectoral muscles on the left (*dashed arrow*).

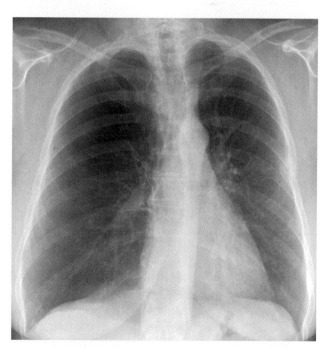

FIGURE 14-6. Left lung transplant. PA chest radiograph of a 62-year-old woman with a left lung transplant shows a hyperlucent right lung. The native right emphysematous lung is hyperlucent and hyperexpanded, causing mediastinal shift to the left.

TABLE 14-1

CAUSES OF UNILATERAL HYPERLUCENT HEMITHORAX

Patient positioning
  Rotation
  Scoliosis

Chest wall defect
  Mastectomy
  Poland syndrome (absent pectoralis muscle)

Pneumothorax

Airway obstruction
  Bronchial compression (hilar mass, cardiomegaly)
  Endobronchial obstruction with air trapping (foreign
    body, tumor)
  Obliterative bronchiolitis
  Swyer-James syndrome
  Pulmonary emphysema (asymmetric)
  Congenital lobar emphysema

Pulmonary vascular cause
  Pulmonary embolism
  Pulmonary artery hypoplasia

AIRWAY OBSTRUCTION AS A CAUSE OF UNILATERAL HYPERLUCENT LUNG

The hallmark of airway obstruction on chest radiographs is the finding of air trapping. An exhalation-phase chest radiograph will show whether air trapping is present; this is manifested as failure of the lung to decrease in volume and failure of the lung to increase in opacity on exhalation compared with inhalation. In some cases, the mediastinum shifts to the side that is not trapping air on exhalational views. Air trapping occurs when an *endobronchial lesion*, usually a foreign body in a large airway, causes a check-valve type of obstruction. The foreign body does not completely obstruct the bronchus in which it is lodged. During inhalation, the bronchial diameter normally increases, allowing air to pass around the foreign body and enter the lung distal to the obstruction. During exhalation, the bronchial diameter normally decreases, and the air is trapped within the lung distal to the obstruction. This allows a foreign body that does not completely obstruct a bronchus during inhalation to do so during exhalation. As a result, the lung, lobe, or segment distal to the foreign body becomes increasingly distended until the pressure within it prevents more air from entering. In children, this type of check-valve obstruction usually results from the aspiration of food, commonly a peanut, or a toy or coin. In adults, this type of obstruction can result from aspiration of foreign bodies but also, more important, from an endobronchial tumor (Fig. 14-7). *Extrinsic masses*, such as

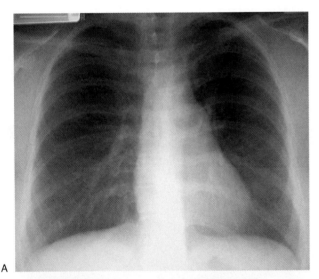

A

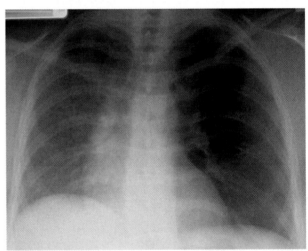

B

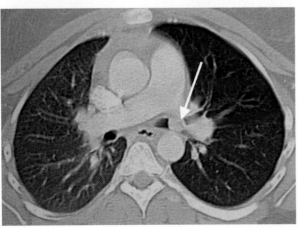

C

FIGURE 14-7. Carcinoid tumor. A: PA inspiratory chest radiograph of a 24-year-old woman with a prolonged history of wheezing, shortness of breath, cough, and recurrent pneumonia appears normal. The patient was treated for asthma with no relief in symptoms. **B:** PA exhalational view shows air trapping in the left hyperlucent lung and mediastinal shift to the right. **C:** CT shows a mass (*arrow*) in the left main bronchus. This mass results in a ball-valve obstruction, where air enters the lung during inhalation but can't exit the lung during exhalation. Note that the left lung is hyperlucent relative to the right lung as a result of air trapping.

enlarged nodes or an enlarged heart, can obstruct a bronchus in a similar fashion.

Obliterative bronchiolitis is a syndrome of airflow limitation caused by bronchiolar and peribronchiolar inflammation and fibrosis, as was discussed in Chapter 13. In adults, it is most often idiopathic in etiology, but is also associated with lung and bone marrow transplantation as well as a variety of other insults to the lung. The *Swyer-James*, or MacLeod, syndrome is a form of obliterative bronchiolitis that occurs following an insult to the developing lung (1). In this syndrome, unlike in large central airway obstruction, small bronchi and bronchioles are affected, and the lung served by abnormal airways remains inflated by collateral air drift. By definition, the airway disease as assessed by the chest radiograph is predominantly unilateral, giving rise to the key finding of unilateral hyperlucent lung. In practice, obliterative bronchiolitis is often bilateral and patchy. The injury to the immature lung, which occurs during the first 8 years of life, commonly follows a viral infection. Bronchi and bronchioles from the fourth generation to the terminal bronchioles have submucosal fibrosis, which causes luminal irregularity and occlusion. Pulmonary tissue is hypoplastic, including the pulmonary artery and its branches, which are reduced in both size and number. Lung distal to diseased airways is hyperinflated and supplied by collateral air drift. Sometimes panacinar emphysematous changes are present. Patients are typically asymptomatic, often presenting as adults with an incidental abnormal chest radiograph.

Chest radiographs show unilateral hyperlucency because of reduced lung perfusion and air trapping (Fig. 14-8). The size and number of vessels in the middle and peripheral lung are reduced on the affected side. The hilum of the involved lung is small, but lung volumes are normal or only slightly decreased. Ipsilateral air trapping on exhalational chest radiography is a key finding of the condition. The air trapping can also be demonstrated on nuclear medicine ventilation studies or paired inhalation/exhalation computed tomography (CT).

The CT findings of Swyer-James syndrome include a patchwork of local low-density and hypovascular areas interspersed with lung of normal density (2). Air trapping can be confirmed on exhalation. Other changes that can be seen on CT include bronchiectasis, bronchiolectasis, atelectasis, and focal scarring (see Fig. 13-26) (3).

Pulmonary emphysema is a pathologic diagnosis that is defined as a condition of the lung characterized by abnormal per-

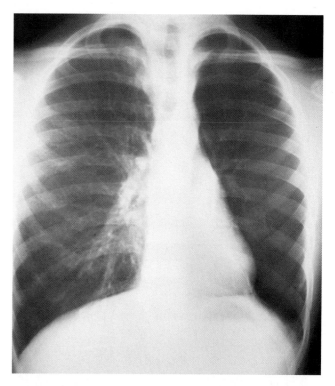

FIGURE 14-8. Swyer-James syndrome. PA chest radiograph of a 12-year-old boy shows hyperlucency of the abnormal left lung. The vessels on the left are diminutive, the hilum is small, and lung volume is slightly decreased.

manent enlargement of airspaces distal to the terminal bronchiole and accompanied by the destruction of their walls and without obvious fibrosis. Although emphysema is usually a diffuse, bilateral process, it can on occasion be asymmetric, with one lung more severely involved than the other. This marked asymmetry in involvement can result in the more severely involved lung appearing hyperlucent compared with the opposite lung (Fig. 14-9). Emphysema is discussed in more detail in Chapter 13.

Congenital lobar emphysema (CLE) usually manifests in the neonatal period, but in some cases the presentation is delayed

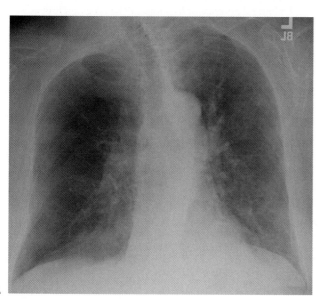

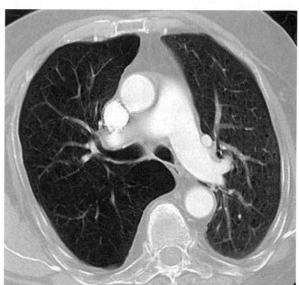

A   B

FIGURE 14-9. Asymmetric pulmonary emphysema. A: PA chest radiograph of a 69-year-old woman with emphysema shows hyperlucency of the right lung. **B:** CT shows the cause of the hyperlucency to be emphysema that more severely involves the right lung compared with the left lung. The vessels in the right lung are diminutive compared with those on the left.

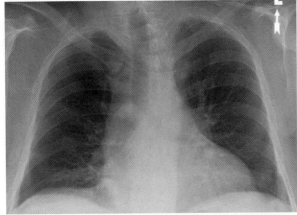

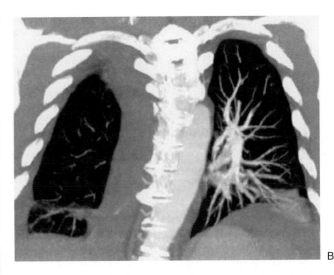

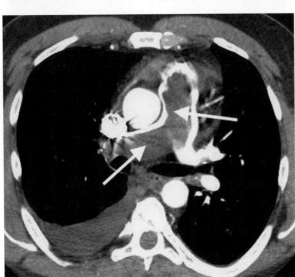

FIGURE 14-10. Pulmonary emboli. A: PA chest radiograph of a man with a lower-extremity soft tissue sarcoma, embolizing to the pulmonary arteries, shows a hyperlucent right lung. B: Coronal reformatted CT shows markedly decreased perfusion to the right lung. C: Axial CT shows low-attenuation filling defect throughout the main and right pulmonary arteries (*arrows*).

until after the first month of life; it can also present in adulthood. Aplasia, hypoplasia, or dysplasia of bronchial supporting structures is postulated as the primary cause of CLE (4). The chest radiographic appearance of CLE is hyperexpansion of an isolated lobe in one lung, usually an upper or middle lobe. The expanded lobe may cause compressive atelectasis of the rest of the lung. Its appearance on chest radiography or CT can be similar to that of obliterative bronchiolitis.

PULMONARY VASCULAR CAUSES OF UNILATERAL HYPERLUCENT LUNG

Pulmonary vascular conditions may result in a hyperlucent lung on chest radiography that is indistinguishable from the lucency associated with airway obstruction. *However, in primary vascular conditions, air trapping is generally not as severe as with airway obstruction.*

One of the chest radiographic signs of pulmonary embolism is oligemia of the lung beyond the occluded vessel (Westermark sign). A large unilateral embolus, whether bland, septic, or neoplastic, can result in a unilateral hyperlucent lung (Fig. 14-10). When seen, the Westermark sign can be very helpful in suggesting further workup for pulmonary embolism in the appropriate patient population; however, this sign is not commonly seen.

A more detailed discussion of radiographic and CT findings of pulmonary embolism is included in Chapter 17.

Unilateral absence or hypoplasia of a lung or a lobe is a congenital abnormality that, surprisingly, may cause few clinical problems when not accompanied by other congenital abnormalities. The chest radiographic findings are those of absent or decreased aeration of the affected side, signs of volume loss, and compensatory hyperaeration of the opposite lung. The decreased perfusion to the affected lung contributes to its relative hyperlucency. Radiographs, and especially CT, show the diminution or absence of a pulmonary artery. Fibrosing mediastinitis, when associated with encasement of a pulmonary artery by fibrous tissue, can produce a similar appearance. In this case, however, CT will show the abnormal fibrous tissue infiltrating the mediastinum and encasing the bronchi and vessels.

References

1. Reid L, Simon G. Unilateral lung transradiancy. *Thorax.* 1962;17:230–239.
2. Moore ADA, Godwin JD, Dietrich PA, et al. Swyer-James syndrome: CT findings in eight patients. *AJR Am J Roentgenol.* 1992;158:1211–1215.
3. Marti-Bonmati L, Perales FR, Catala F, et al. CT findings in Swyer-James syndrome. *Radiology.* 1989;172:477–480.
4. Stovin PGI. Congenital lobar emphysema. *Thorax.* 1959;14:254–261.

CHAPTER 15

NEOPLASMS OF THE LUNG

LEARNING OBJECTIVES

1. Name the four major histologic types of bronchogenic carcinoma and describe the difference between small cell and non–small cell types.
2. Name the type of non–small cell lung cancer that most commonly cavitates.
3. Name the types of bronchogenic cancer that are usually centrally located.
4. Describe the TNM (tumor-node-metastases) classification for staging non–small cell lung cancer, including the components of each stage (I, II, III, IV, and substages), and define each component (T1 to T4, N0 to N3, M0 to M1).
5. Describe the staging of small cell lung cancer.
6. Name the four most common extrathoracic sites of metastases for non–small cell and small cell lung cancer.
7. Name the stages of non–small cell lung cancer that are potentially resectable.
8. Recognize abnormal contralateral mediastinal shift on a postpneumonectomy chest radiograph and state five possible etiologies for the abnormal shift.
9. Name the most common thoracic locations for mucoepidermoid, adenoid cystic, and carcinoid tumors to occur.
10. Describe the role of magnetic resonance imaging in lung cancer staging (e.g., chest wall invasion and brachial plexus involvement).
11. Describe the role of positron emission tomography in lung cancer staging.

Bronchogenic carcinoma, a term referring to tumors originating from the bronchial epithelium, is the leading cause of death from cancer in men and women in the industrialized world. In 1987, bronchogenic cancer surpassed breast cancer as the most common fatal malignancy of U.S. women (1,2). Cigarette smoking is the most important causative factor in the development of bronchogenic carcinoma, and there is a direct link between cigarette smoking and development of bronchogenic cancer (Fig. 15-1), with approximately 85% of deaths directly attributable to tobacco use (2,3). This chapter will focus on the clinical presentation, histologic classification, and staging of bronchogenic carcinoma; this is followed by a brief discussion of postpneumonectomy complications and of carcinoid and salivary gland tumors of the trachea and bronchi.

BRONCHOGENIC CARCINOMA

Clinical Presentation

Bronchogenic carcinoma is relatively uncommon in patients under the age of 30 and typically occurs in 60- to 70-year-old men and women. Patients commonly present with symptoms produced by the primary tumor. Centrally located tumors can cause coughing, wheezing, hemoptysis, and postobstructive pneumonia. Tumors invading the chest wall, pleura, and mediastinal structures can cause pleuritic or local chest pain, dyspnea, cough, the Pancoast syndrome, the superior vena cava syndrome, or hoarseness (from involvement of the recurrent laryngeal nerve). Symptoms can also be related to local or distant metastases (Table 15-1) or paraneoplastic syndromes

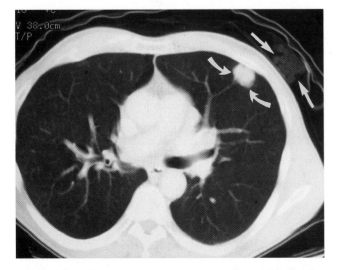

FIGURE 15-1. **Direct link between cigarette smoking and the development of bronchogenic carcinoma.** Note the package of cigarettes within the patient's shirt pocket (*straight arrows*) adjacent to the peripheral adenocarcinoma within the left upper lobe (*curved arrows*).

TABLE 15-1

COMMON EXTRATHORACIC SITES FOR METASTASES OF BRONCHOGENIC CARCINOMA

"LABB"
Liver
Adrenal
Bone
Brain

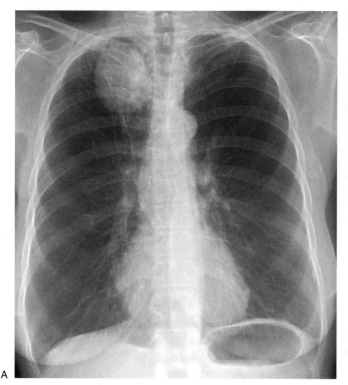
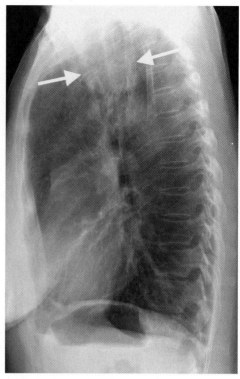

FIGURE 15-2. Poorly differentiated non–small cell lung cancer. A: Posteroanterior (PA) chest radiograph of a 68-year-old woman with emphysema shows a 6-cm mass in the right upper lobe. **B:** The mass is seen superiorly on the lateral view (*arrows*).

(systemic manifestations of the primary tumor unrelated to distant metastases). Paraneoplastic syndromes can cause cachexia of malignancy, digital clubbing and hypertrophic osteoarthropathy, nonbacterial thrombotic endocarditis, migratory thrombophlebitis, and various neurologic and cutaneous syndromes. Paraneoplastic syndromes may also be secondary to secretion of ectopic hormones by tumor cells, which can cause hypercalcemia, the syndrome of inappropriate secretion of antidiuretic hormone, Cushing syndrome from corticotropin secretion, gynecomastia, and acromegaly (4).

Histologic Classification

In 2004, the World Health Organization updated its classification of lung tumors based on histologic features (5). Four cell types account for more than 95% of all primary lung neoplasms: (i) adenocarcinoma (of which bronchioloalveolar carcinoma is a subset), (ii) squamous cell carcinoma, (iii) large cell carcinoma, and (iv) small cell carcinoma. Mixtures of these cell types may occur within the same primary neoplasm, and some tumors are too poorly differentiated to be further classified (Fig. 15-2). Rapid growth, early metastatic spread, and responsiveness to chemotherapy and radiation therapy distinguish small cell carcinoma from the others, which has led to the classification of "small cell" and "non–small cell" carcinoma. Features of the four histologic types are outlined in Table 15-2.

Adenocarcinoma

Adenocarcinoma accounts for 50% of all bronchogenic carcinomas (6), and it is the most common cell type seen in women and nonsmokers. There is a weak association with cigarette smoking and the development of adenocarcinoma. Microscopically, adenocarcinomas are characterized by the formation of glands and papillary structures. Adenocarcino-

mas can arise from pre-existent lung scars, or they can engulf pre-existing scars, giving rise to the term *scar carcinoma*. Like most bronchogenic carcinomas, adenocarcinomas occur most frequently in the upper lobes (Figs. 15-3 and 15-4). They are typically peripheral and subpleural in location, associated with

TABLE 15-2

CLINICAL AND RADIOLOGIC FEATURES OF THE FOUR HISTOLOGIC TYPES OF BRONCHOGENIC CARCINOMA

Non–small cell carcinoma
  Adenocarcinoma
    Most common type
    Weak association with cigarette smoking
    Usually peripheral in location
    Most common type to have air bronchograms
    Bronchioloalveolar carcinoma is a subtype
  Squamous cell carcinoma
    Second most common type
    Strong association with cigarette smoking
    Usually central in location
    Most common type to cavitate
  Large cell carcinoma
    Least common type
    Usually >3 cm in size
    Usually in lung periphery

Small cell carcinoma
  Strong association with cigarette smoking
  Usually central in location
  Often presents with bulky mediastinal adenopathy
  Worst prognosis of all types

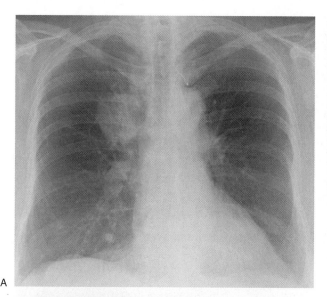

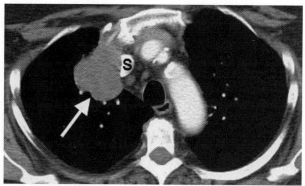

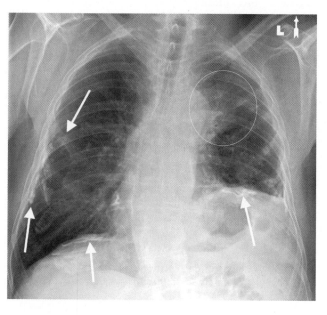

FIGURE 15-3. Adenocarcinoma. A: PA chest radiograph of a 75-year-old woman shows a mass in the right upper lobe abutting the mediastinum. **B:** CT shows the mass (*arrow*) compressing the superior vena cava (*S*). **C:** The mass (*arrow*) is seen on a shoulder radiograph obtained 3 months earlier. Incidental lung cancers can be detected on cervical spine and shoulder radiographs, and review of these studies should include a look at the visualized lungs.

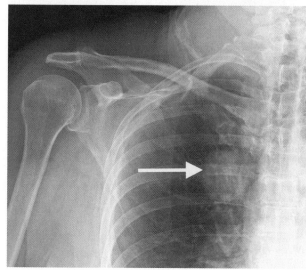

FIGURE 15-4. Adenocarcinoma. PA chest radiograph of a 73-year-old woman with hoarseness and shortness of breath shows calcified pleural plaques (*arrows*) and a poorly defined mass in the left upper lobe (*circle*). The pleural plaques are related to previous asbestos exposure. The hoarseness and elevation (paralysis) of the left hemidiaphragm are related to tumor involvement of the left recurrent laryngeal nerve and left phrenic nerve, respectively, in the aortopulmonary window.

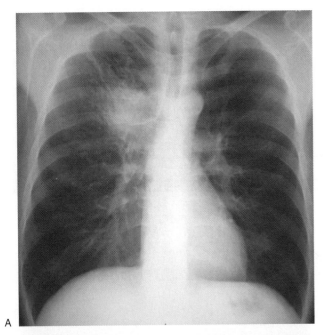

A

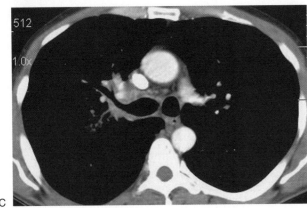

C

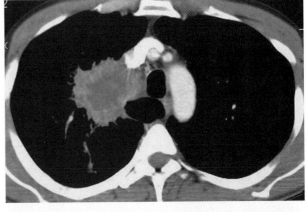

B

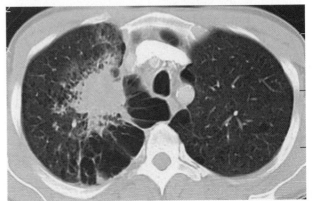

D

FIGURE 15-5. Adenocarcinoma. A: PA chest radiograph of a 48-year-old man shows an irregular mass in the right upper lobe abutting the mediastinum. **B:** CT shows the mass extending into the mediastinum. The center of the mass is of low attenuation, secondary to tumor necrosis. **C:** CT at a more inferior level shows tumor along the posterior wall of the right upper lobe bronchus. **D:** CT with lung windowing shows the spiculated mass and a background of paraseptal and centrilobular emphysema.

retraction of the adjacent pleura, but can also occur centrally (Fig. 15-5). On chest radiography, adenocarcinomas manifest as a solitary pulmonary nodule or mass that can have well-marginated, lobulated, irregular, or spiculated margins. Peripheral adenocarcinomas may directly invade the pleura and grow circumferentially around the lung, mimicking diffuse malignant mesothelioma, metastatic adenocarcinoma of nonlung primary, or malignant thymoma. On computed tomography (CT), adenocarcinomas often have air bronchograms (Fig. 15-6).

Bronchioloalveolar carcinoma (BAC) is a subtype of adenocarcinoma that has a "lepidic" pattern of growth, with cuboidal or columnar cells lining the walls of distal airspaces. The pulmonary interstitium serves as scaffolding for tumor growth. Neoplastic cells can detach from the primary tumor and attach to alveolar septa elsewhere in the lung, resulting in multifocal spread of tumor. The cells can produce abundant mucus, giving rise to "bronchorrhea," the expectoration of large amounts of mucus. The radiologic patterns of BAC are protean. The most common radiologic manifestation of BAC is a well-circumscribed peripheral solitary nodule or mass (7). Actual cavitation is uncommon, although "pseudocavitation" is a well-known feature. Air bronchograms are commonly seen (Figs. 15-6 and 15-7). The lepidic pattern of growth can look like airspace disease on chest radiography, an appearance similar to that of pneumonia (Fig. 15-8). Less common patterns

include multiple nodules or extensive alveolar lung disease involving one or more lobes.

Radiologically, peripheral adenocarcinomas produce a spectrum of ground-glass to solid opacities and can have varying degrees of BAC histology (Fig. 15-9). The greater the solid component, the greater the likelihood of an invasive growth component. A common appearance of adenocarcinoma with a BAC component is a nodule with a central solid component and peripheral ground-glass opacity, the so-called "fried egg" sign (Fig. 15-10). Kodama et al (8) have shown that the radiologic ground-glass component correlates with noninvasive growth (BAC) in pathology specimens. The strict definition of BAC requires that the tumor be composed entirely of a lepidic pattern of growth without evidence of interstitial or stromal invasion (5). In one series, small (<3.0-cm) solitary tumors that comprised an entirely lepidic growth pattern had a 5-year survival rate of 100% (9). BAC can be indolent, growing slowly over many months or years, and should always be considered when serial chest radiographs show chronic alveolar lung disease. It can recur in multiple areas of the lung after resection (Figs. 15-9 and 15-11).

Squamous Cell Carcinoma

Squamous cell carcinoma is the second most common type of bronchogenic carcinoma, and it is strongly associated with

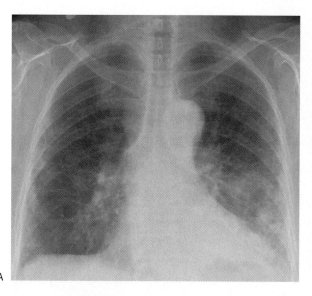

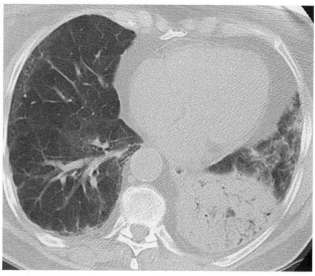

FIGURE 15-6. Adenocarcinoma with bronchioloalveolar carcinoma component. A: PA chest radiograph of a 73-year-old woman with chronic cough and symptoms of pneumonia for 3 months shows airspace disease in the left lower lung. **B:** CT shows numerous air bronchograms within the left lower lobe airspace opacity. The patient was treated with antibiotics for presumed lobar pneumonia before the diagnosis of cancer was made. Adenocarcinoma, particularly bronchioloalveolar carcinoma, should be considered when chest radiographs show chronic airspace disease.

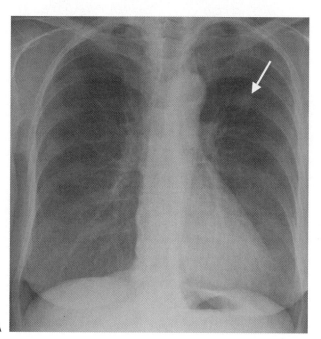

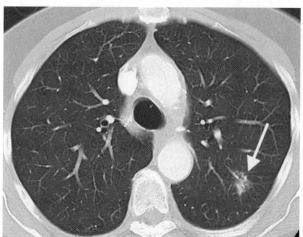

FIGURE 15-7. Bronchioloalveolar carcinoma. A: PA chest radiograph of a 79-year-old woman with a 50–pack-year history of cigarette smoking shows a subtle nodule superimposed on the shadow of the left sixth posterior rib (*arrow*). **B:** CT shows an ill-defined nodule (*arrow*) with air bronchograms in the posterior segment of the left upper lobe.

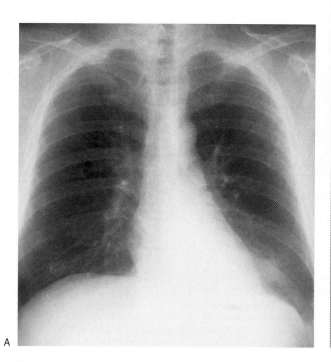

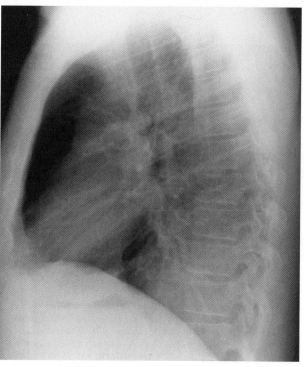

FIGURE 15-8. Bronchioloalveolar carcinoma. A: PA chest radiograph shows focal airspace disease in the left lower lobe, obscuring the medial left hemidiaphragm. B: Lateral view shows increased opacification over the lower thoracic spine (the so-called "spine sign"). The appearance is similar to that of left lower lobe pneumonia.

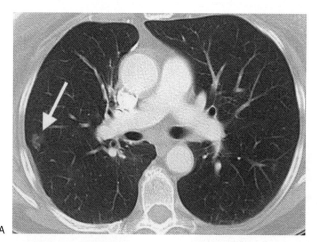

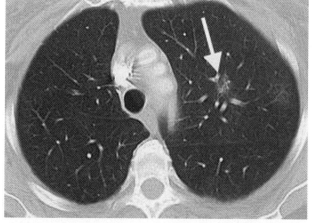

FIGURE 15-9. Bilateral bronchioloalveolar carcinomas. A: CT of a 71-year-old woman with a 30–pack-year history of cigarette smoking and resection of bronchioloalveolar carcinoma in the right upper lobe 4 years earlier shows a ground-glass nodule in the right lower lobe (arrow). B: CT at a more superior level shows a ground-glass nodule in the left upper lobe (arrow). Both nodules were proven to represent bronchioloalveolar cell carcinoma. Ground-glass nodules are very worrisome for bronchioloalveolar carcinoma, especially in a patient with a history of this type of cancer.

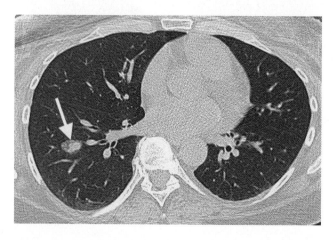

FIGURE 15-10. Bronchioloalveolar carcinoma. CT of a 52-year-old woman with an 11–pack-year history of cigarette smoking shows an incidental right lower lobe nodule (arrow). The nodule has a central dense component and a ground-glass peripheral component, giving rise to the "fried egg" appearance that is characteristic of bronchioloalveolar carcinoma. The patient underwent right lower lobectomy for a stage IA (T1N0M0) cancer.

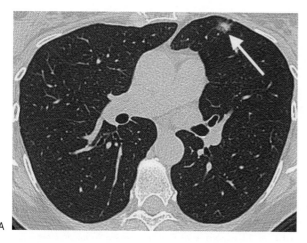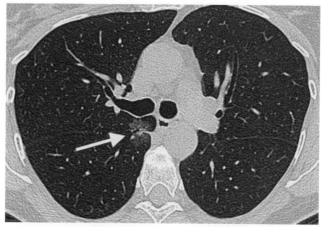

FIGURE 15-11. Recurrent bronchioloalveolar carcinoma. A: CT scan of a 59-year-old woman shows a nodule in the left upper lobe (*arrow*) with a "fried egg" appearance. The patient underwent lingulectomy to remove a stage IA bronchioloalveolar carcinoma. **B:** CT image obtained 2 years later shows a ground-glass nodule with an air bronchogram in the medial right lung (*arrow*). Wedge resection of the right upper lobe and superior segment of the right lower lobe confirmed recurrence of bronchioloalveolar carcinoma.

cigarette smoking. It is the most common type to cavitate and to be associated with hypercalcemia. Microscopically, squamous cell carcinoma is characterized by the presence of intercellular bridges, individual cell keratinization, and formation of keratin pearls. These tumors are most commonly central in location (within the main, lobar, or segmental bronchi), although approximately 25% are peripheral (Figs. 15-12 and 15-13). The typical radiologic manifestations of central squamous cell carcinomas are postobstructive pneumonia and atelectasis because of the total or partial bronchial obstruction produced by these central tumors (Fig. 15-14). The central tumor mass, adjacent to a displaced fissure from obstructive

atelectasis, gives rise to the radiographic Golden S sign (see Chapter 2).

Peripheral squamous cell carcinoma is the most common type of bronchogenic cancer to cause the Pancoast syndrome. In 1924, Henry Pancoast first described a clinical syndrome diagnostic of an apical lung tumor (10). This syndrome is characterized by pain or atrophy of muscles of the ipsilateral upper extremity, caused by involvement of the lower brachial plexus, and Horner syndrome, which results from involvement of the sympathetic chain and the stellate ganglion. Pancoast

(Text continues on page 252)

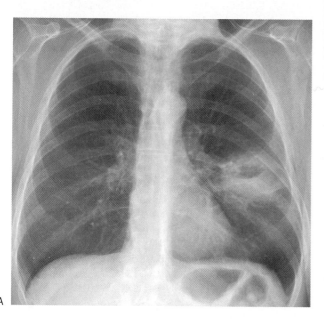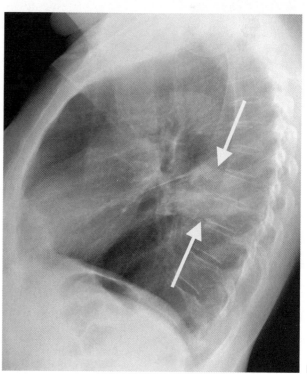

FIGURE 15-12. Squamous cell carcinoma. A: PA chest radiograph of a 62-year-old woman with left chest pain shows an ill-defined mass with central lucency in the left middle lung. **B:** Lateral view confirms that this mass is in the superior segment of the left lower lobe (*arrows*). (*Continued*)

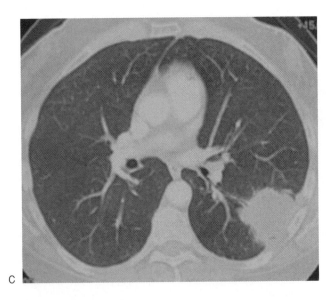

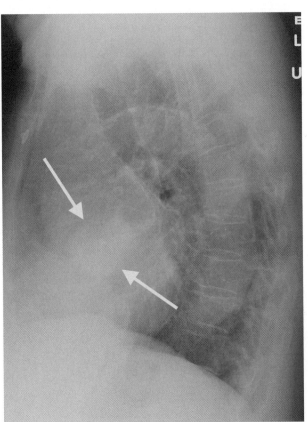

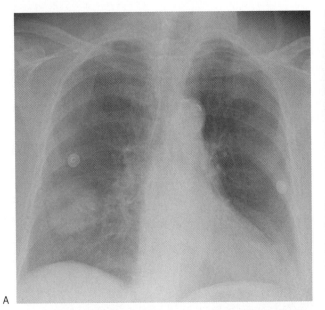

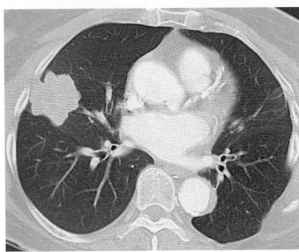

FIGURE 15-12. (*Continued*) C: CT shows a subpleural mass in the superior segment of the left lower lobe, lacking the cavitation that was suggested by the chest radiograph. Approximately 25% of squamous cell lung cancers are peripheral in location.

FIGURE 15-13. Squamous cell carcinoma. A: PA chest radiograph of an 82-year-old woman with a history of cigarette smoking shows a mass in the right lower lung. B: Lateral view shows that the mass is anterior (*arrows*) in the right middle lobe. C: CT shows a lobulated mass in the right middle lobe abutting the major fissure posteriorly.

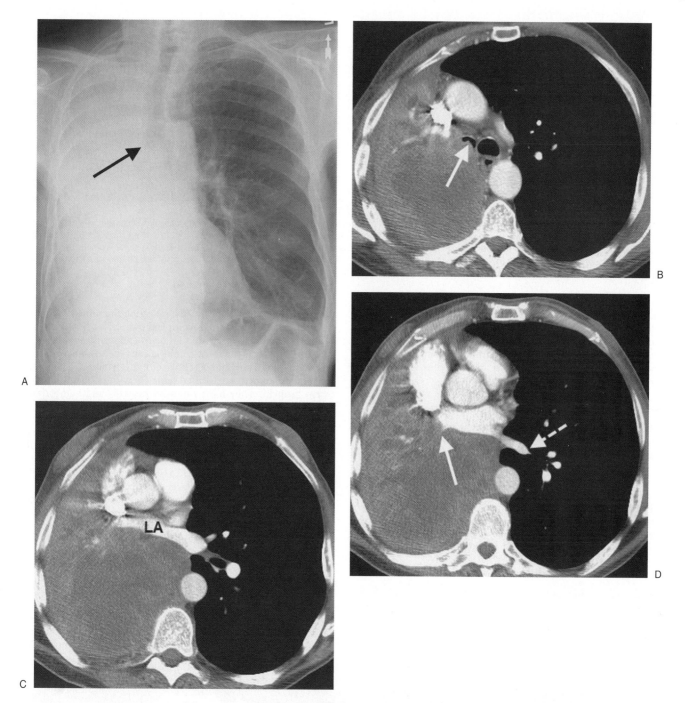

FIGURE 15-14. Squamous cell carcinoma. A: PA chest radiograph of a 63-year-old man with hemoptysis, cough, and dyspnea on exertion shows collapse of the right lung. The right main bronchus appears to be cut off (*arrow*). The right hemithorax is opaque and the mediastinum is shifted to the right. **B:** CT shows a mass that almost completely obliterates the lumen of the right main bronchus (*arrow*). The large, low-attenuation mass extends out into the right lung. **C:** CT at a more inferior level shows anterior compression of the left atrium (*LA*) by the mass. **D:** CT at a level inferior to (**C**) shows obliteration of the right inferior pulmonary vein by tumor (*solid arrow*). Note the normal left inferior pulmonary vein (*dashed arrow*). The appearance of a central tumor with postobstructive pneumonia and atelectasis secondary to total or partial bronchial obstruction is typical of squamous cell carcinoma.

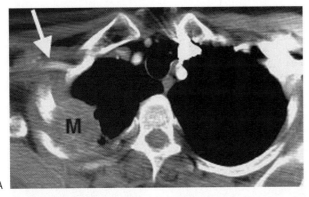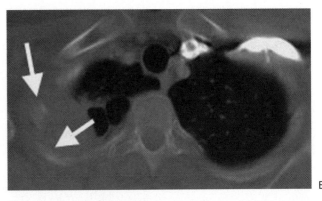

A   B

FIGURE 15-15. Pancoast tumor. A: CT of a 54-year-old man with pain in the right suprascapular area radiating down the medial right forearm, a 60–pack-year history of cigarette smoking, and previous exposure to asbestos shows a right apical mass (*M*) involving the right posterior chest wall and rib. The mass is in close proximity to the right axillary artery (*arrow*), which is suspicious for brachial plexus involvement by tumor. **B:** CT with bone windowing confirms rib involvement by tumor (*arrows*). The patient underwent induction chemotherapy and radiation, followed by right upper lobectomy. At surgery, the tumor was found to be invading the second through the fifth ribs.

tumors can manifest as apical masses or asymmetric apical pleural thickening (Fig. 15-15) and can be associated with bone destruction and soft tissue invasion. Magnetic resonance imaging (MRI) is superior to CT in determining whether there is tumor involvement of the chest wall, brachial plexus, subclavian artery, vertebral bodies, and spinal canal.

Large Cell Carcinoma

These tumors are the least common type of bronchogenic carcinoma. They grow rapidly, metastasize early, and are strongly associated with cigarette smoking. The histologic diagnosis is one of exclusion, given only to bronchogenic carcinomas that lack features of squamous, glandular, or small cell differentiation. Large cell carcinomas are appropriately named: they are usually bulky tumors greater than 3 cm in diameter. They are typically located in the lung periphery, but central lesions are not uncommon (Fig. 15-16). The typical radiologic appearance of these tumors is a large peripheral lung mass (11).

Small Cell Carcinoma

Small cell carcinoma is a rapidly growing neoplasm characterized by early and widespread metastases and by a strong association with cigarette smoking. Histologically, small cell carcinoma is characterized by small, uniform, oval cells with scant cytoplasm. Extensive crushing artifact is frequently seen in bronchial biopsy specimens, reflecting the tumor's scant tumor stroma and lack of desmoplastic reaction. Small cell carcinoma has been classified as a "neuroendocrine neoplasm" of the lung, and it is the most common cell type to cause a clinical hormone syndrome by secreting ectopic hormones. The majority of these tumors are located centrally within lobar and mainstem bronchi. They have extensive necrosis and hemorrhage, invade adjacent structures and lymph nodes, and disseminate along lymphatic routes.

The chest radiograph usually shows a hilar or perihilar mass associated with mediastinal widening; this can be caused by the primary tumor, metastases to hilar/mediastinal lymph nodes, or a combination of both (Fig. 15-17). The primary tumor may not be evident, and nodal enlargement may be the dominant abnormality. Rarely, small cell carcinoma may manifest as a solitary pulmonary nodule or mass (Fig. 15-18). CT usually shows extensive mediastinal lymph node involvement, with soft tissue "infiltration" of the mediastinum similar to that seen with lymphoma (Figs. 15-19 and 15-20). Small cell carcinoma is the most common primary lung cancer to cause superior vena cava obstruction, secondary to extrinsic vascular compression by the tumor, endoluminal thrombosis, or invasion (12). Surgical resection is considered in selected patients with small cell carcinoma only when the tumor manifests as a solitary pulmonary nodule in the absence of metastases. Most patients have disseminated disease at presentation and undergo chemotherapy

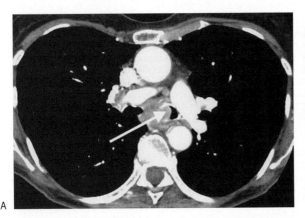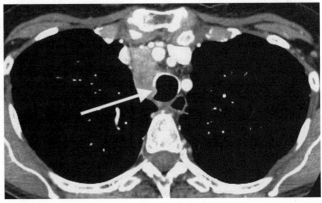

A   B

FIGURE 15-16. Large cell carcinoma. A: CT of an 80-year-old woman with dyspnea, wheezing, cough, fatigue, 12-pound weight loss, and no history of cigarette smoking shows a mass partially obstructing the left main bronchus (*arrow*). **B:** CT at a higher level shows mediastinal lymphadenopathy causing leftward displacement of the trachea (*arrow*).

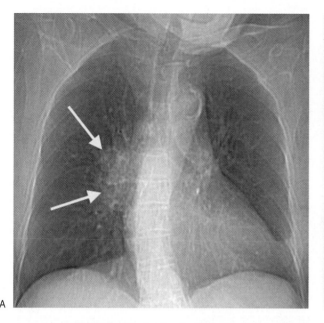
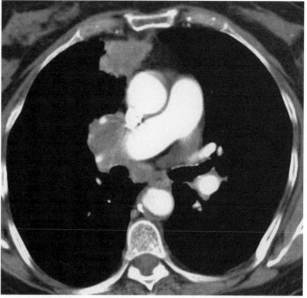

FIGURE 15-17. Small cell carcinoma. A: CT scout image of a 73-year-old woman with a 75–pack-year history of cigarette smoking shows a right hilar mass (*arrows*). **B:** CT shows tumor infiltrating the mediastinum.

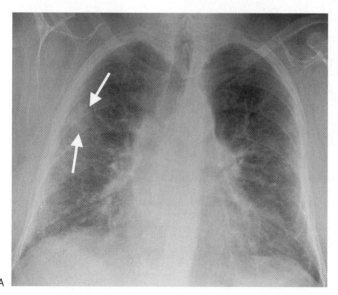
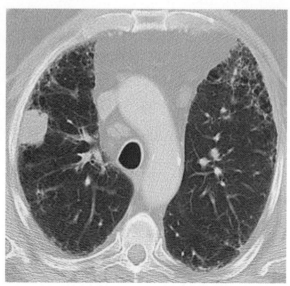

FIGURE 15-18. Small cell carcinoma. A: PA chest radiograph of a patient with pulmonary fibrosis, obtained as part of a workup for lung transplantation, shows a nodule (*arrows*) in the right lung. **B:** CT shows a subpleural nodule in the right lower lobe. Note bilateral subpleural reticular interstitial lung disease. Wedge resection confirmed a stage IB cancer. This is a known but uncommon appearance of small cell lung cancer, which usually presents with extensive lymph node involvement and widespread metastases.

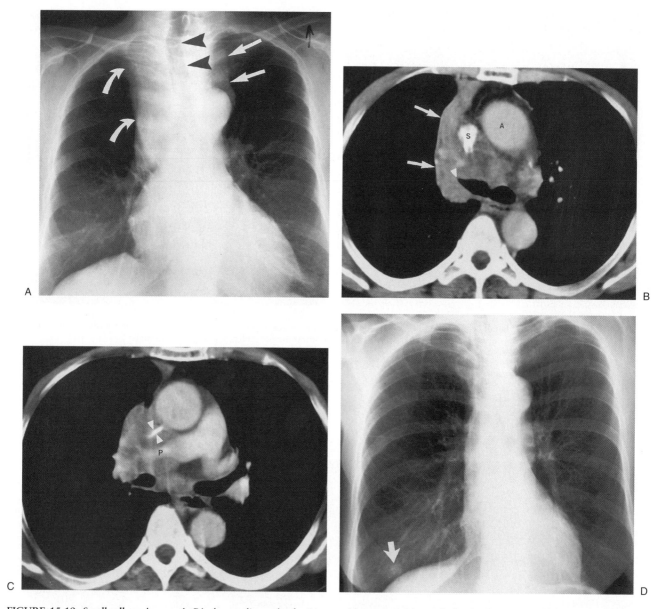

FIGURE 15-19. Small cell carcinoma. A: PA chest radiograph of a 56-year-old woman with weight loss and malaise shows widening of the left mediastinal contour (*straight arrows*), right hilar convexity, and collapse of the right upper lobe, with elevation of the minor fissure (*curved arrows*). The trachea is displaced to the right (*arrowheads*). **B:** CT shows abrupt tapering of the right upper lobe bronchus (*arrowhead*) and collapse of the right upper lobe against the mediastinum (*arrows*). The tumor infiltrates the mediastinum posterior to the ascending aorta (*A*) and superior vena cava (*S*). **C:** CT at a level inferior to (**B**) shows encasement and slitlike compression of the superior vena cava (*arrowheads*) and right pulmonary artery (*P*) by tumor. **D:** PA chest radiograph obtained 4 months later, after chemotherapy and radiation therapy, shows marked regression of tumor. A nipple shadow is incidentally projected over the right lung base (*arrow*).

and radiation therapy. The response to this treatment is usually dramatic, and the mass can disappear in a relatively short period of time, but most patients still die with rapidly recurrent small cell carcinoma (13).

Staging of Bronchogenic Carcinoma

Staging differs between small cell and non–small cell lung cancer. Small cell carcinoma is generally considered inoperable, except in rare cases of small, localized tumors. It is staged as limited or extensive, depending on whether disease is confined to a single radiation port (limited) (Fig. 15-21) or not (extensive) (Fig. 15-22). Patients with limited disease receive radia-

tion therapy and chemotherapy, whereas patients with extensive disease receive only chemotherapy.

The primary goal of staging non–small cell lung cancer is to determine resectability. Revisions to the stage grouping of the TNM (tumor-node-metastases) subsets (Table 15-3) in the International System for Staging Lung Cancer were adopted in 1997 (14). Refinements in the staging system were made to better evaluate treatment strategies for carefully staged groups of patients. Stage grouping involves the concept of combining subsets of patients classified according to TNM descriptors into categories or stages, with each having generally similar treatment options and survival expectations (Table 15-4).

Tumor classification is the most complicated component of the TNM system. Tumors that are classified as anything other

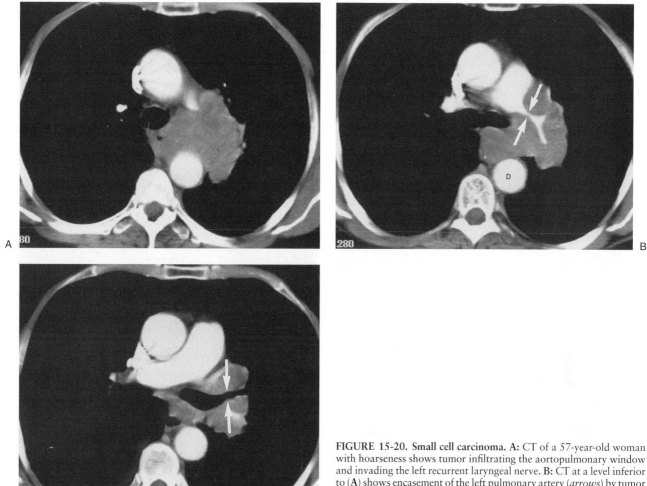

FIGURE 15-20. Small cell carcinoma. A: CT of a 57-year-old woman with hoarseness shows tumor infiltrating the aortopulmonary window and invading the left recurrent laryngeal nerve. B: CT at a level inferior to (A) shows encasement of the left pulmonary artery (*arrows*) by tumor and extension of tumor posterior to the carina, obliterating the fat plane adjacent to the descending aorta (*D*). C: CT at a level inferior to (B) shows encasement of the left upper lobe bronchus by tumor (*arrows*).

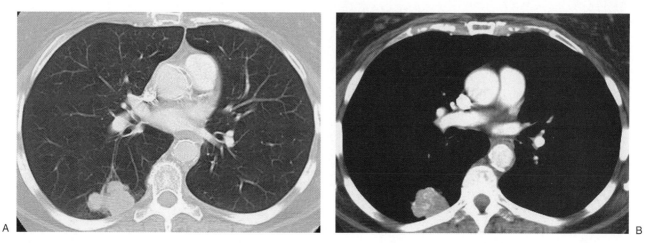

FIGURE 15-21. Small cell carcinoma, limited stage. A: CT of a 64-year-old woman shows a lobulated mass in the right lower lobe. B: CT with mediastinal windowing shows calcification or contrast enhancement within the mass. Mediastinal lymphadenopathy was present in the right paratracheal area (not shown). CT and positron emission tomography showed no evidence of extrathoracic tumor. The patient received radiation therapy and chemotherapy.

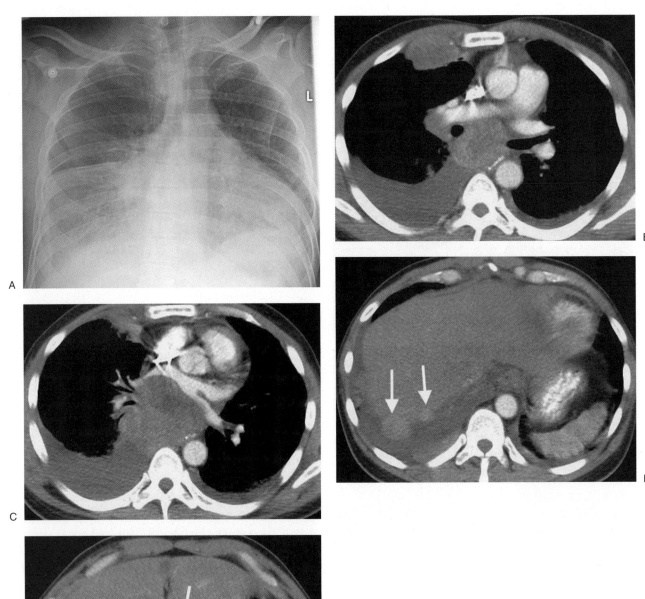

FIGURE 15-22. Small cell carcinoma, extensive. A: PA chest radiograph of a 47-year-old man with abdominal pain and vomiting shows enlargement of the cardiac silhouette, right pleural effusion, and abnormal opacities in the right paratracheal area, right hilum, and both lung bases. **B:** CT shows bilateral pleural effusions, bulky subcarinal lymphadenopathy, and a large pleural mass anteriorly. **C:** CT at a more inferior level shows anterior displacement of the left atrium by bulky tumor. **D:** CT at a level inferior to (C) shows numerous pleural tumor deposits (*arrows*). **E:** CT of the upper abdomen shows bulky celiac lymphadenopathy (*arrow*). The patient received chemotherapy.

TABLE 15-3

TNM DESCRIPTORS FOR STAGING BRONCHOGENIC CARCINOMA

Primary tumor (T)

TX Primary tumor cannot be assessed, or tumor proven, by the presence of malignant cells in sputum or bronchial washing but not visualized by imaging or bronchoscopy

T0 No evidence of primary tumor

Tis Carcinoma in situ

T1 Tumor ≤3 cm in greatest dimension, surrounded by lung or visceral pleura, without bronchoscopic evidence of invasion more proximal than the lobar bronchus[a] (i.e., not in the main bronchus)

T2 Tumor with any of the following features of size or extent:
   >3 cm in greatest dimension
   Involves main bronchus, ≥2 cm distal to the carina
   Invades the visceral pleura
   Associated with atelectasis or obstructive pneumonitis that extends to the hilar region but does not involve the entire lung

T3 Tumor of any size that directly invades any of the following: chest wall (including superior sulcus tumors), diaphragm, mediastinal pleura, parietal pericardium; or tumor in the main bronchus <2 cm distal to the carina, but without involvement of the carina or associated atelectasis or obstructive pneumonitis of the entire lung

T4 Tumor of any size that invades any of the following: mediastinum, heart, great vessels, trachea, esophagus, vertebral body, carina; or tumor with a malignant pleural or pericardial effusion[b] or with satellite tumor nodule(s) within the ipsilateral primary tumor lobe of the lung

Regional lymph nodes (N)

NX Regional lymph nodes cannot be assessed

N0 No regional lymph node metastasis

N1 Metastasis to ipsilateral peribronchial and/or ipsilateral hilar lymph nodes, and intrapulmonary nodes involved by direct extension of the primary tumor

N2 Metastasis to ipsilateral mediastinal and/or subcarinal lymph node(s)

N3 Metastasis to contralateral mediastinal, contralateral hilar, ipsilateral or contralateral scalene, or supraclavicular lymph node(s)

Distant metastasis (M)

MX Presence of distant metastasis cannot be assessed

M0 No distant metastasis

M1 Distant metastasis present[c]

TNM, tumor-node-metastases.

[a] The uncommon superficial tumor of any size with its invasive component limited to the bronchial wall, which may extend proximal to the main bronchus, is also classified T1.

[b] Most pleural effusions associated with lung cancer are caused by tumor. However, there are a few patients in whom multiple cytopathologic examinations of pleural fluid show no tumor. In these cases, the fluid is nonbloody and is not an exudate. When these elements and clinical judgment dictate that the effusion is not related to the tumor, the effusion should be excluded as a staging element and the patient's disease should be staged T1, T2, or T3. Pericardial effusion is classified according to the same rules.

[c] Separate metastatic tumor nodule(s) in the ipsilateral nonprimary tumor lobe(s) of the lung also are classified M1.

Reproduced with permission from Mountain CF. Revisions in the international system for staging lung cancer. *Chest.* 1997;111:1710–1717.

TABLE 15-4

STAGE GROUPING AND CORRESPONDING TNM SUBSETS

Stage	TNM subset	Stage	TNM subset
0	Carcinoma in situ	IIIB	T4N0M0
IA	T1N0M0		T4N1M0
IB	T2N0M0		T4N2M0
IIA	T1N1M0		T1N3M0
IIB	T2N1M0		T2N3M0
	T3N0M0		T3N3M0
IIIA	T3N1M0		T4N3M0
	T1N2M0	IV	Any T Any N M1
	T2N2M0		
	T3N2M0		

TNM, tumor-node-metastases.

Staging is not relevant for occult carcinoma, which is designated TXN0M0.

Reproduced with permission from Mountain CF. Revisions in the international system for staging lung cancer. *Chest.* 1997;111:1710–1717.

than T4 are potentially resectable. T4 tumors invade the mediastinum, heart, great vessels, trachea, esophagus, vertebral body, or carina; or they are associated with a malignant pleural or pericardial effusion or satellite tumor nodules within the ipsilateral primary tumor lobe of the lung. Satellite nodules outside the primary tumor lobe are considered M1 disease (Fig. 15-23). Most pleural effusions associated with lung cancer are malignant, but cytologic proof of malignancy cannot always be obtained. In these cases, the effusion should be excluded as a staging element.

Hilar node involvement is classified as N1. N2 nodes are ipsilateral mediastinal nodes, and N3 nodes are contralateral mediastinal or hilar nodes. N3 nodes also include any ipsilateral or contralateral scalene or supraclavicular lymph nodes. The distant metastases classification is simple. M0 indicates no distant metastases, and M1 is positive distant metastases.

The staging system is complicated and difficult to remember unless one routinely evaluates and stages lung cancer. Patients with T1N0M0 tumors (stage IA) have a significantly better outcome than patients in the other subsets (15,16) (Fig. 15-24). These patients have a tumor that is 3 cm or less in diameter, surrounded by lung or visceral pleura, without bronchoscopic evidence of invasion more proximal than the lobar bronchus, and without nodal involvement or metastases. In other words,

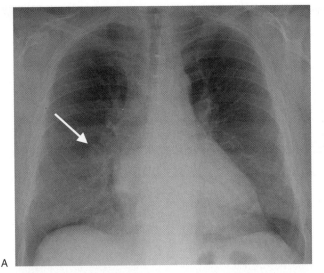

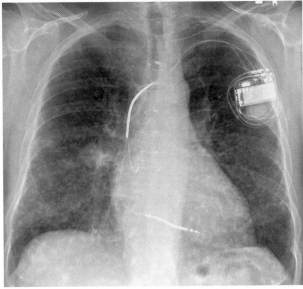

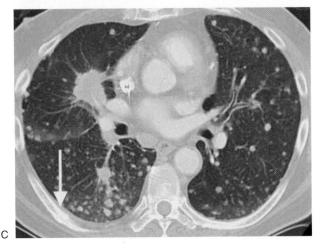

FIGURE 15-23. Adenocarcinoma. A: PA chest radiograph of a 65-year-old man with a 100–pack-year history of cigarette smoking shows a nodule in the right medial lung (*arrow*). B: PA chest radiograph obtained 1 year later shows widespread parenchymal metastases. C: CT shows numerous circumscribed pulmonary metastases involving both lungs. Note a pathologic rib fracture on the right (*arrow*). Other images showed metastases to both adrenal glands, multiple lytic bone lesions, and extensive mediastinal lymphadenopathy.

these are patients with a solitary pulmonary nodule and no spread of tumor. Stage IB tumors also have no nodal or distal metastases, but the primary tumor is either larger than 3 cm in diameter, involves the main bronchus, invades the visceral pleura, or is associated with atelectasis or obstructive pneu-

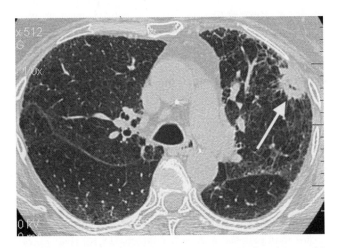

FIGURE 15-24. Adenocarcinoma, stage IA. CT of a 66-year-old woman with pulmonary fibrosis shows a small subpleural nodule (*arrow*) in the left upper lobe, with no evidence of lymphadenopathy or metastatic disease. Nodes removed at surgery were negative.

monitis. Sixty-one percent of patients with clinical stage IA disease and 38% of those with clinical stage IB tumors are expected to survive more than 5 years after treatment. IA and IB subsets have no evidence of lymph node or other metastases and therefore have the best prognosis.

Stage IIA, IIB, and IIIA tumors are potentially resectable, although the prognosis after treatment is poor, especially with IIIA tumors. Some surgeons opt not to resect IIIA tumors for this reason. IIIB staging involves either T4 tumors or N3 nodes, making such tumors unresectable. IIIB tumors are confined to the lung, however, which is an important consideration for radiotherapy. Stage IV tumors are defined by an M1 classification and are therefore unresectable and not confined to the lung. If treated, systemic therapy is required.

CT is commonly used for staging bronchogenic carcinoma prior to surgical resection. Patients with bulky N3 nodes are clearly not surgical candidates, and those patients without evidence of nodal involvement are considered surgical candidates (in the absence of T4 or M1 disease). CT is not perfect in detecting nodal involvement, however. In general, nodes greater than 1 cm in short-axis diameter are considered positive or suspicious, but many of these cases will turn out to be false-positive findings. In addition, nodes that are smaller than 1 cm or not visibly enlarged on CT can be positive histologically. Nodes can be sampled percutaneously, transbronchially, or via transcervical mediastinoscopy (requiring general anesthesia). The Chamberlain procedure involves an anterior thoracotomy, usually with removal of the second anterior rib to allow sampling of lymph nodes in the anterior mediastinum, the aorticopulmonary window, and the hilum. Other limitations of CT include the inability to determine mediastinal or chest wall invasion with certainty. MRI plays a role in evaluating these cases, as well as in evaluating for the presence of brachial plexus invasion.

Whole-body positron emission tomography (PET) imaging with [18]-fluoro-2-deoxy-D-glucose (FDG) has become an integral part of staging non–small cell lung cancer. PET improves the detection of nodal and distant metastases and frequently alters patient management (17). Integrated CT-PET scanners allow for the acquisition of coregistered, spatially matched functional and morphologic data. PET is sufficiently sensitive that a patient with negative mediastinal PET results may proceed directly to surgical resection of the primary tumor without a staging mediastinoscopy (18).

POSTPNEUMONECTOMY COMPLICATIONS

In the United States, the most common indication for pneumonectomy is non–small cell carcinoma of the lung. Most pneumonectomies performed for bronchogenic carcinoma follow an interpleural plane of resection (meaning the parietal pleura is left intact). If there is extension of tumor into the pleural space or parietal pleura, or in the case of malignant mesothelioma, an extrapleural pneumonectomy is generally performed. In this case, the plane of resection is between the parietal pleura and the endothoracic fascia (19).

After pneumonectomy, pleural fluid accumulates in the pneumonectomy space, replacing the normal immediate postoperative air that is resorbed at a variable rate. It is not uncommon for multiple air–fluid levels to be present within the early pneumonectomy space, representing loculation of fluid, and this finding on chest radiography does not necessarily suggest a complication. Most of the air is resorbed by 2 weeks after pneumonectomy; residual air may persist for months, however, or, in a small population of patients, it may never

TABLE 15-5
POSTPNEUMONECTOMY COMPLICATIONS

Early
  Bronchopleural fistula (stump leak)
  Empyema
  Hemothorax (blood within pneumonectomy space)[a]
  Chylothorax (chylous leak into pneumonectomy space)

Late
  Recurrent neoplasm
  Bronchopleural fistula
  Empyema
  Hemothorax
  Chylothorax

[a] There is no true pleural space after pneumonectomy, and the resulting space is referred to as the *pneumonectomy space*.

be completely resorbed. Eventually, the pneumonectomy space will contract, with ipsilateral shift of the mediastinum and elevation of the diaphragm, and the space will fill with fluid and some degree of solid fibrothorax. Shift of the mediastinum away from the operated side indicates a buildup of air or fluid within the pneumonectomy space. Mediastinal displacement away from the operative side suggests one of five diagnoses, depending on the length of time after surgery (Table 15-5). If the air–fluid level has not continued to rise after surgery, the cause of the contralateral mediastinal shift is likely a bronchial stump air leak. If the air–fluid level has continued to rise, the shift can be a result of hemothorax, chylothorax, or empyema, with or without a bronchopleural fistula. A drop in the air–fluid level indicates that fluid is draining through a chest tube, by thoracentesis, through a dehiscence of the incision, through an opening in the bronchial stump (Fig. 15-25), or through a rent in the diaphragm (19). After the postoperative period, shift

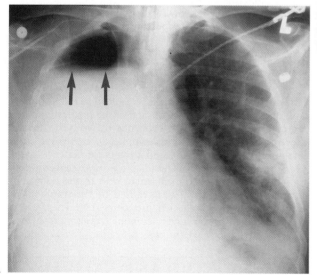
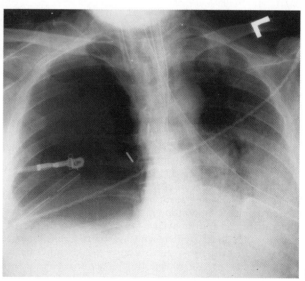

FIGURE 15-25. Postpneumonectomy bronchopleural fistula. A: AP upright chest radiograph of a 52-year-old man after right pneumonectomy shows shift of the mediastinum to the operative side and an air–fluid level within the right pneumonectomy space (*arrows*). There is "postpneumonectomy pulmonary edema" of the left lung. **B:** AP upright chest radiograph obtained 1 day later shows increased air within the right pneumonectomy space and shift of the mediastinum away from the operative side, consistent with a bronchial stump leak and bronchopleural fistula.

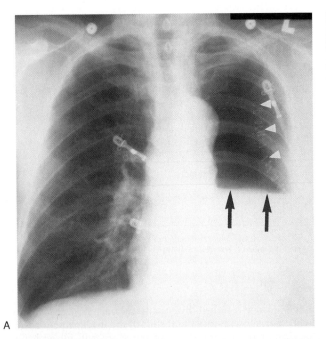

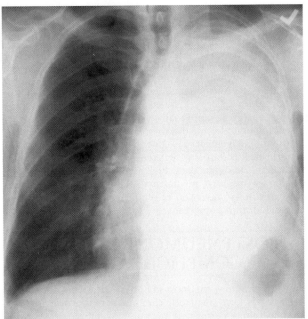

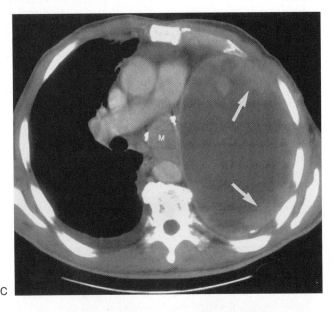

FIGURE 15-26. Recurrence of bronchogenic carcinoma after pneumonectomy. A: PA chest radiograph of a 65-year-old man after left pneumonectomy for bronchogenic carcinoma shows an air–fluid level in the left pneumonectomy space (*arrows*), left skin staples (*arrowheads*), and shift of the mediastinum toward the operative side. **B:** PA chest radiograph obtained 8 months later shows abnormal shift of the mediastinum away from the operative side, an appearance that is consistent with hemothorax, chylothorax, or recurrence of tumor with malignant fluid in the pneumonectomy space. Empyema is less of a consideration in the absence of air within the pneumonectomy space. **C:** CT shows a soft tissue mass (*M*) between the surgical clips and soft tissue deposits studding the surface of the pneumonectomy space (*arrows*). There is malignant fluid within the left pneumonectomy space.

of the mediastinum away from the operative side is also suspicious for recurrent tumor (Fig. 15-26), which can be recognized on CT as a soft tissue mass at the site of surgical ligation and soft tissue deposits studding the periphery of the pneumonectomy space. Recurrence can also be seen in the remaining lung (Fig. 15-27). PET scanning can be very helpful in evaluating for recurrence.

The mortality of pneumonectomy is approximately 6%, with the major causes of death being pneumonia, respiratory failure, pulmonary embolism, myocardial infarction, bronchopleural fistula, and empyema (20,21). The incidence of empyema is 2% to 5%, often with associated bronchopleural fistula (22). In the first postoperative week, empyema is caused by intraoperative soilage or preoperative pleural infection. Delayed onset of empyema is often associated with bronchopleural or esophagopleural fistula. New air within the pneumonectomy space, in a previously opacified hemithorax, with contralateral shift of the mediastinum, is suggestive of empyema or bronchopleural fistula and bronchial stump leak (Fig. 15-28).

A rare complication of right pneumonectomy is obstruction of the left main bronchus, a result of extreme rightward shift and counterclockwise rotation of the mediastinum, causing compression of the left bronchus between the aorta and the left pulmonary artery. This complication is termed the right pneumonectomy syndrome, and it can occur between 1 and 37 years after surgery (23). The diagnosis is suggested on chest radiography by marked mediastinal shift to the right and inversion of the left diaphragm, caused by the trapping of air from a narrowing of the left bronchus (19). There can also be recurrent left lower lobe pneumonia resulting from airway obstruction.

CARCINOID AND SALIVARY GLAND TUMORS

The term *bronchial adenoma* refers to a group of tumors that includes bronchial carcinoid (most common), mucoepidermoid carcinoma, and adenoid cystic carcinoma. This term, however,

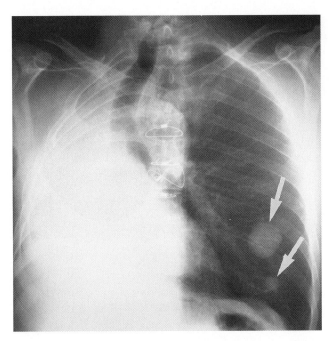

FIGURE 15-27. Metastases after pneumonectomy. PA chest radiograph of a 56-year-old man after right pneumonectomy for bronchogenic carcinoma shows pulmonary metastases within the left lower lobe (*arrows*). Note the normal shift of the mediastinum toward the operative side.

is not accurate, as *adenoma* implies a benign tumor, and many of these tumors are not benign. Additionally, *adeno-* implies glandular elements, which are sometimes lacking in these tumors. Carcinoid tumors have a different cell of origin, and adenoid cystic and mucoepidermoid carcinomas are classified

as salivary gland tumors. Because the term exists in the radiology literature and is still used by some clinicians, it is discussed in this chapter.

There are two forms of *bronchial carcinoid*: typical carcinoid and atypical carcinoid. Atypical carcinoid has cellular and clinical features that are intermediate, between those of typical carcinoid and small cell carcinoma of the lung (24). All three of these tumors are of neuroendocrine origin. Only 15% of typical carcinoids metastasize (25), and the prognosis following surgical resection is excellent. Approximately half of atypical carcinoids metastasize. Most typical bronchial carcinoids arise centrally in the main, lobar, or segmental bronchi and can cause cough and wheezing (symptoms resembling asthma). Recurrent bouts of postobstructive pneumonia are common. Because of their vascularity, bronchial carcinoids can present with hemoptysis (25). "Carcinoid syndrome" is rare with bronchial carcinoids unless liver metastases are present (26).

A bronchial carcinoid tumor can appear on chest radiography as a hilar mass, often with associated atelectasis or postobstructive pneumonia, but when entirely intraluminal it can be very difficult to detect. On CT, the tumor can be seen within a central bronchus, often causing widening of the bronchus (Fig. 15-29). Small tumors in segmental or subsegmental bronchi may result in a bronchocele (mucoid impaction) on chest radiography or CT, resembling bronchial atresia (Fig. 15-30). Approximately 10% to 20% of bronchial carcinoids appear on chest radiography as a solitary pulmonary nodule, usually well defined, round, oval, or lobulated, with occasional calcification (27) (Fig. 15-31). The incidence of calcification is significantly greater in centrally located and larger tumors. It can manifest as multiple nodular and curvilinear configurations, complete calcification, or even ossification of the entire nodule. Contrast enhancement can be marked on CT because of the vascularity of these tumors.

Adenoid cystic carcinoma is the most common salivary gland tumor in the thorax, followed by mucoepidermoid carcinoma. Mucoepidermoid carcinoma is more frequent in the

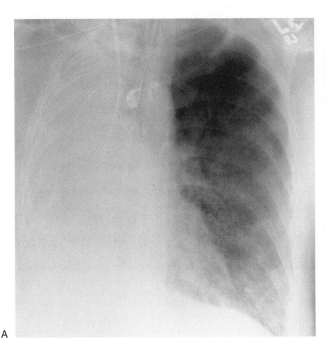
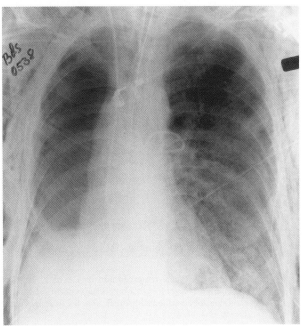

FIGURE 15-28. Bronchopleural fistula after pneumonectomy. A: AP chest radiograph after right pneumonectomy shows complete opacification of the right pneumonectomy space. The air within the pneumonectomy space has resorbed completely. The mediastinum is shifted toward the operative side. There is "postpneumonectomy pulmonary edema" of the left lung. B: AP chest radiograph taken 1 day later shows new air within the right pneumonectomy space, consistent with a bronchial stump leak and bronchopleural fistula. Note the subcutaneous air within the chest wall bilaterally.

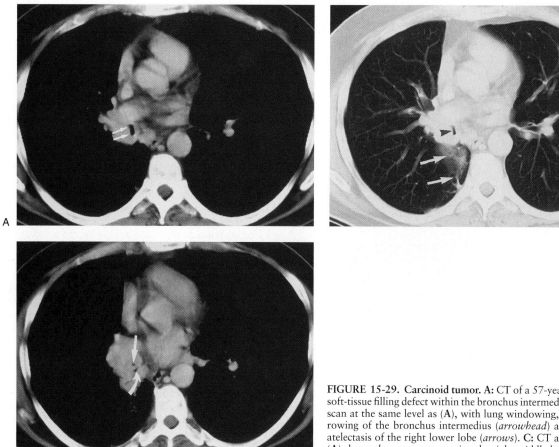

FIGURE 15-29. Carcinoid tumor. A: CT of a 57-year-old man shows a soft-tissue filling defect within the bronchus intermedius (*arrows*). **B:** CT scan at the same level as (**A**), with lung windowing, shows slitlike narrowing of the bronchus intermedius (*arrowhead*) and postobstructive atelectasis of the right lower lobe (*arrows*). **C:** CT at a level inferior to (**A**) shows the mass compressing the right middle lobe (*straight arrow*) and right lower lobe (*curved arrow*) bronchi.

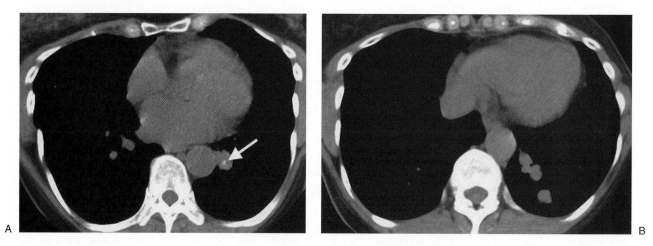

FIGURE 15-30. Carcinoid tumor. A: CT of a 58-year-old woman shows a mass with central calcification in the proximal left lower lobe bronchus (*arrow*). **B:** CT at a more inferior level shows low-attenuation material within the left lower lobe segmental bronchi. Small carcinoid tumors in segmental bronchi may result in mucoid impaction, as shown in this case.

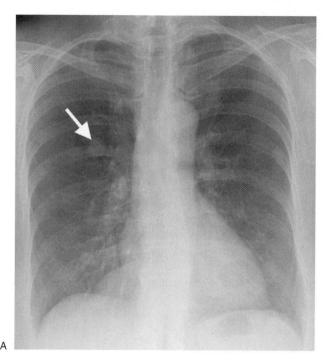

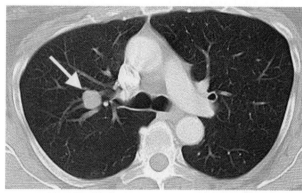

A   B

FIGURE 15-31. Carcinoid tumor. A: PA chest radiograph of a 66-year-old woman shows a solitary pulmonary nodule in the right upper lung (*arrow*). B: CT shows the nodule in the right upper lobe (*arrow*), lateral to the proximal right upper lobe bronchus.

major bronchi than in the trachea, and adenoid cystic carcinomas most commonly involve the posterior wall of the lower two thirds of the trachea (Fig. 13-6). Both are seen on imaging studies as an intraluminal nodule, either polypoid in shape or circumferential. CT can show the extraluminal component, but it is poor at indicating whether mediastinal structures, such as the esophagus and aorta, are invaded (28).

References

1. Stanley K, Stjernsward J. Lung cancer: a world-wide health problem. *Chest.* 1989;96(suppl):1S–5S.
2. Aronchick JM. Lung cancer: epidemiology and risk factors. *Semin Roentgenol.* 1990;25:5–11.
3. Garfinkel L, Silverberg E. Lung cancer and smoking trends in the United States over the past 25 years. *CA Cancer J Clin.* 1991;41:137–145.
4. Boyers MC. Clinical manifestations of carcinoma of the lung. *J Thorac Imaging.* 1991;7:21–28.
5. Travis WD, Muller-Hermelink H-K, Harris CC, et al. *Pathology and Genetics of Tumours of the Lung, Pleura, Thymus and Heart.* Lyon: IARC Press; 2004.
6. Martini N. Operable lung cancer. *CA Cancer J Clin.* 1993;43:201–214.
7. Epstein DM. Bronchioloalveolar carcinoma. *Semin Roentgenol.* 1990;25:105–111.
8. Kodama K, Higashiyama M, Yokouchi H, et al. Prognostic value of ground-glass opacity found in small lung adenocarcinoma on high-resolution CT scanning. *Lung Cancer.* 2001;33(1):17–25.
9. Noguchi M, Morikawa A, Kawasaki M, et al. Small adenocarcinomas of the lung: histologic characteristics and prognosis. *Cancer.* 1995;75(12):2844–2852.
10. Pancoast HK. Importance of careful roentgen ray investigation of apical chest tumors. *JAMA.* 1924;83:1407–1411.
11. Rosado-de-Christenson ML, Templeton PA, Moran CA. Bronchogenic carcinoma: radiologic-pathologic correlation. *Radiographics.* 1994;14:429–446.
12. Müller NL, Miller RR. Neuroendocrine carcinomas of the lung. *Semin Roentgenol.* 1990;25:96–104.
13. Hinson JA Jr, Perry MC. Small cell lung cancer. *CA Cancer J Clin.* 1993;43:216–225.
14. Mountain CF. Revisions in the international system for staging lung cancer. *Chest.* 1997;111:1710–1717.
15. Harpole DH Jr, Herndon JE II, Wolfe WG, et al. A prognostic model of recurrence and death in stage I non-small cell lung cancer utilizing presentation, histopathology and oncoprotein expression. *Cancer Res.* 1995;55:51–56.
16. Prestidge BR, Cox RS, Johnson DW. Non-small cell lung cancer: treatment results at a USAF referral center. *Mil Med.* 1991;156:479–483.
17. Verhagen AF, Bootsma GP, Tjan-Heijnen VC, et al. FDG-PET staging lung cancer: how does it change the algorithm? *Lung Cancer.* 2004;44:175–181.
18. Marom EM, McAdams HP, Erasmus JJ, et al. Staging non-small cell lung cancer with whole-body PET. *Radiology.* 1999;212:803–809.
19. Spirn PW, Gross GW, Wechsler RJ, et al. Radiology of the chest after thoracic surgery. *Semin Roentgenol.* 1988;23:9–31.
20. Harmon H, Fergus S, Cole F. Pneumonectomy: review of 351 cases. *Ann Surg.* 1976;183:719–722.
21. Nagasaki F, Flehinger BJ, Martini N. Complications of surgery in the treatment of carcinoma of the lung. *Chest.* 1982;82:25–29.
22. Shields TW. Pulmonary resections. In: Shields TW, ed. *General Thoracic Surgery.* Philadelphia: Lea & Febiger; 1983:315–330.
23. Shepard JO, Grillo HC, McLoud TC, et al. Right-pneumonectomy syndrome: radiologic findings and CT correlation. *Radiology.* 1986;161:661–664.
24. Choplin RH, Rawamoto EH, Dyer RB, et al. Atypical carcinoid of the lung: radiographic features. *AJR Am J Roentgenol.* 1986;146:665–668.
25. McCaughan BC, Martini N, Bains MS. Bronchial carcinoids: review of 124 cases. *J Thorac Cardiovasc Surg.* 1985;89:8–17.
26. Ricci C, Patrassi N, Massa R. Carcinoid syndrome in bronchial adenoma. *Am J Surg.* 1973;126:671–677.
27. Lawson RM, Ramanathan L, Hurley G, et al. Bronchial adenoma: review of 18-year experience at the Brompton Hospital. *Thorax.* 1976;31:245–252.
28. Spizarny DL, Shepard JAO, McLoud TC, et al. CT of adenoid cystic carcinoma of the trachea. *AJR Am J Roentgenol.* 1986;146:1129–1132.

CONGENITAL LUNG DISEASE

The most common major anomalies of pulmonary development (Table 16-1) span a continuum of maldevelopment involving the pulmonary parenchyma, the pulmonary vessels, or a combination of both (1). At one end of the spectrum, congenital lobar emphysema represents abnormal lung supplied by normal vessels, and at the other end, pulmonary arteriovenous malformation (AVM) consists of abnormal vessels within normal lung parenchyma. Some patients with congenital lung anomalies have mixed features, making exact categorization of the anomaly difficult.

CONGENITAL LOBAR EMPHYSEMA

Congenital lobar emphysema (CLE) is a disorder affecting neonates and young infants and is usually associated with acute or subacute respiratory distress. It may occasionally present as an incidental finding in adults. Various bronchial and alveolar abnormalities can cause this disorder, and in some cases the cause is unknown. The most commonly detected abnormality is absence or hypoplasia of cartilage rings of major and branch bronchi, with resultant bronchial collapse during exhalation. This results in inhalational air entry but collapse of the narrow bronchial lumen during exhalation. The bronchial obstruction leads to progressive hyperinflation and air trapping (Fig. 16-1), usually involving only one pulmonary lobe. The left upper lobe is most commonly involved, followed by the right middle and right upper lobes. CLE has two forms: hypoalveolar (fewer than expected number of alveoli) and polyalveolar (greater than expected number of alveoli). The pulmonary vasculature, although frequently attenuated, is usually normal in structure and distribution. Common chest radiographic findings include a hyperlucent lobe, compressive atelectasis of adjacent parenchyma, and contralateral mediastinal shift (1). In some cases, a subtle hyperlucent lobe may be all that is seen. Computed tomography (CT) best characterizes this abnormality and typically shows a hyperlucent, hyperexpanded lobe;

TABLE 16-1

MAJOR ANOMALIES OF PULMONARY DEVELOPMENT

Congenital lobar emphysema
Bronchogenic cyst
Congenital cystic adenomatoid malformation
Bronchopulmonary sequestration
Pulmonary venolobar syndrome (also called hypogenetic lung syndrome or scimitar syndrome)
Pulmonary arteriovenous malformation
Bronchial atresia

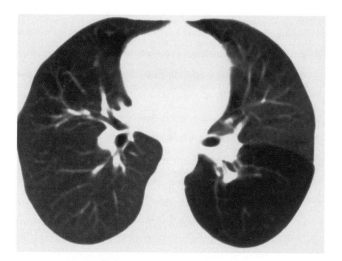

FIGURE 16-1. Congenital lobar emphysema. CT of a 30-year-old asymptomatic woman shows abnormal lucency and diminutive vasculature in the superior segment of the left lower lobe. There was no evidence of endobronchial lesion on CT or bronchoscopy, and the appearance of the left lower lobe was unchanged for 3 years on follow-up CT scans.

attenuated but intact pattern of vascularity; compression of the adjacent lung; and contralateral mediastinal shift.

BRONCHOGENIC CYST

Bronchogenic cysts result from abnormal growth of the lung bud and can be either mediastinal or intrapulmonary. Both types are lined with ciliated columnar epithelium and contain serous or mucous material. No clear-cut predilection for an intrapulmonary or a mediastinal location has been demonstrated. An intrapulmonary bronchogenic cyst often communicates with the bronchial tree, which can result in air–fluid levels and recurrent infections that may damage the cyst wall. Chest radiographs show a nonspecific oval or round, well-circumscribed mass, often as an incidental finding. The most common mediastinal location is subcarinal (Figs. 6-29 to 6-31). CT scans show the mass to have a thin or nearly imperceptible wall and to contain fluid, often of water attenuation. Occasionally, the fluid has a higher attenuation than water because of the presence of proteinaceous material or calcium (see also Chapter 6). The contents of the cyst do not enhance after administration of intravenous contrast material.

CONGENITAL CYSTIC ADENOMATOID MALFORMATION

Congenital cystic adenomatoid malformation (CCAM) is a hamartomatous abnormality of the lung consisting of a multicystic mass of pulmonary tissue in which there is proliferation of bronchial structures at the expense of alveolar development. Three types have been described. Type 1, the most common type, consists of single or multiple large cysts (up to 10 cm in diameter). Type 2 consists of multiple small cysts (1 to 2 cm in diameter), and type 3 (solid form) is a large, noncystic lesion. The prognosis worsens from type 1 to type 3, in part because of associated anomalies that occur with greater frequency with types 2 and 3.

The radiographic appearance varies, depending on the type of lesion. The most common presentation is that of a mass of numerous air-containing cysts that expand the ipsilateral hemithorax and shift the mediastinum to the contralateral side.

Occasionally, one cyst preferentially expands, creating a single large lucent area that is similar in appearance to congenital lobar emphysema. Type 3 lesions present as large homogeneous masses, without cystic spaces. Although most cases of CCAM present in the first month of life, the diagnosis is occasionally delayed until adulthood (2). Adult patients commonly present with persistent or recurrent pneumonia. Chest CT in adults with CCAM shows cystic lesions of variable size, most commonly in a lower lobe, which can mimic cystic bronchiectasis, intralobar pulmonary sequestration, intrapulmonary bronchogenic cyst, or prior infection with pneumatocele formation (3).

BRONCHOPULMONARY SEQUESTRATION

Bronchopulmonary sequestration consists of nonfunctioning lung tissue, usually cystic and often masslike, that has an anomalous systemic blood supply, usually from the aorta, and no normal communication with the tracheobronchial tree. This disorder is classified into two types: intralobar (the more common type) and extralobar (4). Both types occur most commonly in the posterior basal segment of a lower lobe, usually on the left. Intralobar sequestration is contiguous with normal lung parenchyma, has no separate pleural investment, receives arterial supply most commonly from the aorta, has venous drainage most commonly into a pulmonary vein, and is only rarely associated with other anomalies (Figs. 16-2 and 16-3). Extralobar sequestration is related to a hemidiaphragm (usually the left), and it is often situated between the inferior surface of the lower lobe and the diaphragm, or below the diaphragm. It has a pleural investment separate from the rest of the lung; receives arterial supply from the aorta but usually has venous drainage into the systemic venous system (e.g., inferior vena cava, azygos vein, or portal vein); and is often associated with other congenital anomalies (most commonly eventration or paralysis of the ipsilateral diaphragm and left diaphragmatic hernia) (Fig. 16-4). The classic radiographic appearance of pulmonary sequestration is recurrent or persistent abnormal opacity in a lower lobe that never completely clears. The diagnosis can be confirmed by showing the systemic arterial supply, either with magnetic resonance imaging or CT angiography (5). In adults, this disorder is often discovered incidentally.

(Text continues on page 268)

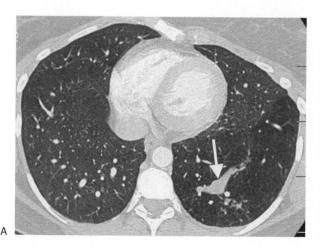
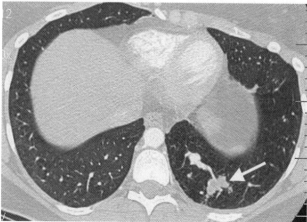

FIGURE 16-2. Intralobar sequestration. A: CT of a 37-year-old woman with chest pain shows a prominent tubular structure in the left lower lobe (*arrow*). The surrounding lung, also part of the sequestration, is hyperlucent. **B:** CT at a more inferior level shows the tubular structure leading to a lobulated mass (*arrow*) in the left lower lobe. (*Continued*)

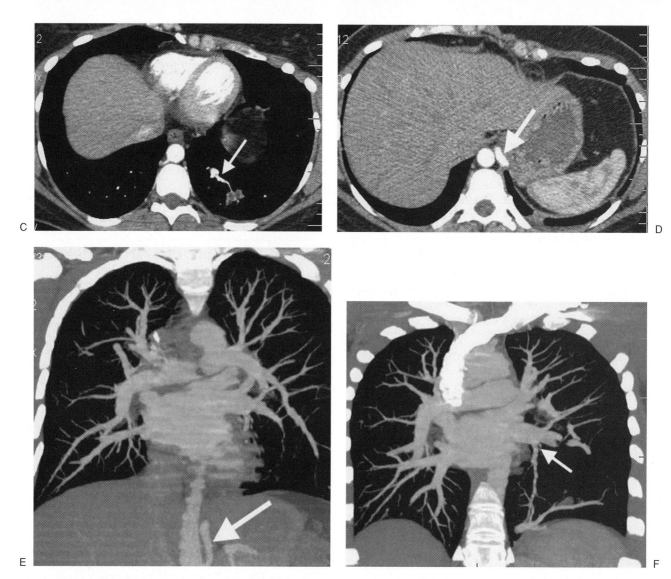

FIGURE 16-2. (*Continued*) **C:** CT with mediastinal windowing shows the tubular structure be a vessel (*arrow*). **D:** CT of the upper abdomen shows a prominent vessel (*arrow*) arising from the abdominal aorta and heading toward the left lower lobe. **E:** Coronal reformatted CT confirms that a vessel arises from the abdominal aorta (*arrow*) and heads superiorly toward the left lower lobe. **F:** Paddlewheel reformatted CT shows drainage from the left lower lobe mass to the left inferior pulmonary vein (*arrow*).

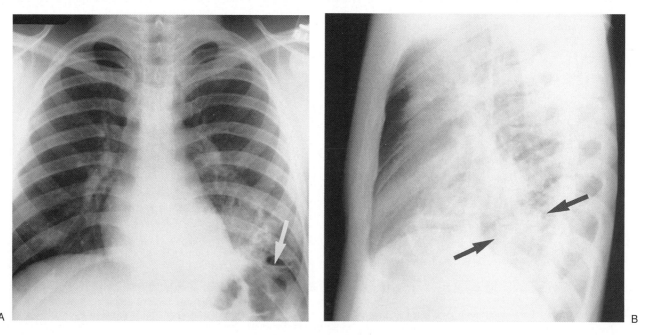

FIGURE 16-3. Intralobar sequestration. A: Posteroanterior (PA) chest radiograph of a 20-year-old man with recurrent left lower lobe pneumonia shows abnormal opacification of the left lower lobe, with obliteration of the left hemidiaphragm shadow, and an air–fluid level (*arrow*). **B:** Lateral view shows left lower lobe opacification involving the posterior segment (*arrows*). (*Continued*)

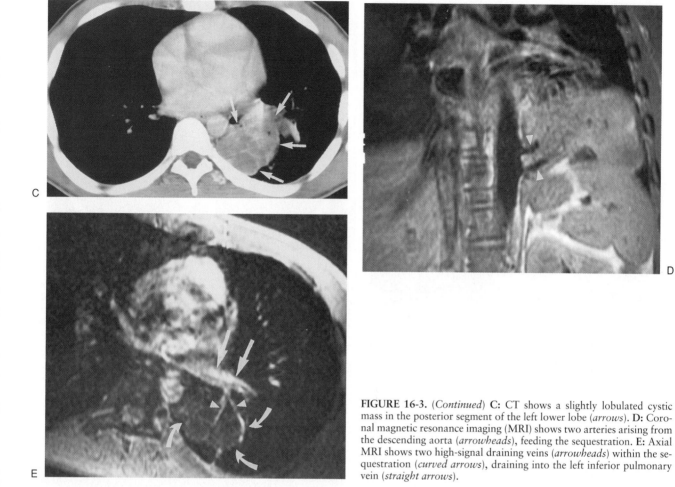

FIGURE 16-3. (*Continued*) **C:** CT shows a slightly lobulated cystic mass in the posterior segment of the left lower lobe (*arrows*). **D:** Coronal magnetic resonance imaging (MRI) shows two arteries arising from the descending aorta (*arrowheads*), feeding the sequestration. **E:** Axial MRI shows two high-signal draining veins (*arrowheads*) within the sequestration (*curved arrows*), draining into the left inferior pulmonary vein (*straight arrows*).

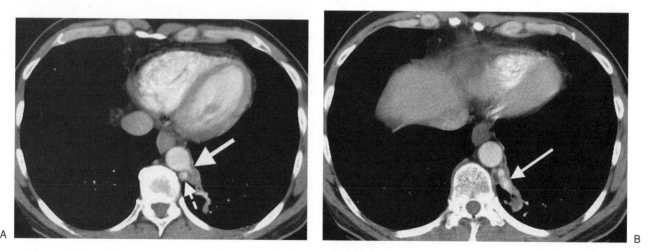

FIGURE 16-4. Extralobar sequestration. A: CT of a 56-year-old man with persistent abnormal opacity in the left lower lobe on chest radiography shows a vascular structure arising from the descending aorta (*solid arrow*) and directed toward a mass in the left lower lobe. The hemiazygos vein is prominent (*dashed arrow*). **B:** CT at a more inferior level shows a large vein arising from the left lower lobe mass and draining into the hemiazygos vein (*arrow*). (*Continued*)

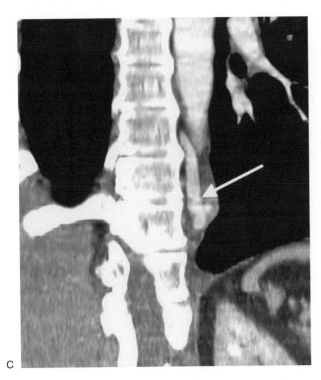

C

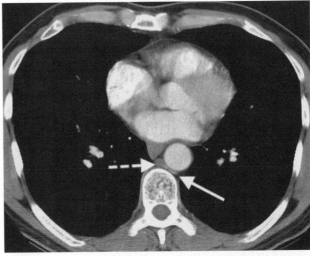

D

FIGURE 16-4. (*Continued*) C: Coronal reformatted CT shows a prominent hemiazygos vein (*arrow*). D: CT at the level of the left atrium shows the hemiazygos vein (*solid arrow*) crossing the midline posterior to the descending aorta to join the azygos vein (*dashed arrow*). Surgical resection of the left lower lobe sequestration confirmed the arterial supply and venous drainage.

PULMONARY VENOLOBAR SYNDROME

Also referred to as the scimitar syndrome or hypogenetic lung syndrome, pulmonary venolobar syndrome is a form of partial anomalous pulmonary venous return that is accompanied by ipsilateral lung hypoplasia. The anomalous venous return is commonly to the inferior vena cava (Fig. 16-5). The hypoplastic lung (which is almost always right sided) is supplied partly or completely by systemic arteries. The ipsilateral pulmonary artery is diminutive. Associated cardiovascular anomalies are frequent, the most common being atrial septal defect (6). Other associated anomalies include pulmonary sequestration, absence of the inferior vena cava, and accessory diaphragm. Less commonly, the syndrome may involve tracheal trifurcation, eventration and partial absence of the diaphragm, phrenic cyst, horseshoe lung, anomalous superior vena cava, and absence of the left pericardium (7). Bronchial anomalies are common, particularly isomerism (identical right and left branching patterns). The anomalous vein is usually visible on frontal chest radiographs as a broad, gently curved shadow descending to the diaphragm just to the right of the heart (Figs. 16-6 and 16-7). The shadow is shaped like a Turkish sword (a scimitar); thus, the designation *scimitar syndrome*. Other radiographic findings include a small ipsilateral hemithorax with diminished pulmonary vascularity, shift of the mediastinum toward the involved side, and, often, indistinctness of the cardiomediastinal border on the involved side. The lateral radiograph usually

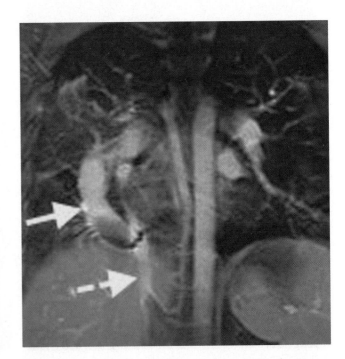

FIGURE 16-5. Pulmonary venolobar syndrome. MRI of a 24-year-old man shows a large venous structure (*solid arrow*) draining into the abdominal inferior vena cava (*dashed arrow*).

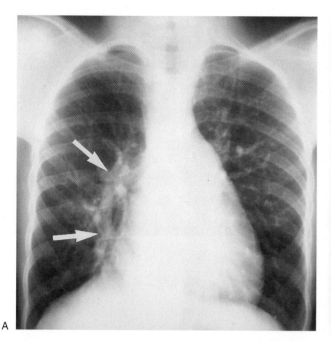
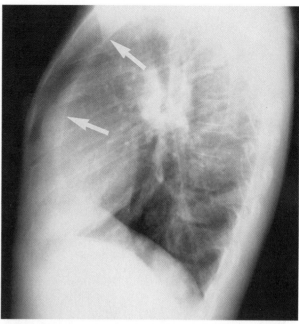

FIGURE 16-6. Pulmonary venolobar syndrome. A: PA chest radiograph of an 11-year-old girl shows a curvilinear band of opacification (*arrows*) adjacent to the right heart border, representing an anomalous pulmonary vein draining into the inferior vena cava. The vein is shaped like a Turkish sword, giving rise to the name "scimitar syndrome," another term used to describe this entity. Hypoplasia of the right lung is not clearly seen on this view. **B:** Lateral view shows a retrosternal band of opacification (*arrows*), created by shortening of the anteroposterior diameter of the right lung, and contact of the anterior right lung with a rotated and shifted mediastinum.

shows a retrosternal band of opacification, which is secondary to the shortening of the anteroposterior diameter of the involved lung, and contact of the anterior involved lung with a rotated and shifted mediastinum (8). Anomalous pulmonary venous return can also be an isolated finding, unassociated with other anomalies (Fig. 16-8).

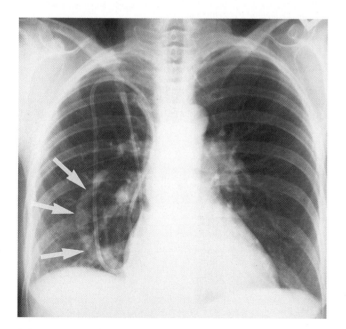

FIGURE 16-7. Pulmonary venolobar syndrome. PA chest radiograph of a 56-year-old woman shows the anomalous draining vein (scimitar; *arrows*), diminutive right pulmonary artery, and relatively small right lung.

PULMONARY ARTERIOVENOUS MALFORMATION

A pulmonary AVM or congenital arteriovenous fistula is an abnormal vascular communication between a pulmonary artery and a pulmonary vein. The etiology is thought to be defective development of the terminal capillary loops, resulting in the formation of thin-walled, dilated vascular spaces, usually supplied by one distended artery and drained by one distended vein. Pulmonary AVMs are multiple in 33% to 50% of patients and are bilateral in 8% to 20% (1). Approximately 60% of pulmonary AVMs occur in patients with Rendu-Osler-Weber disease (also known as hereditary hemorrhagic telangiectasia; see also Chapter 7). Chest radiographs and CT scans show round or oval, well-defined nodules, which can be lobulated, ranging in size from less than 1 cm to several centimeters in diameter, with prominent feeding and draining vessels (see Figs. 7-32 and 7-33). Although typically incidental findings in adults, AVMs can cause physiologic right-to-left shunting if large, which can result in paradoxical septic emboli.

BRONCHIAL ATRESIA

Bronchial atresia is an uncommon focal obliteration of the proximal portion of a segmental bronchus. It occurs most commonly in the left upper lobe, followed by the left lower lobe and the right middle lobe (9). It is thought to be related to a vascular insult early in development. Mucoid impaction in the airway distal to the obliterated portion is usually seen radiologically as an ovoid, round, or branching tubular structure. The distal lung, aerated by collateral air drift, is typically hyperlucent and hyperinflated and has decreased vascular markings. Bronchial

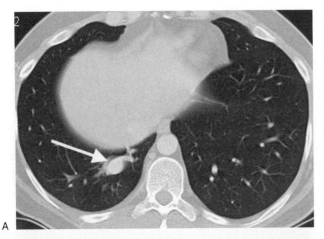

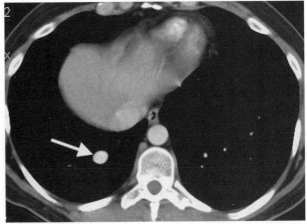

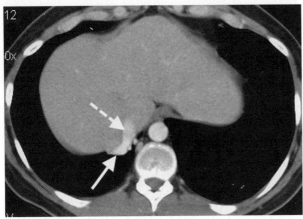

FIGURE 16-8. Anomalous pulmonary venous return. A: CT shows a large tubular structure in the right lower lobe (*arrow*). **B:** CT with mediastinal windowing shows enhancement of the structure (*arrow*), confirming its vascular nature. **C:** CT at a level inferior to (**B**) shows the vascular structure (*solid arrow*) draining into the inferior vena cava (*dashed arrow*).

atresia is often discovered incidentally. Bronchoscopy is usually required to exclude an endobronchial neoplasm.

References

1. Panicek DM, Heitzman ER, Randall PA, et al. The continuum of pulmonary development anomalies. *Radiographics.* 1987;7:747–772.
2. Avitabile AM, Greco MA, Hulnick DH, et al. Congenital cystic adenomatoid malformation of the lung in adults. *Am J Surg Pathol.* 1984;8:193–202.
3. Patz EF Jr, Müller NL, Swensen SJ, et al. Congenital cystic adenomatoid malformation in adults: CT findings. *J Comput Assist Tomogr.* 1995;19:361–364.
4. Savic B, Birtel FJ, Tholen W, et al. Lung sequestration: report of seven cases and review of 540 published cases. *Thorax.* 1979;34:96–101.
5. Mata JM, Caceres J, Lucaya J, et al. CT of congenital malformations of the lung. *Radiographics.* 1990;10:651–674.
6. Kiely B, Filler J, Stone S, et al. Syndrome of anomalous venous drainage of the right lung to the inferior vena cava. A review of 67 reported cases and three new cases in children. *Am J Cardiol.* 1967;20:102–115.
7. Woodring JH, Howard TA, Kanga JF. Congenital pulmonary venolobar syndrome revisited. *Radiographics.* 1994;14:349–369.
8. Ang JGP, Proto V. CT demonstration of congenital pulmonary venolobar syndrome. *J Comput Assist Tomogr.* 1984;8:753–757.
9. Kinsella D, Sissons G, Williams MP. The radiological imaging of bronchial atresia. *Br J Radiol.* 1992;65:681–685.

CHAPTER 17

PULMONARY VASCULATURE DISEASE

LEARNING OBJECTIVES

1. Recognize central and subsegmental pulmonary emboli on chest computed tomography (CT).
2. Define the role of ventilation-perfusion scintigraphy, CT pulmonary angiography, chest magnetic resonance imaging/magnetic resonance angiography, CT venography, and lower-extremity venous ultrasound studies in the evaluation of a patient with suspected venous thromboembolic disease, including the advantages and limitations of each modality depending on patient presentation.
3. Recognize enlarged pulmonary arteries on a chest radiograph and distinguish them from enlarged hilar lymph nodes.
4. Recognize enlargement of the central pulmonary arteries with diminution of the peripheral pulmonary arteries on a chest radiograph and suggest the diagnosis of pulmonary arterial hypertension.
5. Name several causes of precapillary and postcapillary pulmonary arterial hypertension.

Pulmonary vascular disease is a relatively common cause of chest pain and dyspnea. It can be acute, as in pulmonary embolism (PE), or chronic, as in most cases of pulmonary arterial hypertension (PAH). This chapter will review these two conditions and pulmonary artery tumors. Pulmonary arteriovenous malformations are discussed in Chapter 16.

PULMONARY THROMBOEMBOLIC DISEASE

PE is the third most common acute cardiovascular disease, after myocardial infarction and stroke (1). However, there is considerable uncertainty and confusion with regard to accurate diagnosis of this condition. The clinical signs and symptoms associated with PE are nonspecific, as are laboratory investigations, electrocardiograms, and chest radiographs. When PE occurs without infarction, the chest radiograph may be normal, or it may show any or all of the following: oligemia of the affected lung (the Westermark sign; see Fig. 2-21), increase in the size of the main pulmonary artery, elevation of the diaphragm, pleural effusion (usually small and unilateral), or discoid atelectasis. The chest radiograph is usually abnormal in patients with PE, however, with nonspecific subsegmental atelectasis being the most common abnormal finding (2). No chest radiographic sign is specific for pulmonary embolism or infarction, and the sensitivity of chest radiography for these conditions is poor. Even with a large pulmonary artery clot burden, the chest radiograph can be normal (3). The main role of the chest radiograph, therefore, is to exclude other diagnoses that might mimic PE clinically, such as pneumonia or pneumothorax. Because PE often goes undetected, the diagnosis of PE should be considered in any patient who presents with acute shortness of breath and pleuritic chest pain.

Deep venous thrombosis (DVT) originates most commonly in lower-extremity or pelvic veins, where they dislodge and propagate cranially into the pulmonary arterial tree. Radiologic studies used to diagnose thromboembolic disease include chest radiography, ventilation-perfusion (V/Q) scans, computed tomographic pulmonary angiography (CTPA), mag-netic resonance imaging/magnetic resonance angiography (MRI/MRA), CT venography (CTV), MR venography, and lower-extremity ultrasound. Once the gold standard for diagnosing PE, catheter-based pulmonary angiography has largely been replaced by CTPA and is now used mainly when the results of CTPA and V/Q scanning are indeterminate and there is continued high clinical suspicion of PE. The ideal test to diagnose PE should be accurate, direct (objective), rapid, safe, readily available, and of reasonable cost. Because only approximately 30% of patients with clinically suspected PE have the disease (4), a diagnostic test that is able to provide information regarding the presence and significance of other chest disease would also be desirable. None of the common tests in use (other than CTPA) meet all or even most of these criteria. V/Q scintigraphy was the main imaging modality used in the evaluation of patients with suspected PE until the advent of multidetector CT scanning. A high-probability V/Q scan provides sufficient certainty to confirm the diagnosis of PE, while a normal or near normal scan reliably excludes the diagnosis. However, in the Prospective Investigation of Pulmonary Embolism Diagnosis (PIOPED) study (4), indeterminate scans, which were present in 364 (39%) of 931 patients, showed a 30% incidence of PE, and low-probability scans (i.e., two thirds of V/Q scans in the PIOPED study) were not useful in establishing or excluding PE. In many institutions, CTPA has become the test of choice rather than V/Q scintigraphy or catheter-based pulmonary angiography. A suggested diagnostic algorithm for the evaluation of suspected PE is described in Table 17-1.

Recent studies have found the sensitivity of thin-section multidetector CTPA to be 96% to 100% and the specificity to be 89% to 98% for the detection of pulmonary emboli to the level of the subsegmental arteries (5,6). Characteristic findings of acute PE are: (a) partial central filling defect surrounded by a thin rim of contrast material, or (b) complete filling defect with obstruction of an entire vessel section ("vessel cutoff sign") (Figs. 17-1 to 17-5). Pulmonary arteries that are completely obstructed by an acute embolus usually have an increased diameter (Figs. 17-6 and 17-7). Arteries peripheral to a central thrombus may or may not opacify. Central clot does not necessarily completely obstruct the distal flow of contrast. Although nonocclusive clot is depicted by CTPA, false-negative

TABLE 17-1

DIAGNOSTIC ALGORITHM FOR THE EVALUATION OF SUSPECTED PULMONARY EMBOLISM

1. All patients should have a chest radiograph, the main role of which is to exclude abnormalities, such as acute pneumonia, that may mimic pulmonary embolism clinically.
2. Patients with symptoms or signs of DVT should undergo evaluation of the leg veins with Doppler ultrasound. If Doppler ultrasound is positive, the patient can be considered to have acute pulmonary embolism and usually does not require further investigation.
3. Patients who have no symptoms or signs of DVT and symptomatic patients who have a negative Doppler ultrasound examination, and who do not have extensive underlying parenchymal lung disease or COPD, should undergo V/Q scintigraphy.* A high-probability or normal V/Q scan can be considered diagnostic. All other patients should undergo further evaluation with CTPA.
4. Patients who have extensive pulmonary parenchymal disease or COPD and patients who have a nondiagnostic V/Q scan should undergo CTPA.
5. Patients in whom the CTPA scans are suboptimal and patients in whom the CTPA results are negative, but who have a high clinical index of suspicion for acute pulmonary embolism, should undergo catheter-based pulmonary angiography.

DVT, deep venous thrombosis; COPD, chronic obstructive pulmonary disease; V/Q, ventilation-perfusion; CTPA, computed tomographic pulmonary angiography.
*At many institutions, V/Q scanning has been largely eliminated from the diagnostic algorithm, with patients going directly to CTPA instead. In addition, more and more diagnostic algorithms begin with a D-dimer assay.

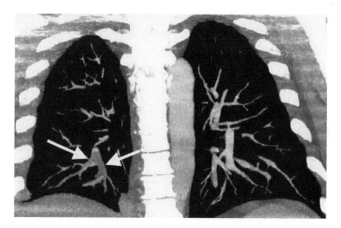

FIGURE 17-2. Acute PE. Coronal CTPA of a 43-year-old man with acute shortness of breath shows extensive intraluminal filling defect within the right lower lobe pulmonary arteries (*arrows*).

scintigraphy in this setting is well known. Acute embolic obstruction of a large degree of the pulmonary circulation increases pulmonary vascular resistance, leading to acute PAH. CTPA findings suggesting this complication include right ventricular enlargement (right ventricle/left ventricle ratio >1) and straightening or leftward bowing of the interventricular septum (Fig. 17-8). Pitfalls to be aware of in diagnosing PE include lymph nodes; impacted bronchi (Figs. 17-9 and 17-10); respiratory motion; vessel bifurcation; unopacified pulmonary veins (Fig. 17-11); periarterial abnormalities (lymph node enlargement or infiltration of the axial interstitium by edema fluid, inflammation, or neoplasm); pulmonary artery catheters; and pulmonary artery sarcoma (7).

CTPA findings diagnostic of *chronic* PE include mural thrombus (adherent to the arterial wall), which may or may not be calcified (Fig. 17-12); webs; stenosis or strictures of the arteries (Fig. 17-13); and a central "dot" of contrast surrounded by circumferential thrombus, which is indicative of recanalization. Ancillary findings include mosaic perfusion with decreased caliber of vessels in the hypoattenuated areas of lung (Fig. 17-14), enlarged pulmonary arteries and right ventricle (Figs. 17-15 and 17-16), and enlarged bronchial arteries (Figs. 17-3 and 17-17). CTPA, like conventional angiography, usually enables distinction between acute and chronic PE; this is not possible with scintigraphy.

The clinical significance of small emboli is unclear, but data suggest that small, untreated clots in patients without impaired cardiopulmonary reserve may not be associated with poor outcome (8). Several investigations have found that the negative predictive value of CTPA ≥97% (9), suggesting that anticoagulants can be safely withheld when CTPA is normal and of good diagnostic quality. In patients without concomitant cardiopulmonary disease, no difference in the incidence of recurrent PE between treated and untreated patients with small clots has been noted (10). However, in patients with limited cardiopulmonary reserve, such small emboli may be fatal. Isolated subsegmental clot on single-detector CT is very unusual, and the risk of anticoagulation may exceed the risk of morbidity and mortality from the suspected clot in this setting (11).

Major advantages of CTPA over V/Q scintigraphy to investigate patients suspected of acute PE include (a) direct visualization of emboli on CTPA; (b) evaluation of the lung parenchyma and mediastinum, which may provide an alternate diagnosis; and (c) capability of acquiring a CTV study without

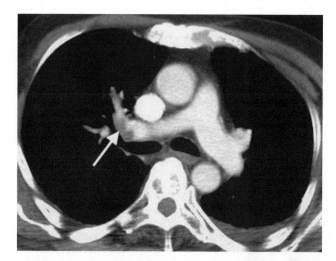

FIGURE 17-1. Incidental PE on CT. CT of a 70-year-old man with colon cancer shows intraluminal filling defect (*arrow*) in the right upper lobe pulmonary artery. The study was performed to assess for metastatic disease. Acute emboli are occasionally detected incidentally on routine CT; such findings illustrate the importance of evaluating the pulmonary arteries on all CT studies.

(Text continues on page 280)

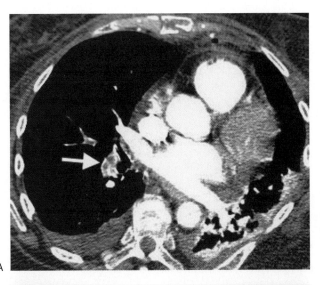

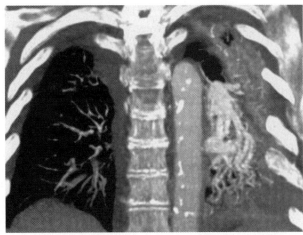

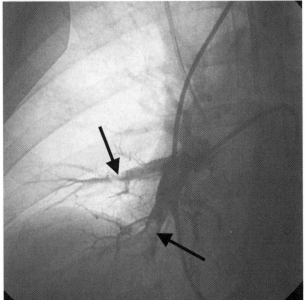

FIGURE 17-3. Acute PE. A: CTPA of a 77-year-old man with shortness of breath shows an intraluminal filling defect, surrounded by a rim of contrast, within the right lower lobe segmental pulmonary arteries (*arrow*). B: Coronal CTPA shows decreased caliber of arteries in the right lung compared with the left and filling defect within right lower lobe vessels. C: Catheter-based pulmonary angiogram confirms clot within right lower lobe vessels (*arrows*).

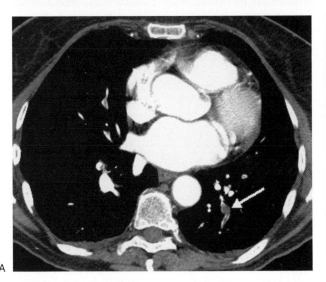

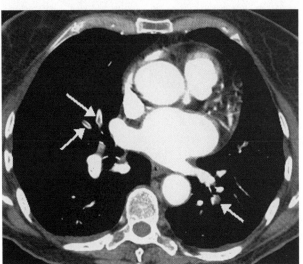

FIGURE 17-4. Acute PE. A: CTPA of a 77-year-old woman with a gastrointestinal bleed and DVT shows an intraluminal filling defect in a left lower lobe segmental pulmonary artery (*arrow*). B: CTPA at a more superior level shows intraluminal filling defects, surrounded by contrast material, in the right middle lobe and left lower lobe pulmonary arteries (*arrows*). (*Continued*)

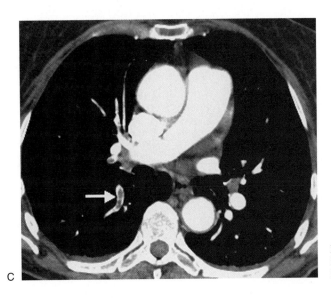

C

FIGURE 17-4. (*Continued*) **C:** CTPA at a level superior to (**B**) shows an intraluminal filling defect, surrounded by a thin rim of contrast material, in a right lower lobe segmental pulmonary artery (*arrow*).

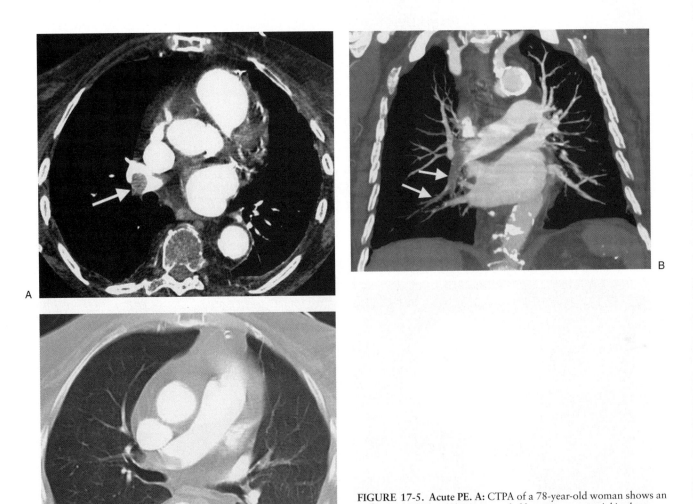

A

B

C

FIGURE 17-5. Acute PE. A: CTPA of a 78-year-old woman shows an intraluminal filling defect surrounded by contrast material in the proximal right lower lobe pulmonary artery (*arrow*). **B:** Coronal CTPA shows that the intraluminal filling defect extends from the proximal right lower lobe pulmonary artery inferiorly to distal branches (*arrows*). **C:** CTPA with lung windowing shows oligemia and diminution of vessels on the right (Westermark sign).

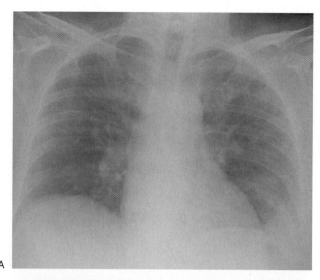

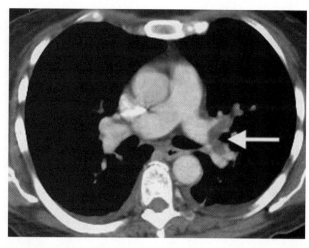

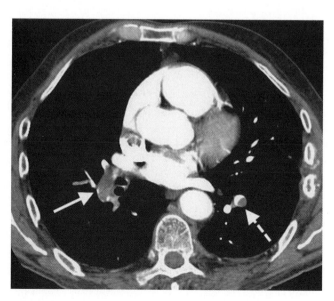

FIGURE 17-6. Acute PE. A: Posteroanterior (PA) chest radiograph of a 52-year-old woman with cholangiocarcinoma shows a rounded opacity at the left costophrenic angle, representing a Hampton hump of pulmonary infarction. B: CTPA shows a saddle embolus bridging the lingular and left lower lobe pulmonary arteries (*arrow*). C: CTPA at a more inferior level shows intraluminal filling defects expanding the proximal lower lobe pulmonary arteries (*arrows*).

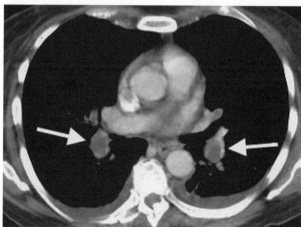

FIGURE 17-7. Acute PE. CTPA of a 76-year-old man with acute shortness of breath shows a large intraluminal filling defect within the proximal right lower lobe pulmonary artery (*solid arrow*) and a smaller intraluminal filling defect within a segmental pulmonary artery to the left lower lobe (*dashed arrow*).

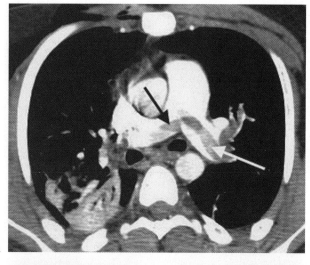

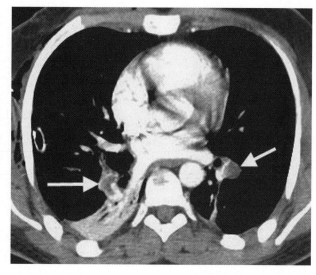

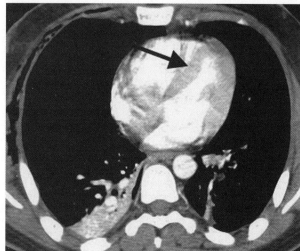

FIGURE 17-8. Acute PE associated with pulmonary arterial hypertension. A: CTPA of a 23-year-old man involved in a motor vehicle crash shows a saddle embolus straddling the right and left main pulmonary arteries (arrows). The central pulmonary arteries are enlarged. B: CTPA at a more inferior level shows thrombus within segmental branches of the lower lobe pulmonary arteries (arrows). C: CTPA at a level inferior to (B) shows leftward bowing of the interventricular septum (arrow).

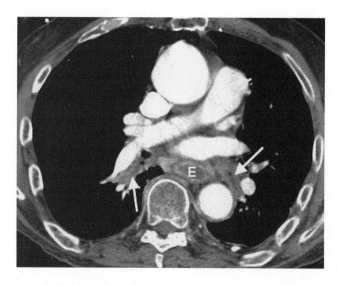

FIGURE 17-9. Mucous plugging. CTPA of a 75-year-old man with an esophageal stricture and gastroesophageal reflux shows a dilated esophagus (E) and low-attenuation material within the lower lobe segmental bronchi (arrows). The adjacent pulmonary vessels enhance normally.

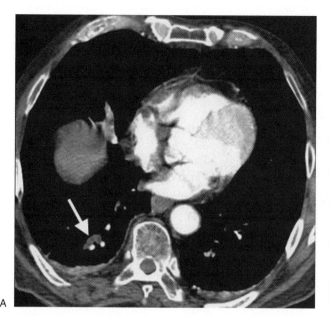

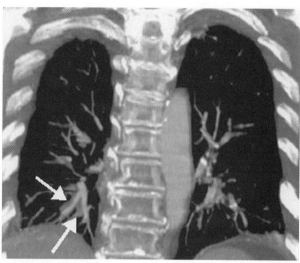

A   B

FIGURE 17-10. Mucous plugging. A: CTPA shows low-attenuation material occluding the right lower lobe subsegmental bronchi (*arrow*). The adjacent pulmonary vessels enhance normally. **B:** Coronal CT shows the impacted right lower lobe bronchi (*arrows*) adjacent to normally enhancing pulmonary vessels.

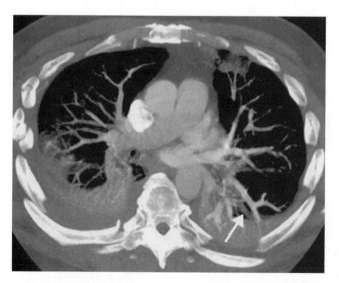

FIGURE 17-11. Pulmonary vein. CTPA shows a nonenhancing pulmonary vein in the left lower lobe (*arrow*). This should not be confused with a pulmonary artery. Pulmonary veins can be traced back to the left atrium on serial images.

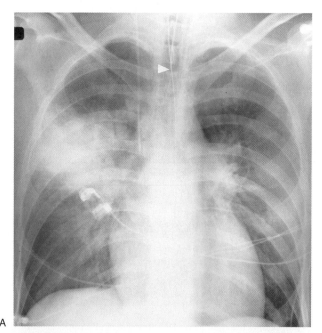

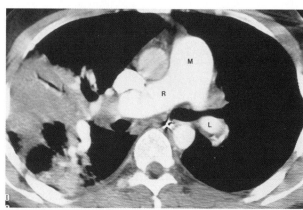

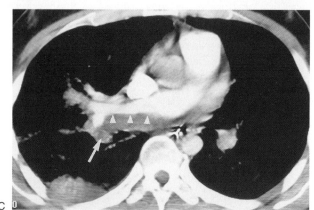

FIGURE 17-12. Acute and chronic PE. A: Anteroposterior recumbent chest radiograph of a 27-year-old man with a history of DVT and acute shortness of breath shows right upper lobe airspace disease, mimicking pneumonia, and fullness of the left hilum, mimicking adenopathy. Endotracheal tube is positioned slightly high (*arrowhead*). **B:** CTPA shows wedge-shaped, pleural-based airspace disease in the right upper and lower lobes. The main (*M*), right (*R*), and left lower lobe (*L*) pulmonary arteries are enlarged, correlating with the measured systolic pulmonary artery pressure of 90 mm Hg. **C:** CTPA at a level inferior to (**B**) shows old low-attenuation clot, eccentrically distributed along the posterior wall of the right pulmonary artery (*arrowheads*), and acute clot filling a right lower lobe basilar segmental pulmonary artery branch (*arrow*).

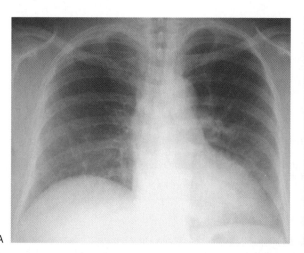

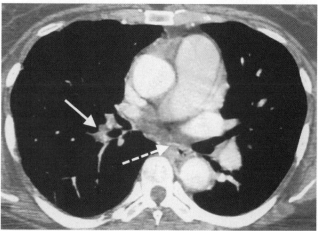

FIGURE 17-13. Chronic PE. A: PA chest radiograph of a 43-year-old woman with recurrent DVT and PE for 20 years shows a small right pulmonary artery and diminutive vessels in the right upper lobe. **B:** CTPA shows a small irregular right pulmonary artery with residual clot and areas of recanalization (*solid arrow*) and bronchial artery collaterals (*dashed arrow*). (*Continued*)

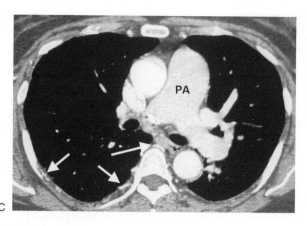

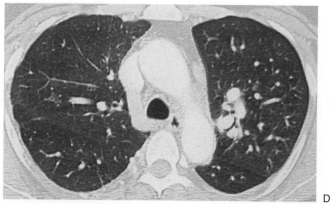

FIGURE 17-13. (*Continued*) **C:** CTPA at a more inferior level shows additional bronchial artery collaterals in a paraspinal and subpleural location (*arrows*). The main pulmonary artery (*PA*) is markedly enlarged. **D:** CTPA with lung windowing shows small right pulmonary arteries and a mosaic pattern of lung attenuation.

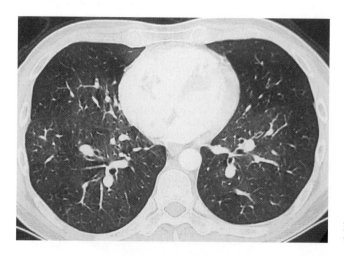

FIGURE 17-14. Chronic PE. CTPA shows a mosaic pattern of lung attenuation. Note diminutive vessels in the areas of hypoattenuated lung.

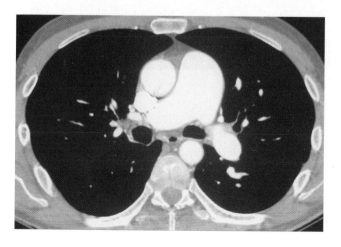

FIGURE 17-15. Chronic PE. CTPA shows marked enlargement of the main pulmonary artery, which is larger in diameter than the adjacent ascending aorta.

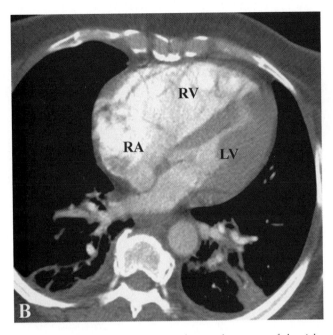

FIGURE 17-16. Chronic PE. CTPA shows enlargement of the right ventricle (*RV*) and right atrium (*RA*). The right ventricle/left ventricle (*LV*) ratio is greater than 1.

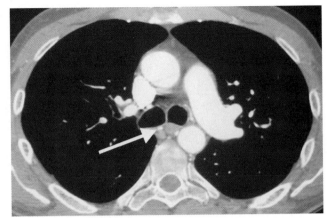

FIGURE 17-17. Chronic PE. CTPA shows enlarged bronchial arteries (*arrow*) adjacent to the esophagus.

additional contrast (Fig. 17-18). Investigators have shown that CTPA provides an alternative diagnosis (e.g., pneumonia, pneumothorax, pleural effusion, pericarditis, aortic dissection, aortic aneurysm, congestive heart failure, rib fracture, lung nodules or mass, mediastinal mass or air, gallstones, chronic obstructive pulmonary disease) in up to two thirds of patients

with an initial suspicion of PE (8). Limitations of CTPA include patients with an allergy to contrast material, impaired renal function, the inability to lie supine, the inability to be transported to the CT scanner, or inadequate intravenous access. Other limitations of CTPA include motion artifact caused by inability of the patient to hold his or her breath or by adjacent cardiac motion, poor contrast bolus enhancement, image noise in large patients, partial volume averaging (Fig. 17-19), parenchymal disease, and streak artifact from lines and tubes or dense contrast material.

PE and DVT are different manifestations of the same clinical disease. One advantage of CTPA is the ability to add CTV, from the iliac crest to the tibial plateau, to detect DVT in the legs

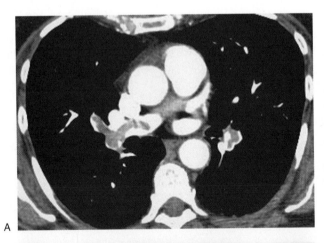

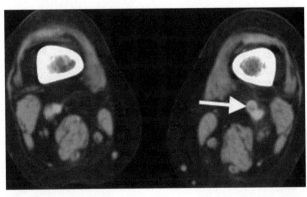

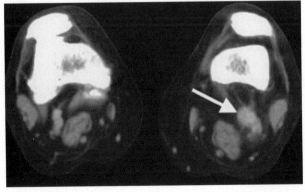

FIGURE 17-18. Deep venous thrombosis and acute PE. A: CTPA of a 66-year-old woman with an endometrial mass and left leg swelling shows bilateral PE. B: CTV performed immediately after the CTPA shows left DVT (*arrow*). C: CTV at a more inferior level shows expansion of the involved left lower-extremity vein and soft tissue stranding of the adjacent fat (*arrow*).

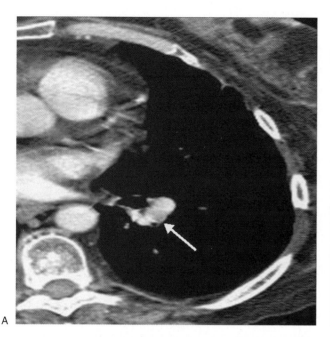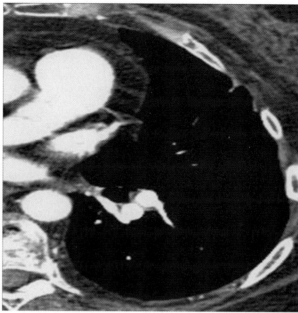

FIGURE 17-19. **Partial volume artifact. A:** CT with 5-mm collimation shows incomplete enhancement of a left lower lobe segmental pulmonary artery (*arrow*). **B:** CTPA on the same day shows homogeneous enhancement of the vessel and no evidence of PE.

and pelvis (Figs. 17-20 and 17-21). Both CTPA and CTV can be accomplished with the same bolus of contrast agent. Unlike lower-extremity ultrasound, CTV can image the external and internal iliac veins. Venous thrombosis can also occur in the upper extremities and in the thorax and can be detected on CTPA (Fig. 17-22).

The D-dimer assay, a test that detects one of the products of fibrin breakdown in the blood, is an important rapid initial test for DVT and PE. Recent studies show that the enzyme-linked immunosorbent assay D-dimer test can accurately rule out DVT and PE in the vast majority of cases (11). However, this test can be falsely positive in postoperative patients, patients on anticoagulation, and patients with recent trauma.

MRI is useful in the evaluation of suspected PE when patients are allergic to iodinated contrast medium. Because it does not involve ionizing radiation, it is also advantageous in children and pregnant women.

Anticoagulant therapy must be considered for DVT as well as for PE; therefore, ultrasound of the deep venous system should have a primary screening role in patients suspected of PE. Ultrasound imaging has the advantages of being readily available and noninvasive. If ultrasound is negative for DVT, depending on the degree of clinical suspicion, further evaluation is generally obtained with a V/Q scan or CTPA.

The diagnostic feature of PE on a V/Q scan is a perfusion defect in a region of normally ventilated lung—the so-called "mismatched perfusion defect." Interpretation of V/Q scans is based on a comparison of the V/Q images and the chest radiograph, which gives rise to a report of "normal" or of low, intermediate, or high probability of PE (4). An abnormal V/Q scan indicating a low probability for recent PE is one in which the individual perfusion defects are smaller than 25% of a segment, regardless of the chest radiographic and ventilation scan appearances; are matched on the ventilation scan; or are accompanied by larger chest radiographic abnormalities. A high-probability scan is one in which there are two or more perfusion defects that are not matched by corresponding ventilation defects or chest radiographic abnormalities, including at least one of segmental or larger size. In the appropriate clinical setting, a high-probability V/Q scan indicates a probability of PE exceeding 90%. An intermediate-probability V/Q scan, also described as an indeterminate scan, is an abnormal scan that does not fit into the low- or high-probability categories. It includes those with perfusion defects that, although matched, correspond in size and shape to an area of opacity on the chest radiograph (and, therefore, may represent infarction or pneumonia) or with perfusion defects in areas of severe obstructive lung disease, pulmonary edema, or pleural effusion.

FIGURE 17-20. **Deep venous thrombosis.** CTV shows intraluminal filling defect within the left femoral vein (*arrow*).

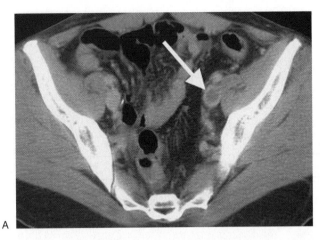

FIGURE 17-21. Deep venous thrombosis. A: CTV of a 42-year-old man with protein C deficiency and recurrent DVT shows a filling defect within a left pelvic vein (*arrow*). **B:** CTV at a more inferior level shows thrombus within the left femoral vein (*arrow*).

Only 15% or fewer of thromboemboli cause pulmonary infarction (12). It is not known why some emboli cause infarction and others do not, but it is likely a result of compromise of both the pulmonary and bronchial arterial circulation. This is most likely to occur with peripheral emboli and in patients with left heart failure or circulatory shock (13). It is known that bronchial circulation alone can sustain the lung parenchyma without infarction occurring (14).

Pulmonary infarction results in airspace opacities that are usually multifocal and predominantly in the lower lungs. They usually appear within 12 to 24 hours after the embolic event.

The opacities are classically peripheral, with a triangular or rounded shape (thus the term *Hampton hump*), and they are always in contact with the pleural surfaces (Figs. 17-23 and 17-24). The apex of the opacity is directed toward the lung hilum. Occasionally, lobar opacity resembling pneumonia can occur. Air bronchograms are rarely present. It is important to note that the opacities can represent a combination of pulmonary hemorrhage and atelectasis without infarction, in which case clearing occurs within a week. Infarction takes several months to resolve, often with residual scarring (Fig. 17-25). As infarcts resolve, they melt away "like an ice cube" (giving rise

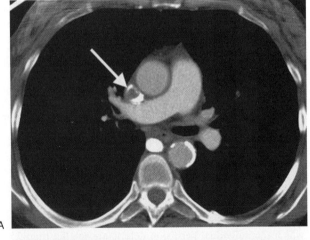

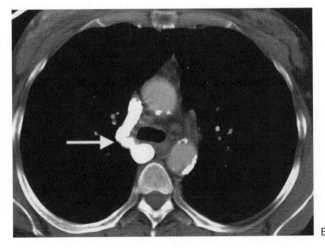

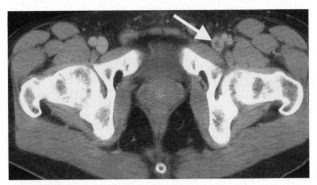

FIGURE 17-22. Superior vena cava thrombus. A: CT of a 47-year-old woman on hemodialysis shows nearly complete occlusion of the superior vena cava with thrombus (*arrow*). **B:** CT at a more inferior level shows collateralization of blood flow through an enlarged right azygos vein (*arrow*). **C:** CT at a level inferior to (**B**) shows enlargement of the azygos (*solid arrow*) and hemiazygos (*dashed arrow*) veins.

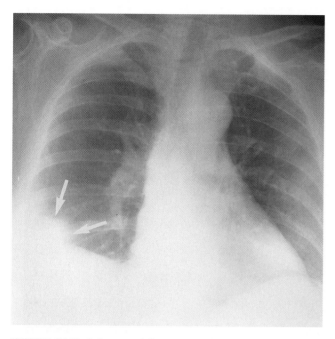

FIGURE 17-23. Pulmonary infarction. PA chest radiograph of a 68-year-old woman with acute shortness of breath shows a pleural-based, rounded opacity at the right costophrenic angle (Hampton hump; *arrows*), representing an acute parenchymal infarct. There is elevation of the right hemidiaphragm from atelectasis and subpulmonic effusion.

to the so-called "melting ice cube sign"; Fig. 2-16). The opacity clears from the periphery first, whereas in pneumonia the opacity clears homogeneously, both centrally and peripherally at the same time. Cavitation can occur within infarcts but is rare without coexisting infection, either secondary infection of an infarct or a result of septic emboli or vasculitis.

PULMONARY ARTERIAL HYPERTENSION

PAH is defined as pulmonary artery pressures above the normal systolic value of 30 mm Hg or above the mean value of 18 mm Hg. There are numerous causes of PAH (Table 17-2),

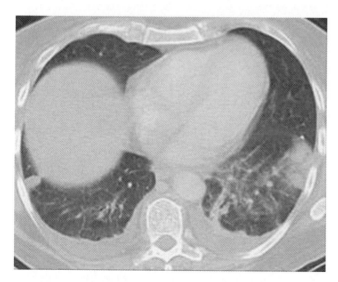

FIGURE 17-24. Bilateral pulmonary infarcts. CT shows bilateral pleural-based opacities characteristic of pulmonary infarcts.

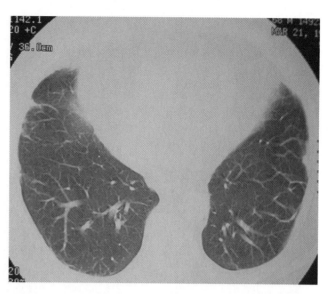

FIGURE 17-25. Old pulmonary infarcts. CT shows bilateral subpleural linear opacities, representing scarring from previous pulmonary infarcts.

which is classically categorized as either precapillary or postcapillary. Regardless of the etiology, the radiologic features are similar and include enlargement of the central pulmonary arteries and narrowing or "pruning" of the peripheral pulmonary artery branches (Fig. 17-26). Right ventricular enlargement is often appreciated on the lateral chest radiograph. However,

TABLE 17-2

CAUSES OF PULMONARY ARTERIAL HYPERTENSION

Precapillary
Primary vascular
Primary pulmonary hypertension
Acute and chronic pulmonary thromboembolic disease
Pulmonary vasculitis
Peripheral pulmonary artery stenoses
Pleuropulmonary
Emphysema
Chronic interstitial lung disease
Bronchiectasis
Postpneumonectomy
Fibrothorax
Chest wall deformity
Alveolar hypoventilation
Obesity/hypoventilation syndrome
Upper airway obstruction
Neuromuscular disease
Postcapillary
Cardiac
Cardiac disease with Eisenmenger physiology
Left atrial myxoma/thrombus
Mitral valve disease
Left ventricular failure
Constrictive pericarditis
Pulmonary venous
Pulmonary veno-occlusive disease
Congenital pulmonary vein stenosis
Anomalous drainage of pulmonary veins
Fibrosing mediastinitis

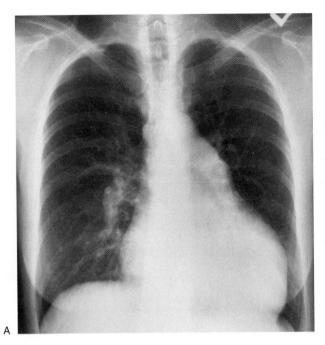
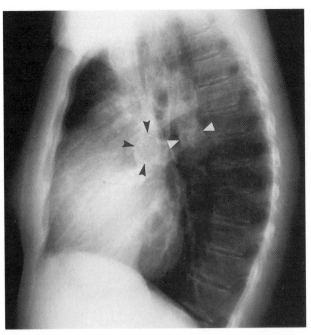

FIGURE 17-26. Primary pulmonary arterial hypertension. PA (**A**) and lateral (**B**) chest radiographs of a 54-year-old woman, obtained as part of a workup for lung transplantation, show enlargement of the central pulmonary arteries and narrowing of the peripheral branches. Fine curvilinear calcification can be seen outlining the central pulmonary arteries on the lateral view (*arrowheads*). There is also enlargement of the right atrium and right ventricle (note increased opacity posterior to the sternum on the lateral view).

substantial PAH may be present in patients with normal chest radiographs. CT more accurately depicts the size of the pulmonary arteries and cardiac chambers. As a general rule, PAH is present when the main pulmonary artery diameter exceeds that of the ascending aorta or is 29 mm or more in diameter (15) (Fig. 17-27). In long-standing and severe PAH, the enlarged central pulmonary arteries may develop thrombus and peripheral calcification. This is most often seen in patients with Eisenmenger physiology, a condition characterized by a rever-

sal in the direction of a long-standing severe left-to-right shunt (i.e., atrial septal defect, ventricular septal defect, patent ductus arteriosus) (Fig. 17-28). In postcapillary and some precapillary disorders, changes of pulmonary venous hypertension may be seen. The most salient finding is cephalization of pulmonary vasculature, which represents recruitment of upper lobe vasculature secondary to a diversion of blood flow. Pericardial effusions, usually small to moderate in size, are commonly associated with PAH.

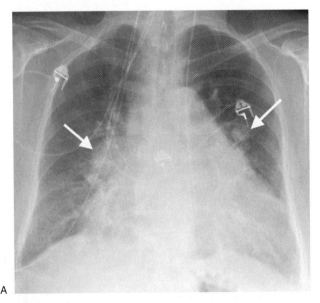
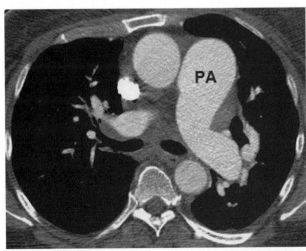

FIGURE 17-27. Primary pulmonary arterial hypertension. A: PA chest radiograph of a 54-year-old woman shows enlargement of the pulmonary arteries (*arrows*) and cardiac enlargement. **B:** CT confirms enlargement of the main (*PA*), right, and left pulmonary arteries. Note that the main pulmonary artery is larger in diameter than the adjacent ascending aorta. Systolic and diastolic pulmonary artery pressures were 97 mm Hg and 53 mm Hg, respectively, with a mean pressure of 70 mm Hg. (*Continued*)

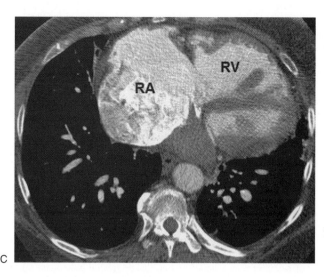

FIGURE 17-27. (*Continued*) **C:** CT at a more inferior level shows enlargement of the right atrium (*RA*) and right ventricle (*RV*).

PULMONARY ARTERY TUMORS

Primary pulmonary artery sarcomas are exceedingly rare. They involve the central pulmonary arteries and often completely occlude the involved vessel. The appearance on CT can mimic massive acute PE. However, when complete occlusion and *expansion* of the main, left, or right pulmonary arteries is seen, tumor should be considered. Even so, it is more common that this appearance is caused by metastatic tumor or invasion of the pulmonary artery by adjacent mediastinal or central bronchogenic carcinoma than by primary pulmonary artery sarcoma.

Tumors most commonly known to embolize through the pulmonary arterial circulation include bronchioloalveolar carcinoma; carcinomas of the breast, kidney, stomach, liver, and prostate; and choriocarcinoma (16). The characteristic CT features are dilatation and beading of peripheral pulmonary arter-

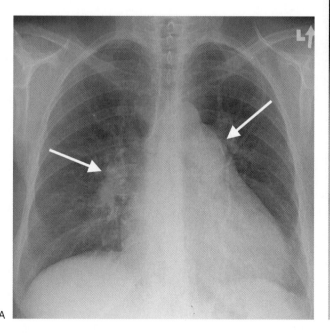

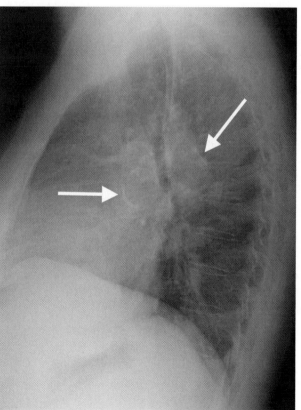

FIGURE 17-28. **Pulmonary arterial hypertension and Eisenmenger physiology. A:** PA chest radiograph of a 47-year-old woman with a long-standing atrial septal defect shows enlargement of the pulmonary arteries (*arrows*) and cardiomegaly. **B:** Lateral view shows rim calcification of enlarged pulmonary arteries (*arrows*).

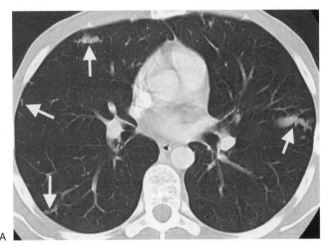
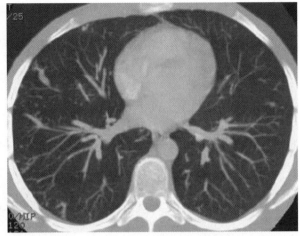

FIGURE 17-29. Tumor emboli. A: CT of a 16-year-old boy with a large pelvic sarcoma shows dilated and beaded peripheral pulmonary arteries (*arrows*). **B:** Maximum-intensity-projection image shows the continuity of these abnormal vessels with the central pulmonary arteries.

ies (Fig. 17-29). The appearance can resemble the "tree-in-bud" appearance of small airway disease (17). Maximum-intensity-projection images can be helpful in showing continuity of the distal vessels with more central pulmonary vessels in cases of tumor emboli. Many more cases of tumor emboli are discovered at autopsy than antemortem.

References

 1. Horlander KT, Mannino DM, Leeper KV. Pulmonary embolism mortality in the United States, 1979—1998: an analysis using multiple-cause mortality data. *Arch Intern Med.* 2003;163:1711–1717.
 2. Worsley DF, Alari A, Aronchick JM, et al. Chest radiographic findings in patients with acute pulmonary embolism: observations from the PIOPED study. *Radiology.* 1993;189:133–136.
 3. Wenger NK, Stein PD, Willis PW. Massive acute pulmonary embolism: the deceivingly nonspecific manifestations. *JAMA.* 1972;220:843–844.
 4. The PIOPED Investigators: value of ventilation-perfusion scan in acute pulmonary embolism. Results of the prospective investigation of pulmonary embolism diagnosis (PIOPED). *JAMA.* 1990;20(263):2753–2759.
 5. Coche E, Verschuren F, Keyeux A, et al. Diagnosis of acute pulmonary embolism in outpatients: comparison of thin-collimation multi-detector row spiral CT and planar ventilation-perfusion scintigraphy. *Radiology.* 2003;229:757–765.
 6. Winer-Muram HT, Rydberg J, Johnson MS, et al. Suspected acute pulmonary

 7. Gotway MB, Yee J. Helical CT pulmonary angiography for acute pulmonary embolism. *Appl Radiol.* 2002;April:21–30.
 8. Hull RD, Raskob GE, Ginsberg JS, et al. A noninvasive strategy for the treatment of patients with suspected pulmonary embolism. *Arch Intern Med.* 1994;154:289–297.
 9. Kavanagh EC, O'Hare A, Hargaden G, et al. Risk of pulmonary embolism after negative MDCT pulmonary angiography findings. *AJR Am J Roentgenol.* 2004;182:499–504.
10. Stein PD, Henry JW, Relyea B. Untreated patients with pulmonary embolism: outcome, clinical, and laboratory assessment. *Chest.* 1995;107:931–935.
11. Perrier A, Roy PM, Sanchez O, et al. Multidetector-row computed tomography in suspected pulmonary embolism. *N Engl J Med.* 2005;352:1760–1768.
12. Moser KM. Pulmonary embolism: state of the art. *Am Rev Respir Dis.* 1977;115:829–852.
13. Tsao MS, Schraufnagel D, Wang NS. Pathogenesis of pulmonary infarction. *Am J Med.* 1982;72:599–606.
14. Dalen JE, Haffajee CI, Alpert JS, et al. Pulmonary embolism, pulmonary hemorrhage and pulmonary infarction. *N Engl J Med.* 1977;296:1431–1435.
15. Kuriyama K, Gamsu G, Stern RG, et al. CT-determined pulmonary artery diameters in predicting pulmonary hypertension. *Invest Radiol.* 1984;19:16–22.
16. Shepard JO, Moore EH, Templeton PA, et al. Pulmonary intravascular tumor emboli: dilated and beaded peripheral pulmonary arteries at CT. *Radiology.* 1993;187:797–801.
17. Franquet T, Gimenez A, Prats R, et al. Thrombotic microangiopathy of pulmonary tumors: a vascular cause of tree-in-bud pattern on CT. *AJR Am J Roentgenol.* 2002;179:897–899.

embolism: evaluation with multi-detector row CT versus digital subtraction pulmonary arteriography. *Radiology.* 2004;233:806–815.

CHAPTER 18

CONGENITAL AND ACQUIRED CARDIAC DISEASE

LEARNING OBJECTIVES

1. Identify and describe the findings of the following on a chest radiograph or computed tomography (CT):
   - Atrial septal defect
   - Ventricular septal defect
   - Patent ductus arteriosus

2. Identify and describe the findings of the following on a chest radiograph:
   - Enlarged left atrium
   - Enlarged right ventricle
   - Enlarged left ventricle

3. Identify and describe the chest radiographic findings and state the most common etiologies of each of the following valvular diseases:
   - Aortic stenosis
   - Aortic insufficiency
   - Mitral stenosis
   - Mitral insufficiency
   - Tricuspid stenosis
   - Tricuspid insufficiency
   - Pulmonic stenosis
   - Pulmonic insufficiency

4. Recognize an enlarged ascending aorta and aortic valve calcification on a chest radiograph and suggest the diagnosis of aortic stenosis when these findings are present.

5. Recognize an enlarged left atrium, vascular redistribution, and mitral valve calcification on a chest radiograph and suggest the diagnosis of mitral stenosis when these findings are present.

6. Describe the radiographic appearance of mitral annulus calcification and name the cardiac diseases associated with mitral annulus calcification.

7. Define the types of cardiomyopathy (dilated, hypertrophic, restrictive) and list the common causes of each.

8. Identify on CT and describe the CT findings and clinical significance of lipomatous hypertrophy of the interatrial septum.

9. Define arrhythmogenic right ventricular dysplasia, describe the role of magnetic resonance imaging (MRI) in its diagnosis, and identify MRI findings that support the diagnosis.

10. Name the most common benign primary cardiac tumors, including myxoma, lipoma, fibroma, and rhabdomyoma.

11. Distinguish cardiac tumor from thrombus on CT and MRI.

12. Name the most common malignancies to metastasize to the heart; describe their appearance on chest radiography and CT.

13. Describe the anatomy of the coronary arteries and identify the following on chest CT:
    - Right coronary artery
    - Left main coronary artery
    - Left anterior descending coronary artery
    - Left circumflex coronary artery

14. Identify on chest CT and describe the clinical significance of aberrant coronary artery origins.

15. Describe the clinical significance of coronary arterial calcification on a chest radiograph.

16. Recognize coronary arterial calcification on CT and describe the current role of coronary artery calcium scoring with CT.

17. Identify the following postoperative findings on chest radiography and CT:
    - Coronary artery stents
    - Coronary artery grafts (normal and aneurysmal)
    - Cardiac valve replacement
    - Poststernotomy infection

18. Describe the difference between a left ventricular aneurysm and pseudoaneurysm and distinguish between the two on chest CT.

19. Recognize pericardial calcification on a chest radiograph and CT and name the most common causes.

20. Identify and describe two chest radiographic signs of a pericardial effusion.

21. Name five causes of a pericardial effusion.

22. Identify and describe the findings of each of the following on a chest radiograph and CT:
    - Constrictive pericarditis
    - Pericardial metastases
    - Pneumopericardium

23. Describe the role of MRI in diagnosing constrictive pericarditis and differentiating constrictive pericarditis from restrictive cardiomyopathy.

Heart disease is the leading cause of morbidity and mortality in industrialized countries. Echocardiography, single photon emission computed tomography (SPECT), scintigraphy, positron emission tomography (PET), and cardiac catheterization with cineangiography have long been used to assess the anatomy and function of the normal and diseased heart. Recent advances in CT and magnetic resonance imaging (MRI) have generated a renewed interest in cardiac imaging, particularly among radiologists. CT in particular is an examination with which radiologists are very comfortable, and it now provides a means to globally assess the heart and lungs simultaneously. This chapter will focus on the chest radiographic and CT findings of common congenital cardiac diseases seen in the adult, normal and abnormal cardiac anatomy, valvular disease, cardiomyopathies, cardiac tumors, complications of myocardial infarction and cardiac surgery, and pericardial disease.

CONGENITAL CARDIAC DISEASE

Whereas congenital abnormalities are the predominant form of heart disease in childhood, in adults, congenital disorders represent only 1% of recognized heart disease (1). In general, adults with newly discovered congenital heart disease are those whose anomalies produced no symptoms or mild symptoms in childhood, or those who were misdiagnosed in childhood only to become symptomatic in adult life. A discussion of all congenital heart defects that can be diagnosed in adults is beyond the scope of this chapter. What will be presented is a brief discussion of common left-to-right shunts that are diagnosed in adulthood and the developmental anomalies of the aorta that can be associated with congenital heart diseases.

Atrial Septal Defect

Atrial septal defect (ASD) accounts for 80% to 90% of congenital left-to-right shunts found in adults (2,3) and is three times more common in women than in men. Almost half of the patients with ASD in all age groups are asymptomatic, and in these cases the ASD is discovered incidentally on a routine chest radiograph. There are different types of ASD, with the ostium secundum type (consisting of an absence or deficiency of tissue in the region of the fossa ovalis) being the most common type seen in adult patients. In uncomplicated ASD, the chest radiograph shows enlargement of the right ventricle and all segments of the pulmonary arteries ("shunt vascularity") (Fig. 18-1). The right atrium is also enlarged, but it is usually not distinguished from right ventricular enlargement on the chest radiograph. Because the radiograph does not accurately reflect the size of the right atrium and ventricle, the overall heart size may appear normal. On the lateral view, right ventricular enlargement results in a filling in of the retrosternal clear space and posterior displacement of the left ventricle toward the spine (4). There is no enlargement of the left heart in a simple ASD. The aorta appears small, relative to the pulmonary artery, and the superior vena cava appears small or "absent" because of rotation of the heart from right-sided cardiac enlargement (Fig. 18-2).

Long-standing large shunts lead to pulmonary arterial hypertension; when pulmonary arterial pressure exceeds systemic arterial pressure, a reversal of shunting of blood from left-to-right to right-to-left occurs (Eisenmenger physiology). In these cases, there is marked central pulmonary artery dilatation and narrowing of peripheral pulmonary artery branches (5). The central pulmonary arteries can become aneurysmal and, rarely, can be calcified (Fig. 18-3).

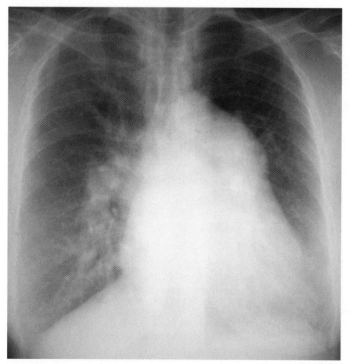

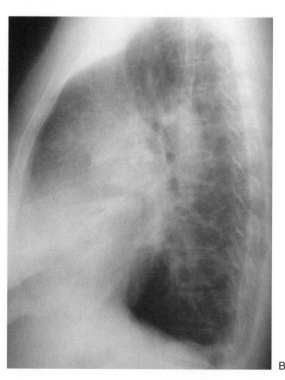

FIGURE 18-1. Atrial septal defect. A: Posteroanterior (PA) chest radiograph shows marked enlargement of the central and all segments of the pulmonary arteries. The cardiac silhouette is enlarged. **B:** Lateral view shows filling in of the retrosternal clear space, secondary to right ventricular enlargement, and pulmonary artery enlargement.

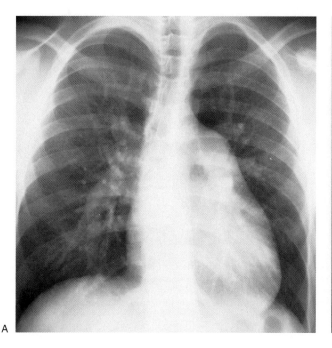

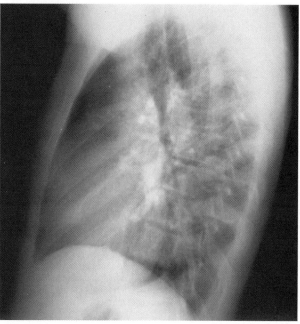

FIGURE 18-2. Atrial septal defect. A: PA chest radiograph of a 17-year-old boy with a heart murmur since birth shows enlargement of the cardiac silhouette, enlarged central and peripheral pulmonary arteries ("shunt vascularity"), a normal- to small-sized aorta, and "absent" superior vena cava shadow. B: Lateral view shows enlargement of the right ventricle, as evidenced by increased opacification posterior to the sternum.

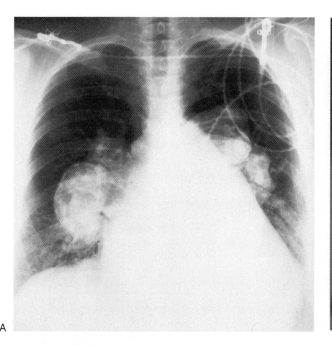

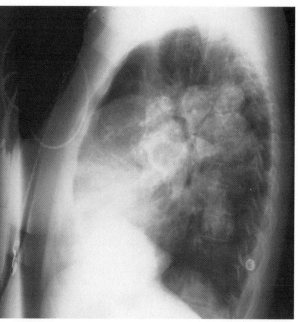

FIGURE 18-3. Atrial septal defect with Eisenmenger physiology. PA (A) and lateral (B) chest radiographs of a 52-year-old woman with a large, long-standing ASD that has resulted in a reversal of shunting of blood and pulmonary arterial hypertension. There is aneurysmal enlargement and calcification of the central pulmonary arteries, enlargement of the right heart, and "absence" of the superior vena cava shadow. (Continued)

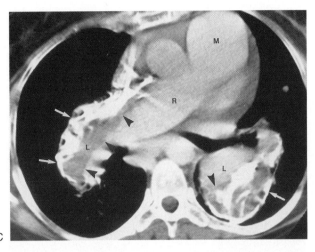
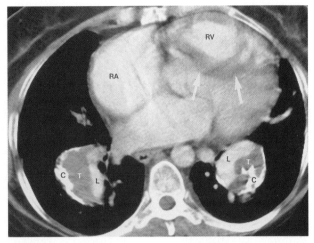

FIGURE 18-3. (*Continued*) **C:** CT shows large main (*M*), right (*R*), and lower (*L*) lobe pulmonary arteries. Long-standing left-to-right shunting of blood has resulted in pulmonary artery aneurysms, which contain low-attenuation thrombus (*arrowheads*), and calcification (*arrows*). **D:** CT at a level inferior to (**C**) shows enlarged lower lobe pulmonary arteries containing thrombus (*T*) and calcification (*C*), enlarged right atrium (*RA*), and enlarged right ventricle (*RV*), causing leftward bowing and hypertrophy of the interventricular septum (*arrows*). The pulmonary artery lumina are outlined by high-attenuation contrast material (*L*).

ASD closure can be accomplished with a variety of percutaneously placed devices. A catheter that is placed via the common femoral vein is fed through the cardiac defect into the left atrium using fluoroscopic and echocardiographic guidance. A commonly used device is the Amplatzer Septal Occluder (AGA Medical Corporation, Golden Valley, MN) (Fig. 18-4). This is a two-part closure device. One of two nitinol mesh disks is pushed out through the catheter into the left atrium; this is followed by release of the second disk into the right atrium to close the defect.

Ventricular Septal Defect

Ventricular septal defect (VSD) is the most common congenital heart disease in childhood, but it represents only 10% of

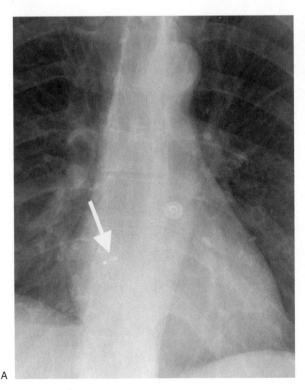
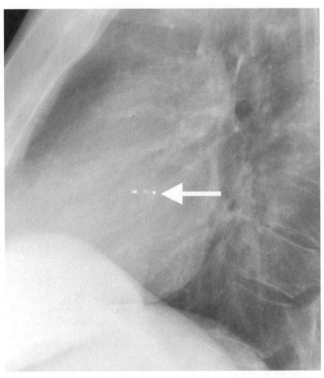

FIGURE 18-4. **Atrial septal defect occluder. A:** PA chest radiograph of a 50-year-old woman with a history of transient ischemic attacks shows an Amplatzer Septal Occluder device (AGA Medical Corporation, Golden Valley, MN) (*arrow*) in the location of the foramen of ovale. **B:** Lateral view confirms appropriate placement of the device (*arrow*).

congenital cardiac lesions in the adult patient. Surgical correction and spontaneous closure of the defect account for the decreased incidence in the adult patient (6). Most patients with VSD who survive into adulthood without intervention have small and physiologically inconsequential defects. Patients who reach adult life with large VSDs have pulmonary arterial hypertension, progressive right-to-left shunting (Eisenmenger physiology), and cyanosis. Small shunts cannot be identified on chest radiography. With large shunts (VSDs with a shunt ratio greater than 2:1) and normal pulmonary vascular resistance, the chest radiograph shows "shunt vascularity," enlargement of the left atrium and both ventricles, a normal or small aorta, and a normal right atrium. The left ventricular apex projects to the left, inferiorly and posteriorly. On frontal chest radiographs, enlargement of the left atrium is seen as a "double density" behind the right atrium, and straightening or focal convexity of the left mediastinal border is seen below the pulmonary artery shadow.

Patent Ductus Arteriosus

The ductus arteriosus is a portion of the sixth aortic arch in the fetus that connects the left pulmonary artery to the descending thoracic aorta. Twelve to 24 hours after birth, the ductus is functionally closed, and anatomic closure occurs 1 to 2 weeks later. However, for unknown reasons, the ductus arteriosus may remain patent, creating a left-to-right shunt and varying degrees of overcirculation to the lungs, left atrium, left ventricle, and the ascending and arch portions of the aorta. If the ductus does not close, Eisenmenger physiology develops when pulmonary vascular resistance exceeds systemic resistance and causes a right-to-left shunt across the ductus arteriosus. The radiographic features of an uncomplicated patent ductus arteriosus (PDA) are similar to those of a VSD, except for the size of the aorta. In PDA, the ascending and arch portions of the aorta can enlarge (with the degree of enlargement dependent on the size of the shunt), indicating that the shunt is extracardiac, as opposed to an intracardiac shunt, such as a VSD, with which the size of the aorta is normal or small. However, aortic size is not always a reliable criterion, and in practice it can be difficult to distinguish VSD from PDA on chest radiography. Another finding of PDA in an adult is calcification of the ductus.

Anomalies of the Thoracic Aorta

Congenital bicuspid aortic valve is a relatively common malformation. As the valve thickens and becomes fibrotic, it becomes stenotic. When this occurs, the valve becomes calcified. A densely calcified aortic valve, as seen on chest radiography or CT in a patient under the age of 55, should prompt consideration of this anomaly.

In left aortic arch with aberrant right subclavian artery, the right subclavian artery, instead of the first branch, takes off as the final branch of the aorta. Patients with this common anomaly are usually asymptomatic but may present with dysphagia as a result of the retroesophageal course of the aberrant artery. The frontal chest radiograph often shows an abnormal mediastinal contour at the level of the aortic arch, where the proximal portion of the aberrant artery is dilated—the so-called "diverticulum of Kommerell." The lateral chest radiograph may show anterior displacement of the trachea.

A right aortic arch occurs when there is interruption of the embryonic left aortic component of the hypothetical double aortic arch. Two types are described: Type 1 is a mirror image of left aortic arch and is associated with cyanotic congenital heart disease in more than 95% of patients, most of whom have tetralogy of Fallot (7). Type 2 right aortic arch—a right aortic arch with an aberrant left retroesophageal subclavian artery—is common, occurring in 1 in 2,500 persons, and is usually found incidentally (1). Additional cardiac anomalies occur in only 5% to 15% of patients with type 2. Chest radiographs of a right aortic arch show that the trachea is bowed to the left at the level of the right aortic arch, producing a convex bulge just above the azygous vein (Figs. 18-5 and 18-6). It is typical for a right-sided arch to be high riding and present as a "mass" in the right paratracheal area. An aortic diverticulum, or proximal arterial dilation, is seen to the left and slightly below the usual site of a left-sided aortic arch. The diverticulum may be of sufficient size to produce a large bulge immediately above the left main pulmonary artery and simulate a left aortic arch or a nonvascular mediastinal mass. Most often, the left mediastinal bulge is a result of the aortic diverticulum rather than the aberrant left subclavian artery itself. As the left subclavian artery crosses from right to left, it will cause a posterior impression on the air-filled esophagus and the trachea, which is seen best on the lateral chest radiograph. The right aortic arch usually crosses to the left side posteriorly, in the middle of the thorax behind the right pulmonary artery, to descend into the abdomen on the left side. A double aortic arch forms a complete vascular ring and on occasion can first present in adulthood.

Pseudocoarctation is a term used to denote a focal narrowing of the aortic arch that has the same morphology as classic coarctation but does not produce obstruction. This anomaly is a buckling of the aorta at the isthmus with little or no pressure gradient across the buckled portion (less than 30 mm Hg) (8). Because there is no obstruction, there is no collateral flow, and there is no rib notching as is seen with classic coarctation. The chest radiograph shows a left "mediastinal mass" that represents an elongated, redundant, and high aortic arch. Sagittally reconstructed CT of the chest can show the high arch with a kink at the isthmus, resembling the numeral 3, in which the midportion of the 3 corresponds to the attachment of the ligamentum arteriosum (Fig. 18-7). A "cervical aortic arch" can resemble pseudocoarctation of the aorta on chest radiographs, but with a cervical arch, the aortic arch lies in the neck, above the clavicles, usually on the right side.

ACQUIRED HEART DISEASE

Valvular Disease

The radiologic signs of uncomplicated valvular lesions are relatively straightforward (Table 18-1). Valve stenosis produces pressure overload and myocardial hypertrophy without dilatation. Dilatation indicates that heart failure has developed. Valve insufficiency produces volume overload and a combination of dilatation and hypertrophy of the involved cardiac chambers. With insufficiency, a dilated heart does not indicate cardiac decompensation.

Aortic Stenosis

Aortic stenosis (AS) can exist at the valvular, subvalvular, or supravalvular level. The chest radiographic abnormalities depend on the age of the patient as well as on the severity of the stenosis. The adult heart is of normal size and the lungs are normal, because left ventricular failure and dilatation occur only in terminally ill patients. Radiographically detectable calcification in the aortic valve occurs in all types of aortic stenosis and marks the stenosis as clinically severe. Dilatation of the ascending aorta is frequent in aortic stenosis but correlates poorly with severity or with the site of the stenosis. Poststenotic dilatation of the ascending aorta is caused by the jet of blood through the stenotic valve striking the lateral aortic wall. The lateral wall

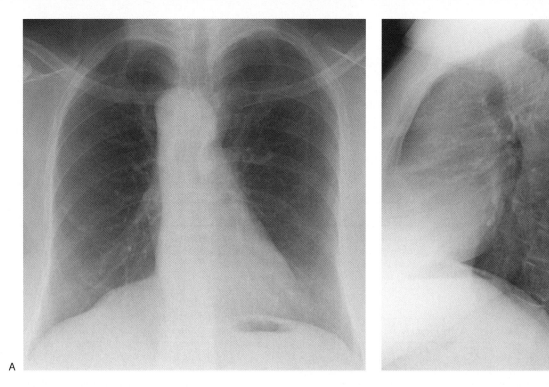

A   B

FIGURE 18-5. Right aortic arch. A: PA chest radiograph shows a right-sided aortic arch and descending aorta. The trachea is not deviated to the right, as is usually seen with a left aortic arch. **B:** Lateral view shows a posterior impression on the tracheal air column, secondary to compression from the aberrant left subclavian artery crossing from right to left.

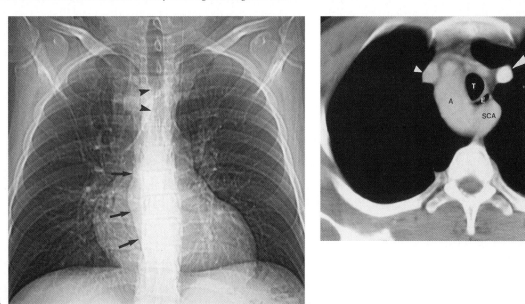

A   B

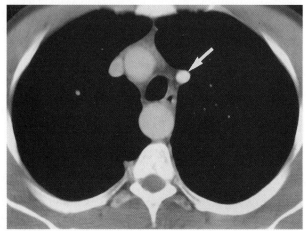

C

FIGURE 18-6. Right aortic arch with aberrant left subclavian artery. A: Scout view from a CT of a 29-year-old man with dysphagia shows deviation of the trachea to the left (*arrowheads*) and a right-sided descending thoracic aorta (*arrows*). **B:** CT shows the right-sided aortic arch (*A*) and an aberrant left subclavian artery (*SCA*) arising from the posterior arch and coursing posterior to the trachea (*T*) and esophagus (*E*). Note the compression of the esophagus from the aberrant vessel, causing the patient's dysphagia. There is also a persistent left superior vena cava (*arrow*), in addition to a right superior vena cava (*arrowhead*). **C:** CT at a level inferior to (**B**) shows the persistent left superior vena cava (*arrow*) coursing in a left paramediastinal location before draining into the coronary sinus more inferiorly. The descending aorta is midline at this level.

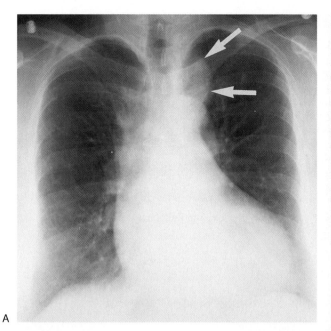

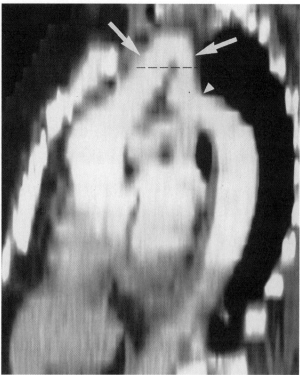

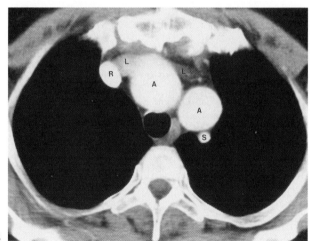

FIGURE 18-7. **Pseudocoarctation of the aorta. A:** PA chest radiograph of a 50-year-old woman shows a left paratracheal "mass" (*arrows*). Sternotomy wires are present from previous coronary artery bypass graft surgery. **B:** CT shows the left subclavian artery (*S*), right (*R*) and left (*L*) brachiocephalic veins, and the high-riding, "buckled" aortic arch (*A*). **C:** Sagittal reconstruction shows the buckled aortic arch (*arrows*) and focal kinking of the aorta at the isthmus (*arrowhead*). This reconstruction shows how an axial view at the level of the aortic arch (*dashed line*) will show "two" rounded, contrast-enhanced structures adjacent to each other.

of the aorta becomes both dilated and elongated, accentuating the rightward displacement of the aorta. In most children and adults with pure, severe aortic stenosis, the left ventricle is a small cavity that is hypercontractile and has the usual signs of hypertrophy. In the absence of other anomalies, left ventricular dilatation in pure aortic stenosis is direct evidence of heart failure.

Calcific AS in the adult can be caused by rheumatic heart disease, a congenital bicuspid aortic valve, or advanced age and degeneration of the valve (8). The average age at which aortic valve calcification is first detected is 25 years for congenital AS, 47 years for rheumatic AS, and 54 years for degenerative AS (9). Valve calcification is best seen on the lateral chest radiograph, because the valve usually projects over the spine in the frontal projection. An important clue to the diagnosis of rheumatic disease in the aortic valve is the presence of mitral stenosis or regurgitation.

AS in elderly patients results from degeneration of the valve leaflets, with subsequent thickening and calcification. These aortic valves are tricuspid and have clumps of calcium within the webs of the leaflets. Some of these elderly patients also have coronary artery calcification and calcification in the mitral annulus and aortic arch.

Aortic Insufficiency

Stenotic aortic valves generally also have some insufficiency. If the aortic insufficiency (AI) is both chronic and severe, the chest radiograph shows left ventricular enlargement and dilatation of the entire aorta. This pattern follows the principle that insufficiency of any of the heart valves enlarges structures on both sides of the insufficient valve. Isolated AI most commonly results from a congenital bicuspid aortic valve. Other rare causes of AI include syphilitic aortitis (presenting between 45 and 65 years of age and associated with calcification of the ascending aortic aneurysm), Marfan syndrome (presenting before age 30 and not associated with calcification of the aneurysm), ankylosing spondylitis, relapsing polychondritis, and traumatic rupture of the aortic valve.

Mitral Stenosis

Most mitral stenosis (MS) is acquired and usually results from rheumatic carditis that occurred at least 5 to 10 years previously. Less common etiologies include left atrial myxoma, thrombus, or a tumor that may prolapse through the mitral orifice during diastole and create functional stenosis. Early in the course of rheumatic MS in the adult, the pulmonary blood flow

TABLE 18-1

RADIOGRAPHIC APPEARANCES OF CARDIAC VALVULAR DISEASE

Valvular disease	Radiographic findings
Aortic stenosis	■ Calcification of aortic valve ■ Dilatation of ascending aorta ■ Dilated left ventricle and pulmonary edema only with left ventricular failure
Aortic insufficiency	■ Calcification of aortic valve ■ Dilatation of ascending aorta ■ Dilated left ventricle ■ Pulmonary edema with left ventricular failure
Mitral stenosis	■ Enlargement of left atrium, right ventricle, and pulmonary trunk ■ Cephalization of pulmonary vasculature ■ Septal (Kerley B) lines ■ Calcification of mitral valve
Mitral insufficiency	■ Markedly dilated left atrium ■ Mildly dilated left ventricle ■ Moderate enlargement of pulmonary trunk and right ventricle
Tricuspid stenosis	■ Systemic venous dilatation ■ Pulmonary oligemia
Tricuspid insufficiency	■ Dilatation of right ventricle and right atrium ■ Dilatation of venae cavae ■ Pulmonary oligemia
Pulmonic stenosis	■ Right ventricular enlargement ■ Poststenotic dilatation of the pulmonary trunk and left pulmonary artery ■ Increased pulmonary blood flow to the left lung and decreased pulmonary blood flow to the right lung
Pulmonic insufficiency	■ Dilatation and hypertrophy of the right ventricle ■ Systolic enlargement of the pulmonary trunk and central pulmonary arteries

redistributes to the upper lobes. Later, the pulmonary arteries enlarge as pulmonary arterial hypertension develops. Later still, the right ventricle fails, from both a pressure overload from pumping into hypertensive pulmonary arteries and from pulmonic insufficiency secondary to a dilated annulus (Fig. 18-8). The chest radiograph in MS physiologically reflects the left atrial hypertension. The left atrium is enlarged, but the left ventricle is normal in size (unless there is coexisting mitral insufficiency). Left atrial enlargement can manifest as straightening of the left heart border or a convex shadow just below the left mainstem bronchus on the posteroanterior chest radiograph (indicating enlargement of the left atrial appendage), splaying of the tracheal carina, and posterior displacement of the pulmonary venous confluence and left lower lobe bronchus on the lateral chest radiograph (Fig. 18-9). The lungs show a diffuse increase in interstitial markings that is likely related to both fibrosis and edema. Patients with severe MS can have hemoptysis caused by bleeding of the engorged plexus of vessels around the middle to smaller bronchi, with a late sequela of pulmonary hemosiderosis, the deposits of which can calcify. The amount of calcium in the mitral valve roughly correlates with the degree of MS, but, unlike the aortic valve, the mitral valve may be severely stenotic and have no radiologically visible calcification. To distinguish aortic from mitral valve calcification on a lateral chest radiograph, one can draw a line from the inferior aspect of the right pulmonary artery along the right middle lobe branch to the tip of the xiphoid; the aortic valve is above this line, and the mitral valve is below this line.

Mitral Insufficiency

Acute mitral insufficiency (MI) can be traumatic, infectious, degenerative, or idiopathic. The pathology is usually a rupture of a chorda, a papillary muscle, or a mitral leaflet. Acute MI leads to acute left ventricular failure with severe pulmonary edema and a normal-sized heart or minimal cardiomegaly.

The major causes of chronic MI are rheumatic fever, mitral valve prolapse, coronary heart disease, and cardiomyopathy. Typical radiographic manifestations include a markedly dilated left atrium, a well-contracting but only mildly enlarged left ventricle, cephalization of the pulmonary vasculature without frank pulmonary edema, and moderate pulmonary trunk and right ventricle enlargement. MI can also be associated with focal edema in the right upper lobe. The pathogenesis for this condition is the vector of the regurgitant jet of blood flow from the left ventricle to the left atrium, toward the right superior pulmonary vein, which locally accentuates the forces for edema formation in the right upper lobe (10) (Fig. 18-10). With coronary heart disease and cardiomyopathy, the left ventricle is usually markedly dilated with poor contractility, with only mild enlargement of the left atrium.

Mitral Annulus Calcification

The mitral valve ring may calcify in individuals over age 60; this occurs more commonly in women than in men. The calcification often forms a pattern resembling the letter "J," the letter "O," or a reverse letter "C" (Fig. 18-11). In most instances, mitral annulus calcification has little clinical significance and is a

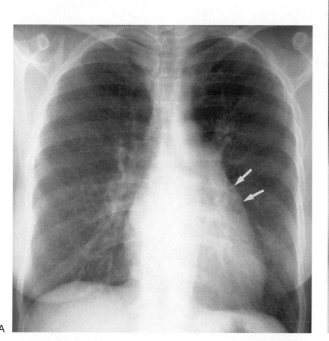
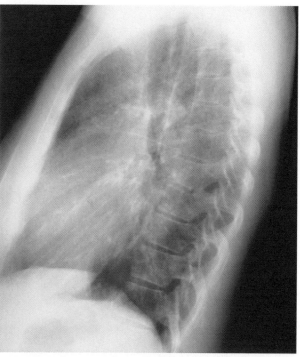

A   B

FIGURE 18-8. Rheumatic mitral stenosis. PA (**A**) and lateral (**B**) chest radiographs of a 40-year-old woman show enlargement of the right ventricle (note increased opacity posterior to the sternum on the lateral view) and left atrium (note the convexity of the left heart border inferior to the left pulmonary artery shadow; *arrows*). The central pulmonary arteries are enlarged from pulmonary arterial hypertension, and there is pulmonary vascular redistribution. Unlike the aortic valve, the mitral valve may be severely stenotic and, as in this case, have no radiographically visible calcification.

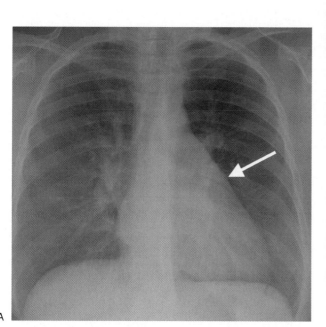
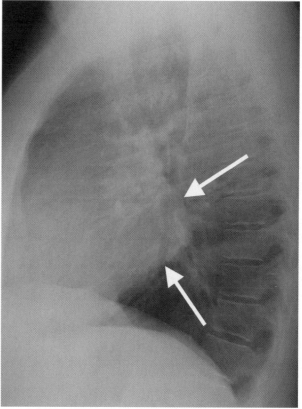

A   B

FIGURE 18-9. Mitral stenosis. A: PA chest radiograph of a 43-year-old woman with atrial fibrillation and a history of rheumatic fever as a child shows abnormal convexity to the upper left heart border, indicating an enlarged left atrial appendage (*arrow*). **B:** Lateral view shows posterior displacement of the pulmonary venous confluence (*arrows*).

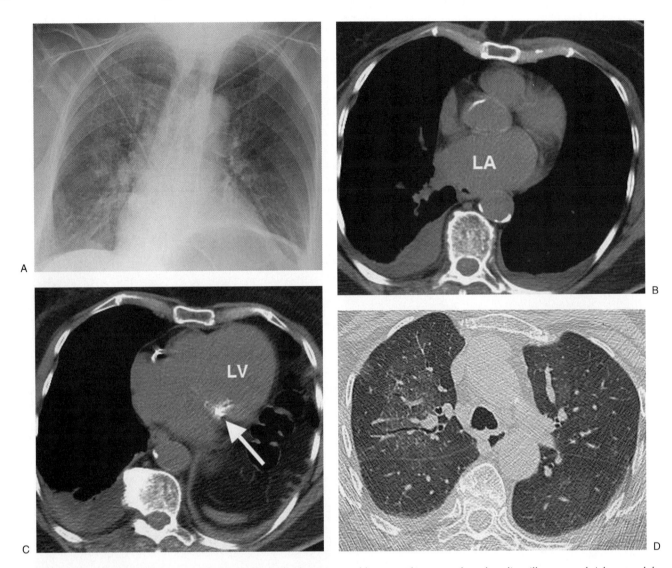

FIGURE 18-10. Mitral insufficiency. A: PA chest radiograph of an 84-year-old woman shows an enlarged cardiac silhouette and right upper lobe pulmonary opacity representing edema. **B:** CT shows an enlarged left atrium (*LA*) and bilateral pleural effusions. **C:** CT at a level inferior to (**B**) shows calcification of the mitral valve (*arrow*) and enlargement of the left ventricle (*LV*). **D:** CT with lung windowing shows ground-glass opacity limited to the right upper lobe. Right upper lobe edema in patients with mitral insufficiency is thought to be caused by the regurgitant jet of blood flow through the mitral valve to the right superior pulmonary vein.

noninflammatory chronic degenerative process. AS and hypertension are associated with mitral annulus calcification, likely as a result of the increased strain exerted on the mitral valve apparatus from the left ventricular pressure overload. If the calcification grows posteriorly into the ventricular myocardium, heart block can occur. If it grows anteriorly into the mitral valve leaflets, MS and MI can occur. Mitral annulus calcification is also associated with increased risk of stroke.

Tricuspid and Pulmonic Valve Disease

Acquired disease isolated to the tricuspid and pulmonic valves is much less common than aortic and mitral valve disease. Primary disease of the tricuspid valve is most commonly caused by rheumatic disease and is associated with disease also involving the left-sided cardiac valves. Pulmonic stenosis is almost always congenital (Fig. 18-12), and pulmonary insufficiency is most commonly a result of severe pulmonic arterial hypertension of any etiology (e.g., severe MS and recurrent pulmonary thromboembolic disease).

Multivalvular Disease

Multivalvular involvement is common in patients with rheumatic heart disease, cardiomyopathies, and connective tissue disorders (Fig. 18-13). In general, the proximal valvular lesions tend to obscure the distal ones, both clinically and radiographically.

Cardiomyopathy

Cardiomyopathies can be classified as dilated, hypertrophic, or restrictive. Each can be further categorized as primary (affecting the myocardium but not other organs) or secondary (myocardial disease as one manifestation of systemic disease). *Idiopathic dilated cardiomyopathy* is characterized by dilatation of both ventricles or only the left ventricle, and it is either idiopathic or, in about half of cases, is thought to have a viral or immune etiology. *Secondary dilated cardiomyopathy* can be caused by ethanol toxicity, chemotherapeutic agents (e.g., doxorubicin), heavy metals, infection, connective tissue diseases, sarcoidosis, neuromuscular diseases, metabolic or endocrine

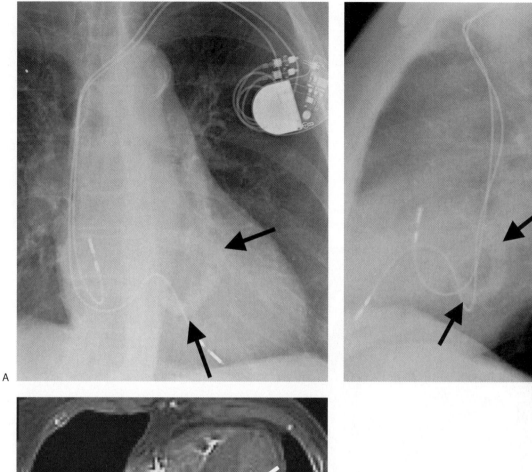

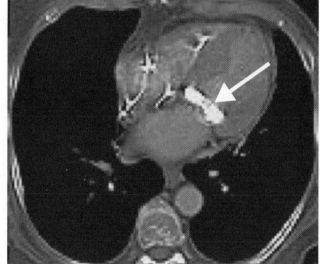

FIGURE 18-11. **Mitral annulus calcification.** PA (**A**) and lateral (**B**) chest radiographs of an 87-year old woman show a C-shaped calcification in the expected location of the mitral annulus (*arrows*) and a dual-lead pacemaker. **C:** CT shows dense calcification of the mitral annulus (*arrow*).

abnormalities (e.g., hypocalcemia or hypothyroidism), nutritional deficiencies (e.g., vitamin B_{12} deficiency), pregnancy, hypertension, or chronic myocardial ischemia; or it may be familial in origin. Chest radiography shows global cardiac enlargement and pulmonary edema.

Genetic hypertrophic cardiomyopathy is characterized by biventricular myocardial hypertrophy without chamber dilatation and is distinguished from acquired hypertensive heart disease. Initially this disease was called idiopathic hypertrophic subaortic stenosis, but it was recognized that subaortic obstruction was only one feature of cardiac hypertrophy. In some cases, the left ventricle or interventricular septum is predominantly involved. The disease is genetically transmitted as an autosomal-dominant trait. The disease can cause sudden death in young patients. Chest radiographs most commonly show

normal heart size. This is because the hypertrophy decreases ventricular capacity but does not increase ventricular size. *Acquired* or *secondary hypertrophic cardiomyopathy* can be caused by essential hypertension, renal and adrenal disease, endocrine diseases, and left ventricular outflow obstruction (i.e., aortic stenosis).

Restrictive cardiomyopathy is characterized by impaired filling of noncompliant ventricles and diastolic dysfunction. Either right- or left-sided symptoms may predominate. Causes include amyloidosis, scleroderma, endomyocardial fibrosis, carcinoid heart disease, sarcoidosis, radiation, and familial or idiopathic origins. Heart size and contour are usually normal on chest radiography. As the disease progresses, a combination of both enlargement and a thick left ventricular wall may develop. Because of the stiff right and left ventricles, the right and left

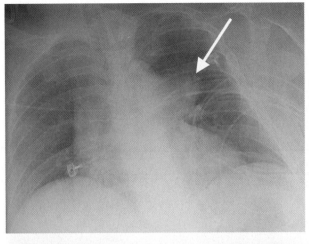

A

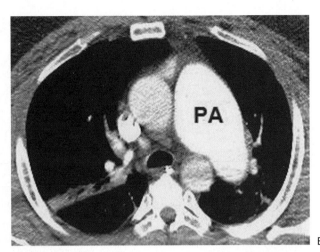

B

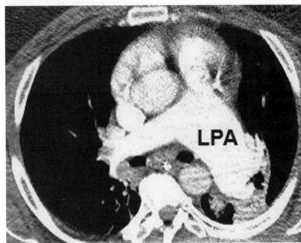

C

FIGURE 18-12. Pulmonic stenosis. A: Anteroposterior chest radiograph of a 52-year-old man shows an abnormal opacity in the expected location of the main and left pulmonary arteries (*arrow*). B: CT shows marked enlargement of the main pulmonary artery (*PA*). C: CT at a level inferior to (B) shows marked enlargement of the left pulmonary artery (*LPA*) and a normal-size right pulmonary artery.

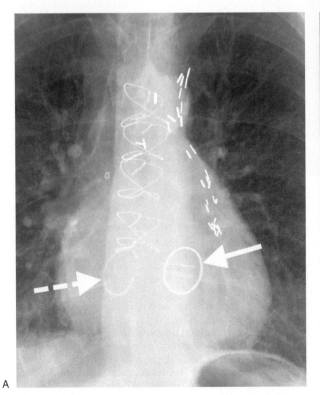

A

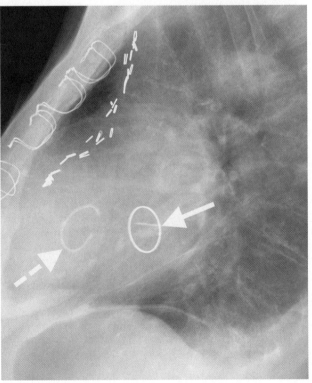

B

FIGURE 18-13. Multivalvular disease. PA (A) and lateral (B) chest radiographs of a 66-year-old woman with a history of rheumatic fever show mitral (*solid arrows*) and tricuspid (*dashed arrows*) valve prostheses.

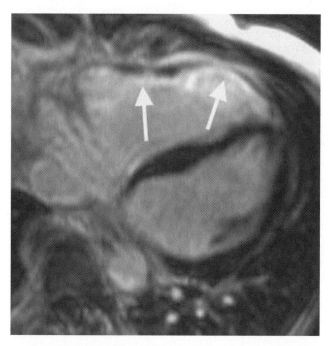

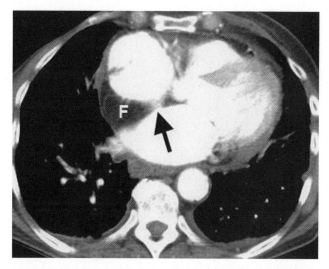

FIGURE 18-15. Lipomatous hypertrophy of the interatrial septum. CT of a 72-year-old woman shows fatty infiltration of the interatrial septum (*F*), which spares the fossa ovalis (*arrow*).

FIGURE 18-14. Arrhythmogenic right ventricular dysplasia. MRI shows delayed hyperenhancement of the right ventricular free wall (*arrows*). (Image courtesy of David Bluemke, MD, PhD, Johns Hopkins Medical Institutions, Baltimore, MD.)

atria dilate in response to filling the ventricles under increased diastolic pressure. Dilated venae cavae, large atria, and small ventricles are also features of constrictive pericarditis, and the two may be difficult to distinguish. The presence of a thickened and calcified pericardium is relatively specific for constrictive pericarditis. However, not all constrictive pericarditis is calcified, and some patients with restrictive cardiomyopathy may have mild thickening of the pericardium.

Arrhythmogenic right ventricular dysplasia (ARVD), an idiopathic cardiomyopathy, is a myocardial disorder of primarily the right ventricle that is more common in males than females and has a frequent familial occurrence (11). The disorder is characterized by transmural or nontransmural infiltration of the right ventricular myocardium with fat or fibrous tissue, diffuse thinning of the right ventricular myocardium, dyskinesia of the right ventricle, and abnormal enhancement on delayed images (12) (Fig. 18-14). MRI is the optimal technique for detection and follow-up of clinically suspected ARVD. Clinically, ARVD is characterized by ventricular arrhythmias with left bundle branch block that may lead to cardiac arrest. It is recognized as a major cause of sudden death in young adolescents. The differential diagnosis of ARVD includes idiopathic dilated cardiomyopathy (usually presenting with a progressive decline in left ventricular function, as opposed to the right ventricular failure seen in ARVD) and the Uhl anomaly (characterized by a paper-thin right ventricle owing to the nearly complete absence of myocardial muscle fibers, with no gender predilection or familial occurrence). The diagnosis of ARVD is based on the presence of structural, histologic, electrocardiographic, and genetic factors. Positive MRI findings serve as an important criterion in the clinical diagnosis of ARVD, although negative MRI findings do not rule out ARVD.

Lipomatous Hypertrophy of the Interatrial Septum

Lipomatous hypertrophy of the interatrial septum (LHIS) is a benign disorder characterized by the accumulation of fat in the interatrial septum. The term is actually a misnomer, as the disorder is caused by an increase in the number, and not hypertrophy, of adipocytes (13). It typically occurs in elderly and obese patients. The thickness of the fatty septum is typically between 2 and 6 mm (14). CT shows a mass of fat attenuation with sharp margins and sparing of the fossa ovalis (Fig. 18-15), resulting in a dumbbell shape. The diagnosis is most commonly made incidentally and is usually unassociated with symptoms, although it can lead to rhythm disturbances such as P-wave abnormalities, atrial fibrillation, and even sudden death.

Cardiac Masses

The most common intracardiac mass is thrombus, which is usually located within the left atrium or the left ventricle and is associated with mitral valve disease, atrial fibrillation, or cardiomyopathy. The distinction between tumor and thrombus is made on MRI by the difference in signal characteristics or on MRI or CT by the presence or absence of enhancement after administration of contrast material. Tumor is usually hyperintense in comparison with myocardium and skeletal muscle (and thrombus) on T2-weighted MRI images and typically enhances with contrast on MRI or CT images (whereas thrombus does not enhance).

In all age groups, benign primary cardiac neoplasms are more common than malignant ones (13). Myxomas are the most common primary cardiac neoplasms, accounting for about 50% of all primary cardiac tumors. They are located in the left atrium in 75% of cases and in the right atrium in 20%. Unlike thrombus, left atrial myxomas are typically attached by a narrow pedicle to the area of the fossa ovalis (Fig. 18-16). They usually have heterogenous low attenuation on CT and are frequently calcified. Rhabdomyomas are the most common cardiac tumors in children, with up to 50% occurring in children with tuberous sclerosis. They typically occur in the left or right ventricle. Other benign cardiac tumors include papillary fibroelastoma (usually attached to the valves by a short pedicle); fibromas (arising in the myocardial walls, commonly calcified, and associated with arrhythmias and sudden death); lipoma; pheochromocytoma (most often located outside the cardiac chamber); and hemangioma.

One fourth of primary cardiac tumors are malignant, with sarcomas representing the largest number, followed by primary

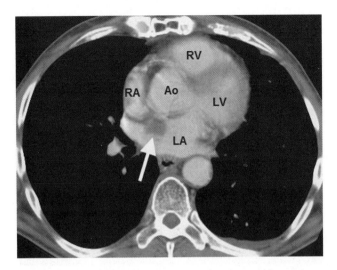

FIGURE 18-16. Left atrial myxoma. CT of a 63-year-old man shows a low-attenuation mass (*arrow*) in the anterior left atrium (*LA*), along the interatrial septum. Note the right atrium (*RA*), aortic outflow track (*Ao*), right ventricle (*RV*), and left ventricle (*LV*).

cardiac lymphomas. Malignant cardiac tumors typically involve more than one cardiac chamber; extend into pulmonary veins, pulmonary arteries, or vena cavae; have a wide point of attachment to the wall of a chamber or chambers; extend outside the heart; and are associated with internal necrosis and hemorrhagic pericardial effusion.

Metastases to the heart and pericardium are much more common than primary cardiac tumors (15). Melanoma, lymphoma, and breast cancer are the most common tumors to metastasize to the heart (Fig. 18-17). Tumors of the lung and mediastinum can locally invade the pericardium and heart (Fig. 18-18). Focal obliteration of the pericardial line with or without effusion indicates extension of tumor into the pericardial sac. If the effusion is hemorrhagic, extension is almost certain.

Coronary Artery Disease

Coronary arteriography is the accepted method used to examine the coronary arteries. However, technological advancements with CT and MRI have dramatically improved the ability to noninvasively image the coronary arteries. Electrocardiography-gated multidetector CT shows promise as

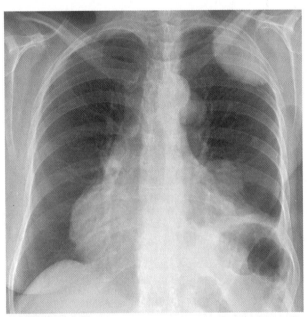

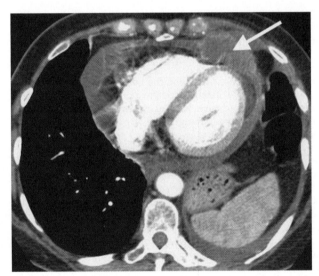

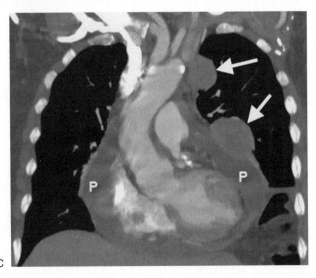

FIGURE 18-17. Pericardial metastases. A: PA chest radiograph of a 76-year-old woman with breast cancer shows an enlarged cardiac silhouette and numerous pleural-based masses. The left hemidiaphragm is elevated, and there is blunting of the left costophrenic angle. B: CT shows pericardial and left pleural effusions, as well as a soft tissue mass infiltrating the anterior pericardium (*arrow*). C: Coronal reformatted CT shows left pleural-based masses (*arrows*) and pericardial effusion (*P*). The more inferior mass involves the pericardium.

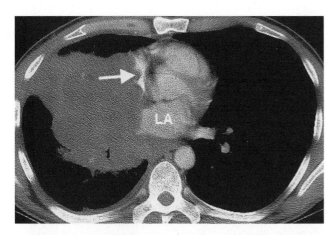

FIGURE 18-18. Carcinoma invading the heart. CT shows a large right lung mass compressing the superior vena cava (*arrow*) and left atrium (*LA*). The right superior and inferior pulmonary veins are obliterated.

a comprehensive method for evaluating cardiac and noncardiac chest pain in stable emergency department patients (16). Among the diagnoses that can be made on CT in addition to coronary artery disease are aortic dissection and pulmonary embolism (the so-called "triple rule-out"). Further hardware and software improvements will be necessary before CT can replace coronary arteriography and become widely used in clinical practice.

Cardiac Anatomy

Multidetector CT, even in routine use to evaluate the lungs, can provide information about the morphology of the heart and coronary arteries. Therefore, it is important to have an understanding of the normal anatomy and CT appearance of these structures. On axial imaging, the right ventricle is anterior and has a triangular appearance, whereas the left ventricle is posterior and more ovoid. The maximum internal diameter of the right ventricle in its small axis should be equivalent to that of the left ventricle (17). The normal myocardial thickness of the right ventricle is 3 to 4 mm, approximately three times thinner than that of the left ventricle. The interventricular septum does not normally measure more than 13 mm in thickness. Anterior and posterior trabecular muscles, and the smaller medial papillary muscle, are connected to the tricuspid valve leaflets via the chordae tendineae in the right ventricle. The moderator band extends from the interventricular septum to the anterolateral aspect of the right ventricle in the region of the ventricular apex, where it inserts at the base of the anterior papillary muscle. It conveys the electrical apparatus of the right bundle of His. Anterior and posterior papillary muscles can also be seen in the left ventricle connecting to the leaflets of the mitral valve via chordae tendineae.

The crista terminalis can be recognized as a muscular prominence on the posterolateral aspect of the right atrium extending from the orifice of the superior vena cava to that of the inferior vena cava, and should not be mistaken for intracavitary tumor or thrombus on CT. The atrioventricular valves are located at the base of each ventricle.

The coronary arteries arise from the right and left coronary cusps, which are anatomic dilations of the ascending aorta at the aortic root, just above the aortic valve. (Figs. 18-19 and 18-20). Each aortic sinus can also be referred to as a sinus of Valsalva. The left main coronary artery arises from the left coronary cusp and passes behind the pulmonary trunk. It divides into the left anterior descending (LAD) and left circumflex (Cx) arteries. Occasionally, the left main coronary artery termi-

nates in a trifurcation, giving rise to an intermediate coronary artery (ramus intermedius) that is directed laterally. The LAD artery courses along the anterior interventricular groove. Diagonal branches arise from the LAD and course at downward angles to supply the anterolateral free wall of the left ventricle. The LAD supplies the anterior two thirds of the septum, the anterior and anterolateral walls, the apex, and the anterolateral papillary muscle. The Cx artery extends laterally and posteriorly in the left atrioventricular groove and gives rise to obtuse marginal branches that extend on the lateral and posterior wall toward the apex. The Cx artery supplies the lateral left ventricular wall and anterolateral papillary muscle.

The right coronary artery typically arises from the right coronary cusp. It passes between the right ventricular outflow tract and the right atrial appendage and then runs in the right atrioventricular sulcus. The right coronary artery supplies the posterior one third of the septum, the inferior surface of the left ventricular and right ventricular free wall and the posteromedial papillary muscle. The distal right coronary artery courses along the diaphragmatic surface of the heart. The right coronary artery branches are the conus branch, the right ventricular branches, the acute marginal branch and the posterior descending artery. The posterior descending artery arises from a dominant right coronary artery in 85% of individuals and it courses in the posterior interventricular sulcus.

Anomalous origin of a coronary artery can occur from the pulmonary artery or aorta (Figs. 18-21 and 18-22). Ectopic origin of coronary arteries from the aorta is found in approximately 1% of the population (18). On occasion, these anomalies are seen incidentally on CT. The most common anomaly is ectopic origin of the Cx artery from the right coronary cusp or right coronary artery. When a major coronary artery such as the left main or LAD passes between the pulmonary artery and the aorta, the patient can suffer from angina pectoris, myocardial infarction, or sudden death.

Coronary Artery Calcification

Electron beam or helical multidetector CT of the coronary arteries is being used increasingly often for the detection and quantification of calcium deposits. A calcium "score" is computed and compared with data normalized by sex and age. An elevated score may be a signal of clinically significant disease. There are several limitations to this test. Not all calcium deposits in the coronary arteries mean that there is a blockage, and not all blocked arteries contain calcium. A high heart rate may interfere with the test. Exactly how the calcium score relates to the likelihood of experiencing angina, myocardial infarction, and sudden cardiac death remains uncertain. Men younger than 35 years of age and women younger than 40 are not likely to benefit from the test unless there are risk factors such as diabetes or a strong family history of heart disease. Men older than 65 years and women older than 70 are not likely to be treated differently as a result of test findings.

Calcification of the coronary arteries is a frequent incidental finding on chest radiography and routine chest CT (Fig. 18-23). In this setting, the observation should not be considered clinically significant unless the patient is under the age of 40.

Cardiac Postoperative Complications

Coronary artery bypass grafting (CABG) and percutaneous coronary intervention have long been the definitive aggressive options for treating patients with coronary artery disease (19). These treatments, particularly CABG, are associated with a variety of acute and chronic postoperative complications. Similar complications are seen after valve replacement, although anticoagulation therapy for valve replacement results in more problems with bleeding. Acute complications resulting

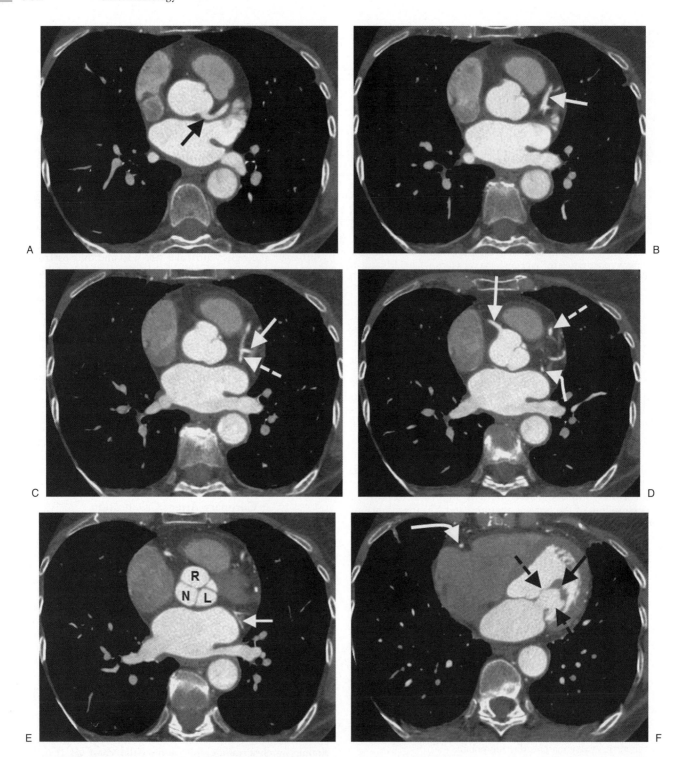

FIGURE 18-19. Cardiac anatomy. A: Electrocardiography-gated multidetector CT shows a normal left main coronary artery (*arrow*) arising from the left coronary cusp. **B:** The left anterior descending coronary artery (*arrow*) arises from the left main coronary artery and courses anteriorly in the interventricular groove. **C:** Occasionally, as in this case, the left main coronary artery terminates in a trifurcation, giving rise to an intermediate coronary artery (ramus intermedius; *solid arrow*), left anterior descending coronary artery (coursing anteriorly), and left circumflex coronary artery (*dashed arrow*). **D:** The right coronary artery arises from the right coronary cusp (*solid arrow*). Note the left anterior descending coronary artery (*dashed arrow*) and circumflex coronary artery (*curved arrow*). **E:** The circumflex coronary artery gives rise to marginal branches (*arrow*). Note the left (*L*), right (*R*), and noncoronary (*N*) cusps. **F:** Papillary muscles (*solid black arrow*) are connected to the mitral valve leaflets via the chordae tendineae (*dashed black arrows*). Note the right coronary artery (*curved white arrow*). (*Continued*)

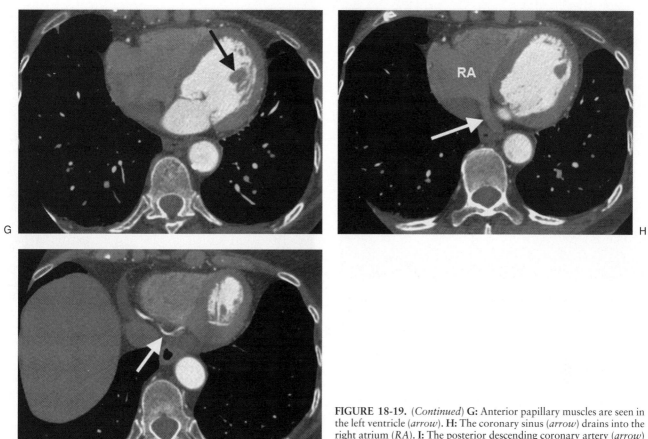

FIGURE 18-19. (*Continued*) G: Anterior papillary muscles are seen in the left ventricle (*arrow*). H: The coronary sinus (*arrow*) drains into the right atrium (*RA*). I: The posterior descending coronary artery (*arrow*) arises from the right coronary artery in 85% of individuals and courses in the posterior interventricular sulcus.

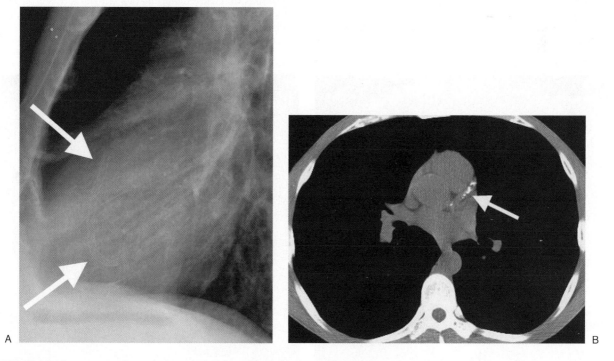

FIGURE 18-20. **Coronary artery stent. A:** Lateral chest radiograph of a 46-year-old man shows a right coronary artery stent (*arrows*). **B:** CT shows calcification in the left main and left anterior descending arteries (*arrow*).

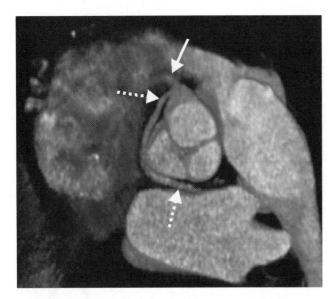

FIGURE 18-21. Anomalous origin of coronary artery. CT shows the right main coronary artery arising from the right coronary cusp (*solid arrow*). The left main coronary artery also arises from the right coronary cusp and courses posterior to the aorta (*dashed arrows*). This is considered a benign anomalous course. (Case courtesy of Cris A. Meyer, MD, and Rhonda Strunk, RT, R(CT), University of Cincinnati 3D Post Processing Lab, University of Cincinnati Medical Center, Cincinnati, OH.)

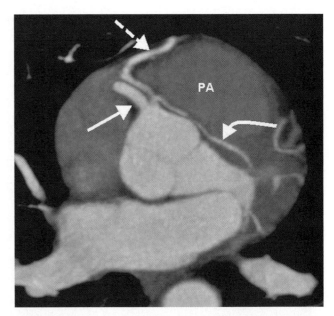

FIGURE 18-22. Anomalous origin of coronary artery. CT shows the right main coronary artery arising from the right coronary cusp (*solid arrow*). The left main coronary artery also arises from the right coronary cusp. The left anterior descending coronary artery courses anterior to the pulmonary artery, a benign course (*dashed arrow*). The circumflex coronary artery (*angled arrow*) courses posteriorly, between the aorta and pulmonary artery (*PA*). This anomaly can result in angina pectoris or myocardial infarction. (Case courtesy of Cris A. Meyer, MD, and Rhonda Strunk, RT, R(CT), University of Cincinnati 3D Post Processing Lab, University of Cincinnati Medical Center, Cincinnati, OH.)

from cardiac surgery include atelectasis, edema, hemorrhage, pericardial effusion, and extrapulmonary air collections (e.g., pneumothorax, pneumomediastinum). Chronic complications include postpericardiotomy syndrome (a febrile illness consisting of various combinations of pericarditis, pleuritis, and pneumonitis); constrictive pericarditis; postoperative infection; pseudoaneurysm; and aortic dissection.

CT is helpful in evaluating poststernotomy complications. Expected postoperative changes, which can persist for 2 to

3 weeks, include minimal presternal and retrosternal soft tissue infiltration with edema and blood, focal retrosternal air and fluid, localized hematoma, postincisional bone defects, minor sternal irregularities or offset, and minimal pericardial thickening (20). After this period of time, these changes should prompt

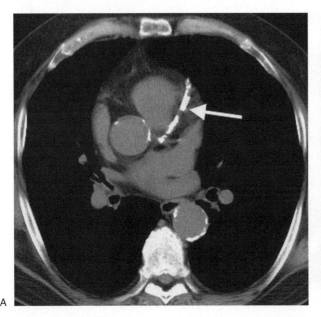

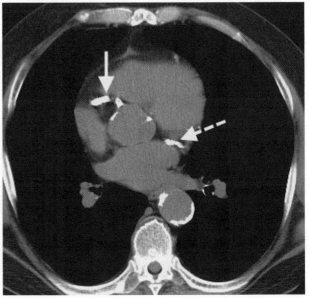

FIGURE 18-23. Coronary artery calcification. A: CT of a 66-year-old man shows dense calcification in the left anterior descending coronary artery (*arrow*). **B:** CT at a level inferior to (B) shows dense calcification of the circumflex coronary artery (*dashed arrow*) and a stent in the right coronary artery (*solid arrow*).

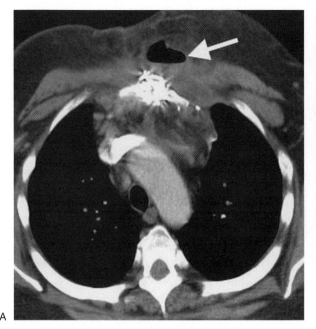
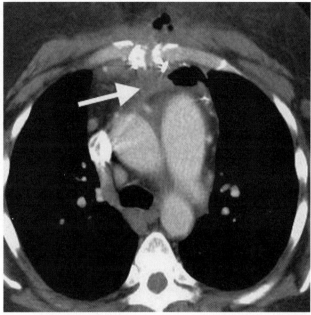

FIGURE 18-24. **Poststernotomy infection. A:** CT of a 47-year-old woman who underwent coronary artery bypass grafting shows fluid in the presternal and retrosternal areas and an air–fluid level in the presternal area (*arrow*). **B:** CT at a level inferior to (**A**) shows abnormal air and fluid in the retrosternal area (*arrow*).

consideration of infection, especially when focal collections of presternal or retrosternal air and fluid are seen (Figs. 18-24 and 18-25). Noninfected mediastinal fluid collections can also be seen at this time, and only bacteriological analysis can differentiate bland from infected fluid collections.

Aneurysms of saphenous vein grafts to coronary arteries are unusual complications of CABG surgery, with only 50 cases reported since 1975 (21). True aneurysms are atherosclerotic in nature and appear as a late postoperative com-

plication more than 5 years after CABG. Pseudoaneurysms may occur early as well as late after initial surgery, at the anastomotic site in most cases. Whenever a new mediastinal mass is seen on chest radiography in a patient who has undergone CABG, a graft aneurysm should be considered, and CT or MRI with intravenous contrast should be obtained. CT shows a round mass adjacent to a graft site with variable degrees of luminal enhancement or thrombus (Fig. 18-26).

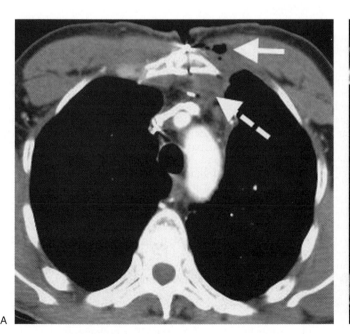
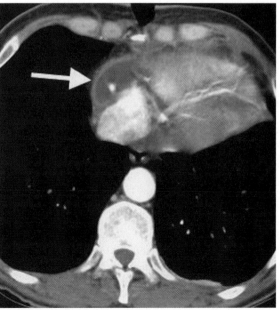

FIGURE 18-25. **Poststernotomy infection. A:** CT performed 13 days after coronary artery bypass grafting shows air in the presternal area (*solid arrow*) and fluid in the retrosternal area (*dashed arrow*). **B:** CT at a level inferior to (**A**) shows a focal fluid collection with an enhancing rim (*arrow*) encasing the right coronary artery.

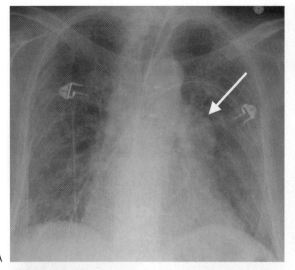

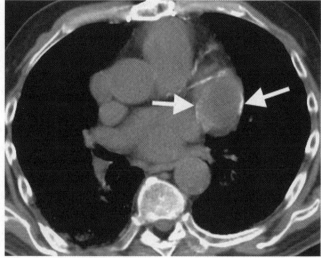

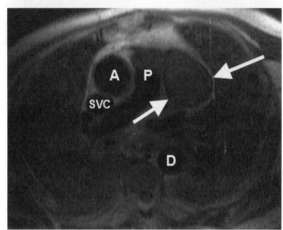

FIGURE 18-26. Coronary artery bypass graft aneurysm. A: PA chest radiograph of a 70-year-old woman with a history of coronary artery bypass grafting shows an abnormal left mediastinal contour (*arrow*). B: CT shows a round mass with peripheral calcification (*arrows*) at a graft site. C: MRI shows the graft aneurysm (*arrows*) adjacent to the main pulmonary artery (*P*). Note the ascending aorta (*A*), superior vena cava (*SVC*), and descending aorta (*D*).

More and more patients are undergoing percutaneous stenting of diseased coronary arteries as an alternative to CABG. These stents can be visualized on routine chest radiography and CT (Figs. 18-20 and 18-23).

Complications After Myocardial Infarction

Ischemic myocardial disease may be associated with a normal chest radiograph, or the radiograph may show nonspecific signs of cardiac failure. Ventricular aneurysm formation can complicate previous myocardial infarction in up to 10% of cases, occurring between 2 weeks and 2 years after ischemic myocardial necrosis and being located most often on the anterior wall of the left ventricle or at the cardiac apex (17) (Fig. 18-27). An abnormal bulge to the lower left heart border on a frontal chest radiograph may be seen. CT can show thinning of the involved myocardium, hypodensity in the abnormal ventricular wall that approaches that of fat, myocardial calcification, or local endoluminal thrombus. True ventricular aneurysms arising from previous myocardial infarction with associated scar formation and thinning of the myocardium should be differentiated from ventricular pseudoaneurysms, which are characterized by actual rupture of the myocardium and containment of the aneurysm by only the thin pericardium and which are at high risk of fatal rupture (17). Pseudoaneurysms are typically inferior in location and have a more discrete, narrower neck than true aneurysms. CT is helpful in distinguishing aneurysm from pseudoaneurysm by demonstrating a narrow orifice or

"neck" leading from the ventricular chamber to a pseudoaneurysm.

Pericardial Disease

The pericardium is outlined by epicardial and pericardial fat, and the two layers of the pericardium together normally measure no more than 3 mm in thickness. It is important to understand the anatomy of the pericardial recesses and not mistake them for enlarged lymph nodes or other masses, especially in the right paratracheal region (Fig. 18-28), in the aortopulmonary window, in the subcarinal region, and around the insertion of the pulmonary veins (Fig. 18-29). When visible, pericardial recesses can usually be recognized as having fluid attenuation on CT.

The more common causes of pericardial effusion are listed in Table 18-2 (8). Cardiac tamponade is a low cardiac output state caused by excess fluid in the pericardial space that compresses the heart (Fig. 18-30). This can occur when as little as 150 to 250 mL of fluid accumulate acutely. In chronic or recurrent pericarditis, pericardial fluid may accumulate slowly, so that several liters may be present without tamponade occurring. Enlargement of the cardiac silhouette on the chest radiograph usually is not apparent until 250 mL of fluid are in the pericardial space. A typical chest radiograph of a patient with a pericardial effusion shows a wide cardiac silhouette with little abnormality in the lungs. The classic appearance is that of a "water bottle–shaped heart," in which both sides of the

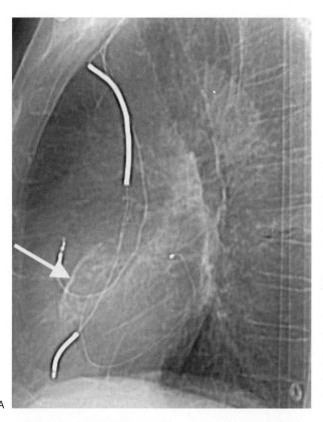
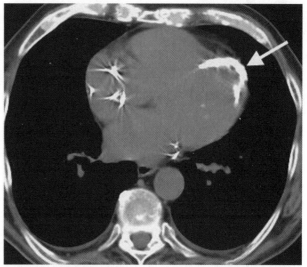

FIGURE 18-27. Left ventricular aneurysm. A: Lateral CT scout image of a 78-year-old man with ischemic cardiomy-opathy and previous anteroseptal and apical septal myocardial infarction shows a curvilinear area of calcification overlying the heart (*arrow*). B: CT shows a focal outpouching of the left ventricular apex with a densely calcified rim (*arrow*). Note the relatively wide aneurysmal neck, which is typical of true aneurysms and distinguishes this from a pseudoaneurysm.

heart appear rounded and displaced laterally. The epicardial "fat pad" sign is produced when the pericardial layers and fluid widen the space between the anterior epicardial fat and substernal fat stripes by more than 4 mm. This is best appreci-ated on the lateral chest radiograph. Pulmonary edema is rarely seen in cardiac tamponade unless another disease, such as left ventricular failure from myocardial infarction, is also present. Diagnostic mimics of large pericardial effusions include pan-chamber cardiac enlargement and a large anterior mediastinal tumor in front of the heart.

In chronic constrictive pericarditis, ventricular filling is im-peded by loss of compliance. The cardiac chambers are con-stricted by the thickened pericardium, and diastolic pressures are elevated. In constrictive pericarditis, the thickness of the pericardial layers typically exceeds 4 mm. The pericardium is calcified on the chest radiograph in about 50% of patients with constrictive pericarditis and presents as a curvilinear opacity conforming to the anatomy of the pericardial sac (Fig. 18-31).

(Text continues on page 310)

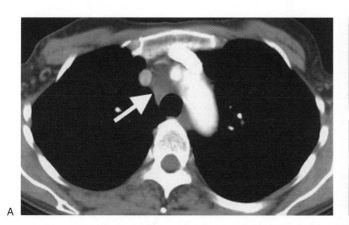
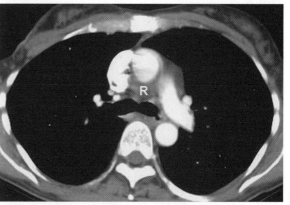

FIGURE 18-28. Right paratracheal pericardial recess. A: CT shows a mass of fluid attenuation in the right paratra-cheal area (*arrow*). This fluid collection should not be mistaken for paratracheal lymphadenopathy. B: CT at a level inferior to (A) shows pericardial recess fluid (*R*) posterior to the ascending aorta.

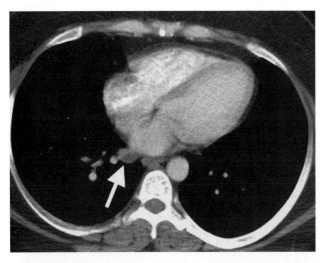

FIGURE 18-29. Right pulmonary vein pericardial recess. CT shows a focal fluid collection (*arrow*) adjacent to the right inferior pulmonary vein. This should not be mistaken for lymphadenopathy or other masses.

TABLE 18-2

COMMON CAUSES OF PERICARDIAL EFFUSION

Serous
Congestive heart failure
Hypoalbuminemia
Collagen vascular disease
Hypothyroidism (myxedema)
Bloody
Acute myocardial infarction
Trauma, including cardiac surgery (postpericardiotomy syndrome)
Neoplasm
Chronic renal failure
Purulent
Bacterial
Viral (especially coxsackievirus)
Mycobacterial
Fungal and parasitic

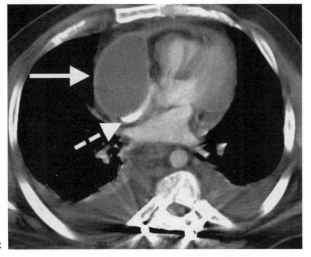

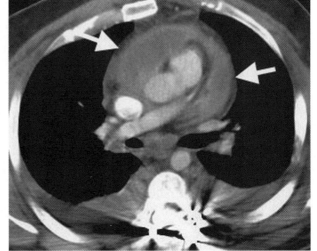

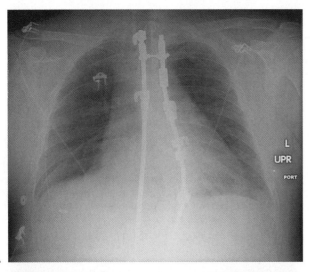

FIGURE 18-30. Acute infectious pericarditis. A: PA chest radiograph of a 26-year-old man with a neck abscess shows an enlarged cardiac silhouette. **B:** CT shows high-density pericardial fluid and thickening and enhancement of the pericardium (*arrows*). **C:** CT at a level inferior to (**B**) shows a focal pericardial fluid collection (*solid arrow*) compressing the superior vena cava (*dashed arrow*) and left atrium. The patient had clinical symptoms of pericardial tamponade.

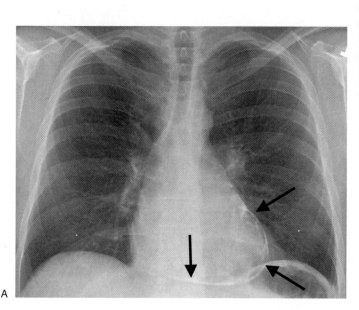
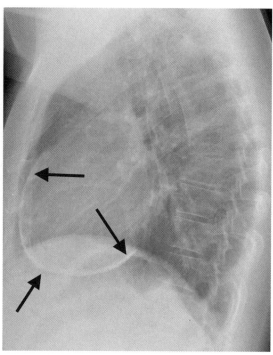

FIGURE 18-31. **Constrictive pericarditis.** PA (**A**) and lateral (**B**) chest radiographs show curvilinear calcification conforming to the anatomy of the pericardial sac (*arrows*).

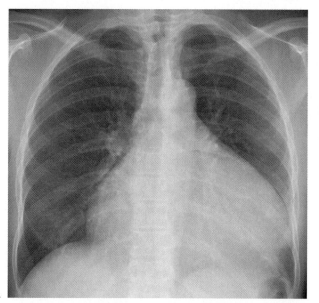
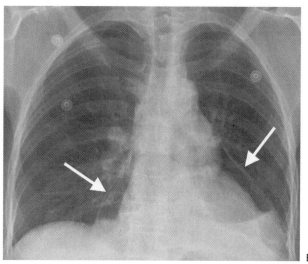

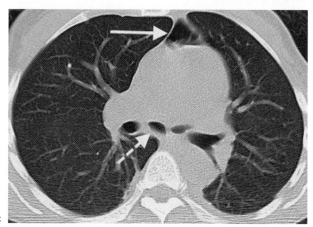

FIGURE 18-32. **Uremic pericarditis. A:** PA chest radiograph of a 33-year-old woman with acute chest pain and a history of human immunodeficiency virus infection–related nephropathy shows a "water bottle"–shaped heart. **B:** After drainage of exudative pericardial fluid, the chest radiograph shows air outlining the pericardial sac (*arrows*). **C:** CT shows pneumopericardium (*solid arrow*), including air in the pericardial recess (*dashed arrow*).

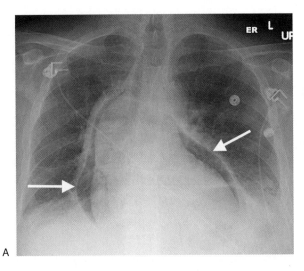
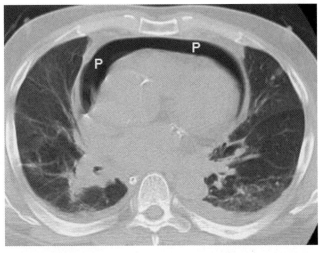

FIGURE 18-33. Purulent pericarditis. **A:** PA chest radiograph of a 61-year-old man with acute chest pain shows pneumopericardium (*arrows*). The air in the pericardial sac does not extend above the aortic arch. **B:** CT shows air confined to the pericardial sac (*P*). One hundred forty milliliters of gas and pus were drained via pericardiocentesis.

When the calcifications are thin and linear, the etiology is usually viral or uremic pericarditis. Other causes include collagen vascular disease, trauma (including postsurgery), and radiation. When shaggy, thick, and amorphous, the calcification has historically been attributed to tuberculosis. Asbestos can also affect the pericardium, creating thick plaques similar to those occurring in asbestos-related pleural disease. MRI does not show calcification but demonstrates pericardial thickening and sometimes can be used to show impaired diastolic function. Because CT will detect minute amounts of calcium and MRI can miss significant deposits, some have advocated the use of MRI for the diagnosis of constrictive pericarditis only in those patients who have contraindications to iodinated contrast material (22). Additional findings seen with constrictive pericarditis include distorted contours of the ventricles (tubular-shaped ventricles), hepatic venous congestion, ascites, pleural effusions, and occasionally pericardial effusion. Often the atria, coronary sinus, inferior vena cava, and hepatic veins are dilated, reflecting elevated central venous pressure. Patients with constrictive pericarditis and restrictive cardiomyopathy can have similar clinical and physiologic findings. The presence of pericardial thickening or other signs of constriction suggests that the abnormality is pericardial in origin. A normal pericardium with thickening of the myocardium suggests cardiomyopathy as the diagnosis.

Numerous congenital abnormalities of the pericardium can occur. Pericardial cysts are discussed in Chapter 6. Absence of the pericardium can be complete but is more often partial, with the defects more often left-sided. When most of the pericardium is absent, the heart axis will usually shift to the left and posteriorly. Partial absence of the left pericardium can result in a prominent-appearing left atrial appendage or pulmonary artery segment. Herniation of the heart through a congenital, traumatic, or surgical pericardial defect is rare but life threatening.

Pneumopericardium is gas in the pericardial sac and can rarely be idiopathic but more commonly results from trauma; infection with a gas-forming organism; increased intrathoracic pressure (e.g., asthma, barotrauma, Valsalva maneuver); adjacent lung cancer or infection; esophageal rupture; forceful coughing; cocaine abuse; gastric perforation; liver abscess; pancreatic pseudocyst; or pregnancy. When a large amount of air

collects in the pericardial sac acutely, the patient can suffer from cardiac tamponade. On chest radiography, pneumopericardium presents as lucency confined to the pericardial sac that does not extend above the aortic arch (Fig. 18-32). CT clearly shows air confined to the pericardial sac, distinguishing it from pneumomediastinum (Fig. 18-33).

References

1. Steiner RM, Gross GW, Flicker S, et al. Congenital heart disease in the adult patient: the value of plain film chest radiology. *J Thorac Imaging*. 1995;10:1–25.
2. Gross GW, Steiner RM. Radiographic manifestations of congenital heart disease in the adult patient. *Radiol Clin North Am*. 1991;29:293–317.
3. Child JS, Perloff JK. Natural survival patterns. In: Perloff JK, Child JS, eds. *Congenital Heart Disease in Adults*. Philadelphia: WB Saunders; 1991:21–52.
4. Boxt LM, Reagan K, Katz J. Normal plain film examination of the heart and great arteries in the adult. *J Thorac Imaging*. 1994;9:208–218.
5. Soto B, Bargeron LM Jr, Diethelm E. Ventricular septal defect. *Semin Roentgenol*. 1985;20:200.
6. Perloff JK. Congenital heart disease in adults. In: Braunwald E, ed. *Heart Disease*. Philadelphia: WB Saunders; 1991:966–990.
7. Stewart JR, Kincaid OW, Titus JL. Right aortic arch: plain film diagnosis and significance. *AJR Am J Roentgenol*. 1966;97:377.
8. Miller SW, ed. *Cardiac Radiology. The Requisites*. St. Louis, MO: Mosby–Year Book; 1994:157, 270, 432.
9. Edwards JE. On etiology of calcified aortic stenosis. *Circulation*. 1962;26:817–818.
10. Gurney JW, Goodman LR. Pulmonary edema localized in the right upper lobe accompanying mitral regurgitation. *Radiology*. 1989;171:397–399.
11. Kayser HWM, van der Wall EE, Sivananthan MU, et al. Diagnosis of arrhythmogenic right ventricular dysplasia: a review. *Radiographics*. 2002;22:639–648.
12. Tandri H, Saranathan M, Rodriguez ER, et al. Noninvasive detection of myocardial fibrosis in arrhythmogenic right ventricular cardiomyopathy using delayed-enhancement magnetic resonance imaging. *J Am Coll Cardiol*. 2005;45:98–103.
13. Araoz PA, Mulvagh SL, Tazelaar HD, et al. CT and MR imaging of benign primary cardiac neoplasms with echocardiographic correlation. *Radiographics*. 2000;20:1303–1319.
14. Heyer CM, Kagel T, Lemburg SP, et al. Lipomatous hypertrophy of the interatrial septum: a prospective study of incidence, imaging findings, and clinical symptoms. *Chest*. 2003;124:2068–2073.
15. Chiles C, Woodard PK, Gutierrez FR, et al. Metastatic involvement of the heart and pericardium: CT and MR imaging. *Radiographics*. 2001;21:439–449.

16. White CS, Kuo D, Kelemen M, et al. Chest pain evaluation in the emergency department: can MDCT provide a comprehensive evaluation? *AJR Am J Roentgenol.* 2005;185:533–540.

17. Bruzzi JF, Remy-Jardin M, Delhaye D, et al. When, why, and how to examine the heart during thoracic CT: part 1, basic principles. *AJR Am J Roentgenol.* 2006;186:324–332.

18. Baltaxe H, Wixson D. The incidence of congenital anomalies of the coronary arteries in the adult population. *Radiology.* 1977;122:47–52.

19. Hannan EL, Racz MJ, Walford G, et al. Long-term outcomes of coronary-artery bypass grafting verus stent implantation. *N Engl J Med.* 2005;352:2174–2183.

20. Templeton PA, Fishman EK. CT evaluation of poststernotomy complications. *AJR Am J Roentgenol.* 1992;159:45–50.

21. Le Breton H, Langanay T, Roland Y, et al. Aneurysms and pseudoaneurysms of saphenous vein coronary artery bypass grafts. *Heart.* 1998;79:505–508.

22. Breen J. Imaging of the pericardium. *J Thoracic Imaging.* 2001;16:47–54.

THORACIC AORTA

This chapter will focus on acquired aortic diseases, expanding on the content provided in Chapters 6 and 18. Chest computed tomography (CT) and magnetic resonance imaging (MRI) have replaced conventional angiography as the primary imaging modalities in the evaluation of thoracic aortic disease. In particular, multidetector CT is able to quickly and accurately provide imaging information regarding the diagnosis (e.g., dissection, aneurysm, intramural hematoma, penetrating ulcer), location, and extent of aortic disease, in addition to providing information regarding alternative diagnoses for the patient's symptomatology. Information provided by CT is also useful in presurgical planning and postsurgical follow-up.

AORTIC DISSECTION

Acute aortic dissection is the most common cause of aortic emergency, exceeding that of thoracoabdominal aortic aneurysm rupture (1). Dissection is a life-threatening condition that requires immediate diagnosis and treatment. Intramural hematoma and penetrating atherosclerotic ulcer, discussed later in this chapter, are considered by some to represent atypical forms of dissection. All three entities can produce chest or back pain in a patient with hypertension. Thoracic aortic dissection is classified as acute if the symptoms last fewer than 2 weeks and chronic if the symptoms last longer (2).

Acute aortic dissection occurs most commonly in the sixth and seventh decades of life. However, it can also occur in patients under 40 years of age, especially those with Marfan syndrome (3). Risk factors for the development of aortic dissection are listed in Table 19-1. The initiating event is usually a tear in the intima of the aortic wall that allows blood to enter the media, resulting in separation of the intima from the adventitia. Dissection can also occur as a sequela of pre-existing intramural hematoma or penetrating atherosclerotic ulcer. The sites of intimal tear are most commonly within a few centimeters of the aortic valve (60%), at the origin of the descending aorta just distal to the left subclavian artery (30%), and in the aortic arch (10%) (2).

Two classification schemes are used to describe aortic dissection. Both define the descending aorta as distal to the left subclavian artery. The most widely used scheme is the Stanford classification, which includes two types, based on whether surgery is required: Type A (60%) involves the ascending aorta

regardless of the site of intimal tear or distal extent (requires immediate repair), whereas type B (40%) does not involve the ascending aorta (treated medically for hypertension unless complications occur) (4). The DeBakey classification is as follows: Type I originates in the ascending aorta and extends distally throughout the aorta, type II is confined to the ascending aorta, and type III originates in the descending aorta and extends distally (5). Complications of type A dissection include rupture into the pericardium (producing cardiac tamponade) and left pleural space, occlusion of coronary artery and aortic arch branches, and severe aortic insufficiency with acute left heart failure. Rupture is less common in type B dissections, which usually progress to a chronic form. However, surgery is indicated for persistent pain or abdominal organ ischemia.

When acute aortic dissection is suspected, unenhanced CT should always precede contrast-enhanced scanning to detect intramural hematoma. The entire aorta must be imaged to assess the extent of disease. Typical aortic dissection is produced by an intimal tear that allows blood to enter the medial layer, giving rise to two lumina—one true and one false (see Fig. 6-28). The main finding on enhanced CT is the presence of an intimal flap separating the true lumen from the false lumen. If the false lumen is thrombosed, the intimal flap may not always be detected. The dissection flap is usually curved in an acute dissection and flat in a chronic dissection. Identification of the two lumens is critical for planning endovascular stent placement. The true lumen tends to lie close to the inner curvature of the aortic arch and anteromedially in the descending aorta, whereas the false lumen commonly lies in the outer portion of aorta (Fig. 19-1). The false lumen usually has a larger cross-sectional diameter than the true lumen and often has intraluminal thrombus, but there is great variability in appearance of the false lumen. Unenhanced CT may show internal displacement of intimal calcifications, if present. The "beak sign" is the cross-sectional imaging manifestation of the wedge of hematoma that cleaves a space for the propagation of the false lumen. Slender, linear areas of low attenuation occasionally appear in the false lumen, known as the "cobweb sign." This sign corresponds to residual ribbons of the media that have been incompletely sheared away by the dissection. Intimointimal intussusception is produced by circumferential dissection of the intimal layer, which subsequently invaginates like a windsock. On CT, this is seen as one lumen wrapped

TABLE 19-1

RISK FACTORS FOR DEVELOPMENT OF AORTIC DISSECTION

Hypertension (most common)
Connective tissue diseases
- Marfan syndrome
- Ehlers-Danlos syndrome
- Turner syndrome
- Familial aortic dissection

Cystic medial necrosis (most commonly associated with Marfan syndrome)
Congenital lesions
- Aortic coarctation
- Bicuspid and unicommissural aortic valve

Trauma
- Cardiac surgery or catheterization
- Blunt trama

Pregnancy
Aortitis
- Aortic aneurysm
- Aortic infection

Cocaine abuse

around the other in the aortic arch, with the inner lumen invariably being the true lumen. Other findings on enhanced CT include delayed enhancement of the false lumen and mediastinal and/or pericardial hematoma. Fluid around the aorta may be a sign of ongoing penetration or perforation.

The key information required for treatment is the extent of the dissection and whether branch vessels originate from the true lumen or the false lumen. When the dissection flap extends into the lumen of a branch vessel and narrows it, treatment is usually angioplasty, with or without deployment of an endovascular stent. Surgical treatment of type A dissection consists of replacement of the ascending aorta, aortic root, and aortic valve and reimplantation of the coronary arteries into the graft (Fig. 19-2).

INTRAMURAL HEMATOMA

Intramural hematoma (IMH) is caused by a spontaneous hemorrhage of the vasa vasorum of the medial layer. Unlike dissection, it is not associated with an intimal tear. The median age of patients with IMH is 68 years, and a common predisposing factor is hypertension (3). IMH, thought to account for approximately 13% of acute aortic dissections (6), is classified according to the Stanford system. It is generally considered to have a more favorable prognosis than classic aortic dissection.

On unenhanced CT, IMH appears as a crescent-shaped area of high attenuation in the aortic wall that corresponds to a hematoma in the medial layer. The hematoma may or may not compress the aortic lumen. Intimal calcifications may be displaced. It is important to perform unenhanced CT prior to

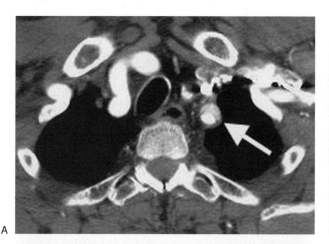

A

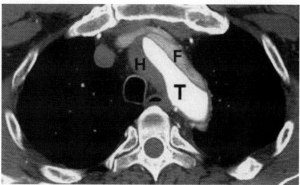

B

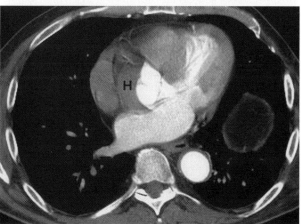

C

FIGURE 19-1. Acute ascending aortic dissection. A: CT of a 50-year-old man with chest pain, numbness of the left hand, and a history of hypertension shows a dissection involving the left subclavian artery (*arrow*). B: CT of the aortic arch shows dense enhancement of the true lumen (*T*), less dense enhancement of the false lumen more laterally (*F*), and medial hematoma (*H*). C: CT at the level of the aortic root shows periaortic hematoma (*H*).

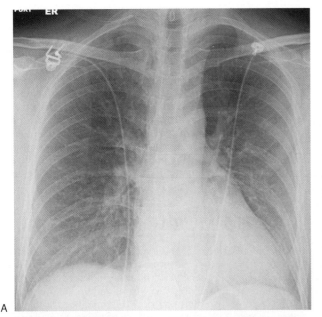

A

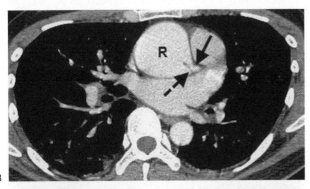

B

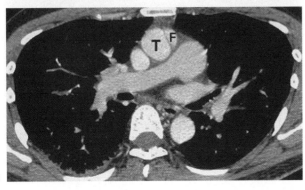

C

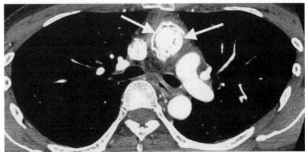

D

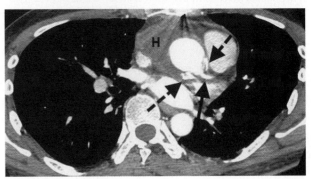

E

FIGURE 19-2. Acute ascending aortic dissection. A: Posteroanterior (PA) chest radiograph of a 31-year-old man with chest pain and shortness of breath shows a normal appearing aorta. Note that a normal appearing aorta on chest radiography does not exclude disease of the ascending aorta. **B:** CT shows a dilated aortic root (*R*). The origin of the left coronary artery is seen (*solid arrow*) and was noted to be involved at the time of surgery. The linear area of low attenuation near the left coronary artery is artifact (*dashed arrow*). **C:** CT at a level inferior to (**B**) shows an intimal flap in the ascending aorta and enhancement of the true (*T*) and false (*F*) lumens. **D:** CT after replacement of the ascending aorta, aortic root, and aortic valve and reimplantation of the left coronary artery shows a "ribbon" of high attenuation surrounding the repair (*arrows*). This is a normal postoperative appearance and should not be mistaken for a contrast leak. **E:** CT at the level of the aortic root, after repair, shows Teflon felt (Meadox Medical Inc., Oakland, NJ) (*dashed arrows*) around the reimplanted left coronary artery (*solid arrow*). A normal postoperative hematoma is seen (*H*).

enhanced CT, as IMH is usually more difficult or impossible to detect on enhanced scans. Unlike the false lumen in aortic dissection, IMH remains unenhanced after administration of contrast. Whereas dissection tends to spiral longitudinally around the aorta, IMH tends to maintain a circumferential relationship with the aortic wall. A type A IMH greater than 5 cm in diameter is at high risk for subsequent aortic dissection or aneurysm formation (3).

PENETRATING ATHEROSCLEROTIC ULCER

Penetrating atherosclerotic ulcer (PAU) is defined as an ulceration of atheromatous plaque that has eroded the inner, elastic

layer of the aortic wall; reached the medial layer; and produced a hematoma in the media (7). Unlike typical aortic dissection, PAU most often occurs in elderly patients with severe underlying atherosclerosis. PAU may lead to aortic dissection, pseudoaneurysm formation if it penetrates through the media, or transmural aortic rupture if it extends through the adventitia (3). The most common location of PAU is the middle or distal third of the descending thoracic aorta, although any portion of the aorta can be involved. Surgical intervention with grafting of the affected area is indicated in patients with hemodynamic instability, persistent or recurrent pain, expanding hematoma, aortic rupture, distal embolization, and development of pseudoaneurysm, pericardial effusion, or bloody pleural effusion.

In patients with PAU, extensive atherosclerosis is usually seen on CT. On unenhanced CT, IMH and displacement of intimal calcification are commonly seen. Enhanced CT shows a collection of contrast material outside the aortic lumen, similar in appearance to a peptic ulcer, with adjacent subintimal hematoma. PAU lesions can be single or multiple. The aortic wall is often thickened. Care should be taken in making a diagnosis of PAU if the lesions are discovered incidentally in an asymptomatic patient and focal IMH is absent. Atheromatous ulcers that are confined to the intimal layer sometimes resemble PAU on enhanced CT. PAU is usually treated medically. Surgery is indicated when symptoms of chest or back pain persist, IMH expands, or there are other signs of impending rupture. Surgery involves local incision of the ulcerated portion of the aorta and replacement with an interposition graft. In nonsurgical can-

didates, an endovascular stent graft is placed or the PAU is percutaneously embolized.

THORACIC AORTIC ANEURYSM

Thoracic aortic aneurysm is defined as an aortic diameter greater than 4 cm and is classified as to location, morphology, integrity of the aortic wall, and etiology (Fig. 19-3). The most common etiology is atherosclerosis. The most common location is at the junction of the aortic arch and descending aorta (Fig. 19-4). Aneurysms that involve the ascending aorta are usually caused by cystic medial necrosis, connective tissue

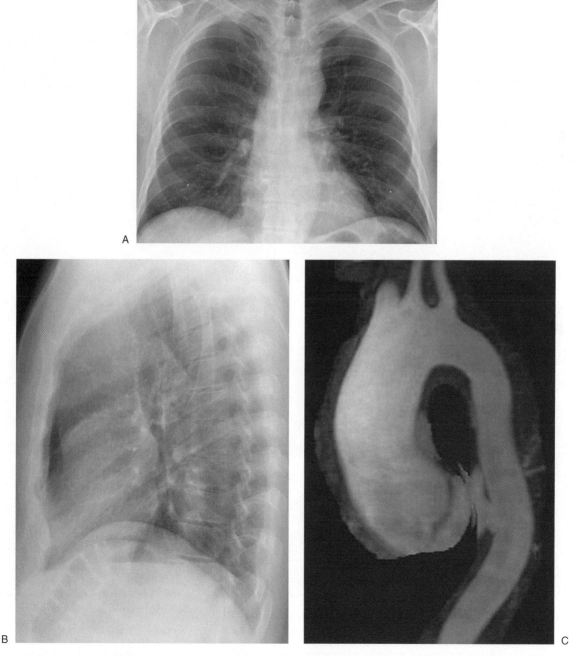

FIGURE 19-3. Ascending aortic aneurysm. A: PA chest radiograph of a 54-year-old man with a heart murmur shows a tortuous-appearing aorta. **B:** Lateral view shows a markedly dilated ascending aorta. **C:** White-blood sagittal MRI shows fusiform dilation of the ascending aorta.

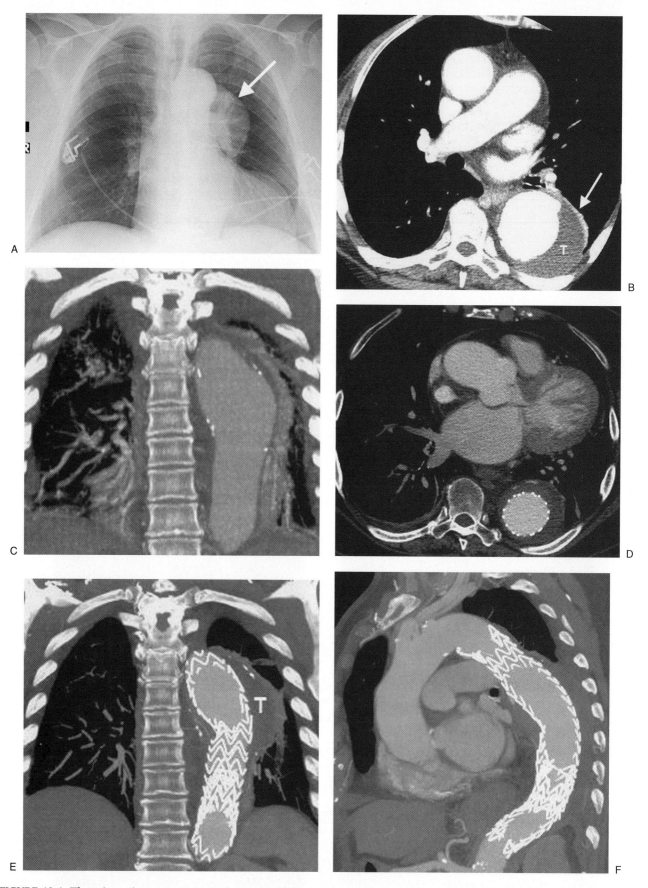

FIGURE 19-4. Thoracic aortic aneurysm. A: PA chest radiograph of a 77-year-old woman shows a left mediastinal mass contiguous with the contour of the aorta (*arrow*). **B:** CT shows an aneurysm of the proximal descending aorta with extensive mural thrombus (*T*). Adjacent rim of high attenuation represents atelectatic lung (*arrow*). **C:** Coronal CT shows a fusiform aneurysm involving the junction of the aortic arch and descending aorta; this is the most common location of atherosclerotic thoracic aortic aneurysms. **D:** CT after placement of endovascular stent graft shows the metallic stent, enhancing aortic lumen, and surrounding low-attenuation thrombus. There is no evidence of leak. **E:** Coronal CT shows overlapping stents. Note persistent thrombus (*T*). **F:** Sagittal CT shows normal appearance of overlapping stents.

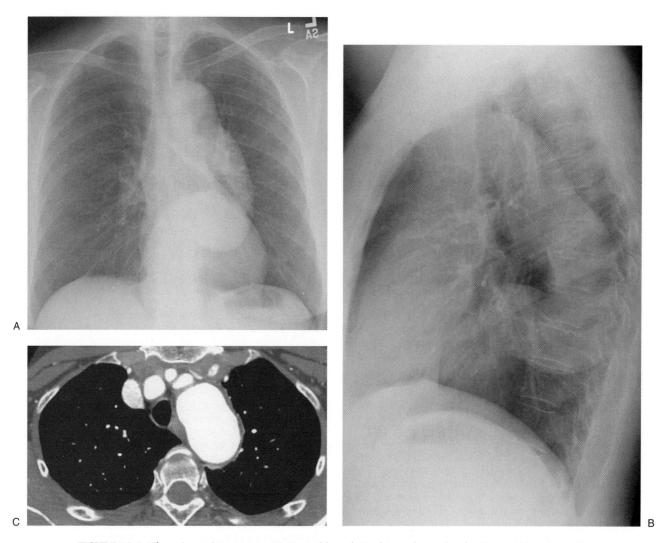

FIGURE 19-5. Thoracic aortic aneurysm. PA (**A**) and lateral (**B**) chest radiographs of a 56-year-old woman with back pain show tortuosity and dilation of the thoracic aorta. **C:** CT shows fusiform dilation of the aortic arch and minimal low-attenuation mural thrombus. (*Continued*)

disorders such as Marfan and Ehlers-Danlos syndromes, and syphilis (now rare). Aneurysms involving the descending aorta are usually atherosclerotic, posttraumatic, infectious (mycotic), or inflammatory (rheumatoid arthritis and ankylosing spondylitis). *Fusiform* aneurysms are those with general enlargement of the entire aortic circumference (Fig. 19-5), whereas *saccular* aneurysms are sharply delineated and usually involve a localized segment of the aorta, which often appears as an eccentric outpouching. Regarding aortic wall integrity, aneurysms can be classified as *true* (having an intact aortic wall that is composed of intima, media, and adventitia) or *false* (also called *pseudoaneurysm*, characterized by a disrupted aortic wall contained by the adventitia, perivascular connective tissue, and organized blood clot). Atherosclerotic and connective tissue disorder–related aneurysms are true aneurysms. Posttraumatic and infectious (mycotic) aneurysms are usually false aneurysms.

Imaging assessment of aneurysms includes size, location, and relationship with branch vessels, as well as the morpho-

logical type of aneurysm and the presence or absence of findings that suggest impending rupture. The risk of rupture increases with size and with rapid expansion. Surgical repair should be considered when thoracic aneurysms reach a diameter of 5 to 6 cm (3). Characteristic CT findings include focal or diffuse aortic dilations and deformity, peripheral curvilinear and plaque-like intimal calcification at the edge of the aorta or near the aortic margin, thickened aortic wall, filling of the patent portion of lumen by contrast media, intraluminal thrombus that may be circumferential or crescentic, displacement of mediastinal structures, bone erosions, periaortic hematoma, or pleural fluid. Other complications include aortobronchial fistula, compression of the right pulmonary artery, aortoesophageal fistula, and distal embolization. The aorta may rupture into the mediastinum, pericardium, pleural sac, or extrapleural space. The presence of pleural or extrapleural blood on the left and contained aortic leak are signs of impending or actual rupture (see Fig. 6-27). A contained leak can be found when the aneurysm is in close contact with the spine, with lateral draping of the

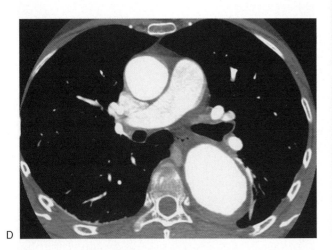
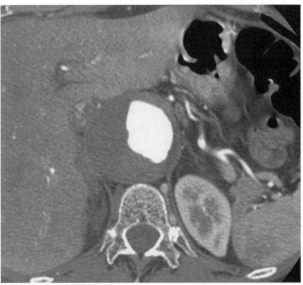

FIGURE 19-5. (*Continued*) **D:** CT at a level inferior to (**C**) shows dilation of the descending aorta and mural thrombus. **E:** CT of the abdominal aorta shows extension of the aneurysm into the abdomen, atherosclerotic plaque, and mural thrombus.

aneurysm around the vertebral body with a deficient posterior aortic wall.

IMAGING THE REPAIRED AORTA

Both CT and MRI can be used to evaluate the postprocedural aorta and monitor for complications. Numerous types of surgical repairs are performed, and the normal appearance on CT will depend on the type of repair made. Portions of the aorta may be resected, grafts may be sewn end to end or end to side, and branch vessels may be reimplanted or grafted using synthetic interposition grafts. A continuous suture, graft inclusion procedure involves aortotomy, graft inclusion, and enclosure of the graft within the native aorta. This procedure creates a space between the graft and native aorta that can fill with bland or infected fluid, blood/thrombus, or contrast material. A small amount of fluid and air in this space is normal immediately after surgery. Fluid seen 6 weeks after surgery and gas seen 2 weeks after surgery are reliable signs of infection.

Felt pledgets and strips are often used to reinforce sutures, which should not be mistaken for contrast material leaking from a graft. A small portion of the native aorta next to the coronary ostium is often implanted onto a coronary artery graft. This is called a coronary button and should not be mistaken for a pseudoaneurysm.

Endoluminal stent grafts are being used increasingly frequently to treat many aortic diseases. Imaging after stent graft deployment can be used to confirm complete exclusion of the aneurysm, assess patency of the stent graft and aortic branches, and evaluate sequential shrinkage of an aneurysm (Fig. 19-6) (3). An *endoleak* is defined as continued flow within an

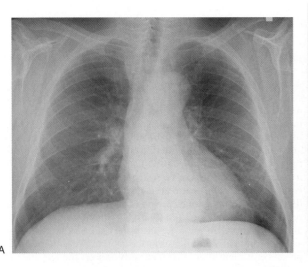
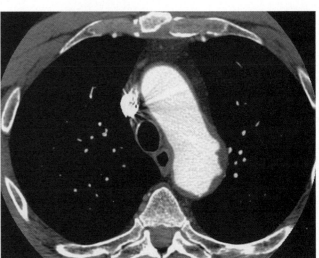

FIGURE 19-6. Thoracic aortic aneurysm. A: PA chest radiograph of a 58-year-old man with hypertension shows a tortuous and dilated descending aorta. **B:** CT at the junction of the aortic arch and descending aorta shows atheromatous plaque and mural thrombus. (*Continued*)

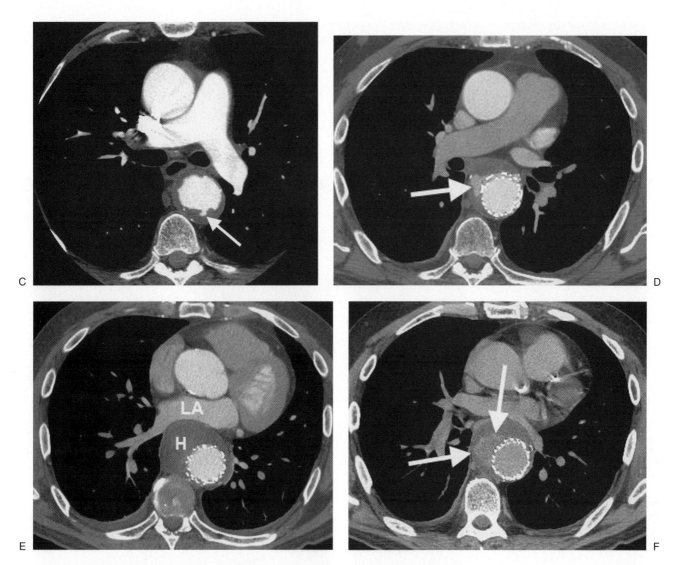

FIGURE 19-6. (*Continued*) **C:** CT at a level inferior to (**B**) shows atheromatous ulcers (*arrow*) confined to the intimal layer, which should not be mistaken for penetrating atherosclerotic ulcers. Note that there is no displacement of intimal calcifications. **D:** CT after placement of overlapping endovascular stent grafts shows a focal leak (*arrow*) and surrounding hematoma. **E:** CT at a level inferior to (**D**) shows that the hematoma (*H*) is compressing the posterior left atrium (*LA*). **F:** Delayed CT at the same level as (**E**) shows high-attenuation contrast leaking from the stent (*arrows*).

aneurysm sac after deployment of a stent. Type I endoleaks are leaks at the proximal or distal attachment sites of the stent and correlate with aneurysmal enlargement and late aneurysmal rupture. Type II endoleaks are caused by patent aortic side branches, including lumbar, inferior mesenteric, and accessory renal arteries.

References

1. Castaner E, Andreu M, Gallardo X, et al. CT in nontraumatic acute thoracic aortic disease: typical and atypical features and complications. *Radiographics.* 2003;23:S93–S110.

2. Prete R, Von Segesser LK. Aortic dissection. *Lancet.* 1997;349:1461–1464.

3. Takahashi K, Stanford W. Multidetector CT of the thoracic aorta. *Int J Cardiovasc Imaging.* 2005;21:141–153.

4. Crawford ES, Svensson LG, Coselli JS, et al. Surgical treatment of aneurysm and/or dissection of the ascending aorta, transverse aortic arch, and ascending aorta and transverse aortic arch. Factors influencing survival in 717 patients. *J Thorac Cardiovasc Surg.* 1989;98:659–674.

5. DeBakey ME, Cooley DA, Creech O. Surgical treatment of dissecting aneurysm. *JAMA.* 1995;162:1654–1657.

6. Nienaber CA, von Kodolitsch Y, Peterson B, et al. Intramural hemorrhage of the thoracic aorta: diagnostic and therapeutic implications. *Circulation.* 1995;92:1465–1472.

7. Stanson AW, Kazmier FJ, Hollier LH, et al. Penetrating atherosclerotic ulcers of the thoracic aorta: natural history and clinicopathologic correlations. *Ann Vasc Surg.* 1986;1:15–23.

CHAPTER 20

SELF-ASSESSMENT

Directions: For questions 1-30, choose the most likely diagnosis from the alternatives listed, given the history and radiologic findings.

1. History: Asymptomatic

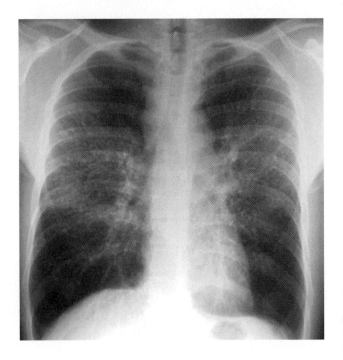

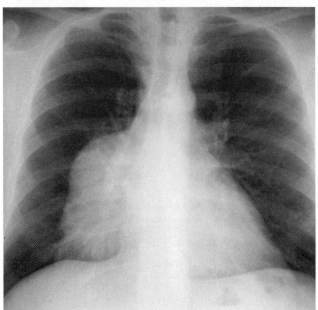

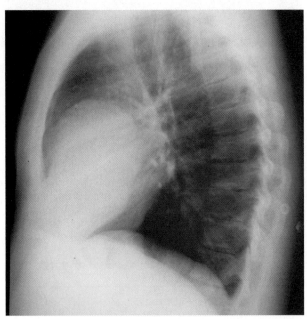

    A. Tuberculosis
    B. Sarcoidosis
    C. Lymphoma
    D. Langerhan cell histiocytosis
    E. Asbestosis

2. History: 46-year-old-man
    A. Teratoma
    B. Thyroid neoplasm
    C. Thymoma
    D. Malignant mesothelioma
    E. Metastatic prostate carcinoma

See Figures in Right Column

3. History: Blunt trauma to the chest

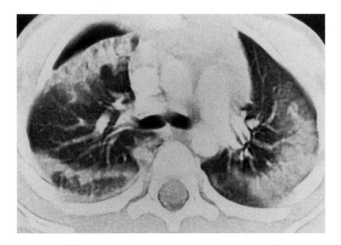

   A. Eosinophilic pneumonia
   B. Pulmonary contusions
   C. Alveolar sarcoidosis
   D. Cryptogenic organizing pneumonia
   E. Pulmonary infarcts

4. History: 53-year-old man with right chest pain

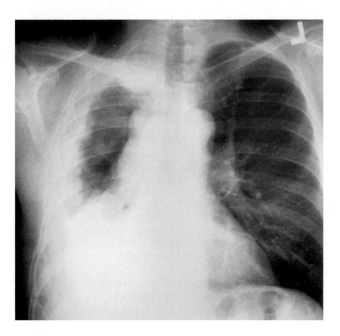

   A. Empyema
   B. Metastatic colon cancer
   C. Acute hemothorax
   D. Chylothorax
   E. Malignant mesothelioma

5. History: Withheld

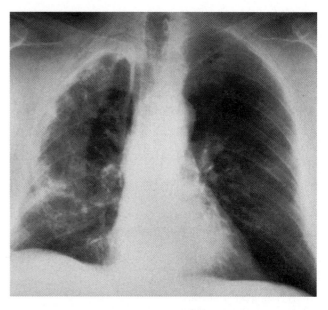

   A. Previous tuberculous empyema
   B. Benign asbestos-related pleural disease
   C. Malignant mesothelioma
   D. Scleroderma
   E. Multifocal pneumonia

6. History: Bone marrow transplant

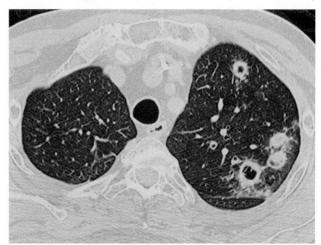

   A. Wegener granulomatosis
   B. Rheumatoid nodules
   C. Invasive pulmonary aspergillosis
   D. Staphylococcal pneumonia
   E. Primary bronchogenic carcinoma

7. History: 28-year-old man with mild shortness of breath

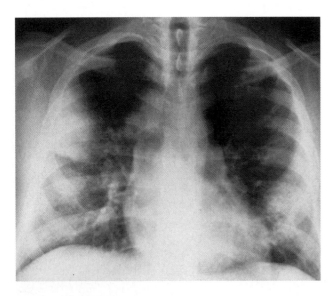

A. Hodgkin lymphoma
B. Eosinophilic pneumonia
C. Pulmonary contusions
D. Sarcoidosis
E. Reactivation tuberculosis

8. History: Dyspnea on exertion and clubbing

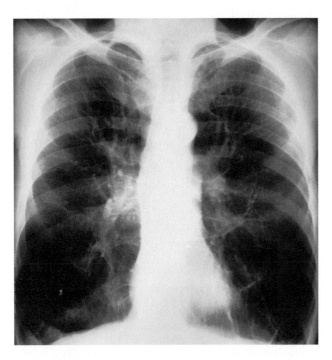

A. Bilateral pneumothoraces
B. Asthma
C. Cystic fibrosis
D. Obliterative bronchiolitis
E. Alpha-1-antitrypsin deficiency

9. History: Cough and fever

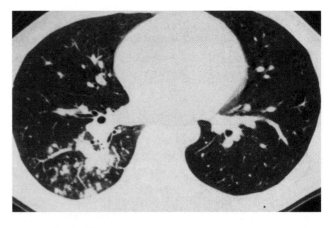

A. Cystic fibrosis
B. *Mycobacterium kansasii* infection
C. Silicosis
D. Langerhan cell histiocytosis
E. Pulmonary hemorrhage

10. History: Shortness of breath

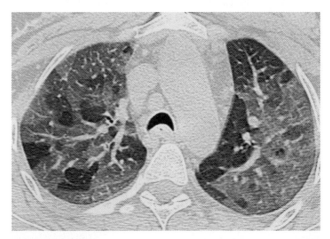

A. Obliterative bronchiolitis
B. *Pneumocystis jiroveci* pneumonia
C. Pulmonary hemorrhage
D. Desquamative interstitial pneumonitis
E. Acute respiratory distress syndrome

11. History: Left pneumonectomy for bronchogenic carcinoma 1 year ago

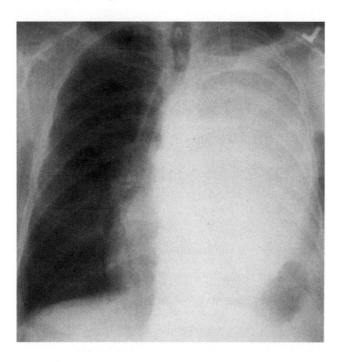

A. Bronchopleural fistula
B. Recurrent tumor
C. Hemothorax
D. Empyema
E. Normal

12. History: 52-year-old asymptomatic woman

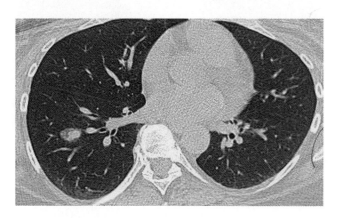

A. Asbestosis
B. *Mycobacterium* tuberculosis
C. Sarcoidosis
D. Bronchioloalveolar carcinoma
E. Silicosis

13. History: Cough and shortness of breath

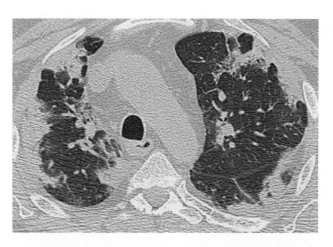

A. Pulmonary hemorrhage
B. Pulmonary edema
C. Pulmonary alveolar proteinosis
D. Bronchioloalveolar carcinoma
E. Eosinophilic pneumonia

14. History: Asymptomatic 34-year-old man

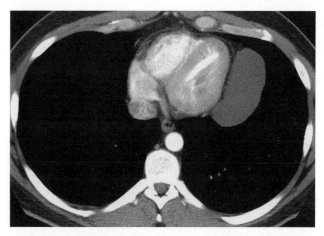

A. Mediastinal abscess
B. Thymoma
C. Lymphoma
D. Pericardial cyst
E. Teratoma

15. History: Recent upper endoscopy

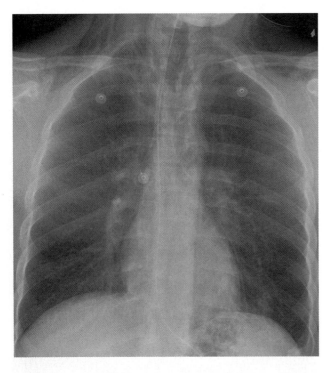

A. Pneumomediastinum
B. Pneumothorax
C. Mediastinal abscess
D. Pulmonary emphysema
E. Empyema

16. History: 75-year-old man

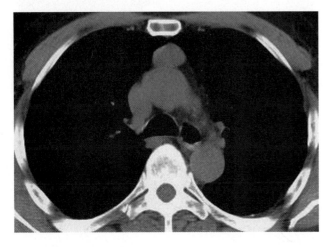

A. Bronchogenic carcinoma
B. Germ cell tumor
C. Thymoma
D. Mediastinal abscess
E. Sarcoidosis

17. History: 37-year-old man with cough

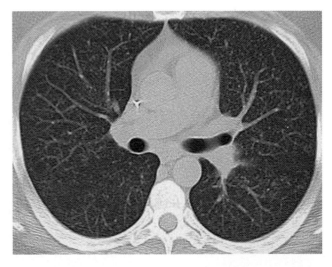

A. Metastatic prostate cancer
B. Asbestosis
C. Mycobacterial pneumonia
D. Pulmonary alveolar proteinosis
E. Pulmonary lymphoma

18. History: 25-year-old man with chronic cough

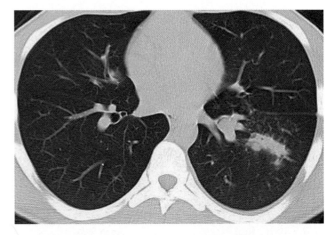

A. Carcinoid tumor
B. Mucoepidermoid carcinoma
C. Mycobacterial pneumonia
D. Bronchial atresia
E. Sarcoidosis

19. History: 58-year-old woman with chronic cough

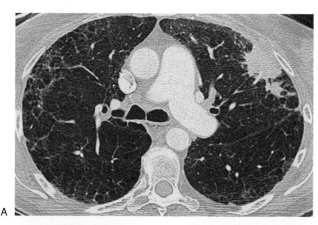

A

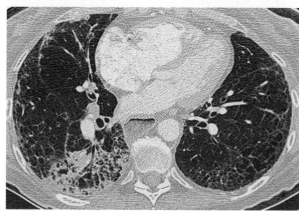

B

A. Idiopathic pulmonary fibrosis
B. Metastatic breast cancer
C. Silicosis
D. Scleroderma
E. Cryptogenic organizing pneumonitis

20. History: 46-year-old man with a bone marrow transplant (note: second image acquired 3 weeks after first image)

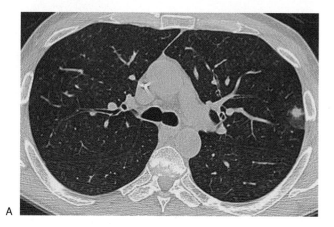

A

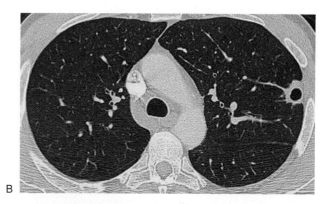

B

A. Bronchogenic carcinoma
B. Mycobacterial pneumonia
C. Posttransplant lymphoproliferative disease
D. Invasive pulmonary aspergillosis
E. Septic emboli

21. History: Acute shortness of breath

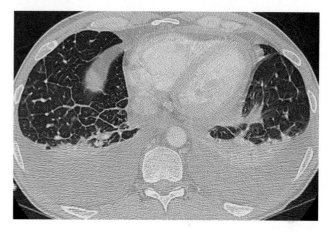

A. Cardiogenic pulmonary edema
B. Lymphangitic carcinomatosis
C. Sarcoidosis
D. Kaposi sarcoma
E. Pulmonary infarct

22. History: 61-year-old woman with Sjögren syndrome

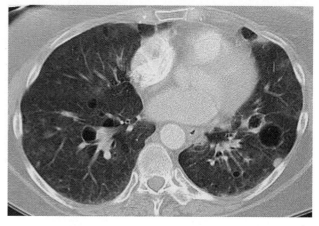

A. Fungal pneumonia
B. Metastatic breast cancer
C. Cryptogenic organizing pneumonia
D. Wegener granulomatosis
E. Lymphocytic interstitial pneumonia

23. History: 53-year-old woman with fever and pleuritic chest pain

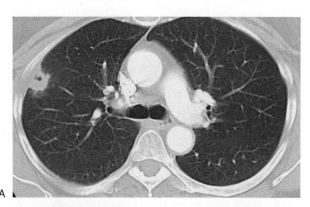

A

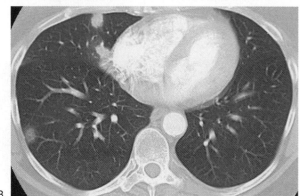

B

A. Pulmonary infarcts
B. Cryptogenic organizing pneumonia
C. Eosinophilic pneumonia
D. Langerhan cell histiocytosis
E. Septic emboli

24. History: 74-year-old man with poor dentition

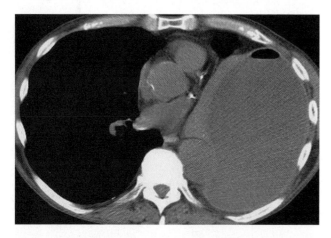

A. Pulmonary abscess
B. Empyema
C. Bronchogenic carcinoma
D. Asbestos-related pleural disease
E. Chylothorax

25. History: 34-year-old woman

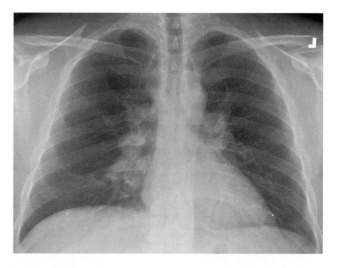

A. Asbestosis
B. Sarcoidosis
C. Pulmonary artery aneurysm
D. Silicosis
E. Hamartoma

26. History: 51-year-old woman with severe hypoxia

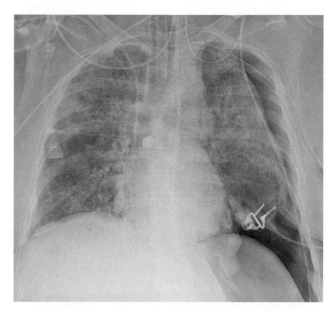

A. Silicosis
B. Scleroderma
C. Acute respiratory distress syndrome
D. Cryptogenic organizing pneumonia
E. Lymphangioleiomyomatosis

27. History: 65-year-old man with shortness of breath

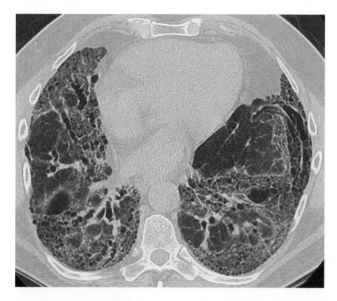

A. End-stage sarcoidosis
B. Chronic hypersensitivity pneumonitis
C. Idiopathic pulmonary fibrosis
D. Complicated silicosis
E. Cryptogenic organizing pneumonia

28. History: 46-year-old woman

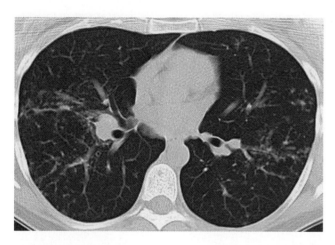

A. Sarcoidosis
B. Langerhan cell histiocytosis
C. Wegener granulomatosis
D. Asbestosis
E. Acute hypersensitivity pneumonitis

29. History: 49-year-old asymptomatic man

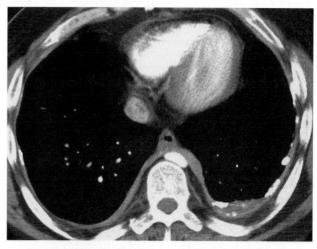

A. Complicated silicosis
B. Tuberculous empyema
C. Metastatic bronchogenic carcinoma
D. Chronic congestive heart failure
E. Asbestos-related pleural disease

30. History: 38-year-old woman

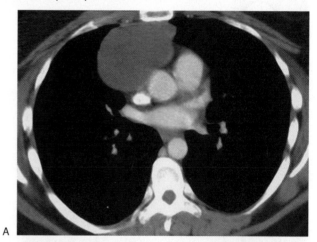

A

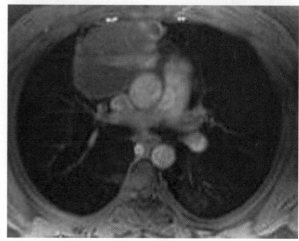

B

A. Pericardial cyst
B. Mediastinal abscess
C. Bronchogenic cyst
D. Bronchogenic carcinoma
E. Cystic teratoma

Directions: For questions 31 to 36, one radiographic image is shown for each question; each image represents an "Aunt Minnie" (meaning that the appearance alone suggests a specific diagnosis). Write the most likely diagnosis, based on the image shown, on the blank line next to each number.

31. _____

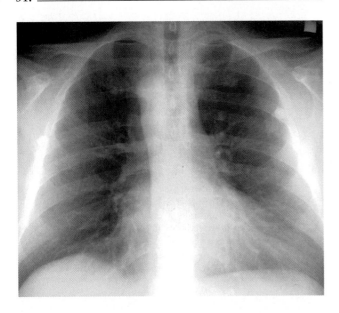

32. _____

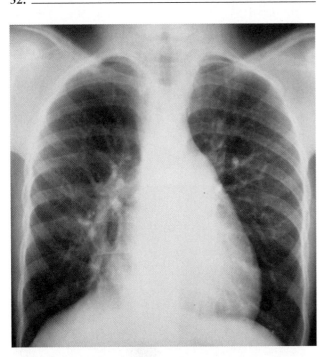

33. _____

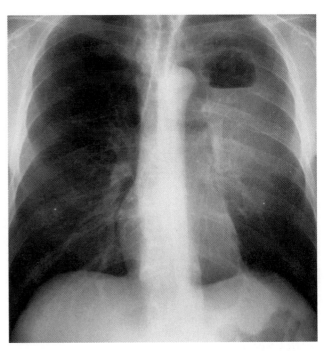

34. _____

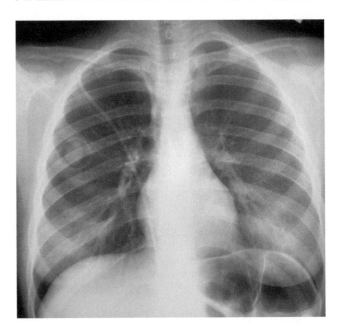

35. _____

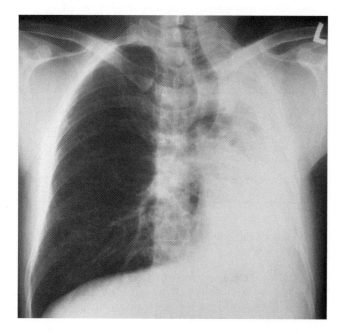

36. _____

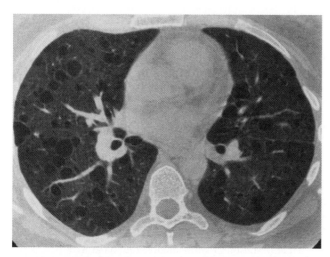

Directions: For questions 37 to 41, match each of the following radiographic descriptions (37–41) with the anatomic term (A–E) with which it is most closely associated.

A. Accessory azygos fissure
B. Inferior accessory fissure
C. Minor fissure
D. Phrenic nerve
E. Aortic "nipple"

_____ 37. Separates medial basal segment from other basal segments
_____ 38. Four pleural layers
_____ 39. Left superior intercostal vein
_____ 40. Separates right upper lobe from right middle lobe
_____ 41. Traverses the prevascular space

Directions: For questions 42 to 46, match each of the following radiographic descriptions (42–46) with the radiographic sign (A–E) with which it is most closely associated.

A. Halo sign
B. Gloved finger sign
C. Fallen lung sign
D. Luftsichel sign
E. Flat waist sign

_____ 42. Bronchial laceration
_____ 43. Invasive pulmonary aspergillosis
_____ 44. Left upper lobe collapse
_____ 45. Left lower lobe collapse
_____ 46. Allergic bronchopulmonary aspergillosis

Directions: For questions 47 to 51, match the following radiographic findings or patient history (47–51) with the most closely associated cause of interstitial lung disease (A–E).

A. Lymphangioleiomyomatosis
B. Lymphocytic interstitial pneumonia
C. Silicosis
D. Scleroderma
E. Asbestosis

_____ 47. Chrysotile
_____ 48. Sjögren syndrome
_____ 49. Chylous pleural effusion
_____ 50. Progressive massive fibrosis
_____ 51. Recurrent pneumothorax

Directions: Questions 52 to 55 consist of four lettered headings followed by a set of numbered items. For each numbered item, select

A if the item is associated with (A) **only**
B if the item is associated with (B) **only**
C if the item is associated with **both (A) and (B)**
D if the item is associated with **neither (A) nor (B)** and write the correct letter on the blank line next to the appropriate number.

A. Atrial septal defect
B. Ventricular septal defect
C. Both
D. Neither

_____ 52. Enlarged left atrium
_____ 53. Enlarged central and peripheral pulmonary arteries
_____ 54. Enlarged thoracic aorta
_____ 55. Small thoracic aorta

Directions: For questions 56 to 81, write **T** for *true* or **F** for *false* on the blank line next to each number.

_____ 56. An air crescent sign can be seen in invasive or semi-invasive forms of *Aspergillus* lung disease.
_____ 57. Silicosis, asbestosis, sarcoidosis, and Langerhan cell histiocytosis are all causes of upper lung disease.
_____ 58. Both adenopathy and parenchymal disease are associated with stage II sarcoidosis.
_____ 59. Sarcoidosis, cryptogenic organizing pneumonia, eosinophilic pneumonia, and pulmonary infarcts are all causes of peripheral pulmonary opacities.
_____ 60. Both Swyer-James syndrome and endobronchial foreign body can produce a hyperlucent lung and air trapping on exhalation.
_____ 61. The presence of N2 nodes and bronchogenic carcinoma implies nonresectability.
_____ 62. A T3 bronchogenic cancer is within 2 cm of the carina but does not invade the carina.
_____ 63. N2 nodes include ipsilateral supraclavicular nodes.
_____ 64. A stage IIIA bronchogenic cancer is potentially resectable.

_____ 65. Pleural effusion and adenopathy are commonly associated with pulmonary infection from *Pneumocystis jiroveci* pneumonia.

_____ 66. *Pneumocystis jiroveci* pneumonia is associated with lung cysts and spontaneous pneumothorax.

_____ 67. The most common location of an intrapulmonary sequestration is the superior segment of the left lower lobe.

_____ 68. On a lateral chest radiograph, the right upper lobe bronchus is normally higher than the left upper lobe bronchus.

_____ 69. On a properly positioned lateral chest radiograph, the right hemidiaphragm and ribs extend more posteriorly than the left hemidiaphragm.

_____ 70. The azygos vein is an anterior mediastinal structure.

_____ 71. The "aortic nipple" represents the left superior intercostal vein.

_____ 72. On a posteroanterior chest radiograph, the right hilum is normally higher than the left.

_____ 73. The most common cause for abnormal thickening of the posterior wall of the bronchus intermedius is pulmonary edema.

_____ 74. Calcified pleural plaques are a manifestation of asbestosis.

_____ 75. Small nodules are the prominent feature of complicated silicosis.

_____ 76. The ideal radiographic position for the radiopaque portion of an intra-aortic balloon pump is at the level of the aortic arch, just distal to the takeoff of the left subclavian artery.

_____ 77. Of patients with sarcoidosis and hilar adenopathy (stage I disease), 60% will have complete resolution of hilar adenopathy.

_____ 78. Silicosis can be a progressive disease, despite the cessation of dust exposure.

_____ 79. The majority of cases of postprimary tuberculosis occur in the apical/posterior segment of an upper lobe.

_____ 80. The incidence of pulmonary hemorrhage in leukemic patients is approximately 40%.

_____ 81. The most common malignancy in patients with AIDS is Kaposi sarcoma.

Directions: For questions 82 to 99, write the one best correct answer on the blank line.

82. Into which sinus does a persistent left superior vena cava drain?_____

83. What vein drains into the posterior aspect of the superior vena cava at the level of the tracheobronchial angle?_____

84–88. Name five general causes of chronic alveolar lung disease ("BALLS").

84. _____

85. _____

86. _____

87. _____

88. _____

89–92. Name four general causes of an anterior mediastinal mass ("4 Ts").

89. _____

90. _____

91. _____

92. _____

93–96. Name four general categories of causes of a large unilateral pleural effusion.

93. _____

94. _____

95. _____

96. _____

97–99. Name the three components of Kartagener syndrome.

97. _____

98. _____

99. _____

Directions: For questions 100 to 108, circle the letter of the one best response.

100. The smallest discrete portion of the lung that can be appreciated on thin-section CT of the chest in normal healthy lungs is
    A. Primary pulmonary lobule
    B. Secondary pulmonary lobule
    C. Pulmonary acinus
    D. Pulmonary alveolus
    E. Terminal bronchiole

101. Which of the following is **NOT** a named segment of the right lung?
    A. Apical segment, right upper lobe
    B. Anterior segment, right upper lobe
    C. Superior segment, right lower lobe
    D. Anterior basal segment, right lower lobe
    E. Superior segment, right middle lobe

102. Which of the following is a manifestation of AIDS, especially in children?
    A. Cryptogenic organizing pneumonia
    B. Usual interstitial pneumonia
    C. Desquamative interstitial pneumonia
    D. Lymphoid interstitial pneumonia
    E. Giant cell interstitial pneumonia

103. Which of the following is **NOT** a characteristic chest CT manifestation of lymphangioleiomyomatosis?
    A. Nodules
    B. Pneumothorax
    C. Cysts
    D. Chylothorax
    E. Hyperinflation

104. Which of the following is **NOT** typically associated with honeycomb lung (pulmonary fibrosis)?
    A. Scleroderma
    B. Hypersensitivity pneumonitis
    C. Asthma
    D. Asbestosis
    E. Sarcoidosis

105. Which of the following is **NOT** characterized by multiple small 1- to 5-mm pulmonary nodules?
    A. Langerhan cell histiocytosis
    B. Tuberculosis
    C. Asbestosis
    D. Silicosis
    E. Metastases

106. Which of the following is **NOT** associated with Swyer-James syndrome?

   A. Adenovirus infection
   B. Bronchiectasis
   C. Absent pectoralis muscle
   D. Air trapping
   E. Small ipsilateral hilum

107. Which of the following is associated with centrilobular emphysema?

   A. Alpha-1-antitrypsin deficiency
   B. "Swiss cheese" appearance on thin-section CT
   C. Involvement of the entire secondary pulmonary lobule
   D. "Lung simplification" appearance on thin-section CT
   E. Lower lung–predominant distribution

108. Which of the following is typically associated with *intralobar* sequestration?

   A. Venous drainage to pulmonary veins
   B. Separate pleural sheath
   C. Venous drainage to systemic veins
   D. Lining of columnar respiratory epithelium
   E. Most commonly occurs in posterior segment of left upper lobe

Directions: For questions 109 to 113, circle **ALL** of the correct responses for each statement or question.

109. Potential complications of central venous catheter placement include the following:

   A. Pneumothorax
   B. Cardiac perforation
   C. Arrhythmia
   D. Air embolization
   E. Clot formation

110. Concerning a left ventricular assist device:

   A. The left arm is secured into the left atrium.
   B. The right arm is sutured into the ascending aorta.
   C. The pump is positioned in the left upper quadrant of the abdomen.
   D. The device does the work of both ventricles.
   E. The device is used as a bridge to heart transplantation.

111. Which of the following can suggest the diagnosis of tracheobronchial tear?

   A. Fallen lung sign
   B. Pneumomediastinum
   C. Persistent pneumothorax with chest tubes in place
   D. Missing diaphragm sign
   E. Overdistended endotracheal tube cuff

112. Which of the following stages of bronchogenic cancer are potentially resectable?

   A. I
   B. II
   C. IIIA
   D. IIIB
   E. IV

113. Which of the following chest radiographic appearances suggest the diagnosis of acute aortic injury?

   A. Widened mediastinum
   B. Apical cap
   C. Widening of the left paraspinous line
   D. Displacement of the nasogastric tube
   E. Fracture of the first and second ribs

SELF-ASSESSMENT ANSWERS

1. **B**—Sarcoidosis, stage II. There are bilateral small nodules in an upper and middle lung–predominant distribution, along with mediastinal and hilar adenopathy. Patients with tuberculosis and lymphoma and these radiographic findings are almost always symptomatic, with fever, night sweats, cough, and so forth. This much adenopathy would be very unusual for Langerhan cell histiocytosis. Asbestosis is not associated with this degree of adenopathy or interstitial nodules; it is associated with reticular/linear interstitial opacities, typically in a bibasilar and subpleural distribution.

2. **C**—Thymoma. This is an anterior mediastinal mass (note the very smooth contours that result from the mass abutting the mediastinal pleura). The patient's age (over 40) makes this mass much more likely to be a thymoma than a teratoma. The mass does not extend to the neck and does not cause tracheal deviation, and, therefore, a thyroid mass would not be considered. Although the mass could represent a focal pleural mass, malignant mesothelioma typically involves the lateral pleura as well as the medial pleural surface, and it tends to be much more lobulated. Metastatic prostate carcinoma tends to produce blastic bony lesions, well-circumscribed pulmonary nodules, and, on occasion, mediastinal adenopathy.

3. **B**—Pulmonary contusions. All the choices are disorders that can result in peripheral opacities on the chest radiograph and CT scan. The right pneumothorax and history of trauma support the correct diagnosis of pulmonary contusions. Eosinophilic pneumonia, alveolar sarcoidosis, and cryptogenic organizing pneumonia would otherwise all be reasonable choices. Pulmonary infarcts, although peripheral in location, seldom result in such diffuse peripheral opacification, and they do not result in opacities with central sparing, as is seen in the right lower lobe.

4. **E**—Malignant mesothelioma. There is extensive right pleural opacification, which is lobulated in contour and wraps around the entire pleural surface. The mediastinum is "fixed," not shifted to the left, as is often seen with large pleural fluid collections. These findings are classic for malignant mesothelioma. Although metastatic colon adenocarcinoma can produce pleural metastases, it would be uncommon to see such extensive *unilateral* involvement, especially in the absence of pulmonary metastases. Empyema, chylothorax, and hemothorax usually have more mass effect, causing contralateral shift of the mediastinum, and they do not typically produce such a lobulated contour to the entire pleural surface.

5. **A**—Previous tuberculous empyema. There is right pleural opacification extending from the lung apex to the costophrenic angle, a result of pleural thickening and fibrosis. The "hazy" appearance of the right lung is caused by pleural fibrosis involving the anterior and posterior pleural surfaces, not by pulmonary disease, so this is not multifocal pneumonia. There is also dense pleural calcification, especially apicolaterally. Although these findings can all be seen with benign asbestos-related pleural disease, the *unilateral* involvement makes either previous hemothorax or previous tuberculous empyema the likely diagnosis. Malignant mesothelioma does not result in dense pleural calcification (although bilateral pleural calcification may be seen in patients with underlying benign asbestos-related pleural disease). Collagen vascular diseases, such as scleroderma, can uncommonly result in calcified pleural thickening, but the extensive *unilateral* involvement again makes this diagnosis unlikely.

6. **C**—Invasive pulmonary aspergillosis. There are multiple cavitary nodules, some with a halo of ground-glass attenuation and some with an "air crescent" sign; this is very suggestive of invasive pulmonary aspergillosis in a patient with a bone marrow transplant. All the other choices are causes of cavitary nodules, but they are less likely etiologies given the patient history. Also, rheumatoid nodules are quite rare, staphylococcal pneumonia uncommonly produces multiple cavitary nodules (septic emboli from staphylococcal septicemia would be more likely), and primary bronchogenic carcinoma typically presents with one dominant cavitary nodule or mass.

7. **D**—Sarcoidosis. The mediastinal adenopathy and bilateral peripheral areas of parenchymal opacification are typical disease patterns seen in "alveolar" sarcoidosis. The fact that the patient is only mildly symptomatic makes lymphoma and tuberculosis unlikely. Also, reactivation tuberculosis does not typically result in adenopathy, except in patients with AIDS. Bulky adenopathy is also not typical of eosinophilic pneumonia, although the peripheral opacities are consistent with the diagnosis. Without a history of trauma, pulmonary contusions would not be in the differential diagnosis, especially given the presence of adenopathy.

8. **E**—Alpha-1-antitrypsin deficiency. There is marked hyperinflation and lucency of the lungs and diminution of pulmonary vasculature; these signs are most marked in the lower lungs, a distribution that is typical of pulmonary emphysema secondary to alpha-1-antitrypsin deficiency. Asthma does not cause such striking diminution of pulmonary vasculature on the chest radiograph. Cystic fibrosis is associated with bronchiectasis, bronchial wall thickening, and mucous plugging, none of which are evident in this case. Obliterative bronchiolitis can result in hyperinflation and increased lucency of the lungs, but it rarely has such striking radiographic findings as seen in this case, and it does not typically have a lower lung–predominant distribution on chest radiography. This case does not represent bilateral pneumothoraces, as some vascular markings are seen within the lucent lower lungs; however, in some cases, large bullae can be difficult to distinguish from pneumothoraces on chest radiography.

9. **B**—*Mycobacterium kansasii* infection. There are nodular and linear branching opacities (so-called "tree-in-bud"), representing bronchiolar disease in the right lower lobe. This appearance is most often the result of an infectious process. Cystic fibrosis can result in a "tree-in-bud" pattern, but it is typically a bilateral, diffuse process, not focal, as this case is. Although silicosis and Langerhan cell histiocytosis can produce small interstitial nodules, the nodules do not represent endobronchial disease and the "tree-in-bud" pattern is not produced. Pulmonary hemorrhage does not typically produce a dominant nodular pattern on chest CT.

10. **A**—Obliterative bronchiolitis. Note the anterior bowing of the posterior membranous trachea, indicating that the CT scan was obtained during exhalation. There is a mosaic pattern of lung attenuation, which in this case is secondary to air trapping. This pattern of disease is most likely to represent asthma or obliterative bronchiolitis. The other choices all produce "infiltrative" lung disease, in which the more opaque areas of lung are abnormal. In this case, where there are patchy areas of air trapping, the more opaque areas of lung are normal and the lucent areas represent abnormal lung with air trapping.

11. **B**—Recurrent tumor. There is opacification of the left hemithorax, which is a normal finding after pneumonectomy, but the mediastinum is shifted to the contralateral side, which is abnormal. All the choices except **E** (normal) can produce contralateral shift of the mediastinum after pneumonectomy. With bronchopleural fistula, and often with empyema, however, there is also air within the pneumonectomy space. Both hemothorax and empyema tend to occur earlier after surgery.

12. **D**—Bronchioloalveolar carcinoma. CT shows a small dense nodule in the right lower lobe with a halo of ground-glass opacity, the so-called "fried egg" sign, which is characteristic of bronchioloalveolar carcinoma. This type of cancer can appear as solid, ground glass, or mixed. The "fried egg" appearance demonstrates both solid and ground-glass components. Asbestosis presents as reticular and linear interstitial lung disease with a basilar-predominant distribution. Mycobacterial disease is typically multifocal, and the findings can include nodules with or without cavitation, ill-defined dense airspace opacities, and small nodular and linear branching opacities in a bronchiolar distribution (so-called "tree-in-bud"). The findings vary depending on the type of mycobacterial infection and the patient's immune status. The characteristic features of sarcoidosis are multiple small nodules in a perilymphatic distribution. In silicosis, CT typically shows multiple small nodules in the upper lungs that often progress to larger masses (so-called "progressive massive fibrosis").

13. **E**—Eosinophilic pneumonia. CT shows dense airspace opacities in a subpleural or peripheral distribution, typical of eosinophilic pneumonia. Cryptogenic organizing pneumonia, although not an option in this case, often has the same appearance. Pulmonary hemorrhage and pulmonary edema can present as multifocal dense airspace opacities but do not typically have a peripheral distribution. Bronchioloalveolar carcinoma can be multifocal but also does not typically have a predominantly peripheral distribution. Pulmonary alveolar proteinosis typically presents as areas of ground-glass opacity with a background of septal thickening (so-called "crazy paving").

14. **D**—Pericardial cyst. CT shows a circumscribed mass of homogeneous fluid attenuation, contiguous with the pericardium, with no perceptible wall or evidence of enhancement. A mediastinal abscess typically has an enhancing wall of varying thickness. Most thymomas are solid, although they may have prominent cystic components. A thymoma that is largely cystic usually has a perceptible wall that often enhances with contrast material. Although lymphoma can have cystic components, it typically has a solid component. A teratoma may be largely cystic but will usually demonstrate wall enhancement or enhancement of a mural nodule.

15. **A**—Pneumomediastinum. Note air outlining the cardiomediastinal borders and extending up into the neck as linear lucencies. The pneumomediastinum was secondary to an esophageal tear that occurred during an endoscopic procedure to retrieve a pill stuck in the esophagus. Pneumothorax does not extend into the neck. A mediastinal abscess presents as a mass in the mediastinum that has varying degrees of fluid and air. Pulmonary emphysema is a parenchymal process that results in abnormal parenchymal lucency. Empyema presents as a pleural fluid collection that is often large and loculated.

16. **C**—Thymoma. CT shows a homogeneous solid mass in the anterior mediastinum, in the expected location of the thymus gland. The thymus is typically fatty replaced in a 75-year-old person. This would be an atypical location for lymphadenopathy associated with bronchogenic carcinoma or sarcoidosis, and there is no evidence of lymphadenopathy in other visualized areas of the mediastinum. Germ cell tumors can have this appearance but generally occur in younger patients (typically under age

40). A mediastinal abscess typically appears as a fluid-filled mass with varying degrees of wall thickness and internal air.

17. **C**—Mycobacterial pneumonia. CT shows a diffuse random distribution of 1- to 2-mm nodules (so-called "miliary" pattern). This is typical of hematogenous mycobacterial disease. Metastatic prostate cancer could have this presentation but would be unusual in a 37-year-old patient. Asbestosis is characterized by reticular and linear interstitial lung disease in a bibasilar-predominant distribution. The characteristic CT appearance of pulmonary alveolar proteinosis is that of multifocal ground-glass opacities with a background of septal thickening (so-called "crazy paving"). Although pulmonary lymphoma can uncommonly present as a miliary pattern, it more commonly presents as larger nodules and/or areas of dense airspace disease, often with lymphadenopathy.

18. **A**—Carcinoid tumor. CT shows a mass almost completely occluding a left lower lobe segmental bronchus. A small crescent of air is seen around the anterior edge of the mass. Postobstructive pneumonia is seen distal to the obstructed airway. Mucoepidermoid carcinoma could have this appearance but is much less common than carcinoid tumor. Obstructing endobronchial masses are not common features of mycobacterial pneumonia or sarcoidosis. The tubular opacity in the left lower lobe is similar to the appearance of bronchial atresia, but in the latter there is no obstructing endobronchial mass and the surrounding parenchyma is typically hyperlucent.

19. **D**—Scleroderma. The first image shows bilateral reticular interstitial lung disease in a predominantly subpleural distribution, with areas of honeycombing, typical of the appearance of pulmonary fibrosis associated with scleroderma. Patients with pulmonary fibrosis, either idiopathic or from a specific cause, have an increased risk of developing bronchogenic carcinoma, which is shown in this case in the periphery of the left upper lobe. The second image shows a fluid–debris level in a dilated esophagus, another feature of scleroderma. Associated with this is dense airspace disease in the right lower lobe, representing aspiration (also related to esophageal disease). Although idiopathic pulmonary fibrosis presents with similar findings, the presence of esophageal disease suggests the diagnosis of scleroderma. Metastases from breast cancer can present as modular septal thickening and pulmonary nodules and masses but would not be associated with honeycombing and traction bronchiectasis. The typical CT features of silicosis are multiple small nodules in an upper lung distribution that often coalesce into larger masses. Although cryptogenic organizing pneumonia can present as peripheral lung disease, it is not associated with honeycombing.

20. **D**—Invasive pulmonary aspergillosis. The first image shows a solid nodule with a surrounding halo of ground-glass opacity, the so-called "halo" sign, which is characteristic of invasive pulmonary aspergillosis. The second image, acquired 3 weeks later, shows the typical progression to a cavitary nodule. These findings are highly suggestive of invasive pulmonary aspergillosis in patients with bone marrow transplants or who are otherwise immunocompromised. The cavitation of the nodule indicates recovery of the patient's immune system. Bronchogenic carcinoma is less likely given the patient history and the rapid progression of the solid nodule to a cavitary nodule. Mycobacterial disease is typically more profuse and is often associated with "tree-in-bud" opacities of bronchiolitis. The typical CT features of posttransplant lymphoproliferative disease are multiple circumscribed nodules in a subpleural or bronchovascular distribution. The rapid progression from solid to cavitary nodules would be atypical. The appearance of septic emboli can be similar to that of invasive pulmonary aspergillosis, but it tends to be more profuse than what is shown in this case, and the "halo sign" suggests the latter diagnosis.

21. **A**—Cardiogenic pulmonary edema. CT shows the typical features of pulmonary edema: smooth septal thickening, pleural effusions, and scattered ground-glass opacities. Lymphangitic carcinomatosis can have a similar appearance, but with this diagnosis, the septal thickening tends to be nodular. Sarcoidosis typically presents as nodular thickening of bronchovascular bundles and subpleural nodules (a perilymphatic distribution). Kaposi sarcoma typically presents with nodules or masses in a bronchovascular distribution and is often associated with pleural effusion. Pulmonary infarcts present as subpleural airspace opacities, often wedge-shaped.

22. **E**—Lymphocytic interstitial pneumonia. CT shows multiple thin-walled cystic lesions and scattered small nodules (note a prominent nodule in the subpleural left lower lobe). These findings are characteristic of lymphocytic interstitial pneumonia, which is associated with Sjögren syndrome. The thin-walled cystic lesions are not characteristic features of fungal pneumonia, metastatic breast cancer, or cryptogenic organizing pneumonia. The cavitary nodules seen with Wegener granulomatosis typically have thicker walls.

23. **E**—Septic emboli. The first image shows a subpleural cavitary nodule in the right upper lobe. The second image shows additional subpleural nodules. The location (subpleural), ill-defined margins, cavitation, and multiplicity of nodules are typical of septic emboli. Multiple other similar nodules were present at other levels (not shown). A pulmonary infarct can be associated with pleuritic chest pain and pulmonary embolism but is usually more wedge-shaped in the acute stage, and cavitation is uncommon. The opacities associated with cryptogenic organizing pneumonia and eosinophilic pneumonia are often peripheral but also do not typically cavitate. The characteristic CT features of Langerhan cell histiocytosis are multiple small nodules and often bizarre-shaped cysts with an upper lung–predominant distribution.

24. **B**—Empyema. CT shows a large round left pleural fluid collection associated with mild thickening and enhancement of the pleural layers (so-called "split pleura" sign), a fluid–fluid level posteriorly, and a small air–fluid level anteriorly. There is associated passive atelectasis of most of the left lung. Some cases of pulmonary abscess can be difficult to distinguish from empyema, but in this case the clear distinction of the pleural layers and compression rather than infiltration of the adjacent lung allows a confident diagnosis of empyema to be made. Bronchogenic carcinoma can present with a large cavitary mass, but it is usually clearly seen to be a parenchymal and not a pleural process. The typical CT features of asbestos-related pleural disease are calcified and noncalcified pleural plaques and diffuse pleural thickening, with varying amounts of pleural fluid. Large pleural fluid collections are uncommon and when seen should raise suspicion of mesothelioma. A chylothorax can present as a large unilateral pleural effusion but is less commonly associated with thickening and enhancement of the pleural layers or fluid–fluid levels than is empyema. The history of poor dentition makes an infectious process more likely. The air in the pleural space suggests one of three possibilities: (a) recent thoracentesis, (b) empyema secondary to a gas-forming organism, or (c) bronchopleural fistula.

25. **B**—Sarcoidosis. The chest radiograph shows bilateral hilar lymphadenopathy, right greater than left. The lungs

appear clear. These features are characteristic of sarcoidosis. Other diagnoses to be considered, although not options in this case, include histoplasmosis, lymphoma, and metastases from an extrathoracic primary or bronchogenic carcinoma. Although it can be difficult to distinguish pulmonary artery enlargement from hilar lymphadenopathy, the diagnosis of pulmonary artery aneurysm is much less common and in this case the hilar enlargement is bilateral. On the right, there are multiple enlarged hilar nodes, which create a lobulated contour. This would be an unusual appearance for pulmonary artery enlargement. Hilar lymphadenopathy, often calcified, is commonly seen in patients with silicosis but is associated with parenchymal disease. This degree of hilar lymphadenopathy is not a feature of asbestosis or hamartoma. A hamartoma typically presents as a circumscribed nodule or mass in the lung with varying degrees of fat and calcium.

26. **C**—Acute respiratory distress syndrome (ARDS). The chest radiograph shows bilateral diffuse parenchymal disease, a large left pneumothorax (note the deep sulcus), a left chest tube, and an endotracheal tube. These findings suggest the diagnosis of ARDS. The pneumothorax is a result of barotrauma, which results from high positive pressure ventilation in the setting of stiff lungs. The presence of an endotracheal tube suggests an acute severe respiratory condition, which makes the diagnoses of silicosis, scleroderma, and lymphangioleiomyomatosis less likely. Cryptogenic organizing pneumonia is typically more multifocal and not as homogeneously diffuse in distribution, and uncommonly results in respiratory compromise requiring intubation.

27. **C**—Idiopathic pulmonary fibrosis. The CT shows bibasilar honeycombing, traction bronchiectasis, and architectural distortion. With these findings, the diagnosis of pulmonary fibrosis can be made with a high degree of confidence. Any end-stage lung disease can result in similar findings of fibrosis, although with sarcoidosis and hypersensitivity pneumonitis, the findings typically predominate in the upper lungs and not the lung bases. Asbestosis and any collagen vascular disease can result in a similar appearance, although these options were not offered. The typical CT features of complicated silicosis are conglomerate masses in the upper lungs, small nodules, hilar retraction, architectural distortion, and peripheral emphysema. Cryptogenic organizing pneumonia does not typically progress to pulmonary fibrosis.

28. **A**—Sarcoidosis. CT shows small nodules in a bronchovascular and subpleural (perilymphatic) distribution, the characteristic features of sarcoidosis. Although Langerhan cell histiocytosis, Wegener granulomatosis, and acute hypersensitivity pneumonia can also present with nodules, they do not typically have a perilymphatic distribution. The typical CT features of asbestosis are reticular and linear interstitial lung disease in a predominantly subpleural and bibasilar distribution, subpleural bands, and varying degrees of honeycombing and traction bronchiectasis. There is often associated asbestos-related pleural disease.

29. **E**—Asbestos-related pleural disease. CT shows diffuse calcified pleural thickening and a small left pleural effusion. The bilaterality of these findings is very characteristic of asbestos-related pleural disease. Tuberculous empyema is typically a unilateral process. Bronchogenic carcinoma can be associated with pleural metastases that are typically nodular, associated with larger pleural effusions, and not calcified. The typical CT features of complicated silicosis are described in the answer to question #27. Although pleural thickening can occasionally result from recurrent pleural effusions related to chronic congestive heart failure, it is typically not diffuse, bilateral, and calcified.

30. **E**—Cystic teratoma. CT shows a circumscribed, homogeneous, fluid-attenuation mass in the anterior mediastinum. Note the small lobulation to the medial margin and a hint of high attenuation around the medial margin. MRI with intravenous contrast shows enhancement of the capsule and a small enhancing nodule medially. Both bronchogenic and pericardial cysts will typically have no demonstrable capsule and show no contrast enhancement. Bronchogenic carcinoma and mediastinal abscess will typically have a larger soft tissue component and changes in the adjacent lung. Other diagnoses to consider, which were not offered as options, are cystic thymoma and cystic lymphoma.

31. **Right aortic arch.** Note that the trachea is slightly shifted to the left and there is no aortic arch on the left.

32. **Pulmonary venolobar syndrome.** Note the scimitar-shaped anomalous pulmonary vein on the right.

33. **Left upper lobe collapse.** There is hazy opacification of the left lung, elevation of the left hemidiaphragm, shift of the mediastinum to the left, and lucency around the aortic arch (the luftsichel sign), all of which indicate left upper lobe collapse. The most common reason for left upper lobe collapse in an adult patient, especially one over the age of 40, is bronchogenic carcinoma. There is an air–fluid level in the left upper lobe, indicating a cavitary mass. This is a case of squamous cell bronchogenic carcinoma, the most common bronchogenic carcinoma to cavitate.

34. **Mycetoma.** There is a thin-walled cavity in the right upper lobe that contains a central mass. This is the classic appearance of a fungus ball (mycetoma).

35. **Collapse of the left lung.** There is shift of the mediastinum into the left hemithorax (note marked tracheal deviation). The left hemithorax is completely opaque, except for subtle lucency in the upper left hemithorax which represents hyperexpanded right lung. Although the left lung collapse could be caused by a mucous plug or foreign body within the left main bronchus, in this case it was caused by a remote tear of the left bronchus, the result of a motor vehicle crash.

36. **Lymphangioleiomyomatosis.** Thin-section CT shows numerous thin-walled cysts of homogeneous round shape. Langerhan cell histiocytosis, which can have a similar appearance, tends to be associated with both cysts and nodules, and the cysts tend to have more bizarre shapes.

37. **B** (see Chapter 1)
38. **A** (see Chapter 1)
39. **E** (see Chapter 1)
40. **C** (see Chapter 1)
41. **D** (see Chapter 1)
42. **C** (see Chapter 2)
43. **A** (see Chapter 2)
44. **D** (see Chapter 2)
45. **E** (see Chapter 2)
46. **B** (see Chapter 2)
47. **E** (see Chapter 3)
48. **B** (see Chapter 3)
49. **A** (see Chapter 3)
50. **C** (see Chapter 3)
51. **A** (see Chapter 3)
52. **B** (see Chapter 18)
53. **C** (see Chapter 18)
54. **D** (see Chapter 18)
55. **C** (see Chapter 18)
56. **True** (see Chapter 10)
57. **False** (see Chapter 10, Table 10-1)
58. **True** (see Chapter 10, Table 10-2)
59. **True** (see Chapter 12, Table 12-1)
60. **True** (see Chapter 14)
61. **False** (see Chapter 15, Tables 15-3 and 15-4)

62. **True** (see Chapter 15, Table 15-3)
63. **False** (see Chapter 15, Table 15-3)
64. **True** (see Chapter 15)
65. **False** (see Chapter 10)
66. **True** (see Chapter 10)
67. **False** (see Chapter 16)
68. **True** (see Chapter 1)
69. **True** (see Chapter 1)
70. **False** (see Chapter 1)
71. **True** (see Chapter 1)
72. **False** (see Chapter 1)
73. **True** (see Chapter 1)
74. **False** (see Chapter 3)
75. **False** (see Chapter 3)
76. **True** (see Chapter 5)
77. **True** (see Chapter 10)
78. **True** (see Chapter 10)
79. **True** (see Chapter 10)
80. **True** (see Chapter 10)
81. **True** (see Chapter 10)
82. **Coronary sinus** (see Chapter 1)
83. **Azygos** (see Chapter 1)

84.–88. **Bronchioloalveolar carcinoma, alveolar proteinosis, lymphoma, lipoid pneumonia, sarcoidosis** (see Chapter 4, Table 4-4)
89.–92. **Terrible lymphoma, teratoma, thyroid mass, thymoma** (see Chapter 6, Table 6-1)
93.–96. **Hemothorax, chylothorax, empyema, malignant effusion** (see Chapter 9)
97.–99. **Situs inversus, sinusitis, bronchiectasis** (see Chapter 13)
100. **B** (see Chapter 1)
101. **E** (see Chapter 1)
102. **D** (see Chapter 10)
103. **A** (see Chapter 3)
104. **C** (see Chapters 3, 13)
105. **C** (see Chapters 3, 10)
106. **C** (see Chapter 14)
107. **B** (see Chapter 13, Table 13-6)
108. **A** (see Chapter 16)
109. **A, B, C, D, E** (see Chapter 5, Table 5-1)
110. **B, C, E** (see Chapter 5)
111. **A, B, C, E** (see Chapter 8)
112. **A, B, C** (see Chapter 15)
113. **A, B, C, D, E** (see Chapter 8, Table 8-1)

Note: Page numbers followed by *f* denote figures and *t* denotes tabular material.